Eighth Edition

Haimann's

Healthcare
Management

Eighth Edition

Haimann's

Healthcare Management

Rose T. Dunn

Health Administration Press
Chicago, Illinois

Your board, staff, or clients may also benefit from this book's insight. For more information on quantity discounts, contact the Health Administration Press Marketing Manager at (312) 424-9470.

Library of Congress Cataloging-in-Publication Data

Dunn, Rose.
    Haimann's healthcare management / Rose T. Dunn.—8th ed.
      p. ; cm.
    Includes bibliographical references and index.
    ISBN 978156793255X—ISBN 1-56793-255-X
    1. Health facilities—Administration. I. Title: Healthcare management. II. Haimann, Theo. III. Title.
    [DNLM: 1. Health Facilities—organization & administration. 2. Personnel Management. WX 150 D923ha 2006]
    RA971 .H22   2006
    362.11068—dc22

                                        2005046782

The paper used in this publication meets the minimum requirements of American National Standard for Information Sciences—Permanence of Paper for Printed Library Materials, ANSI Z39.48–1984. ∞™

Acquisitions editor: Janet Davis; Project manager: Melissa Rompesky; Cover design: Robert Rush

Health Administration Press
A division of the Foundation of the
   American College of Healthcare Executives
1 North Franklin Street, Suite 1700
Chicago, IL 60606-3424
(312) 424-2800

Contents

Preface

The challenge to today's healthcare organizations is stronger than ever. They must keep pace with revolutionary and sophisticated breakthroughs in medical science and technology, a demanding public, a growing aging population, and federal regulators imposing new rules every day that may further burden the organization.

At the center of all these changes is the supervisor, who has to bring and hold together the human resources, physical facilities, professional expertise, technology, information systems, and other support systems necessary to deliver and monitor the care and services rendered. In addition, these tasks have to be accomplished within the fiscal constraints of a more efficient healthcare system. Therefore, healthcare managers and supervisors must understand the complexities of organization life, behavior, development, and climate.

The hardest job in any organization is clearly that of the supervisor. The supervisor is responsible for motivating the team to achieve organizational goals as set by the board of trustees or senior administration. The supervisor must be able to translate the goals into understandable and achievable terms for his or her team members and gain their buy-in; without the buy-in, the organization could fail.

However, thousands of middle- and first-level management positions, such as departmental managers, supervisors, and group leaders, are filled by health professionals, technicians, and others who have limited or no formal education or training in administration, management, and supervision.

This book is intended for these departmental managers and supervisors in all types of healthcare organizations. These people became supervisors primarily because they did an outstanding job in their chosen healthcare professions. Yet they often find themselves in increasingly demanding jobs and have little or no familiarity with the administrative and management aspects of their newly attained rank.

The book is introductory in that it assumes no previous knowledge of the concepts of supervision. As such, this book is also written for students taking an introductory course in management and will acquaint them with their future roles in any organization. It can be used in any course in which managerial, supervisory, and leadership concepts are studied.

Because this book is intended to aid people with their supervisory tasks, it serves as a reference to those individuals who already hold supervisory positions. Its purpose is to demonstrate that proficiency in supervision better equips them to cope with the ever-increasing demands of getting the job done. Because non-healthcare entities have had success dealing with change and implementing efficient and effective practices, this book draws on many sources for its content to permit the supervisor to choose from the lessons learned by others, regardless of whether they were experienced in a healthcare environment.

To create a framework in which management knowledge can be organized in a practical way, I have chosen to use the functions of management as the primary framework: planning, organizing, staffing, influencing, and controlling. Each function is thoroughly dealt with by breaking it down and explaining its relationship to the material already presented. This approach allows any new knowledge, from behavioral and social sciences, quantitative approaches, or any other field, to be incorporated at any point.

The supervisor's job—to get things done with and through people—has its foundation in the relationship between the supervisors and the people with whom they work. For this reason, the supervisor must have considerable knowledge of the human aspects of supervision—that is, the behavioral factors that motivate employees. This book attempts to present a balanced picture of such behavioral factors in the conceptual framework of managing.

This edition of Haimann's Healthcare Management is sure to be a welcome addition to any manager's library. In this eighth edition, much new material has been added, but the book retains the basic concepts and the emphasis on the five managerial functions. I have attempted to respond to each of the recommendations offered by readers and text reviewers when I incorporated the revisions. In doing so, the eighth edition includes an expansion of the performance improvement concepts, including Six Sigma, incorporates the concept of collaboration in the coordination and cooperation discussion, and now presents contemporary theories on authority and span of control. Ethics concepts have been added and appear throughout the book. Two of the organizing chapters have been consolidated to permit the creation of a reorganizing chapter, which includes process and performance improvement concepts. Additionally, mechanistic and organic organizations are described, along with communicating change techniques. Finally, the controlling section of the book includes some additional budget scenarios and a discussion on benchmarking and dashboards. Prior editions have given attention to how the behavioral sciences affect the management of human resources. Expanded coverage of management theories has been incorporated to speak to cybernetics, chaos, and entrepreneurial theories.

With the many changes taking place in healthcare today, I was not at a loss to find new management challenges to discuss. I was assisted by several well-qualified contributors, including Michael Troncone, M.P.H., CHE. Robert Sutter, R.N., M.B.A., M.H.A., Six Sigma Master Black Belt, provided the content on performance improvement and Six Sigma. The chapters on unions and grievances have been updated by a respected and experienced labor attorney, Marc Leff, Esq. Neither chapter is intended to be a substitute for legal advice from an organization's legal counsel.

In writing this edition, I attempted to retain the enthusiasm for effective management exhibited by Theo Haimann, the professor for whom this book is named. Theo Haimann served as the Mary Louise Professor of Management Sciences at Saint Louis University until his death in November 1991. He always incorporated current management issues into his teachings. By doing so, he was able to keep the students' attention. This edition attempts to carry on the Haimann tradition.

No book is ever the product of one person's efforts. Many individuals contributed to its development, editing, formatting, and publishing. I was fortunate to have some of the best working with me on this edition. Janet Davis, acquisitions editor for Health Administration Press, thoroughly reviewed the manuscript and offered many valuable suggestions. Melissa Rompesky and Helen-Joy Lynerd kept the production running smoothly and crossed the Ts and dotted the Is. James Niebruegge of First Class Solutions assisted with capturing figures electronically. These and many other behind-the-scenes individuals made the book happen.

Many healthcare organizations allowed me to reproduce documents, policies, and other figures. For these, I extend special thanks.

As always, I welcome your comments—good or bad—so that I can make the ninth edition better.

Rose T. Dunn, RHIA, CPA, FACHE
Chief Operating Officer
First Class Solutions, Inc.^{sm}
St. Louis, Missouri
Rose@FirstClassSolutions.com

PART I

Stepping into Management

CHAPTER ONE

The Supervisor's Job, Roles, Functions, and Authority

CHAPTER OBJECTIVES

After you have studied this chapter, you should be able to do the following:

1. Provide an overview of the rapidly changing healthcare environment and the challenges it poses for managers and supervisors.

2. Discuss the dimensions of the supervisor's job.

3. Review the aspects of the supervisor's position and the skills necessary to be successful.

4. Discuss the managerial role of the supervisor.

5. Enumerate and discuss the meaning, interrelationships, and universal nature of the five managerial functions.

6. Discuss the concept of authority and its meaning as the foundation of the formal, organizational, and positional aspects of authority.

THE HEALTHCARE PERSPECTIVE

The needs and demands for the highest-quality management in all healthcare delivery activities are intensifying to such a degree that survival has become an issue for some of today's healthcare organizations. No letup is in sight: the current market pressures are demanding new delivery methods. For example, in the past, patients came to the healthcare center; now, healthcare services are conveniently located near the patient's home and accessible through satellite outpatient services, Wal-Mart, mobile mammography units, and health fairs at the grocery store.

Other trends affecting healthcare management include managed care contracting, an increasingly difficult issue for every healthcare institution. The further growth of managed care seems inevitable, and many healthcare centers are lacking the data they need for successful managed care contracting. Medical practice arrangements are also changing greatly, and the traditional fee-for-service concept is undergoing radical rethinking. Fee schedules, or limits on fees for certain services, are defined by insurers, and some managed care organizations have capitated the amount they pay for the care rendered to a given insured during a period by paying the physician a fixed fee at the beginning of the month for services to the insured; this fee is flat regardless of the amount of care rendered by the physician to the patient during the month.

Finances are being affected by regulation as well. The Balanced Budget Act (BBA) of 1997 and various prospective payment (PPS) regulations have resulted in significant cuts in compensation for capital expenditures, teaching programs, and outpatient services in the form of the ambulatory payment classification (APC). The BBA, PPS, and Health Insurance Portability and Accountability Act (HIPAA) regulations have imposed major changes in the operations of such areas as information technology, patient financial services, ancillary services, home health, rehabilitation, and health information management.

New breakthroughs in science and technology are likely to change key services, such as in the fields of cardiology, oncology, orthopedics, neurology, and women's health. Insurers are identifying a few hospitals to which the insured are sent to receive high-tech care such as lung, heart, and pancreas transplants. Hospitals, in turn, are creating centers of excellence to focus limited resources on the growth of more profitable service areas and niche markets. Another challenge comes from healthcare facilities providing more and more services in the outpatient setting that are geographically spread out across a region.

Faced with a shortage of nurses whose expertise and assistance are crucial to high-quality healthcare, healthcare providers have attempted to guard against closing patient care units and clinics due to nurse staff shortages by training other staff to perform many of the nonregulated functions previously performed by nurses. These individuals—sometimes called multiskilled professionals, nurse extenders, or certified nurse assistants—record temperatures; pass medications; draw blood; collect specimens; and perform some patient care services such as turning, exercising, and assisting patients when ambulating. Not only are these individuals readily employable, but their hourly rates are lower than those of nurses, thus reducing labor costs for the healthcare provider. This well-intended safeguard has lead to unionization activities by nursing professionals and unions to protect nursing jobs at some organizations. A shortage of nurses, low unemployment rates, and work attitudes of Generation Xers[1] have hampered the hiring efforts of even the best-intentioned healthcare providers.

In addition to these factors, many other changes from all directions are affecting healthcare delivery. Challenges such as those considered below will continue to impose constraints on healthcare services and set higher expectations.

To pool labor, clinical, and capital resources and expertise, many facilities are merging with nearby hospitals, prior competitors, or other strategically located facilities to allow them to benefit from the larger, merged entity image. Mergers, in some cases, have actually closed facilities. In fact, according to the

Healthcare Financial Management Association's (HFMA 2000) CFO Forum, the total number of hospitals dropped to 5,890 in 1999, falling below 6,000 for the first time in nearly 80 years. The Office of Inspector General (OIG 2005) issued reports in May 2004 stating that 5,091 hospitals remained opened at the end of 2000, a 12 percent decline from the earlier report by the HFMA.

Mergers are not an activity limited to hospitals. Physicians, laboratories, and home health agency mergers have been similarly prevalent. This type of activity requires extensive and sophisticated long-range planning and good control over internal affairs. In turn, all this radical reshaping of the healthcare field calls for more and better management. Managers, from chief executive officers (CEOs) down to first-line supervisors, are needed to help implement these changes and make their organizations function effectively.

The organization is the most important and critical element in the change process, providing the means for bringing the resources together. Managing is the process by which healthcare organizations fulfill this responsibility. Thus, the manager is responsible for acquiring and combining the resources to accomplish the goals. As scientific, economic, competitive, social, and other pressures change, it is not the nurse or the technologist on whom the organization depends to cope with the change; it is the manager. Management has emerged as a potent force in our society since the turn of the twentieth century and has become essential to the life of all healthcare endeavors.

Today's health services are almost exclusively delivered in organizational settings.[2] Only an organizational setting can bring together the physical facilities, professional expertise, skills, information systems, technology, and myriad other supports that today's health services delivery requires, whether these services are curative, rehabilitative, or preventive. However, the "physical" confines in which healthcare staff work are changing. In the past, all staff came to a physical location to perform the tasks assigned. Today, some radiology interpretations (teleradiology) and some physician evaluation services (telemedicine) are being performed remotely or through robots, while non–patient-care functions such as billing, information systems, financial services (e.g., managed care contracting, reimbursement), purchasing, clinical coding, and transcription are being performed at home (telecommuting) or in remote campus locations through the use of wireless and other high-tech hardware and software paths to the Internet, known as broadband.[3] Therefore, it is absolutely necessary that those involved in the delivery of healthcare services as well as those managing the remotely located functions understand the complexities of organizational life, behavior, development, and climate and the importance of expert administration in addition to their own professional areas of expertise.

Because the delivery of healthcare largely means providing a service, which is by nature people intensive, approximately 57 percent of the total expenditures within the field are for wages and benefits (PriceWaterhouseCoopers 2005). Therefore, much criticism has naturally centered around employee productivity to justify such large labor expenditures and increased interest in outsourcing, even off-shoring, services whenever possible to cap rising labor costs. The

United States needs better and more effective administration of healthcare activities; that is, ultimately better supervision throughout the entire healthcare industry. It is the frontline management—the supervisor of the department, regardless of the title and nature of work—who is responsible for the department functioning smoothly and efficiently. It is essential, therefore, that due emphasis be placed on the need for the managerial development of effective supervisors within all phases of the healthcare field.

THE DEMANDS OF THE SUPERVISORY POSITION

The supervisory position within any administrative structure has long been acknowledged as a difficult and demanding one. You have probably learned this from your own experience or by observing supervisors in hospitals and related institutions as they perform their daily tasks. The supervisor, whether a manager of printing and mail services or a chief technologist in the clinical laboratory, can be viewed as the person in the middle of a pyramid structure, for example. He or she serves as the principal link between higher administration (the top of the pyramid shown in Figure 1.1) and the employees (the base of the pyramid).

Looking carefully at the job of almost any supervisor, regardless of whom or what he or she supervises, we can see that it involves four major dimensions, or four areas of responsibility. First, the supervisor must be a good boss, a good manager, and a team leader of the employees in the unit. This includes having the technical, professional, and clinical competence to run the department smoothly and see that the employees carry out their assignments successfully. The supervisor's first responsibility, not given in any order of importance, is to the employees of the department. Second, the supervisor must be a competent subordinate to the next higher manager: in most instances, this person is an administrator, an associate administrator, a center executive, or a director of a service. This responsibility answers to administration and the "owners" of the organization.

Third, the supervisor must act as a connecting link between the administration and the employees. For example, employees such as laboratory scientists (formerly technologists), technicians, and clerical support staff see their supervisor—who is perhaps the chief technologist—as the "administration." The supervisor is the primary contact, through whom the employees communicate their concerns to the administration at large and from whom come the goals and policies established by senior administration for hospital-wide management. The supervisor serves as a filter in this third area in that he or she sorts the expressed concerns into categories (i.e., those that the supervisor should address, those that the supervisor's boss should address, and those that should be pushed further up the ladder and may represent concerns shared by employees outside of the department). Similarly, the supervisor receives information from multiple levels in the hierarchy and must decide which items should be passed on to his or her immediate subordinates and from there to those working on the front line. Goal and policy communications are items that must be shared

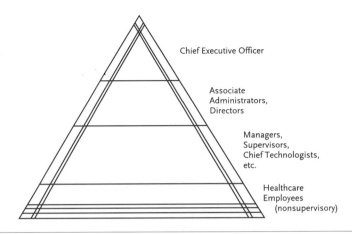

with all staff because the supervisor is that member of the administration who must make certain that the work gets done to achieve the goals established by the organization.

Fourth, the supervisor must maintain satisfactory working relationships with the heads, leaders, and peer supervisors of all other departments and services. The supervisor must foster a good-colleague relationship, being willing and eager to coordinate the department's efforts with those of other departments to reach the overall objectives and goals of the institution and providing the best possible service and patient care regardless of which department or service gets credit.

The four dimensions of the supervisor's job are shown in Figure 1.2. The supervisor must be successful in vertical relationships downward with subordinates and upward with his or her superior. In addition, the supervisor must be skillful in handling horizontal relationships with other supervisors because this facilitates getting the job done for the benefit of the client.

Henry Mintzberg (1973) depicts these dimensions in ten roles common to the work of all managers. A role is an organized set of behaviors, and Mintzberg categorized the ten roles into three groups: interpersonal, informational, and decisional (see Figure 1.3).

The interpersonal roles link all managerial work, as discussed in the fourth dimension above, satisfying relationships with other supervisors. This role group includes serving as a figurehead, leader, and liaison and sharing information as necessary to maintain effective two-way communication with peers, subordinates, superiors, and individuals outside of the organization. The informational roles ensure that information is provided and processed. In this role the manager uses information collected during monitoring activities, disseminates information to others, and reacts to information received. The decisional

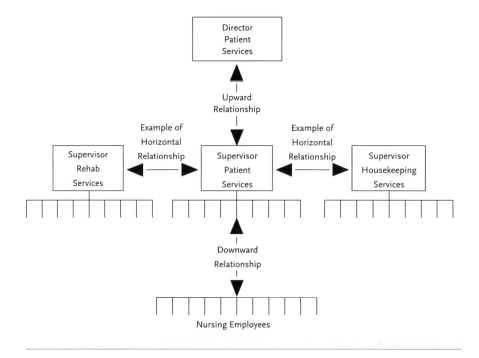

roles make significant use of the information for decision making. In this role the manager or supervisor may implement change based on the information, thus being considered an "entrepreneur," according to Mintzberg. Alternatively, the information could be used as an alert or to recognize when the organization may be threatened. In this situation, the role being played is one of "disturbance handler." The final two roles of the decisional group include resource allocator and negotiator. In both, the manager is using information to determine where resources can be best utilized and how to most economically and effectively obtain and use these resources.

Because of the complexity of these relationships, the role of the first-line supervisor in any organization is commonly acknowledged to be the most difficult. It is even more difficult for supervisors within the healthcare field because their activities directly or indirectly affect people, the quality of patient care, and the smooth overall functioning of the institution. In addition to their many professional obligations, healthcare supervisors must always bear in mind the needs and desires of patients and their relatives, who may be physically drained and emotionally upset. Thus, the supervisor should be informed of any interaction problems among medical staff members and patients. All these considerations make the job of the healthcare supervisor particularly demanding and challenging.

FIGURE 1.3: MINTZBERG'S MANAGERIAL ROLES

Information Task

Interpersonal:	figurehead, leader, liaison (provide information)
Informational:	monitor, disseminator, spokesperson (process information)
Decisional:	entrepreneur, disturbance handler, resource allocator, negotiator (use information)

Source: Mintzberg, H. 1973. *The Nature of Managerial Work*, 55–58. New York: HarperCollins Publishers.

For example, consider the long list of demands made on a charge nurse of a nursing unit. Whether the institution practices team nursing, primary care, or total patient care, the charge nurse's duty is still to provide for and supervise the nursing care rendered to the patients in the unit. She does this partly by delegating a certain amount of her authority for the care of patients and the supervision of personnel to subordinate nursing team leaders within her area. Still, the charge nurse must plan, direct, and control all activities within the nursing unit. She must make the rounds with medical and nursing staff. She is also expected to make rounds to personally observe the safety, condition, and behavior of patients and to assess the need for and quality of continued nursing care. She may even have to assume general nursing functions in the care of patients who have complex problems or when vacancies exist.

Furthermore, the charge nurse must interpret and apply the policies, procedures, rules, and regulations of the facility in general and of nursing services in particular. She must provide 24-hour coverage of the unit by scheduling staff properly at all times. She is to communicate and report to her immediate nursing superior all pertinent information regarding patients in her unit. She must orient new personnel to the unit and acquaint them with the general philosophies of the institution. She is also responsible for continued in-service education in her unit, teaching personnel new patient care techniques and patient safety initiatives. Likewise, she participates in the evaluation of her subordinates.

In addition, it is part of the charge nurse's job to coordinate her patient care with the care and therapeutic procedures of the various departments throughout the institution. Furthermore, she is involved in the design and regular reevaluation of the budget. She serves on a number of committees, in addition to attending all patient care management meetings. She may also be expected to help in the supervision and instruction of student nurses and medical housestaff when necessary. Many additional duties are often assigned to a charge nurse, depending on what the particular healthcare facility specifies in its description of this very demanding position.

Although it is difficult, if not impossible, to forecast when and how a new scientific or technological event will affect the supervisory position, every supervisor must keep abreast of those changes affecting his or her profession. It is important that supervisors prepare themselves and their employees professionally, scientifically, technologically, and psychologically for changes that occur inevitably in the delivery of healthcare. In addition to the medical and scientific breakthroughs, increased automation and its concomitant benefits and challenges will continue to affect all supervisors. Adaptations and uses for personal, wireless, handheld (e.g., PDA or personal digital assistant), and point-of-care computers will grow, and supervisors and staffs will have to be familiar with this technology as part of their daily routines. Access to the latest information on virtually any subject is just a click away on the Internet. Supervisors, however, must be attentive to the time that subordinates spend on the Internet so as to not lose valuable work time and guard against misuse for personal purposes.

With a growing, complex society and increasing demands for more sophisticated and better healthcare, the job of any supervisor in the field is likely to become even more challenging. This is true whether his or her title is health information manager, operating room supervisor, decision support analyst, foreman of the electricians, or food service supervisor. The one factor that helps the supervisor cope with all of this responsibility is the continued advancement of his or her knowledge and skill in the managerial part of the job.

This supervisory position is usually the first in a long career of administrative positions that increasingly demand demonstrated competent management skills from the individual moving up the administrative ladder. For instance, a programmer analyst may begin his ascent into management as applications manager. After serving in this capacity for some time, he is promoted to network administrator, then to associate administrator, information technology services, and eventually to the organization's vice president or chief information officer (CIO).

One may also move up the ladder in a less traditional way. For example, consider the staff nurse selected to manage the preregistration and scheduling activities. After serving successfully in this capacity for some time and establishing good relations with a managed care company, the staff nurse is recruited by that managed care organization to oversee the precertification unit and given the title of precertification manager. She is then promoted to director of benefit determinations and eventually to assistant vice president for customer service and medical management.

Most of the tens of thousands of managerial positions in healthcare today are filled by healthcare professionals who have not had any formal administrative training or studied management or administration. Therefore, it is essential that the supervisor, department head, or leader learn as much as possible about the meaning of being a competent first-line manager because it is likely his or her first step in the climb up the managerial and administration ladder.

THE MANAGERIAL ASPECTS
OF THE SUPERVISORY POSITION

The job of a supervisor can be viewed in terms of three essential skills. First, the good supervisor must possess technical skills. These skills are primarily concerned with systematic procedures to ensure that the supervisor knows the clinical and technical aspects of the work to be done. In addition, two more skills are needed, human relations skills and conceptual skills. Human relations skills are those that concern working with and motivating people and understanding individual and group feelings. Conceptual skills enable the supervisor to visualize the big picture and to understand how all parts of the organization contribute and coordinate their efforts. These human and conceptual skills are essential to the managerial aspects of a supervisor's job. The relative degree of importance of all three skills depends on the level of the position within an organization; however, all levels of management require these skills at one time or another.

Some supervisors on different occasions appear frequently harassed, disorganized, and overly involved in doing the job at hand; they are muddling through and are knee-deep in work. Such supervisors put in long hours and are never afraid of doing anything themselves. They are working exceedingly hard but never seem to have enough time left to actually supervise. On the other hand, some supervisors seem to be on top of the job, and their departments function smoothly and in an orderly fashion. They have found time to sit at their desks at least part of each day and keep their desk work up-to-date. Why is there such a difference between these two types of managers?

Some supervisors are more capable or proficient than others, whereas others are inept. If you compare two health information managers in two hospitals to discover why one is on top of the job and the other is constantly fixing things himself or herself, you will probably find that one understands his or her job better than the other and has developed subordinate staff to whom he or she can delegate or entrust assignments. Assume that both are equally good professionals, both have graduated from health information management programs in the same community and have similar staffing ratios and technology available, and the conditions under which they perform are similar. The results of one health information manager are significantly better than those of the other because one is simply a better manager. He or she is able to supervise the functions of his or her department in a manner that allows him or her to get the job done through and with the people of his or her department. The difference between a good supervisor and a poor supervisor, assuming everything else is equal, is the difference in each person's managerial abilities.

However, the managerial aspect of the supervisor's position has long been neglected. Rather, the emphasis has always been placed on clinical and technical competence. Consider your own job, for example. It is very likely that you were appointed to this job from the ranks of one of the various professional services or crafts. As a result of your ingenuity, initiative, and personal drive, you were promoted to the supervisory level and were expected to assume the responsibilities of managing your unit. Little was probably done, however, to acquaint you with these responsibilities or to help you cope with the managerial aspects of your new job. More or less overnight, you were made a part of administration without having been prepared to be a manager. Since your promotion, you have done the best you could by imitating and learning from your predecessors, and your department is probably functioning reasonably well. Still, some problems are likely. These may be dealt with by a better understanding of the supervisory aspects of your job so that you are running the department instead of the department running you.

The aim of this book is to show the supervisor how to become a better manager. This does not mean that one can neglect or underestimate the actual work involved in getting the job done. Often, the supervisor is actually the most skilled individual in the department and can do a more efficient and quicker job than anyone else. He or she must not be tempted, however, to step in and take over the job, except for purposes of instruction, during extended vacancies, or in case of an emergency. Rather, the supervisor's responsibility is to ensure adequate staffing and to see that the employees can do the job and do so properly. As a manager, the supervisor must plan, guide, and supervise. A discussion of these managerial requirements of the supervisory position follows.

THE MEANING OF MANAGEMENT

The term *management* has been defined in many ways, generally as a process of coordinating and integrating human, technical, and other resources to accomplish specific results. A more meaningful definition for our purposes is the process of getting things done through and with people by directing and motivating the efforts of individuals toward common objectives. You have undoubtedly learned from your own experience that in most endeavors one person alone can accomplish relatively little. For this reason, people have found it expedient and even necessary to join with others to attain the goals of an enterprise. In every organized activity, the manager's function is to achieve the goals of the enterprise with the help of subordinates, peers, and superiors.

Achieving goals through and with people is only one aspect of the manager's job, however; creating a working atmosphere—that is, a climate or a culture in which subordinates can find as much satisfaction of their needs as possible—is also necessary. In other words, a supervisor must provide a climate conducive for the employees to fulfill such needs as recognition, achievement, and companionship. If these needs can be met on the job, employees are more likely to strive willingly and enthusiastically toward the achievement of departmental objectives as well as the overall objectives of the institution. Thus, we must add to our earlier definition of management: the manager's job is getting things done through and with people by enabling them to find as much satisfaction of their needs as possible while motivating them to achieve both their own objectives and the objectives of the institution. The better the supervisor performs these duties, the better the departmental results are.

You may have noticed by this time that the terms supervisor, manager, and administrator have been used interchangeably. The exact meaning of these titles varies with different institutions, but the terms administrator and executive are generally used for top-level management positions and manager and supervisor usually connote positions within the middle or lower levels of the institutional hierarchy. Some theoretical differences may be considered, but for the purposes of this book, these terms are used interchangeably. Furthermore, the use of gender terms—he or she—are not meant to the exclusivity of the other.

As you read this book and review your situation, you will discover that the managerial aspects of all supervisory jobs are the same. This is true regardless of the supervisor's department, section, or level within the administrative hierarchy. Thus, the managerial content of a supervisory position is the same whether the position is director of case management, head of environmental services, chief engineer in the maintenance department, or lead clinical dietitian. By the same token, the managerial functions are the same for the first-line supervisor, mid-level management, or top administrative group. In addition, the type of organization in which you work does not matter; managerial functions are the same for a commercial or industrial enterprise, not-for-profit or for-profit organization, professional association, government agency, and hospital or other healthcare facility. Regardless of the activities of the organization, department, or level, the managerial aspects and skills are the same. The difference is in the extent to which or frequency by which a supervisor performs each of the tasks.

MANAGERIAL SKILLS AND TECHNICAL SKILLS

These managerial skills must be distinguished from the professional, clinical, and technical skills that are also required of a supervisor. As stated before, all supervisors must also possess special technical skills and professional know-how in their field. Technical skills vary between departments, but any supervisory position requires both professional technical skills and standard managerial skills. Mere technical and professional knowledge is not sufficient.

It is important to note that as a supervisor advances up the administrative ladder, he or she will rely less on professional and technical skills and more on managerial skills. Therefore, the top-level executive generally uses far fewer technical skills than those who are employed under him or her. In the rise to the top, however, the administrator has had to acquire all the administrative skills necessary for the management of the entire enterprise.

Consider the following real-life example; the real name of this supervisor has been disguised. John Andrews, an English major in college, taught junior high school. When his teaching salary became inadequate to support his growing family, John joined an insurance company as a claims adjudicator (a base-level position). He noticed abnormalities in some claims from some providers and researched these for his superior. Eventually he was promoted to the fraud investigations unit and ultimately directed that operation until he was promoted to oversee all claims and investigations functions. John interacted well with physicians and insurance representatives alike. As he gained more experience, he began negotiating arrangements with physician groups and hospitals for preferred provider organizations (PPOs) and health maintenance organizations (HMOs). He was selected to be CEO of an HMO, which was national in scope and very successful. At each step of his advancement, John built on prior experience and knowledge, but he did not need to personally perform all activities to ensure the success of the HMO. He left the details to his proficient subordinates.

Similarly, the CEO of a hospital is concerned primarily with the overall management of hospital activities; his or her functions are almost purely administrative. In this endeavor, the chief executive depends on the managerial and technical skills of the various subordinate administrators and managers, including all the first-line supervisors, to get the job done. The CEO, in turn, uses managerial skills in directing the efforts of all these subordinate managers toward the common objectives of the hospital.

MANAGERIAL SKILLS CAN BE LEARNED

How does a supervisor acquire these very important managerial skills? First, she must understand that standard managerial skills can be learned. Although good managers, like good athletes, are often assumed to be born, not made, this belief is not based in fact. We cannot deny that people are born with different physiological and biological potentials and that they are endowed with differing amounts of intelligence and many other characteristics; a person who is not a natural athlete is not likely to run 100 yards in record time. Many individuals who are natural athletes, however, have not come close to that goal either.

A good athlete is made when a person with some natural endowment develops it into a mature skill by practice, learning, effort, sacrifice, and experience. The same holds true for a good manager; by practice, learning, and experience he or she develops this natural endowment of intelligence and leadership into mature management skills. The skills involved in managing are as able to be learned and practiced as the skills involved in playing tennis.

If you currently hold a supervisory position, you likely have the necessary prerequisites of intelligence and leadership and you are now ready to acquire the skills of a manager. Developing these skills takes time and effort; they are not acquired overnight. The supervisor has ample opportunity to apply the principles and guidelines discussed in this book to the daily work, and by applying its content, the supervisor certainly prevents many difficulties from occurring and before too long reaps the many benefits from practicing good supervision.

The most valuable resource of any organization is the people who work there, or the human resources. The first-line supervisor is the person to whom this most important resource is entrusted in the daily working situation. The best use of an organization's human assets depends greatly on the managerial ability and understanding of the supervisor, as manifested by his or her expertise in influencing and directing them. The supervisor's job is to create a climate of motivation, satisfaction, leadership, and continuous further self-development and self-improvement. This is a challenge to every supervisor because it ultimately means the need for his or her own further self-development as a manager.

The supervisor's managerial role rests on two foundations: managerial functions and managerial authority. *Managerial functions* are those that must be performed by a supervisor for him or her to be considered a true manager. The concept of authority inherent in the supervisory position is briefly discussed later in this chapter and more extensively throughout the book.

Five managerial functions are described in this book: planning, organizing, staffing, influencing, and controlling the resources of the organization. The resources include people, positions, technology, physical plant, equipment, materials, supplies, information, and money. (The labels used to describe managerial functions vary somewhat in management literature; some textbooks list one more or one less managerial function. Regardless of the terms or number used, the managerial functions collectively are interrelated and goal driven and constitute one of the two major characteristics of a manager.) A person who does not perform these functions is not a manager in the true sense of the word, regardless of title. The following explanation is introductory; most of the book is devoted to the discussion, meaning, and ramifications of each of these five functions.

Planning

The act of planning determines in advance what should be done in the future. Planning involves developing a systematic approach for attaining the goals of the organization. This function consists of determining the goals, objectives, policies, procedures, methods, rules, budgets, and other plans needed to achieve the purpose of the organization. In planning, the manager must contemplate and select a course of action from a set of available alternatives.

Thus, planning is mental work that involves thinking before acting, looking ahead, and preparing for the future. In other words, planning is laying out in advance the goals to be achieved and the best means to achieve these objectives. It is the collection of information and data from various sources to make decisions, and its purpose is to prepare the organization for what is to come in the future.

You may have observed supervisors who are constantly confronting one crisis after another. The probable reason is that they did not plan or look ahead. It is every manager's duty to plan; this function cannot be delegated to someone else. Certain specialists may be called on to assist in laying out various plans, but as the manager of the department, the supervisor must make departmental plans. These plans must coincide with the overall objectives of the institution as laid down by higher-level administration. Within the overall directives and general boundaries, however, the manager has considerable leeway in mapping out the departmental course.

Planning must come before any of the other managerial functions. Even after the initial plans are laid out and the manager proceeds with the other managerial functions, the function of planning continues in revising the course of action and choosing different alternatives as the need arises. Therefore, although planning is the first function a manager must tackle, it does not end at the initiation of the other functions. The manager continues to plan while performing the organizing, staffing, influencing, and controlling tasks.

Organizing

Once a plan has been developed, the manager must determine how the work is to be accomplished—that is, arranging the necessary resources to carry out the plan. The manager must define, group, and assign job duties. Through organizing, the manager determines and enumerates the various activities to be accomplished and combines these activities into distinct groups (e.g., departments, divisions, sections, teams, or any other units). The manager further divides the group work into individual jobs, assigns these activities, and at the same time provides subordinates with the authority needed to carry out these activities.

In short, to organize means to design a structural framework that sets up all the positions needed to perform the work of the department and to assign particular duties to these positions. Organizing encompasses the following elements:

- *Specialization*: a technique used to divide work activities into easily managed tasks and assign those tasks to individuals based on their skills.
- *Departmentalization*: a technique used to divide activities and people according to the needs of the organization or its customers.
- *Span of management*: a concept that defines the optimum number of subordinates a supervisor can effectively manage.
- *Authority relationships:* a set of theories concerning individuals' rights to decide, make assignments, direct activities, and so on in managing people, materials, machinery, expenses, and revenues.
- *Responsibility*: the obligation to perform certain duties.
- *Unity of command:* the concept that each individual should have one person to report to for any single activity.
- *Line and staff*: the theory of authority that defines whether one has the authority to direct (a line capacity) or advise (a staff capacity).

These and other factors are discussed throughout the book. The result of the organizing function is the creation of an activity-authority network for the department, which is a subsystem within the total healthcare organization.

Staffing

Staffing represents the manager's responsibility to recruit and select employees who are qualified to fill the various positions needed based on the organization of duties to achieve the plan. The manager must also remain within the budgeted labor amount for the department.

Besides hiring, staffing involves training employees, appraising their performance, counseling them on how to improve their performance, promoting them, and giving them opportunities for further development. Staffing also includes compensating employees appropriately. In most healthcare institutions, the department of human resources helps with the technical aspects of staffing. The basic authority and responsibility for staffing, however, remain with the supervisor.

Influencing

The managerial function of influencing means issuing directives and orders in such a way that staff respond to these directives to accomplish the job. Influencing also means identifying and implementing practices to help the members of the organization work together. This function is also known as leading, directing, or motivating.

It is not sufficient for a manager to plan, organize, and staff. The supervisor must also stimulate action by giving directives and orders to the subordinates, then supervising and guiding them as they work. Moreover, it is the manager's job to develop the abilities of the subordinates by leading, teaching, and coaching them effectively. To influence is to motivate one's employees to achieve their maximum potential and satisfy their needs and to encourage them to accomplish tasks they may not choose to do on their own.

Thus, influencing is the process around which all performance revolves; it is the essence of all operations. This process has many dimensions such as employee needs, morale, job satisfaction, productivity, leadership, example setting, and communication. Through the influencing function, the supervisor seeks to model performance expectations and create a climate conducive to employee satisfaction while achieving the objectives of the institution. As you may know from personal experience, much and perhaps most of your time is spent influencing and motivating subordinates.

Controlling

Controlling is the function that ensures plans are followed, that actual performance matches the plan, and that objectives are achieved. A more comprehensive definition of controlling includes determining whether the plans are being carried out, whether progress is being made toward objectives, and whether other actions must be taken to correct deviations and shortcomings. Again, this relates to the importance of planning as the primary function of the manager. A supervisor could not check on whether work was proceeding properly if there were no plans to check against. Controlling also includes taking corrective action if objectives are not being met and revising the plans and objectives if circumstances require it.

The Interrelationships of Managerial Functions

It is helpful to think of the five managerial functions as the management cycle. A cycle is a system of interdependent processes and activities. Each activity affects the performance of the others. As shown in Figure 1.4, the five functions flow into each other, and at times there is no clear line indicating where one function ends and the other begins. Because of this interrelationship, no manager can set aside a specific amount of time each day for one or another function. The effort spent on each function varies as conditions and circumstances change. The planning function, however, undoubtedly must come first. Without plans the manager cannot organize, staff, influence, or control. Throughout this book, therefore, we shall follow this sequence of planning first, then organizing, staffing, influencing, and controlling.

Although the five managerial functions can be separated theoretically, in the daily job of the manager these activities are inseparable. The output of one provides the input for another, all as elements of a system.

Universality of the Managerial Functions
and Their Relation to Position and Time

Whether as chair of the board, president of the healthcare center, vice president for patient care, or supervisor of the telephone operators, a manager performs all five functions. This idea is known as the principle of *universality of managerial functions*. The time and effort that each manager devotes to a particular function vary, however, depending on the individual's level within the administrative hierarchy.

The CEO is likely to plan, for example, one year, five years, or even ten years ahead. A supervisor is concerned with plans of much shorter duration. At times, a supervisor has to make plans for 6 or 12 months ahead but more frequently just makes plans for the next month, the next week, or even the next day or shift. In other words, the span and magnitude of plans for the supervisor are smaller.

The same is true of the influencing function. The CEO normally assigns tasks to subordinate managers, delegates authority, depends on them to accomplish tasks, and spends a minimum of time in direct supervision. As a first-time supervisor, however, you are concerned with getting the job done each day, so you have to spend much time in this influencing or directing function. Similar observations can be made for organizing, staffing, and controlling (Figure 1.4).

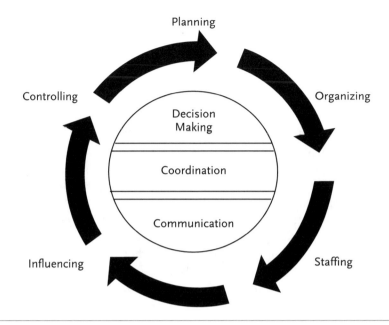

MANAGERIAL AUTHORITY

The second major characteristic of the managerial position is the presence of authority. Authority is the lifeblood of any managerial position; a person in an organizational setting cannot be a manager without it. Why is authority the primary characteristic of the managerial position? Briefly, authority is legal or rightful power—the right to act and to direct others. It is the power by which a manager can ask subordinates to do or not to do a certain task that he or she deems appropriate and necessary to realize the objectives of the department.

One must realize that this kind of organizational authority is part of the formal position a manager holds and is not given to the manager as an individual. This concept of authority must also include the possession of power to impose sanctions when necessary. Without such power to enforce an order, the enterprise could become disorganized and chaos could result. If a subordinate refuses to carry out the manager's directive, managerial authority includes the right to take disciplinary action and possibly to discharge the employee.

This aspect of authority obviously has many restrictions, including legal restrictions; union contracts; organizational policies; or considerations of morals, ethics, and human behavior. For example, legal restrictions and organizational procedures require fulfilling many disciplinary and documentation steps before an employee can be dismissed. Also, every successful manager must take into consideration human behavior in the workplace: to influence and motivate subordinates to perform required duties, it is best not to depend on this formal managerial authority but to use other persuasive ways and means to accomplish the job. In other words, it is far better not to depend on the negative aspects of dominance and authority.

In practice, most managers do not speak of authority at all; they prefer to speak of the responsibility, tasks, or duties they have. Such managers are right in saying that they have the responsibility for certain activities instead of saying that they have the authority to get the job done. For a supervisor, however, having authority means having the power and right to issue directives. Once you accept responsibility to oversee a certain project and achieve a certain outcome, you can delegate authority to lower-level staff to complete the project, but you cannot delegate the responsibility. The responsibility lies with you to accomplish the task through proper planning, organizing, staffing, influencing, and controlling.

The discussion in Chapter 12 on the meaning and various other bases of authority sheds additional light on this concept. Chapter 14 looks at how subordinates and workers react to authority and how authority is delegated. Delegation of authority means the process by which a supervisor receives authority from the superior manager as well as the process by which some of the authority assigned to this position is delegated to subordinates. Just as authority is the foundation of any managerial position, delegating authority to the lower ranks within the managerial hierarchy makes it possible to build an organizational structure with effective managers on every level.

Authority is discussed more fully throughout this book because it plays such an important role in supervisory management. This concept of formal positional authority eventually becomes a part of an entire spectrum of influence and power. At this point, however, you need only remember that authority is one of the basic characteristics of the managerial job. Without authority, managerial functions and the supervisor-subordinate relationship are weakened and become meaningless.

BENEFITS OF BETTER MANAGEMENT

The benefits that you as a supervisor derive from learning to be a better manager are obvious. First, you are given many opportunities to apply managerial principles and knowledge to your present job. Good management by a supervisor makes a great deal of difference in the performance of your department: it functions more smoothly, work gets done on time, staying within your budget is easier, and your team members or subordinates more willingly and enthusiastically contribute toward the ultimate objectives.

The application of management principles puts you on top of your job, instead of being "swallowed up" by it. You also have more time to be concerned with the overall aspects of your department, and in so doing, become more valuable to those to whom you are responsible. For example, you are more likely to contribute significant suggestions and advice to your superiors, perhaps in areas about which you have never before been consulted but that ultimately affect your department. In these times of rapid change and facility mergers and acquisition, you may also find that you see more easily the complex interrelationships of the various departments and organizations throughout the evolving healthcare system. This, in turn, helps you work in closer harmony with your colleagues who are supervising other departments. In short, you are able to do a more effective supervisory job with much less effort.

In addition to the direct benefits of doing a better supervisory job for your healthcare organization, you may gain other benefits. As a supervisor applying sound management principles, you will grow in stature. As time goes on, you will be capable of handling more important and more complicated assignments. You will advance to better and higher-paying jobs. You will move up within the administrative hierarchy and will naturally want to improve your managerial skills as you advance.

As stated earlier, an additional, satisfying thought is that the functions of management are equally applicable in any organization and in any managerial or supervisory position. That is, the principles of management required to produce memory chips, manage a retail department, supervise office work, or run a repair shop are all the same. Moreover, these principles are applicable not only in the United States but in other parts of the world as well. Aside from local customs and questions of personality, it would not matter whether you are a supervisor in a textile mill in India, a supervisor in a chemical plant in Italy, a department foreman in a steel mill in Pittsburgh, or a supervisor of the patient-focused care unit for trauma care in a hospital in San Francisco. By being a manager, you are more mobile in every direction and in every respect.

Therefore, there are great inducements for learning the principles of good management. Again, however, you cannot expect to learn them overnight. You can only become a good manager by actually managing—that is, by applying the principles of management to your own work. You will undoubtedly make mistakes occasionally but will, in turn, learn from those mistakes. The principles and guidelines of management discussed in this book can be applied to most situations, and your efforts to become an outstanding manager will pay substantial dividends. As your managerial competence increases, you will be able to prevent many of the errors and difficulties that make a supervisory job a burden instead of a challenging and satisfying task.

SUMMARY

The demands on good management in healthcare activities are increasing rapidly, making the role of the supervisor most challenging. To employees in the department, the supervisor represents management. To supervisors in other departments, he or she is a colleague, coordinating efforts with theirs and sharing information to achieve the organization's objectives. The supervisor must possess technical, human, and conceptual skills; he or she must have the clinical and technical competence for the functions to be performed in the department and at the same time must manage that department. Good managers are made; they are not born.

Management is the function of getting things done through and with people. The way a supervisor handles the managerial aspects of the job makes the difference between running the department and being run by the department. The managerial aspects of any supervisory job are the same, regardless of the particular type of work involved or the position on the administrative ladder. As a supervisor climbs this ladder, the managerial skills increase in importance and the technical and professional skills gradually become less important. The five managerial functions of planning, organizing, staffing, influencing, and controlling comprise one of the two benchmarks of the manager's job. Each blends into another, and each affects the performance of the others. The output of one provides the input for another. These five functions are universal for all managers, regardless of position in the managerial hierarchy and the nature of the enterprise. The time and effort involved in each function vary, depending on the manager's position on the administrative ladder.

The second benchmark of the managerial job is authority; it makes the managerial position real. This organizational, formal authority is delegated to positions within the organization, permitting those who hold it to make decisions, issue directives, take action, and impose sanctions. To be successful, a manager must embrace the managerial functions and, with the authority he or she has been given, use these functions to achieve the goals for which he or she is responsible. A supervisor benefits greatly both professionally and personally if he or she takes the time to study and acquire managerial expertise and excellence.

NOTES

1. Members of Generation X (born 1965–1979) have embraced free agency over company loyalty. Ambitious, technologically adept, and independent, Gen Xers strive to balance the competing demands of work, family, and personal life (Holiday Inn Express Navigator 2000/2001).

2. Organizational settings include hospitals, nursing homes, clinics, surgical centers, group model HMOs, physician offices, rehab centers, and home care programs.

3. Broadband encompasses a variety of modalities, including, T-1 or T-3 lines, cable, and digital subscriber lines.

REFERENCES

Healthcare Financial Management Association (HFMA). 2000. "Number of Hospitals Dipped Below 6,000 in 1999." CFO Forum Mailing, 3. Westchester, IL: HFMA.

Holiday Inn Express Navigator. 2000/2001. "Talkin' 'Bout My Generation." Holiday Inn Express Navigator, 10.

Mintzberg, H. 1973. *The Nature of Managerial Work*, 55–58. New York: HarperCollins Publishers.

Office of Inspector General (OIG). 2005. [Online information; retrieved 8/30/05.] http://oig.hhs.gov/oei/reports/oei-04-02-00610.pdf and http://oig.hhs.gov/oei/reports/oei-04-02-00611.pdf.

PriceWaterhouseCoopers. 2005. "Cost of Caring: Key Drivers of Growth in Spending on Hospital Care." [Online information; retrieved 8/30/05.] http://www.aha.org/aha/press_room-info/content/PwCcostsReport.pdf.

CHAPTER TWO

The Theories and History of Management

CHAPTER OBJECTIVES

After you have studied this chapter, you should be able to do the following:

1. Identify the major schools of management theory.

2. Discuss the impact of the Industrial Revolution on management and employee relations.

3. Discuss the features and benefits of organizational development.

4. Distinguish among rational authority, positional authority, and charismatic authority.

5. Explain the terms *organization, motion study, time study, Hawthorne effect*, and *method*.

CHAPTER 1 DISCUSSED the definition of management as getting activities efficiently accomplished through people. "Efficiently" implies using the least amount of resources to achieve the goal. Chapter 1 encouraged new supervisors to learn as much about management as possible. Although much learning will occur while you are on the job, some advantages can be gleaned from studying various schools of management thought. This chapter provides an overview of some significant management theories.

These theories touch on each of the five managerial functions of planning, organizing, staffing, influencing, and controlling. New theories are introduced every day, and each serves as a building block for the next. Because of this, management theory will continue to evolve to meet the needs of society. However, management is not a new theory. Egyptian leaders managed thousands of laborers to build the great pyramids. The Chinese built the Great Wall, and the Romans built aqueducts. To be achieved, these projects each required planning, organizing, staffing, influencing, and controlling.

INDUSTRIAL REVOLUTION (1700s–1800s)

No two countries were more responsible for the Industrial Revolution than the United States and England. In his article, "The Two Countries that Invented the Industrial Revolution," Curt Anderson (2001) points out that during the eighteenth and nineteenth centuries, England had no shortage of skilled labor. Rather than replacing English workers, their machines made work more precise. By contrast, in the sparsely populated United States, the needs of a new nation required rapid and simple means of production. Machines augmented the scant workforce. Whereas in England machines served to make talented artisans better, machines in the United States served to make entrepreneurs more productive.

The Industrial Revolution changed the manager's job from owner-manager to professional, salaried manager.[1] This eighteenth century phenomenon transformed the United States from an agricultural society to one that manufactured goods at small mills, shops, and factories. The shops became our early organizations—that is, two or more people working together in a structured, formal environment to achieve a common goal. As the twentieth century opened, many small shops grew into factories as the inventions, machines, and processes used to manufacture goods and products advanced, division of labor concepts were applied, and electricity and the internal combustion engine were developed. Ford Motor Company, the Radio Corporation of America (RCA), and Bell Telephone and Telegraph all grew from this era of advancing technological growth and bringing together people to create and build products and services for others.

The church and the military served as models for the management and organization structures of these new entities. Today's managers can find terms (e.g., superior, subordinate, strategy, hierarchy, and mission) in the Bible and in ecclesiastical and military writings that date back to the late 1500s.

Raymond E. Miles's (1978) book, *Theories of Management: Implications for Organizational Behavior and Development*, describes the U.S. management theory evolutional model as one that includes classical, human relations, and human resources management.

CLASSICAL SCHOOL (1800s–1950s)

The *classical school of management* thought began in the late 1800s and continued through the 1950s. It included such theorists as Fayol, Follett, Gantt, and Weber; these theorists believed that money motivated employees. During this era, the concept of "economic man" surfaced. This management school focuses on efficiency and includes bureaucratic, scientific, and administrative management. According to Allen (2000)[2], "Bureaucratic management relies on a rational set of structured guidelines, such as rules and procedures, hierarchy, and a clear division of labor. Scientific management focuses on the 'one best way' to do a job." Administrative management emphasizes the essential roles of management.

Bureaucratic Management Theory (1930–1950)

Max Weber (1864–1920), known as the father of modern sociology, analyzed bureaucracy as the most logical and rational structure for large organizations. He defined three types of authority: (1) *rational authority* is based on law, procedures, and rules; (2) *positional authority* of a superior over a subordinate stems from legal authority; and (3) *charismatic authority* stems from the personal qualities of an individual. Weber believed that efficiency in bureaucracies came from the following (Allen 2000):[3]

- clearly defined and specialized functions,
- use of legal authority,
- hierarchical form of the organization,
- written rules and procedures,
- technically trained bureaucrats,
- appointment to positions based on technical expertise,
- promotions based on competence, and
- clearly defined career paths.

Scientific Management (1890–1940)

Several large and industrialized organizations had emerged by the turn of the twentieth century. Often they included an assembly line method for manufacturing products. *Scientific management* focuses on the relationship between workers and machinery and defines how to organize tasks for people. It was believed that organization productivity would increase by increasing the efficiency of production processes or the production line. Those who have seen Charlie Chaplan's *Modern Man* will recognize how the employees may have perceived some of the 'enhancements' made by management. The efficiency perspective is concerned with creating jobs that economize time, human energy, and other productive resources. Jobs are designed so that each worker has a specified, definitive task for which he or she is responsible and that can be performed as instructed. Workers were not expected to "think" but rather to follow the specific procedures and methods for each job with no exceptions. This school of management theory includes four well-known theorists: Frederick Taylor (1856–1915), Frank (1868–1924) and Lillian (1878–1972) Gilbreth, and Henry Gantt (1861–1919).

Frederick Taylor

Many of Frederick Taylor's studies were performed at Bethlehem Steel Company in Pittsburgh, Pennsylvania. To improve productivity, Taylor examined the time and motion details of a job; developed a better method for performing that job; scientifically selected, trained, and developed the worker to perform the job (specialization); supported the premise that management and worker would cooperate; and divided work and responsibility equally between managers and workers. Furthermore, Taylor offered piece rates, incentives, and bonuses to increase workers' production.

Taylor, known as the father of scientific management, published *Principles of Scientific Management* in 1911. In his book, he spoke of breaking a job down into its smallest constituent movements, timing each one with a stopwatch and then redesigning the job with a reduced number of motions as well as effort and risk of error. Various incentives, including rest periods and a differential pay scale, were recommended to improve output. He also supported the need to develop specialization. Specialists in a task would perform the same duties every day and throughout each day, giving rise to dramatic productivity increases.

Frank and Lillian Gilbreth

Frank and Lillian Gilbreth also studied motions used in work. Utilizing motion picture technology, they studied the elemental motions, the way these motions were combined, and the time each motion took. They believed it was possible to design work processes for which times of completion could be estimated in advance.[4] Frank Gilbreth is probably best known for his experiments in reducing the number of motions in bricklaying. While Frank Gilbreth captured the title of Father of Time and Motion Studies, his wife, Lillian Gilbreth garnered the title "The First Lady of Engineering." The Gilbreths believed that there was only one best way to perform a process. This belief was later refuted by an administrative management theorist, Mary Parker Follett, whose Law of Situation emphasized that there is no one best way to do anything, but that it all depends on the situation.

From the Gilbreths came the term *motion study*, defined as the division of work into the most fundamental elements. These elements are studied separately and in relation to one another, and from these studied elements, when timed, methods of least waste are built. Furthermore, the Gilbreths defined *time study* as a scientific analysis of methods and equipment used or planned in doing a piece of work, development in practical detail of the best way of doing it, and determination of the time required.

When the Gilbreths designed a task, they depicted with symbols 17 hand motions (e.g., select, grasp, transport, hold) associated with a task. These symbols were called *therbligs* ("gilbreth" spelled backwards). Interestingly, unions resisted some of Gilbreths' efforts, leaving their union members to use the old, more fatiguing approaches to completing their work.

Henry Gantt

Henry Gantt developed a scheduling approach that allowed management to view overlapping tasks that needed to occur over a given time to reach the end product. The chart that evolved from this approach became known as a *Gantt chart*. His management approach focused on motivating employees with rewards for good work through incentive and bonus systems. He also believed in quality leadership and building effective management skills: the organization would benefit as a result of two forces—motivated employees and skilled leaders working together.

Administrative Management (Late 1800s–1920s)

Administrative management describes how to structure an organization for high performance. The man known as the father of modern management was Henri Fayol (1841–1925). Theo Haimann embraced Fayol's management theory and structured this textbook around it. While other theorists were studying the worker, Fayol was studying the manager. Fayol identified five functions of management: planning, organizing, commanding, coordinating, and controlling. He further categorized the features of management into 14 principles:

1. division of work/labor through specialization,
2. authority and responsibility (including expertise and ability to lead),
3. discipline,
4. unity of command,
5. unity of direction,
6. subordination of individual interests to the organization's needs (pursue only work-related activities at work),
7. employee compensation (Hoffman 2005, 107),
8. centralization (authority based on experience),
9. scalar chain (line of authority),
10. order (all materials and personnel have a designated location)(Hoffman 2005, 107),
11. equity (fair, impartial treatment),
12. personnel stability,
13. initiative (acting without direction from a superior), and
14. esprit de corps (shared devotion to a common cause).

Many of these principles are discussed further in the chapters that follow. Both Fayol and Taylor were task- and thing-oriented. Similarly, the Gilbreths were process-oriented, and Weber focused on structure and rules. Little attention focused on the needs of people—that is, the workers (Hoffman 2005).

Human Relations Movement (1930–Present)

This management theory, also known as behavioral management, emerged in the 1920s and emphasized how managers should behave and recognized workers as "social men." The Hawthorne Studies were undoubtedly the catalyst and most significant contribution to the *human relations movement*. The Hawthorne studies were conducted from 1924 to 1933 at the Hawthorne plant of the Western Electric Company in Cicero, Illinois (Allen 2000).

The Hawthorne studies are important to today's management because they emphasize the effect that other humans have on worker productivity. These studies were conducted by several Harvard Business School researchers, among them were T. N. Whitehead, Elton Mayo, George Homans, and Fritz Roethlisberger. It was Elton Mayo who identified the *Hawthorne effect* as the change that occurs when people know they are being studied.

The studies included interviews with the workers to determine the effects that various working conditions might have on productivity. One decision was to raise the level of lighting; this indeed resulted in an increase in productivity. However, for the control group of this study, the level of lighting was decreased, which resulted in an increase in productivity as well. The conclusion was that the lighting had no influence on productivity whatsoever. Instead, the increased attention from the interviewers to the employees was the catalyst for the increased productivity.

Other studies were pursued with varying degrees of interviewing, direct supervision from the research team, team projects, and involvement of the employees in the design of the activities to be studied, leading to similar conclusions that essentially defined worker attitude as a key element in productivity. Giving attention to employees is much more effective for increasing productivity than changing the working condition. The studies also showed that informal leadership exists and that work groups informally establish acceptable output levels for all workers within the group, regardless of monetary incentives offered. These findings encourage supervisors to recognize the informal organization within the formal organization and to listen to employees' complaints as they are probably a symptom of some underlying problem on the job, at home, or in the person's past. In short, Elton Mayo discovered through the Hawthorne studies that the informal organization and sentiments of the group determine work behavior.

Another theorist, Chester Barnard (1886–1961) is best known for his acceptance theory and strategy planning emphasis. Barnard taught that the three top functions of the executive were to (1) establish and maintain an effective communication system, (2) hire and retain effective personnel, and (3) motivate those personnel. His *acceptance theory of authority* states that managers only have as much authority as employees allow them to have. This suggests that authority flows downward but depends on acceptance by the subordinate, which depends on four conditions: (1) employees must understand what the manager wants them to do, (2) employees must be able to comply with the directive, (3) employees must think that the directive is in keeping with organizational objectives, and (4) employees must think that the directive is not contrary to their personal goals (Allen 2000).[5]

HUMAN RESOURCES SCHOOL (1950–PRESENT)

Beginning in the early 1950s, the introduction of the human resources school of management theory represented a substantial progression from the human relations, or behavioral, school. The behavioral approach did not always increase productivity. Thus, motivation and leadership techniques became a topic of great interest. The *human resources school* understands that employees are very creative and competent and that much of their talent is largely untapped by their employers. Employees want meaningful work; they want to contribute; and they want to participate in decision making and leadership functions (Allen 2000).[6] Maslow's studies were inspired by this school of thought. The fundamental notion of human resources theory whereby there is a reciprocal relationship between organization prosperity and worker prosperity served as the impetus for human resources departments in many organizations.

Both the human relations and human resources theories were encouraged by unions and government regulations that reacted to the rather dehumanizing effects of the earlier scientific management and bureaucratic theories. These later theories spawned further schools based on McGregor's Theories X and Y, and Theory Z, which are discussed in further detail in chapters 11, 22, and 24. Briefly, these theories hold the following beliefs:

> *Theory X*: People are lazy and irresponsible, inherently dislike work, must be controlled to do work, and prefer to be directed.
>
> *Theory Y*: People are responsible, enjoy work, view it as natural as play and rest, exercise self-direction, seek responsibility, and work well if rewarded.
>
> *Theory Z*: Group consensus and decision making are necessary to have a productive workforce; employees are ensured long-term employment; and a continued emphasis on quality improvement is nurtured.

CONTEMPORARY MANAGEMENT THEORIES (1940s–PRESENT)

Three contemporary management theories have developed during the latter half of the 1900s due to the rapidly changing nature of today's organizational environments.

Contingency Theory (mid-1960s)

This theory's roots are from the Classical School era and is espoused by Mary Parker Follett's Law of the Situation, which states that there is no one best way to do anything, but that "it [the method of doing] depends" on the situation. The more contemporary version of this theory, the *contingency theory*, was argued by Fred E. Fielder in 1965: management selects an approach that takes into account all aspects of the current situation and factors faced by the organization at that time. These factors or variables include organization size, task complexity, environmental uncertainty, and individual differences. Still today, some call the contingency theory the "It Depends" theory.

Systems Theory (1940–early 90s)

The *systems theory* depicts the organization as a collection of open systems that constantly interact with the external environment and receive resources and inputs from that environment, transforming them into goods and products or services that are put back into the environment for consumption. Systems provide feedback to the inputs, processes, outputs, and outcomes. A functioning automobile, for example, is a system. The engine's spark plugs create a spark that ignites the gasoline. This ignition creates an explosion, which pushes the piston down, propelling the various components that create the movement of the vehicle. The failure of any of these actions serves as "feedback" to the driver as well as to the automobile "system." Thus, a car that has no gasoline cannot operate.

Applying this scenario to the healthcare environment, we find many systems to consider, such as the emergency department. At the emergency room, patients arrive, register for services, are triaged based on their condition, and are treated. If registration or triaging (inputs) are delayed, treatment (output) is delayed, and the patient's condition may deteriorate (outcome). If the registration information does not pass correctly to triage (process), the triage (process) cannot occur. Patients return to the registration desk and complain (feedback), or physicians complain that patients were not appropriately triaged (feedback).

Systems theory was first surfaced in the 1940s by the biologist Ludwig von Bertalanffy and has served as a foundation for more advanced theories, including general systems theory and cybernetics. *Cybernetics* studies the flow of communication within a complex organization. Systems theory also is closely related to chaos theory, which may have gotten its launch from a systems theory cousin known as catastrophe theory. Wikipedia (2005) defines *catastrophe theory* as a branch of mathematics that deals with dynamical systems and was originated with the work of the French mathematician René Thom in the 1960s. It studies and classifies phenomena characterized by sudden shifts in behavior that arise from small changes in circumstances, analyzing how the qualitative nature of equation solutions depends on the parameters that appear in the equation. For example, the timing and magnitude of a landslide are seemingly unpredictable.

Management by Objective (1940s–Present)

Peter Drucker has held a visible position in the field of management theory for more than 60 years. He stressed management fundamentals such as strategic planning and management by objective (MBO) or by results and asserted that management is a discipline, not a science. His concept of MBO should be credited for some of the emphasis on quality improvement because it established objectives or targets for employees to achieve measurements or matrices often tied to performance. It kept people focused on producing results (Hoffman 2005, 122).

Chaos Theory (1960s–Present)

The roots of *chaos theory* are found in the study of astronomy and mathematics circa 1850. Management theorists, such as Tom Peters, picked up the thoughts of these early times in the 1960s. Chaos theory recognizes that the world is unorganized and filled with unpredictable events; therefore, organizational events cannot always be controlled and managers must recognize that they will be faced with unusual challenges. Consider what healthcare managers faced when Hurricane Katrina devastated the Gulf Coast. Chaos theory depicts the organization as a living adaptive system of highly random movements that are robust and interact in a narrow space between stability and disorder or poised at "the edge of chaos."

Chaos theory is also known as "sensitive dependence." The environment is sensitive to changes in initial conditions. Just a small change in the conditions in which people work or live may result in drastically different long-term behavior of a group of employees or a community. Many long-term employees who lived in New Orleans, Biloxi, and other Gulf Coast communities never returned to work, but instead left the area permanently to find a safer environment for themselves and their families. Chaos theorists suggest that systems naturally go to more complexity, and as they do so, these systems become more volatile and must expend more energy to maintain that complexity. As hospitals attempted to reopen and rebuild following Katrina's disaster, these facilities were not only faced with huge capital outlays but also human resources replacement.

Under chaos theory, as organizations or systems expend more energy, they seek more structure to maintain stability. This trend continues until the system splits, combines with another complex system, or falls apart entirely. Sound familiar? This trend is what many see as they go through life, in organizations, and the world in general (McNamara 1999).

Consider the energy that is being spent on airport and building security post September 11, 2001, when the World Trade Center Twin Towers in New York and the Pentagon in Washington, DC, were attacked with hijacked American airplanes. The increased efforts have been implemented to maintain the sense of security that Americans enjoy and have come to expect. Unfortunately, the level of security in the United States prior to 9/11 failed with devastating results, creating chaos, and increased security measures (imposed by both citizens and the federal government) causing chaos of a different kind—that which comes with a change in procedures.

According to Petree (2001), "For thousands of years humans have noted that small causes could have large effects and that it was hard to predict anything for certain." Because chaos theory is so broad and can be applied to situations every day, supervisors must recognize that even slight changes to a work environment may create chaos. Consider the replacement of a program application on a computer. If no one was told to expect the change, regardless of how minimally different it is, staff will be confused initially, possibly bringing work to a standstill.

Organizational Development (Late 1950s–Present)

Organizations bring two or more people together in a formal, structured environment to achieve a common goal. By bringing individuals together, the organization serves as a social system wherein its participants use technology and work processes to achieve the goals of the organization. Thus, the long-term health and performance of the organization is directly related to enriching the environment and lives of the organization's participants. As a result, the participants are encouraged to provide input and suggestions on how to improve the environment.

Organizational development (OD) works by increasing the "health" of social and technical systems such as work processes, communication, rewards, and shared goals. The key to the OD focus is the organization culture: shared beliefs, values, and behaviors (Zatz 2004).

What particularly characterizes the OD approach is a systems viewpoint, emphasis on the culture, and the use of methods. Methods are planned interventions based on research to increase motivation, remove obstacles, facilitate change, and maximize the value of each individual (Zatz 2004).

OD focuses on people issues, because people drive systems; in turn, systems affect people. Consider the motivation level of an employee who takes drive-up orders at a fast-food restaurant, the communications system of which is malfunctioning, crackling, and squawky. Will that employee be motivated to provide superior customer performance when the systems he has to work with are inadequate?

Organizational development allows people to influence systems that influence them. Employee suggestions are encouraged and implemented, often dramatically increasing quality by changing the system and allowing the individual to reach optimal effectiveness. Younger workers who were raised in an environment that encouraged participation in decision making about what to wear, what kinds of gifts are desired, where to go on vacation, and so on will continue to expect this approach in their work environment. OD accommodates the younger workforce by nurturing a participatory workforce. Furthermore, OD helps organizations in the following way (Zatz 2004):

- empowering leaders and individual employees,
- creating a culture of continuous improvement and alignment around shared goals,
- making change easier and faster,
- putting the minds of all employees to work,

- enhancing the quality and speed of decisions,
- making conflict constructive instead of destructive, and
- giving leaders more control over results by giving employees more control over how they do their jobs.

The outcomes of organizational development may include increases in the following (Zatz 2004):

- profits (or cost reduction for nonprofit organizations);
- innovation;
- customer satisfaction;
- product and service quality;
- cost effectiveness;
- organization flexibility;
- personal feelings of effectiveness; and
- job, work, and life satisfaction.

Many theorists have contributed ideas to enhance your understanding of the role of manager. Later chapters explore these and other schools of thought. It should be apparent that events will vary and the needs of the organization will guide you to select some components of one theory and some components of another to address the situation at hand.

ENTREPRENEURIAL SCHOOL (1970s–PRESENT)

One should be able to see that throughout one's workday, many different personalities and situations will be encountered. The healthcare supervisor needs to apply the contingency theory approach to management, possibly applying scientific management to one situation, while using chaos theory to address another. A supervisor should not assume that he or she must use just one of these theories all the time—that will not work.

Coupling the age range of today's worker, a department may have a seventeen year old and a sixty year old working side by side. The younger employee may enjoy working within a self-directed team, while the older worker may prefer to do his or her job as he or she has loyally done for many years.

When we discuss the traits of our X, Y, and millennial generations, we see greater appreciation of teams and self-recognition. As larger firms fail to provide opportunities for autonomy or to reward individual contributions, the organization will lose some of its best thinkers and workers. These individuals will seek the intimacy of teams (Lins 2005); break away from the mold of "we've always done it that way"; and establish their own, smaller, innovative subcultures within the organization or their own entities outside the organization—enter the entrepreneurial school of management.

My definition of entrepreneurial theory may differ from others who espouse this theory such as C.B. Handy or W.H. Bergquist. I base my description of this theory on experience and tend to side with F.A. Lins. My work with healthcare organizations for 30 years has shown that there is always one (or more) individual who is slightly ahead of the curve. Ignored by their superiors, the individual has two choices—conform with the status quo or break away. I have seen too much talent lost by healthcare organizations that are not willing to consider a new approach.

In the 1980s, I met a gentleman who thought the then quality assurance rage was a waste of time because it monitored what had happened and then retrospectively studied trends rather than demanded excellence and required an explanation as well as modification of the process to achieve excellence. The process might have been chicken-egg, but the reaction was, "we're human, we can't expect excellence." His position was that we should expect excellence because we are human, allowing us to think before blindly doing. Of course, today, the Six Sigma approach to quality is exactly what my 1980s gentleman was espousing.

Within each of our organizations are entrepreneurs waiting to be heard. When they are not, they will leave and create privately owned organizations that are small enough to allow an environment marked by personal interaction and brainstorming. They will not be held back by complex bureaucracies. In healthcare, we see this happen when clinicians get frustrated with burdensome scheduling processes. Rather than continue to deal with it, they join together and open their own facility such as clinician-owned surgery centers or MRI services. Talented supervisors quit their jobs to start billing and consulting companies. Tired of not being listened to, these individuals take the entrepreneurial leap and are often successful at doing so.

So what does entrepreneurial management theory tell us? It suggests that we encourage team building but not necessarily force its development; foster sharing and testing of new ideas; listen to our customers, which include our employees; and recognize that we must be willing to accept and possibly financially support some of these ideas or find ourselves buying the services from former employees in the future.

SUMMARY

The Industrial Revolution changed the way we work and live; it brought together technology and people. By doing so, organizations were created. As organizations developed, so did their structures and their members' roles.

The classical school of management thought began in the late 1800s and focuses on efficiency, including bureaucratic, scientific, and administrative theories of management. Bureaucratic management relies on a rational set of structured guidelines, whereas scientific management focuses on the "one best way" to do a job. Administrative management emphasizes the flow of information within the organization.

The human relations and human resources schools of management recognize the need to involve employees in decision making; those employees must also have talents that should and must be tapped to further the organization's goals. Ironically, these schools spawned opposite theories (Theory X and Theory Y) of the worker's attitude toward work.

Contemporary management theories recognize the rapidly changing environment in which organizations do business and that these organizations may cross multiple continents, many cultures, and various languages, all of which must come together to keep the system functioning. As these organizations expand, a manager must understand that by bringing individuals together, the organization serves as a social system in which its participants use technology and work processes to achieve the goals of the organization. Organizational development has been successful in recent times because management and employees improve work processes, communicate, participate in rewards, and share goals. However, if organizations become so large that their bureaucracy stifles innovation, the innovators will leave and seek smaller, less complex environments within which they can achieve intimacy and incubate new ideas.

NOTES

1. As viewed 2/8/06 at http://www.telecollege.dcccd.edu/ mgmt1374/contents.html Supervision 3E Gemmy Allen 2002.

2. As viewed 2/8/06 at http://www.telecollege.dcccd.edu/ mgmt1374/book_contents/1overview/management_history/mgmt_ history.htm Supervision 3E Gemmy Allen 2002.

3. As viewed 2/8/06 at http://www.telecollege.dcccd.edu/ mgmt1374/book_contents/1overview/management_history/mgmt_ history.htm Supervision 3E Gemmy Allen 2002.

4. As viewed 2/8/06 at http://www.telecollege.dcccd.edu/ mgmt1374/book_contents/1overview/management_history/mgmt_ history.htm Supervision 3E Gemmy Allen 2002.

5. As viewed 2/8/06 at http://www.telecollege.dcccd.edu/ mgmt1374/book_contents/1overview/management_history/mgmt_ history.htm Supervision 3E Gemmy Allen 2002.

6. As viewed 2/8/06 at http://www.telecollege.dcccd.edu/ mgmt1374/book_contents/1overview/management_history/mgmt_ history.htm Supervision 3E Gemmy Allen 2002.

REFERENCES

Allen, G. 2000. *Supervision, Second Edition.* [Online edition; retrieved 02/08/06.] http://ollie.dcccd.edu/mgmt1374/book/contents/1overview /management/ history/mgmt/history.htm.

Anderson, C. 2001. "The Two Countries that Invented the Industrial Revolution." [Online article; retrieved 02/08/06]. Darex Corporation Newsletter. http://www.darex.com/new/articles/brittool.html.

Hoffman, H. F. 2005. "Organizations through the Eyes of a Project Manager." [Online article, pp. 93–146; retrieved 08/31/05.] http://www.tcicampus.net/userfolder/hhoffman/MOT-.

Lins, F. A. 2005. "Analysis and Synthesis of Industrial Era Organizational Theory." [Online student paper, University of Phoenix; retrieved 02/08/06.] http://www.stkhi.com/falwork/O700_p2.htm.

McNamara, C. 1999. "Brief Overview of Contemporary Theories in Management." [Online article, Authenticity Consulting, LLC; retrieved 02/08/06.] www.managementhelp.org/library/mgmnt/cntmpory.htm.

Miles, R. E. 1978. *Theories of Management: Implications for Organizational Behavior and Development.* New York: McGraw-Hill.

Petree, J. 2001. "Part 1: History of Chaos Theory." [Online article; retrieved 12/12/01.] http://www.wfu.edu/petrejh4/HISTORYchaos.htm.

Taylor, F. 1911. *Principles of Scientific Management.* New York: Harper Bros.

Wikipedia (The Free Encyclopedia). 2005. [Online information; retrieved 02/08/06.] http://en.wikipedia.org.

Zatz, D. A. 2004. "Organizational Development Toolpack." [Online information; retrieved 02/08/06.] http://www.toolpack.com.

PART II

Connective Processes

CHAPTER THREE

Decision Making

CHAPTER OBJECTIVES

After you have studied this chapter, you should be able to do the following:

1. Discuss the importance of decision-making skills.

2. Discuss how problem solving and decision making are the essence of all managerial activities.

3. Explain the difference between programmed and nonprogrammed decisions.

4. Discuss five basic steps of the decision-making process.

5. Describe different decision-making approaches.

I F PRACTICING MANAGERS were asked to define in one or two words the essence of their jobs, they probably would reply "making decisions." This process of decision making is the core of all managerial activities; in fact, it is a substantial part of everybody's daily activities. All of us have to solve problems at one time or another; decision making is a basic human activity that begins in early childhood and continues through life. Therefore, the concept of decision making should not be a foreign one.

Decision making can be defined as the process of selecting one alternative from a number of other alternatives. Decisions are an integral part of all five managerial functions, but they are most closely associated with the planning function. Although the manager acts within an organizational environment, in this book managerial decision making is considered an individual process.

At the heart of this process is the individual manager, whose decisions are influenced by many other persons; various departments; the total organization; and a multitude of other factors such as the economy, the state of the arts and technology, governmental requirements, and politics.

PROGRAMMED AND NONPROGRAMMED DECISIONS

Many decision-making situations that confront us in our daily lives are not difficult to resolve because we are familiar with the issues and have a standard solution for them. These decisions are called *programmed decisions* because they refer to repetitive, structured, routine problems that have fixed answers, standardized operating procedures, methods, rules, and regulations.

For instance, a staff nurse finds that a patient in postoperative care has an elevated temperature. To verify this, the nurse measures the temperature again with a different thermometer and determines that the patient just had a cup of hot coffee. The thermometer registers the same degree. Reinforced with these facts, the nurse resolves the problem procedurally by checking the patient's temperature again after a period of time; the results come up the same. The next step in this decision-making process is to determine whether the attending surgeon left orders to cover this problem; if not, the nurse automatically decides to consult the physician for further action or use the designated treatment protocol for such a situation. The staff nurse had to make several decisions up to this point—programmed decisions based on standard procedure.

For other decision-making situations, operations research has greatly aided in developing programmed decisions. *Operations research* is closely aligned with systems analysis and is defined as the use of mathematical models, analytical methods, or structured inquiry to analyze a complex situation to identify a better approach for improving or optimizing performance. For instance, a purchasing agent has the ability to determine the reorder point of items as well as the quantity to be ordered by using a computer program that has been designed for this particular problem. In some advanced organizations, the purchasing agent may not even be involved with this order; it may be electronically transmitted to the preferred vendor or to a vendor that offers the lowest current bid price.

However, supervisors are frequently confronted with new or unusual problems—decision-making situations for which no standard solutions exist and no program has been designed. These new problems, the dimensions and ramifications of which are not known or obvious, call for the making of *nonprogrammed decisions*. Although programmed decision situations occur more frequently than nonprogrammed problems, the supervisor is constantly called on to come up with a solution for each.

In all instances, the manager should use a logical, rational, and consistent decision-making process. When the problem being presented could affect other departments or areas, the supervisor should involve colleagues from those areas if time permits for such team decision making. The following discussions are directed to these nonprogrammed decision-making situations.

THE IMPORTANCE OF DECISION-MAKING SKILLS

Problems arise when an unintended occurrence takes place. As a supervisor, you are constantly called on to find practical solutions to problems that are caused by changing situations or unusual circumstances. Normally you are able to arrive at a satisfactory decision. One reason that you are in a supervisory position is that you have made many more correct decisions than wrong decisions about problems.

All managers at all levels make decisions. Also, decisions are not made in a vacuum because each one affects the entire system. Consider the CEO of a large healthcare system who has seen the system grow and add a broad array of services—a comprehensive continuum of care—only to find his system experiencing significant losses as a result of new prospective payment systems and managed care arrangements. He (and his board of trustees and administrative team) must now make some very difficult decisions under the axiom "better shed than red" (Gee 2000, 152).

All managers go through the same process of decision making. The only difference is that the decisions made at the top of the administrative hierarchy are usually more far reaching and affect more people and areas than those decisions made by a first-line supervisor. Thus, decision making is an essential process that permeates the entire administrative hierarchy and all five managerial functions (planning, organizing, staffing, influencing, and controlling). This is why it is included in this section on connective processes (see Figure 1.4).

As with managerial skills, decision-making skills can be learned and, once learned, provide great benefits for the manager. Moreover, it is important to note that your managerial job involves not only making decisions yourself but also seeing that members of your team make and understand decisions effectively.

Obviously, a supervisor cannot make all the decisions necessary for running the department. Thus, you will delegate many of the daily decision-making activities for which you are responsible as a supervisor. This requires you to teach your team members the process of making decisions.

Steps in the Decision-Making Process

The decision-making process involves several steps, which must be taken in the following sequence:

1. Define the problem.
2. Analyze the problem.
3. Develop alternatives.
4. Evaluate the alternatives, and select the best.
5. Take action, and follow up.

Decision making is a continuous process. Each manager learns something new from each decision made. Each decision opens up a wide array of new factors and questions that managers can stow away in their "programmed" databases for use in making the next decision.

Define the Problem

You may have heard more than one supervisor say, "I wish I had the answer." Instead of seeking an answer, however, the supervisor should be looking for the real problem.

The first task in decision making is always to find the problem in a particular situation; only then can one work toward the solution or the answer. As the saying goes, "There really is nothing as useless as having the right answer to the wrong question." In most cases, defining the problem is not an easy task. What often appears to be the problem might be merely a symptom; thus, it is necessary to dig deeper to locate the real problem and define it. For example, a supervisor is confronted with a problem of conflicting personalities within the department. Two employees often quarrel and cannot get along. On checking into this situation, however, the supervisor finds that the problem is not one of personalities but that the functions and duties of each employee have never really been defined or delineated.

Thus, what appeared on the surface to be a problem of personality conflict is actually a problem of organization and structure. Only after the true nature of the problem has been realized can the supervisor do something about it. In the case of the quarreling coworkers, the chances are good that once the activities and duties of the two employees are delineated, the friction between them will stop.

A common problem in health information management (HIM) departments is the accumulation of reports arriving late. When the HIM supervisor studies the situation, however, she discovers that lateness is not the problem but rather a symptom of several conditions: (1) unit staff fail to file results in patient charts when received on the floor; (2) the HIM's process for filing materials is inadequate; (3) the space for the files is insufficient, forcing clerks to avoid filing so as to not hurt their hands; or (4) any combination of these situations. In this scenario, the supervisor needs to take a three-pronged approach to resolve the problem:

1. Address the issue and appropriate procedures with the patient care managers,
2. Redesign the process in HIM, and
3. Loosen the files by purging older records or expanding the file system.

Defining a problem such as this may be a time-consuming chore, but it is time well spent. The process of decision making cannot proceed further until the problem or problems are clearly defined. Clearly defining the problem cannot always be done from an office. Supervisors need to query staff and study processes to identify the problem completely.

Analyze the Problem

After the problem, not just the symptom, has been defined, the manager can set out to analyze it. The first step in this analysis is to assemble the facts. After finding a clear definition of the problem, the supervisor can decide how relevant certain data are and what additional information may be needed. The supervisor then gathers as much information as possible. In the HIM example, the supervisor may need to receive and review all late reports for a period of time to determine the source of each piece (e.g., patient care units; ancillary service areas; external sources such as physician offices, other hospitals, home health agencies) before deciding on a pathway for correction.

Many supervisors complain, however, that they never have enough facts. This complaint is often just an excuse to delay a decision, because a manager can never have all the facts. Therefore, it is necessary to make decisions on facts that are available and also on additional facts that the supervisor can gather without undue delay in time or without incurring excessive costs.

It is also wise to consider the behavioral impact on problem definition and to remember that what is believed to be a fact may be colored by subjectivity. As much as we may want to exclude prejudice and bias, we are only human, and subjectivity creeps into any assessment, especially because employees are involved. Of course, we should make an effort to be as objective and impersonal as possible.

This process of analysis, however, requires the supervisor to think not only of objective considerations but also of intangible factors that may be involved. These factors are difficult to assess and analyze, but they do play a significant role, especially in healthcare institutions. Such intangibles may be factors of reputation, quality of patient care, morale, discipline, perception, or ethics. It is hard to be specific about such factors, but they should nevertheless be considered in analyzing the problem. The HIM scenario displays an excellent example of intangible factors. If a blood test was run on a patient and the results were sent to the patient care unit but not posted on the record, the physician may be unable to find the results and reorder the test. The patient is stuck twice with a needle, the lab incurs twice the cost, care is delayed, and the payer is charged two times. Worse yet, under the Office of the Inspector General's (OIG) compliance initiative this occurrence may be considered "waste" and therefore could result in a monetary fine to the organization.

You should understand that no one person can have all the answers; you will be wise to seek input from others such as peers, subordinates, and your boss. "Top performance demands the joint effort of many people, working together toward a common goal. When an individual works together with others, effectiveness grows, creating greater productivity for everyone involved," says Gemmy Allen (2000) in her writings on consensus building. This approach to making decisions is imperative, especially when the decisions may affect another department.

Develop Alternatives

After defining and analyzing the problem, the manager's next step is to search for and develop various alternative courses of action and solutions. An absolute rule is to develop as many alternatives as possible. Always bear in mind that the final decision can only be as good as the best of the alternatives you have considered. Any given situation should offer at least several alternatives. These choices, however, may not always be obvious, but it is the duty of the decision maker to search for them. Also, some of the alternatives may not be desirable, but the manager should not decide this until all of them have been carefully considered. If this is not done, an either-or style of thinking may prevail. The type of manager who thinks this way is too easily inclined to see only one of two alternatives as the right one to follow.

Consider the following situation. A patient billing policy states that patient accounts with a balance of $5 or less will be written off after 90 days, and three notices will be sent to the patient asking for payment. Balances in excess of $5, however, will be turned over to a collection agency after the 90-day/three-notice course. A patient with a balance of $5.02 receives an aggressive call from a collection agency and in return calls the surgi-center's CEO. Even in this unpleasant dilemma, several alternatives exist, although none of them is completely desirable.

First, the surgi-center could insist on having the patient cooperate with the collection agency to pay the bill, although this would cause ill will. Second, a payment arrangement could be agreed on with the patient to pay the center directly and possibly cause some ill will with the collection agency. Third, the center could write off the charge and use this occurrence to implement a process to review accounts that may be within a certain window of the collection agency referral threshold, say 10 percent, and handle these with a personal call before transferring them to a collection agency.

It is not enough for you as a supervisor to decide among the various alternatives presented by subordinates. The routine alternatives your staff normally suggest may not include all the possible choices. It is your job as a manager to think of more, and possibly better, alternatives. Even in the most discouraging situations several choices exist, and although none of them may be desirable, the manager still has an obligation to find the least-objectionable solution.

Brainstorming is a tool often used to increase creativity in problem solving (Osborn 1963; Aldag and Stearns 1991; Holt 1990). If the problem is particularly vexing and if time permits, a brainstorming session with other supervisors or employees is a good method for coming up with as many alternatives as possible. This session is likely to result in novel, unusual, and unorthodox alternative solutions.

Brainstorming is discussed later in this book. Note, however, that in any brainstorming session the participants must feel free to contribute as many alternatives as possible, no matter how extreme and wild these may seem. Even the wildest idea may have a grain of usefulness; the participants can build, or "hitchhike," on ideas presented by others. Criticism and ridicule, or even the appearance of them by, for instance, nonverbal gestures, during brainstorming cannot be allowed so as to promote the suggestion of all possible ideas; such negative actions can kill a brainstorming session.

This creative problem-solving process is likely to increase the number of alternatives. The process also encourages dialog among coworkers, which may build team spirit, and gives credence to the old adage, "two heads are better than one." Even a supervisor alone can mentally brainstorm a problematic situation to find additional alternatives.

An alternative to brainstorming in person is using the Internet. Many discussion groups exist on the Internet and enrollment in such groups is easy. Peers throughout the United States and around the world actively participate in discussion groups by sharing their experiences and outcomes to inquiries. The advantage to using this resource is that alternative points of view are obtained from a variety of backgrounds.

Evaluate the Alternatives, and Select the Best

The purpose of decision making is to select from various courses of action the one that can provide the greatest number of desired consequences and the smallest number of unwanted consequences. After developing the alternatives, the manager should test each of them by imagining that each has already been put into effect. Each alternative must be examined to determine whether it is feasible and satisfactory and what the consequences are if it is chosen.

Once the supervisor has thought through the alternatives and appraised them along these lines, he or she as the decision maker is now in a position to select one. In this process, the supervisor should bear in mind the degree of risk involved in each course of action. No decision is without risk; one alternative will simply have more or less risk than another. It is also possible that the time factor makes one alternative preferable to another. There is usually a difference in the amount of time required to carry out each alternative, and this should be considered by the supervisor. For example, consider the time factor in a more personal situation. You are driving along the interstate at 65 miles per hour and suddenly the car in front of you blows its rear tire and starts to swerve across the lanes. You rapidly brainstorm your alternatives and take decisive action, considering in a few swift seconds the risk of each option.

In this process of evaluating different alternatives, the supervisor should also bear in mind the resources, facilities, know-how, equipment, and data that are available. Lastly, the manager should not forget to judge the different alternatives along the lines of economy of effort—in other words, which action yields the greatest result for the least amount of effort and expenditure.

The decision must be of high quality, but it must also be acceptable to the group affected by it. If the highest-quality decision is not acceptable to the group, its effectiveness is diminished because it will be carried out grudgingly at best or might even be quietly sabotaged. In such a situation, the supervisor may be advised to choose a more acceptable decision that is not of the highest quality. Acceptability is one more consideration in this process of choice.

Another consideration that plays a role in evaluating one alternative against others is ethics. Most organizations are extremely sensitive to business ethics— that is, what is morally right and wrong as applied to executive behavior and decision making (Valasquez 1988; Munson 1992). In evaluating the alternatives, the manager must make certain that he or she complies with established corporate and professional ethical codes.

Using these criteria of feasibility, risk, timing, acceptability, ethics, resources, and economy, the manager often can see that one alternative clearly provides a greater number of desirable consequences and fewer unwanted consequences than any other. In such cases, the decision is relatively easy. The best alternative, however, is not always so obvious; occasionally, two or more alternatives may seem equally desirable. The choice then becomes simply a matter of the manager's personal preference. On the other hand, the manager also may believe that no single alternative far outweighs any of the others or is sufficiently stronger. In this case, it might be advisable to combine two of the better alternatives and come up with a compromise solution.

What about a situation in which the manager finds that none of the alternatives is satisfactory and that all of them have too many undesirable effects? As a supervisor, you might have faced a situation in which the undesirable consequences of all the alternatives were so overwhelmingly bad that they paralyzed any action. You might have thought that the only available solution to the problem was to take no action at all. Such a solution, however, is deceptive. A supervisor is wrong to believe that taking no action is as much a decision as deciding to take a specific action, although few people are aware of this. Most people think that taking no action relieves them of making an unpleasant decision. The only way for the manager to avoid this pitfall is to try to visualize the consequences of inaction. The manager needs only to think through what would happen if no action were taken and will probably see that in so doing, an undesirable alternative is chosen.

Having ruled out inaction in most cases, all alternatives may still seem undesirable. In such a case, you should search for new and different alternatives. Be a bit creative, and try to develop at least a couple of new solutions. Also, check to see that all the steps of the decision-making process have been followed. Has the problem been clearly defined? Have all the pertinent facts been gathered and analyzed? Have all possible alternatives been considered? Have you tried brainstorming? Chances are that some new alternatives will come up, and you can make a good decision. However, if a good solution does not present itself at this point, you might have to employ some additional factors such as experience, intuition, and actual testing or resort to scientific decision making.

Experience   The manager's final selection from the various alternatives is frequently influenced and guided by past experience (experiential decision making). Wisely, managers often decide based on their own experience or that of other managers. Managers can apply knowledge gained by past experience to new situations, and no manager should ever underestimate the importance of such knowledge. On the other hand, it is dangerous to follow past experience blindly.

Experiential decision making is often seen in medicine. For example, a person appears at a urologist's office with lower back pain, and the urologist may diagnose it as a bladder infection. An orthopedist looking at the same problem may consider it a spur on a lumbar vertebra, while a neurologist may consider it a pinched nerve. Each physician is basing this initial impression on his or her experience. Before proceeding to treat the initial impression, however, the physician gathers more facts because he or she knows that blindly accepting the first impression could result in the actual condition becoming more serious.

Therefore, whenever the manager calls on experience as a basis for choice among alternatives, he or she should examine the situation and conditions that prevailed at the time of the past decision. Current conditions may still be very similar to that of the previous occasion. More often than not, however, conditions from one case to the next are considerably different, and the underlying circumstances and assumptions are no longer valid. In these cases, of course, the decision made may not be the same.

Previous experience can also be helpful if the manager is called on to substantiate the reasons for making a particular decision. Experience is a good defense tactic, and many superiors use it as valid evidence. Past experience must always be viewed with the future in mind; that is, the underlying circumstances of the past, present, and future must be considered. Only within this framework is experience a helpful approach to selecting an appropriate alternative.

Hunches and Intuition   Managers can admit at times that they have based their decisions on hunches and intuition. At first glance, certain managers may seem to have an unusual ability for satisfactorily solving problems by intuitive means. A deeper search, however, will disclose that the "intuition" on which the manager thought a decision was based was actually past experience or knowledge. In reality, the manager is recalling similar situations from the past that are now stored in his or her memory; this type of recall is labeled having a hunch or gut feeling.

No superior looks favorably on a subordinate who continually justifies decisions based on intuition or hunch alone. These factors may come into play occasionally, but they must always be supplemented by more concrete considerations.

Experimentation   The avenue of experimentation, or testing, is a valid approach to decision making in the scientific world; reaching conclusions through laboratory tests and experimentation for many types of decisions is essential. In management, however, experimenting to see what happens is inappropriate and often too costly and time consuming. Moreover, it is difficult to maintain controlled conditions and to test various alternatives fairly in a normal work environment. There may be certain instances, however, when a limited amount of testing and experimenting is admissible, as long as the consequences are not too disruptive. For example, a supervisor might decide to test different work schedules or different locations for a new desktop computer. In this small, restricted sense, experimentation may at times be valid. In a supervisory situation, however, experimentation usually is at best an expensive way of reaching a decision.

Scientific Decision Making   During the last five decades, a new group of highly sophisticated tools has been available to aid the manager in decision making. These tools are quantitative, involving linear programming, operations research, probability, model building, and simulation. They are mathematical techniques applied by mathematicians, statisticians, programmers, systems analysts, and other scientists who work with computers. The overall process is known as *scientific decision making*, or operations research. A full discussion of these tools is beyond the scope of this book, and a short description could not do justice to this important, large, and well-documented field of scientific decision making. To gain additional information, one can visit many sites on the Internet as well as read journals and texts available at the library.

Only certain types of management problems lend themselves to this type of quantitative analysis and solution. In a healthcare situation, for example, it could be applicable to situations such as scheduling to minimize patient waiting times or maximize use of operating room resources, optimizing inventory stocking levels, and evaluating outcomes data to define the most effective clinical pathway. Often these analyses are performed to assist in reengineering a process, in the context of an operational or performance improvement activity. After the project is completed, the organization can establish performance metrics or scorecards. Such scientific problem solving is complicated and may be costly; however, when the magnitude of a problem warrants considerable effort and expenditure, it may be the best solution.

The problems confronting a line supervisor usually are not of this magnitude. If a major problem is affecting the entire organization, however, or if similar problems are found in several departments, it may be advisable for top management to employ the quantitative approach. Because most healthcare organizations today have access to computer systems or decision-support departments, it should not be difficult to utilize these techniques.

Take Action, and Follow Up

Effective execution of the decision is every bit as important as making the decision. Decision making is not complete without evaluating the effectiveness of the decision. This is the manager's control function. If all is well and the results are as expected and satisfactory, the supervisor has reached his or her goal. If the results are not as expected or if unanticipated consequences arise, the supervisor should look at the situation as a new problem and go through all the steps of the decision-making process from a new point of view.

Action and follow-up are impossible without two other essential processes— communication and coordination. Unless a decision is clearly communicated to the people who must carry it out and unless it is coordinated with other decisions and other departments, it is meaningless. Thus, these two additional connective processes, discussed in the next two chapters, are vital to management's overall task of getting things done through and with people.

SUMMARY

Selecting the best alternative by facts, study, and analysis of various proposals is still the best way to make a managerial decision. If an objective, rational, systematic method is used in this selection process, the manager is likely to make better decisions. The first step in such a method is to define the problem; the second step is to analyze it. Third, develop all the alternatives you possibly can, think them through as if you had already put them into action, and consider the consequences of each. By following this method, you will likely select the best alternative—that which has the greatest number of desired consequences and the least number of unwanted consequences.

Not only can you learn this sound method of decision making, but you, as a supervisor, can teach the same systematic approach to your subordinates. In doing so, you are assured that whenever subordinates are confronted with a decision, they can also arrive at a solution in a systematic and rational manner. Although this process is not always a guarantee for arriving at the best decisions, it is likely to produce more good decisions than would otherwise be the case.

Scientific decision making, or operations research, is an approach to problem solving that involves quantitative analysis, models, and computer applications. If the problem is of sufficient magnitude to warrant such an expensive effort, sophisticated scientific decision-making techniques that involve mathematicians, statisticians, systems analysts, or other specialists should be used.

REFERENCES

Aldag, R. J., and T. M. Stearns. 1991. *Management, Second Edition*, 696. Cincinnati, OH: South-Western Publishing Co.

Allen, G. 2000. *Supervision, Second Edition*. [Online revision; retrieved 02/08/06.] http://www.telecollege.dcccd.edu/mgmt1374/book_contents/4directing/ consensus/consbldg.

Gee, E. P. 2000. "Leaner Is Greener." *Journal of Healthcare Management* 45 (3): 151–54.

Holt, D. H. 1990. *Management Principles and Practices, Second Edition*, 116. Englewood Cliffs, NJ: Prentice Hall.

Munson, R. 1992. *Intervention and Reflection—Basic Issues in Medical Ethics, Fourth Edition*. Belmont, CA: Wadsworth Publishing Company.

Osborn, A. F. 1963. *Applied Imagination, Third Edition*, 151–63. New York: Charles Scribner's Sons.

Valasquez, M. G. 1988. *Business Ethics Concepts and Cases, Second Edition*. Englewood Cliffs, NJ: Prentice Hall.

CHAPTER FOUR

Coordinating Organizational Activities

CHAPTER OBJECTIVES

After you have studied this chapter, you should be able to do the following:

1. Explain the increasing need for coordination as a result of increased work specialization and fragmentation of patient care.

2. Define the meaning of coordination as linking together a multitude of activities.

3. Differentiate between cooperation and coordination.

4. Discuss the obstacles inherent in achieving coordination.

5. Discuss how managers should not treat coordinating as a separate managerial function but as a byproduct of the five managerial functions.

6. Discuss the importance of good decision making and communication in achieving coordination.

7. Describe the internal and external dimensions of coordination.

DIVISION OF WORK, or *work specialization*, means to break down a job into smaller, more specialized tasks. Division of work and specialization, as discussed in Chapter 13, involves separating employees into departments, divisions, units, sections, and so on based on their shared expertise. This method of work specialization is particularly common in the healthcare field. Having many specialized departments leads to large and complex organizational structures. This proliferation of specialties is necessary to ensure the best possible care of patients as well as high standards of medical expertise. However, it creates additional problems for the management of healthcare facilities and even more difficulties within an integrated healthcare system—namely, the need for coordination, the process of linking together the activities of all units in each of the affiliated organizations.

The reason for coordination is that all these healthcare entities depend on each other for services, resources, information, and communications. Patient care data are created and exchanged among patient service areas (e.g., from blood bank to surgery, from surgery to intensive care, from intensive care to radiology) and with affiliated entities to ensure continuity of care (e.g., from the hospital to the home health agency, from the home health agency to the durable medical equipment company, from the primary care physician's office to the consulting specialist). When many different specialized areas are interdependent on patient care data, more attention must be devoted to coordination.

Coordination of information in non-patient-care areas is as important as in patient care entities. If data are not accurately captured, reported, and assessed by management, workflow and support of patient care services are negatively affected and goals are not achieved.

THE MEANING OF COORDINATION

Supervisory management was defined earlier as the process of getting things done through and with people by directing their efforts toward common objectives. This means that management involves coordination of the efforts of all the members of an organization. Some authors have even defined management as the task of achieving coordination or, more specifically, of achieving the orderly synchronization of employees' efforts to provide the proper amount, timing, and quality of execution so that their unified efforts lead to the stated objectives. Other management experts have preferred to look at coordination as a separate managerial function.

Organization, as defined earlier, is two or more people working together in a structured, formal environment to achieve a common goal. Coordination, then, is the linking together of the activities in the organization to achieve the desired results. It is the connective process by which entities, departments, and tasks are interrelated to reach the objectives.

Thus, for the purposes of this book, coordination is viewed not as a separate function of the manager nor as the defining characteristic of management, but as a process by which the manager achieves orderly group effort and unity of action in pursuit of the common purpose. The manager engages in this process while performing the five basic managerial functions of planning, organizing, staffing, influencing, and controlling. The resulting coordination should be one of the goals that the manager keeps in mind when performing each of the five managerial functions. Coordination, therefore, is a byproduct of the appropriate execution of the five managerial functions; it is a part of everything the manager does.

The task of achieving coordination is much more difficult at the top administrative level than at the supervisory level. The CEO must achieve the synchronization of efforts throughout the entire organization, whereas the supervisor of a department only has to be concerned with coordination primarily within her own department and its relation to other divisions. However, you should also keep coordination at the forefront of your mind whenever you plan, organize, staff, influence, and control. Finally, you should recognize that those activities that affect other departments result in a more complex maze of coordination efforts.

COORDINATION AND COOPERATION

The term coordination must not be confused with cooperation. *Cooperation* merely indicates the willingness of individuals to help each other. It is an informal action that requires no structure or planning, and authority is retained by each party in the process. Coordination is much more inclusive, requiring more than the mere desire and willingness of the participants. It is formal, requiring some planning and role and relationship delineation.

For example, consider a group of people attempting to move a heavy object. They are sufficient in number, willing and eager to cooperate with each other, and trying to do their best to get the job done. They are also fully aware of their common purpose. In all likelihood, however, their individual efforts are of little avail until one of them, the manager, gives the proper orders to apply the right amount of force at the right place and time. Only then will the group's efforts be sufficiently coordinated to move the object. This example introduces a third concept—*collaboration,* whereby individuals who see different aspects of a problem work together to achieve a common goal. Collaboration requires both cooperation and coordination to build substantive agreement.

Ensuring timely and accurate billing is a common activity in healthcare today that requires not only cooperation among several units but also, primarily, coordination of data. Clearly, if correct insurance and patient-identifying information is not collected at the time of admission or registration, the final billing function is hindered. Regardless of the accuracy and completeness of the reports prepared by the physician and the coding applied by the health information coding staff, if this information links to an incorrect insurance number or patient name, the bill may not be paid. The coordination of information gathering is dependent on each cooperating party performing his or her function with precision and transmitting the results to those other parties who rely on the information to achieve the intended goal.

To help differentiate between coordination, cooperation, and collaboration, Dave Pollard (2005) created Table 4.1.

It is possible that, by coincidence, mere cooperation can bring about the desired result, but no manager can afford to rely on coincidence. Although cooperation is always helpful and its absence can prevent all possibility of coordination, its presence alone does not necessarily yield results. Coordination is therefore superior to cooperation in order of importance. Coordination is a conscious effort to tie activities together.

TABLE 4.1: COORDINATION, COOPERATION, OR COLLABORATION?

	Coordination	Cooperation	Collaboration
Preconditions for success ("must-haves")	Shared objectives; need for more than one person to be involved; understanding of who needs to do what by when	Shared objectives; need for more than one person to be involved; mutual trust and respect; acknowledgment of mutual benefit of working together	Shared objectives; sense of urgency and commitment; dynamic process; sense of belonging; open communication; mutual trust and respect; complementary, diverse skills and knowledge; intellectual agility
Enablers (additional "nice-to-haves")	Appropriate tools (see below); problem-resolution mechanism	Frequent consultation and knowledge sharing between participants; clear role definitions; appropriate tools (see below)	Right mix of people; collaboration skills and practice collaborating; good facilitator(s); collaborative "four practices" mind-set and other appropriate tools (see below)
Purpose of using the approach	Avoid gaps and overlap in individuals' assigned work	Obtain mutual benefit by sharing or partitioning work	Achieve collective results that the participants working alone are incapable of accomplishing
Desired outcome	Efficiently achieved results that meet objectives	Same as for coordination, plus savings in time and cost	Same as for cooperation, plus innovative, extraordinary, breakthrough results and collective *"we did that!"* accomplishment
Optimal application	Harmonizing tasks, roles, and schedules in *simple* environments and systems	Solving problems in *complicated* environments and systems	Enabling the emergence of understanding and realization of shared visions in *complex* environments and systems

(continued)

TABLE 4.1: *(Continued)*

	Coordination	Cooperation	Collaboration
Examples	Project to implement off-the-shelf IT application; traffic flow regulation	Marriage; operating a local community-owned utility or grain elevator; coping with an epidemic or catastrophe	Brainstorming to discover a dramatically better way to do something; jazz or theatrical improvisation; cocreation
Appropriate tools	Project management tools with schedules, roles, critical path (CPM), PERT and GANTT charts; "who will do what by when" action lists	Systems thinking; analytical tools (root cause analysis, etc.)	Appreciative inquiry; open-space meeting protocols; four practices; conversations; stories
Degree of interdependence in designing the effort's work products (and need for physical colocation of participants)	Minimal	Considerable	Substantial
Degree of individual latitude in carrying out the agreed-on design	Minimal	Considerable	Substantial

Source: Dave Pollard, *Meeting of Minds* Innovation Consultants, Published March 25, 2005 in *How to Save the World* weblog. Used with permission.

DIFFICULTIES IN ATTAINING COORDINATION

Coordination is not easily attained, and it is becoming increasingly difficult as the various duties in the healthcare field become more complex. As an organization grows and more departments become decentralized, the task of synchronizing daily activities becomes more and more complicated. As the number of employees grows, rotates shifts, and telecommutes, the need for coordination and synchronization to secure the unified result increases. Not only can specialization cause problems of coordination, but human nature can present problems as well. Your employees are generally preoccupied with their own work because their evaluations are based on how they perform their jobs. Thus, they may have a narrow perspective and hesitate to become involved in other areas.

Coordination can be both hindered and helped by the use of automation. Some readers can acknowledge the difficulties they encountered when a new computer system was installed, which may have failed to interface adequately with other existing systems. Equally devastating is when an organization has become reliant on a proprietary information system sold by one manufacturer that does not permit the integration of new technologies from another manufacturer. The organization's investment is substantial, and it cannot walk away from the asset, but it also cannot afford to do without the new technologies that may result in labor or other resource savings. This may be why *open architecture systems* are preferred; they allow different yet compatible (nonproprietary) systems from a variety of manufacturers to be used without causing a loss of coordination of data.

COORDINATION AND MANAGERIAL FUNCTIONS

Coordination cuts through each of the managerial functions. The manager's planning stage is the ideal time to incorporate coordination. As a supervisor, you must see that the various plans within your department are properly interrelated. You should discuss these plans and alternatives with the employees who are to carry them out so that they have an opportunity to express any doubts, objections, or suggestions for improvement. Furthermore, if the plans affect other departments, it is imperative that you discuss the plans with those departments' supervisors. By including employees and colleagues in the process while plans are still flexible, you increase your chances for effective coordination and collaboration.

The same concern for coordination should exist when the manager organizes. Indeed, the whole purpose of organizing is to ensure coordination. Thus, whenever a manager groups activities and assigns them to various subordinates, coordination should be in his or her mind. By placing related activities that need to be closely synchronized within the same administrative area, coordination is facilitated.

Moreover, in the process of organizing, management should define authority relationships in such a way that coordination will result. Often poor coordination is caused by lack of understanding of who is to perform what, or by the failure of a manager to delegate authority and exact responsibility clearly. Such vagueness can easily lead to duplication of efforts instead of synchronization.

Coordination should also be an aspect of the staffing function. Having the right number of employees in various positions is important to ensure that the functions are properly performed. Equally as important is that the manager should see that they have the proper qualifications and training.

When a manager directs and influences, he or she is also concerned with coordination. The essence of giving instructions, coaching, teaching, and supervising subordinates is to coordinate their activities so that the overall objectives of the institution are reached in the most efficient way. As some experts have stated, coordination is that phase of supervision devoted to obtaining the harmonious and reciprocal performance of two or more subordinates' responsibilities.

Finally, coordination is directly connected with the controlling managerial function. By checking whether the activities of the department are proceeding as planned and directed, any discrepancy is discovered and immediately corrected to ensure coordination after that point. Frequent evaluation and correction of departmental operations help to synchronize not only the efforts of employees but also the activities of the entire organization. Thus, by its nature, controlling is the last process to bring about the overall coordination.

COORDINATION AND DECISION MAKING

Because the process of decision making is at the heart of all managerial functions, achieving coordination must be foremost in every manager's mind whenever he or she is making decisions. When choosing from the various alternatives, the manager must never forget the importance of achieving synchronization of all efforts. At times, a certain alternative taken by itself may seem to constitute the best choice. A second choice, however, may result in better coordination. This is why Chapter 3 stresses the importance of the solution's acceptability as one of the supervisor's considerations in choosing from alternatives. The supervisor is better advised to follow the second solution because achieving coordination is an important, if not overriding, objective.

COORDINATION AND COMMUNICATION

In all coordination efforts, good communication is imperative. It is not enough for a manager to make decisions that are likely to bring about coordination; having decisions carried out effectively is at least as important. To achieve successful execution, the supervisor must first communicate the decisions effectively to the subordinates so that they understand them correctly (the importance of this is discussed in Chapter 5).

Personal, face-to-face contact is probably the most effective means of communicating with others to obtain coordination. Other means, however, such as written reports, minutes, procedures, rules, and newsletters or electronic methods such as faxes and e-mails also ensure the speedy dissemination of information to employees. Many organizations use e-mail or other web-based technology, allowing immediate response in written form and often facilitating communication between divisions that are geographically separated. Intranets assist geographically dispersed healthcare systems to communicate within seconds new policies, services, and reports to all locations. Remote access to e-mail or intranet permits individuals at home or out of town to coordinate activities without delay.

Internal Communication in Healthcare Centers

Because of the proliferation and specialization of medical sciences and technologies, healthcare centers have become large and complex organizational structures. More and more positions have had to be created, and this increasing specialization and division of work has generated a need for more and better coordination. Because of such specialization, however, the synchronization of daily activities has become extremely complicated and coordination has become harder to attain. As the number of positions in your department and in the facility increases and as more specialized and sophisticated tasks are performed, the greater your need and effort becomes for coordination and synchronization to secure the unified result—namely, the highest-quality patient care.

Of course, the process of bringing about total coordination of all divisions and levels within a healthcare facility is ultimately the concern of the chief administrator. The CEO must deal with the fact that each department, and each facility within a system, is likely to favor one route over another, depending on its particular functions and experience. Considerable thoughtfulness and understanding is required of all managerial and supervisory personnel to coordinate the working relationships of the groups above, below, and alongside each department. Even with cooperative attitudes, self-coordination, and self-adjustment by most members of the healthcare organization, duplication of actions and conflicts of efforts may still result unless administration carefully synchronizes all activities. Only through such coordination can management bring about total accomplishment that exceeds the sum of the individual parts. Although each part is important, the result can be of greater significance if management achieves coordination. Good communications act as necessary lubricants in all these processes.

DIMENSIONS OF COORDINATION

The need for coordination exists in three directions: vertically, horizontally, and diagonally.

Vertical Coordination

Coordination between different levels of an organization can be considered as vertical coordination, such as between the CEO and the vice president of facilities or between the vice president of facilities and the director of housekeeping. *Vertical coordination* is achieved by delegating authority, assigning duties, and supervising and controlling. Although authority carries great power, effective vertical coordination is better achieved by performing the managerial functions wisely instead of relying on the weight of formal authority (see Figure 15.2).

Horizontal Coordination

Horizontal coordination exists among persons and departments on the same organizational level and must be present to solve problems that affect different areas. For example, one goal of many healthcare facilities is to achieve a shorter average length of stay (LOS). To do this, identifying the diagnosis-related group (DRG) as early as possible in the admission process has been targeted as the solution by both the management and medical staffs. As a result, new arrangements have to be made among the various managers of the activities affected, and each has reviewed the plan with his or her staff. The admissions registrar, together with the health information management coding specialist, case manager, patient care manager, chief of diagnostic services, skilled nursing unit manager, and home health coordinator try to coordinate their activities to achieve this goal (see Figure 4.1).

Each individual involved manages his or her own department and has no authority over other managers. Horizontal coordination obviously cannot be ordered by any one of them. It is achieved by a policy and procedure stating that when necessary, the departments must interact, cooperate, and adjust their activities to achieve coordination. If coordination cannot be achieved, then this problem must be referred to a higher level in the managerial hierarchy with authority over all these departments. In all likelihood, this is the CEO or COO (chief operating officer), who will issue the necessary directives to facilitate the shorter length-of-stay program efforts. Obviously, if those who must deal with the problems on a daily basis can gain consensus on the solution to the coordination barrier, implementation, future coordination, and cooperation will be enhanced.

Diagonal Coordination

Diagonal coordination cuts across the organizational arrangements, ignoring positions and levels. In a small day-surgery center, for example, close working relationships and short lines of communication make diagonal coordination easier than in a large organization. Even in this case, expectations must be reasonable. For instance, in an organization, all departments need access to the engineering and maintenance department, a centralized service. However,

FIGURE 4.1: SHORTENING LOS PROJECT

Departments/Services	Actions
Admissions	Registrar checks list of targeted conditions usually requiring discharge planning
Health Information Management	Coding specialist assigns working DRG for case manager
Case Management	Selects appropriate clinical pathway for condition and begins discussions with patient care, alternative care facilities, and attending physician relative to the anticipated services for this DRG, the DRG's average LOS, and reimbursement
Medical Staff	Places orders for treatment, discusses needs with family, places orders for alternative care
Diagnostic Services	Expedites scheduling to diagnostic testing and ancillary services
Patient Care	Ensures testing is completed and patient is informed and cared for
Skilled Nursing Unit	Identifies bed availability for patient care to expedite transfer
Home Health Agency	Coordinator confers with SNF and physician to provide services at home post-discharge

Note: SNF = skilled nursing facility

engineering cannot be everywhere at once. This access has to be coordinated by negotiations between the users and the provider (see Figure 4.2). Furthermore, coordination cannot be accomplished simply by referring the problem up the chain of command because tension may build between the two departments and eventually your boss will question why you are unable to work with other departments to achieve a harmonious solution.

The techniques and methods used in an organizational setting vary with the dynamics of the environment and the degree of specialization. If the manager cannot achieve coordination because of the dynamic nature of the environment or if a project is so broad (e.g., construction of a new hospital), an individual in a liaison role may be called on to facilitate and coordinate. Some organizations engaged in high-performance and dynamic industries have even had to introduce an entire coordinating department into the organizational structure.

Because the task of securing harmonious action and internal coordination within a healthcare center belongs primarily to those in managerial positions, the task should not be assigned to a specialist, who also may be called a coordinator. The managers are in a far better position than a specialist to view the

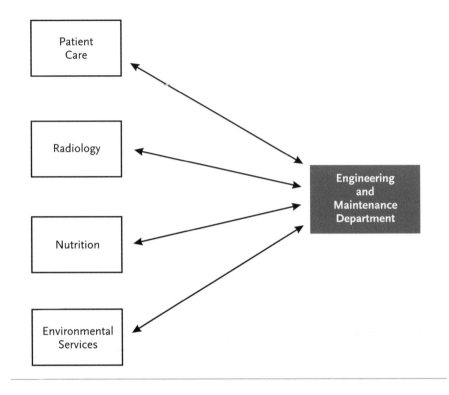

FIGURE 4.2: DIAGONAL COORDINATION

Patient Care

Radiology

Nutrition

Environmental Services

Engineering and Maintenance Department

various functions and to determine how they should be coordinated to bring about the desired objective, and these managers carry the authority to get the job done. Again, all managers must coordinate as they perform their five managerial functions. While some industries have found the coordinator or liaison position helpful, it is questionable whether the task of securing internal coordination within the healthcare center can be shifted or assigned to a special department or a number of individuals (Lawrence and Lorsch 1969).

THE COORDINATOR AS A MISNOMER

Some healthcare entities do have positions labeled "coordinator"; often, however, these are traditional managerial and supervisory jobs and should have been named as such. In these cases, the title "coordinator" is a misnomer. For instance, instead of having a professional known as performance improvement manager, the position may be called "performance improvement coordinator." This position, regardless of the title, is likely to be managerial to the extent that the coordinator manages some staff and activities that cut across many levels of the organization. Some healthcare centers simply prefer the word coordinator to that of supervisor, as, for example, shift coordinator. The federal government uses the term "coordinator" loosely as well. Dr. David Brailer was the former U.S. National Coordinator for Health Information; he managed a staff and resources. On the other hand, some staff professionals who are advisory in nature carry the title coordinator and rightly so.

COORDINATION WITH EXTERNAL ENTITIES

A need for coordination with entities external to the institution also exists. A special coordinator or liaison may be used in situations in which a hospital is trying to coordinate some activities with other healthcare institutions (e.g., joint venture between the hospital, a long-term healthcare facility, surgical center, and home health agency) or with external funding or regulatory agencies (e.g., division of family services, disability determinations, social security administration, workers compensation, health maintenance organization, Medicaid). Such persons should be thoroughly familiar with the conditions and thinking of their institution, be able to explain them to others, and communicate the findings and intentions back to their institution. The coordinator may or may not have been granted authority to commit the institution to action. However, in most instances, the person responsible for coordinating with external factions must check with an administrator or other executive to determine how far the institution will go to support the chosen action. In this situation, the coordinator is not a manager as defined in this book.

Nevertheless, the importance of such external coordination should not be underestimated. The greater the degree of coordination among healthcare centers and related institutions, the better the overall healthcare system is. Indeed, much is being said today about improving healthcare through regional health information organizations and comparative profiling.

SUMMARY

Coordination, the orderly synchronization of all efforts of the members of the organization to achieve the stated objectives, plays a part in every function of a manager. It is not a separate managerial function but cuts across each of the five functions and is a byproduct of these functions. Coordination should not be confused with cooperation: cooperation is always helpful in achieving coordination, but coordination is more encompassing.

As a supervisor plans, organizes, staffs, influences, and controls, he or she must remember that the ultimate goal is to achieve coordination of all efforts. The same thought should be foremost in the manager's mind whenever he or she makes decisions and communicates them to the employees. Achieving coordination is a valid consideration for all managers, regardless of their position, level within the administrative hierarchy, or type of enterprise in which they work. Proliferation and specialization of the medical sciences and technologies have made coordination more difficult.

Coordination with entities external to the institution, such as government agencies, local health councils, users, and other provider groups, is also important. To achieve external coordination, facilities can use a liaison or special coordinator to provide the necessary contacts between the institution and outside entities.

REFERENCE

Lawrence, P. R., and J. W. Lorsch. 1969. *Organization and Environment: Managing Differentiation and Integration.* Homewood, IL: Richard D. Irwin, Inc.

CHAPTER FIVE

Communicating

CHAPTER OBJECTIVES

After you have studied this chapter, you should be able to do the following:

1. Describe the communication model and the roles of the senders and receivers.
2. Discuss how communication affects organizational performance.
3. Identify and discuss communication networks, channels, and barriers.
4. Describe how managers can ensure more effective communication by overcoming roadblocks.
5. Explain the operation of the grapevine and its importance.

FROM THE MANAGER'S point of view, communication is the process of exchanging information in such a way that mutual understanding is achieved between two or more people about work-related issues. In general terms, it is a psychological process of sharing information to achieve a common understanding between ourselves and others. Communication is the third process that serves to link the managerial functions in an organization (see Figure 1.4). Employees look for and expect communication because it is a means of motivating and influencing people. Communication is vital to them not only for purposes of social satisfaction but also for doing their jobs effectively. Thus, the communication process fulfills both human needs and institutional needs. Fundamentally, it is a process of pulling together the employees of the department.

Almost all daily managerial activities involve communication—that is, giving and receiving information. Because communicating involves two or more persons, behavioral processes such as motivation, attitudes, perception, leadership, experience, and feelings play important roles. When the supervisor sends a message by speaking, by writing, or by electronic means, he or she encodes a message from a unique perspective. It is influenced by perceptions of the sender's world, making assumptions about the receiver's perspectives and how the message will be received. Backgrounds, perceptions, attitudes, values, and

65

other factors may differ widely among the individuals involved, all of which make achieving a mutual understanding of others' ideas difficult.

As with all organizations, valid information is needed by a healthcare facility to function effectively. Communication provides the key to this important resource. A hospital devotes much activity to gathering and processing information from the moment the patient enters the facility until the patient is discharged. Serious consequences can arise when communications are minimal, become misunderstood, break down, or do not exist.

You already know that as a supervisor your job is to plan, organize, staff, influence, and control the work of the employees and to coordinate their efforts for the purpose of achieving departmental objectives. To accomplish these goals, you must articulate plans and organize the arrangement of the work, give directives, describe to each subordinate what is expected of her or him, and speak to each regarding his or her performance. All this is done by communicating.

As you continue supervising employees, you probably will realize that your skill in communication determines your success. Communication is the most effective tool for building and keeping a well-functioning team. Communication is the only means a supervisor has to take charge of and train a group of employees, direct them, motivate them, and coordinate their activities. This ability to communicate is the essence of leadership. Is there any area of responsibility within your job as a supervisor that you could fulfill without communicating? No. Without effective communication, the organizational structure cannot survive.

THE NATURE OF COMMUNICATION

Fundamental and vital to all managerial functions, communication is a means of transmitting information and making oneself understood by another or others. The exchange is successful only when mutual understanding results. Agreement is not necessary as long as the sender and receiver have successfully exchanged ideas and understand each other and the message received represents the meaning the message intended.

As a supervisor, you spend most of your time in either sending or receiving information. One cannot assume, however, that real communication is occurring in all these exchanges. Also, being constantly engaged in encoding and decoding messages does not ensure that a supervisor is an expert in communicating.

Communication always involves two persons: a sender and a receiver. One person cannot communicate. For example, a person stranded on a deserted island who shouts for help does not communicate because no one receives the message. This example may seem obvious, but think of the manager who sends out a large number of e-mail memos. Once a memorandum has been sent, many are inclined to believe that communication has occurred. However, communication does not occur until information and understanding have passed between the senders *and* the intended receivers.

Making oneself understood then is an important part of this definition of communication. A receiver may hear a sender but still may not understand what the sender's message means. Understanding is a personal matter between people, and different people may interpret messages differently. If the idea received is not the one intended, communication has not taken place; the sender has merely spoken or written.

In an article, dietitian Carol M. Coughlin (2000) states that "people remember 10% of what they read, 20% of what they hear, 30% of what they see, and 70% of what they see, hear, and read." Supervisors who use only one form of communication are not as effective in sending messages as those who communicate the same message in a variety of ways. Take the staff meeting, for example. This method of communicating allows attendees to hear your voice inflections, have eye contact, and engage in two-way communication because questions can be posed and comments can be made. However, if the messages communicated at the meeting are not written down and posted in the form of minutes, they may easily be forgotten. To take this example even further, consider employees who have special needs, such as those who are deaf and may not read lips. For these employees, communication during a staff meeting does not occur at all without written material that covers the points of the meeting or without a sign language interpreter. Perhaps you hold the meeting in English and several of the attendees only speak Spanish; again, communication does not occur in this case.

Similarly, some staff may lack the capability to read and understand memoranda or minutes. According to the National Adult Literacy Survey, 42 million adult Americans cannot read and 50 million can recognize few printed words. The number of functionally illiterate adults is increasing by approximately two-and-one-quarter million persons each year, including nearly 1 million young people who drop out of school before graduation; 400,000 legal immigrants; 100,000 refugees; 800,000 illegal immigrants; and 20 percent of all high school graduates (National Right to Read Foundation 2005). These individuals require oral communication. Others may find both the written and oral methods difficult to understand or retain. For these individuals, pictures, graphs, and charts may be a more meaningful method of communication. In summary, supervisors must try communication alternatives and use more than one method to ensure maximum communication.

Only through effective communication can policies, procedures, and rules be formulated and carried out. Furthermore, only with such communication can misunderstandings be ironed out, long-term and short-term plans achieved, and activities within a department coordinated and controlled. The success of all managerial functions depends on effective communication. The discussion that follows focuses on the methods of communication in more detail.

COMMUNICATION NETWORK

Organizational structure affects organizational communications. Chapters 12 through 17 discuss the formal organizational structure, and Chapter 18 demonstrates that every organization also has an informal structure. The communication network in each of these structures has distinct but equally important formal and informal channels, usually called the *grapevine*. Each channel carries messages from one person or group to another in downward, upward, horizontal, and diagonal directions (see Figure 5.1).

Formal Channels

The formal channels of communication are established by the organizational hierarchy and formal reporting relationships. These channels follow the lines of authority from the chief administrator to the employees. You are probably familiar with the expression that messages and information "must go through proper channels." This refers to the formal flow of communication through the organizational hierarchy.

Downward Communication

The downward flow of communication begins with someone at the top issuing a message and the next person in the hierarchy passing it along to those who report to him or her, and the flow goes on down the line. The downward direction is the one that management relies on most for its communication. Management devotes much time to communicating with subordinates through e-mails, memos, posters, meetings, and letters to explain objectives, policies, plans, and so forth. Supervisors send messages about these to their subordinates; they instruct employees through directives; inform them about work methods, procedures, and rules; and give feedback about performance and performance expectations. Generally, *downward communication* starts action by subordinates; that is, its content is mostly of a directive nature. The manager's position of higher authority requires effective downward communication. The manager should transmit the right amount of information, neither too little nor too much.

Reading a manager's communication focus takes some practice. Managers typically communicate in one of two ways—either "thing" focused or people focused. An e-mail from your manager that asks, "How is the conversion coming?" differs in style from the query, "How is your conversion team doing?" Knowing whether your manager is often thing-oriented will allow you to focus and structure your communications to him or her on "things" rather than people. Study how your manager reacts under stress to gauge his or her coping limits. By doing so, you find out when, how often, and specifically what should be communicated to him or her when stressful situations arise.

Downward communication helps tie the levels of the organizational structure together and to coordinate activities.

Upward Communication: Initiated by the Subordinate

Upward communication is a second and equally important direction in which messages flow through the official network, but it goes from subordinates to

FIGURE 5.1: THE DIRECTIONS OF INFORMATION ALONG FORMAL COMMUNICATIONS CHANNELS

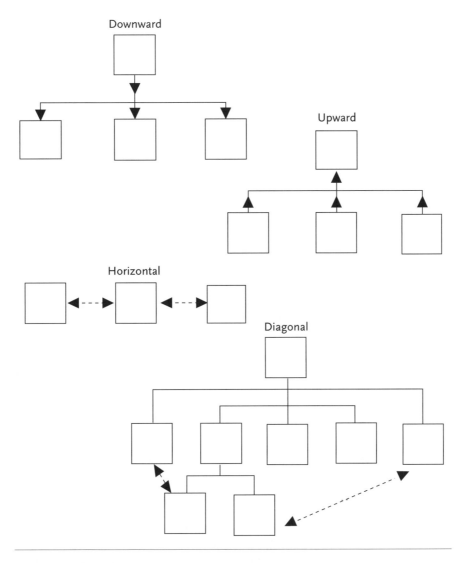

supervisors. Any person charged with supervisory authority also accepts an obligation to keep the superior informed. Subordinates must feel free to convey their opinions and attitudes to their superior and to report on activities and actions regarding their work. Usually, employees report on work progress, activities, and problems they have with their jobs; air complaints; and provide responses to inquiries. Much of this exchange is predetermined and routine. Management should encourage a free flow of upward communication because this is the only means by which supervisors can determine whether their messages have been transmitted and received properly and whether appropriate action is taking place. In addition to following prescribed reporting procedures, an effective manager develops additional systems to encourage an upward flow of information.

As a supervisor, you should encourage and maintain upward communication channels and pay proper attention to the information transmitted through them. You must show that you want the facts and want them promptly. Unfortunately, the reaction of many managers to upward communication may be reluctance; after all, ancient tyrants executed the bearer of bad news. In your supervisory capacity, you must make a deliberate effort to encourage upward communication by (1) showing a genuine desire to obtain and use the ideas and reports of your subordinates, (2) being approachable, (3) truly listening, and (4) recognizing the importance of upward communication. Lack of an effective upward flow throttles the will of your employees to communicate; leads to frustration; and ultimately causes them to seek different outlets such as the grapevine, complaint lines, human resources, or union organizers.

Upward Communication: Initiated by the Supervisor

As stated at the outset of this book, supervisors are the people in the middle. They are not only responsible for providing good communication downward to their employees, they are also responsible for stimulating good communication upward from their workers and then passing this and other information to the next higher level in the administrative hierarchy. However, most supervisors can agree that it is much easier for them to "talk down" to their subordinates than to "speak up" to their superior. This is especially true when supervisors have to tell their boss that they did not meet a deadline or that they forgot to carry out an order.

Nevertheless, it is the supervisor's job to keep his or her superior informed of the department's activities and climate. Be brief. Express your conclusion, findings, or recommendation on the first line. Do not use jargon that is specific to your profession, use short paragraphs, and be timely. The supervisor should inform the superior of any significant developments as soon as possible after they occur, even if the information reveals errors. Recall Chapter 1's discussion of the dimensions of supervision—the supervisor must be a competent subordinate. The boss learning of such news elsewhere is an indication that proper upward communication was not allowed, the supervisor was not providing it, or the supervisor was not on top of the job (incompetent). It is one of the fastest ways to lose credibility in the eyes of your superior. One of management's unwritten rules is, "Never allow your boss to be surprised." Superiors have a right to complete information because they are still responsible if anything goes wrong. An example of a poorly written and well-written memo to a supervisor appears in Exhibit 5.1.

Your superiors may have to act on what you report. Therefore, they must receive the information at a time and in a format that enable them to take the necessary action. As a supervisor, you must assemble all facts that are needed and check them carefully before passing them on to your boss. Bear in mind that upward messages are subject to more distortion than are downward messages. Choose your words wisely, and try to be as objective as possible. This may be difficult at times because all subordinates want to appear favorably in the eyes of their boss. Although you may want to soften the information so that facts do not look as bad as they are, you must remember that sooner or later the full extent of the problem probably will be discovered. When difficulties arise, it is best to report the event to your superior completely, even if it means admitting mistakes. Always remember that your boss depends on the supervisors for upward communication, just as you depend on your employees to pass along information to you.

Horizontal Communication

Horizontal, sideward, or lateral communication is concerned mainly with communication across departments or among peer managers, departments, and coworkers in charge of different activities. *Horizontal communication* is frequently used to coordinate activities, inform others on the same level, and persuade them. Horizontal communication occurs more among managers than among nonmanagerial personnel. For example, lateral communication for an admission from the emergency room (ER) often occurs between the recovery room supervisor and the head nurse on the surgical floor or between the ER physician and the floor physician. This lateral channel is necessary to ensure coordination and to avoid misunderstandings. Horizontal communication also plays an important role in matrix and project organizations, as discussed in Chapter 13.

Diagonal Communication

Diagonal communication, on the other hand, is the flow of messages between positions that are on different lateral planes and activities of the organizational structure. For example, diagonal communication occurs between line groups, such as nursing personnel and staff groups such as the human resources department, or between nursing management and nonmanagerial members of other departments, such as the food service tray delivery person or the phlebotomist (Figure 5.1). To achieve coordination among the various functions in any organization, especially in a healthcare organization, a free flow of diagonal communication is essential. Without it, good patient care is difficult to achieve. The "Shortening LOS Project" example (Figure 4.1) shows how important horizontal and diagonal communication is.

COMMUNICATION MEDIA

The media used most frequently for communication are verbal (oral and written words), visual media (graphs, charts, pictures), and nonverbal (action and behavior). Although spoken and written words are the most widely used media, the power of visuals and nonverbal communication cannot be ignored or underestimated.

Verbal Communication

Words are the most effective and most widely used tools of communication. *Verbal communication* can be a real challenge to the supervisor because words can be tricky, and messages that mean something to one employee can have a completely different meaning to another. Take for example the message Patricia received in The Dilbert Principle (see Figure 5.2). The confusion that can sometimes result from verbal communication relates to the issue of semantics. *Semantics* is concerned with the multiple meaning of words and phrases and how they are used in the context of messages. Supervisors must make an effort to improve their skills in speaking, writing, listening, and reading so that they are aware of the many possibilities of misunderstanding that can occur because of people's different semantic fields. You may have heard the story about the maintenance foreman who asked a new worker to paint the porch behind the Medicine Clinic. When the foreman checked on the job an hour later, he found that the clinic physician's Porsche had been painted.

Oral Communication

The most prevalent form of communication in any organization is oral communication. *Oral communication* with your subordinates is more effective than the written medium because it usually saves time and achieves better understanding. This is true of both face-to-face and telephone communication. In daily performance, face-to-face discussions between the supervisor and subordinate are the principal means of two-way communication. Such daily contacts are at the heart of an effective communication system. Face-to-face discussions are the most frequently used channel for the exchange of information, points of view, instructions, and motivation. Some cautionary guidance is provided in Exhibit 5.2.

Oral communication is simple and can be done with little preparation and without pencil, paper, or computer; therefore, effective supervisors use this medium more than any other. They know that subordinates like to see and hear their boss in person. Also, oral communication is usually well received because most people prefer talking with their supervisor to ensure that they understand what is being said and to express themselves more easily and completely.

Aside from these factors, the greatest single advantage of oral communication is that it provides immediate feedback, even if the feedback is only an expression on the listener's face. By merely looking at the receiver, the sender can often judge the reaction to what is being said. Oral communication thus may enable the sender to find out immediately what the receiver is hearing or not hearing. Oral communication also allows the receiver an opportunity to ask questions immediately if the meaning is not clear. Then the sender can explain the message more thoroughly and clarify unexpected considerations. Moreover, the manner and tone of the human voice can endow the message with meaning and shading that even long pages of written words often cannot convey. The manner and tone create the atmosphere of communication, and the response is influenced accordingly.

There are some minor drawbacks to oral communications. No permanent record of what has been said exists. The sender may forget part of the message, or some noise or random disturbance may interfere. The many benefits, however, far outweigh these shortcomings.

Voicemail

Voicemail generally provides an effective means with which to communicate to others. It has replaced "pink-slip" telephone messages and the staff who once relayed those messages. In addition, it has allowed the caller to call anytime—day, night, or weekend—and leave a message with important facts that may be needed by the supervisor to manage. However, it can also be a barrier to effective communication. Voicemail can be frustrating, especially if its system is poorly configured and does not provide easy access to the message system for either leaving or retrieving messages. Some supervisors have found that voicemail serves as a screening tool and never answer a call directly. This tactic does not result in effective communication. Hiding behind voicemail is annoying to your callers and your staff. It may give your boss the impression that you are not at work. Furthermore, you may miss a caller to whom you wish, or need, to speak. Following are six rules for the supervisor's effective use of voicemail:

1. If you are not in the office, make sure your voicemail is activated.
2. If you are in the office and not involved in a meeting or another call, answer your telephone.
3. Always acknowledge a call received on voicemail.
4. Leave enough information in your messages to others on their voicemail so that the receiving party knows why you are calling and can prepare in advance for returning your call.
5. Do not forward a caller's message to another person's voicemail without the caller's knowledge.
6. Always repeat your return telephone number.

Written Communication

Regardless of the speed and effectiveness of oral communication, a well-balanced communication system includes both written and oral media. Although oral communication is used more frequently, written messages are indispensable and are especially important in healthcare activities. Often, detailed and specific instructions are lengthy and cumbersome; they must be put into writing so that they can be studied over a longer period. Also, using the written medium for widespread dissemination of information that may concern a number of people is advised. Furthermore, a degree of formality, as well as legality, is conveyed by "putting it in writing," which spoken messages may not carry.

Letters are appropriate for external correspondence. Allen (2000) and Kelleghan (1999) suggest the following guidelines for written communication:

- Written communication should be used when the situation is formal, official, or long term or when the situation affects several people in related ways.
- Interoffice memos are internal communication tools used for recording information, inquiries, or replies.
- Letters are formal in tone and addressed to an individual. They are used for official notices, external correspondence, formally recorded statements, and lengthy communications.
- Reports are more impersonal and more formal than a letter. They are used to convey information, analyses, and recommendations.

Communication formalities have lessened with the rising use of e-mail. A supervisor should remember, however, that writing leaves an impression with the receiver. Regardless of how lax your organization may be, you should always try to use the spell-check function on your word processing program and reread your e-mail for correct grammar and sentence structure as well as appropriate word usage before clicking on the send icon. E-mail can be dangerous because it only takes a simple click to send a message to many, leaving the sender with no "out basket" from which to retrieve a perhaps heated and hastily prepared response. You will be wise to close those messages that irk you until you have had time to gather your thoughts, choose the right words to convey your response, gather the facts to support your position, and determine if the response should be handled in person or orally over the phone. If you draft a response in haste, do not send it until you have had a chance to reread it the next day. Time tends to temper our responses.

Written messages have many advantages. They provide a permanent record that can be referred to as often as necessary. The spoken word, in contrast, generally exists only for an instant. Written communications are typically more accurate. The sender can take the necessary time to choose precise terminology, reread, and revise it before sending it. Written communication is preferable when important details are involved and a permanent record is needed, perhaps literally as "evidence." Many situations arise in the healthcare field for which the written form of communication is absolutely necessary, such as in the following:

MEMO
Date: 12-20-01
To: John Smith, CEO
From: Helen Harpin, Human Resources Director
  Per our hallway conversation, I will issue a merit increase for Ned Warner, Nuclear Medicine Manager, even though you have not yet had a chance to finish his evaluation. The increase will be 4.2 percent as instructed. Please advise me if I've misunderstood your instructions. Thank you.

Applying the guidance given in Exhibit 5.1 will enhance your written communication skills.

Visual Media

Sometimes managers also make use of visual aids as a way to communicate. Pictures are particularly effective when used with well-chosen words to complete a message. Even without any words, however, visual media are a useful tool to convey a message. Many enterprises make extensive use of the pictorial language in such forms as blueprints, charts, graphs, models, posters, cartoons, PowerPoint presentations, and overhead projections.

Coughlin (2000) shares an illustration of the benefit of visual media in the following exercise: Two people sit back to back and are given five wooden blocks. The person on the left builds a structure from the blocks and then verbally instructs the person on the right to build the same structure. Working merely from the verbal instructions, the person on the right has difficulty duplicating the structure. However, if the person on the right were given a visual aid, perhaps a drawing of the design, this would be an exercise in simplicity.

Furthermore, Coughlin adds, "visuals can make your presentation more clear, colorful, and interesting. When done properly, visual aids will clarify information, emphasize your major points, and help people visualize concepts. . . . Watch speakers at continuing professional education meetings. The most enjoyable presentations do not have notes: they have great slides."

Nonverbal Communication

Purposeful silence, gestures, a handshake, a shrug of the shoulder, body movements, eye contact, a wink, interpersonal distance, a smile, or a frown can all carry a lot of meaning. These are examples of nonverbal communication, sometimes also referred to as body language. Communication is affected by facial expression, inflection, and tone of voice. By the same token, a manager's inaction also is a way of communicating, just as an unexplained action can often communicate a meaning that was not intended. Suppose, for example, that a piece of equipment has been removed from the laboratory for overhaul and no explanation was given to the employees. The technologists, who may be apprehensive of a staff reduction or change in procedures, may interpret such unexplained action in a way that the supervisor probably had not intended.

Actions (or inaction) and behavior then are two media that play a part in nonverbal communication. As managers, supervisors must not forget that everything they do may be interpreted as symbolic or seen as a model by their subordinates, and those actions often say more about their expectations than the words they speak. What message is sent when employees see the supervisor surfing the Internet for travel locations and reading joke e-mails while his or her work is delegated to subordinates? The employee may receive the message that spending company time and using the organization's resources (in this case, the computer and Internet access) to conduct personal business is acceptable when in fact it is not. Because of their managerial status, all observable acts communicate something to employees, whether supervisors intended them to or not. Employees often mimic the actions of their supervisors, especially if they see positive results. A supervisor who takes on a loud, unhappy customer by speaking softly, using an apologetic approach, and eventually ending the conversation with a smiling customer provides the perfect example for staff on how to diffuse this situation in the future.

The setting for the communication also can play a role as a nonverbal medium, expressing symbols of familiarity or power. For example, consider the manager sitting in a reclining, comfortable office chair behind the desk and the receiver of his or her communication either standing up or sitting in the stiff, unyielding chair across the desk; this setting displays the power and control of the supervisor. The manager's body position and facial expression also convey meaning, whether the expression used is accessible and accommodating or closed off and condescending. Managers who wish to convey "equality" meet around a table, over lunch in the cafeteria, or at the employee's cubicle where the turf is neutral.

The supervisor must always realize that nonverbal communication reinforces or contradicts what is expressed verbally. These hidden messages are often subtle and ambiguous and must be read with caution. They are, however, an important medium for the communicator.

THE MANAGER'S ROLE IN COMMUNICATION

Because organizational effectiveness largely depends on its communication network functioning successfully, all managers must become aware of communication problems and learn how to minimize them to ensure its success. Most organizational structures today have many levels of supervision and long lines of communication. Breakdowns and distortions of communication can occur at any level of supervision.

We have all seen the confusion, friction, and inconvenience that arise when communication breaks down. These breakdowns are not only costly in terms of money, but they also create misunderstandings that may hurt teamwork, morale, and even patient care. Indeed, many managerial problems are caused by faulty communication. Moreover, most human relationship problems grow out of poor or nonexistent communication.

The way you, as a supervisor, communicate with your subordinates is the essence of your relationship. Always remember that no communication occurs until and unless the meaning received by the listener is as close as possible to the meaning the sender intended to convey. The effective communicator must realize that the speaker and the listener are two individuals with separate backgrounds, experiences, values, attitudes, and perceptions. Both live in different worlds, and many factors can interfere with the messages that pass between them.

BARRIERS TO COMMUNICATION

The supervisor must realize that there are many barriers to effective communication, sometimes referred to as "noise" in the system. The more important barriers can be grouped into three general categories: language barriers, status and position barriers, and general resistance to change.

Language

Normally, words serve us well and we generally understand each other. Sometimes, however, the same words suggest different meanings to different persons so that the words themselves create a barrier to communication (see Exhibit 5.2). This can result in the feeling that two people "are just not speaking the same language," although both participants are conversing in English. The term *language barrier* here does not refer to a difference in native tongue but a breakdown in communication as a result of the communicator not speaking in terms, or in a style, the receiver understands. The sender should speak a language to which the receiver is accustomed. It is not a question of whether the receiver should understand it; the question is simply whether he or she understands the language as the sender intended. Toward this end, the supervisor must use plain, simple words and direct, uncomplicated language.

In the healthcare field, concern about the language barrier is heightened. The many levels of unskilled and skilled positions in a healthcare facility range from, for example, the food service worker to the cardiothoracic surgeon. All of these people must communicate in an understandable language to ensure patient care is delivered as planned.

This is difficult at times because one word in the English language may have several meanings. This problem is one of *semantics*. For example, the word *round* has many meanings. We speak of round as a ball, a circle, a sphere, or a globe; he walks round and round, round robin, a round trip, a round of beef, a round of boxing, roundtable, in round numbers, and so forth. Applied to the healthcare setting, when administration speaks of "increased productivity," these words may have a positive, goal-oriented meaning for the manager, whereas the employees may receive this term in a less positive way—that is, "more work ahead." When using words that can carry such different semantic understanding, the communicator must clarify the exact meaning intended. The sender should not just assume that the receiver will interpret the word in the same way he or she does.

Many words in the English language have similar meanings, but they convey different messages, as shown in the following lists (adapted from Altman, Valenzi, and Hodgetts 1985):

List A	List B
Firm	Unreasonable
Aggressive	Mean
Compassionate	Weak
Detail oriented	Nit-picking/Anal
Confident	Cocky
Easygoing	Unconcerned
Selective	Unfair
Respects line of authority	Bureaucratic
Independent	Rebellious
Direct	Rude

For most people, the words in List B convey a less favorable message than those in List A. When describing someone you care for, you are likely to use the words in List A. However, the listener tends to listen and interpret the language based on his or her own experience and frame of reference, not yours.

Workplace Diversity

Healthcare organizations often employ individuals from different cultures, backgrounds, lifestyles, educational levels, and experiences. Many are bilingual, which allows them to translate for patients and staff members who are not. With this diversity comes the possibility that some employees may not fully understand English or are unable to read English. To accommodate these barriers, you must alter your communication approaches and if needed, use a translator or use words or examples that are familiar to the individuals. For some instructions, the supervisor may be able to show the individual how to do the task or draw a picture. The degree to which you are able to communicate in these environments and accommodate workplace diversity while still focusing on producing results for the organization contributes to your success.

An organization's workforce often reflects the community it serves. Taking advantage of one's diverse citizenry may serve an organization well. Having individuals with bilingual skills facilitates communication with patients as well as coworkers and allows you to identify with their experiences. A supervisor would be wise to cultivate an atmosphere where differences are appreciated. Such an atmosphere encourages dialog and understanding of each other's opinion.

Status and Position

An organizational structure and its administrative hierarchy create a number of different status levels among the members of the organization. Status refers to how the members of an organization regard a particular position and its occupant. A difference in status certainly exists between the level of the president and that of the supervisors and between the level of the supervisors and that of their employees. This difference in status or position often creates barriers that distort the sending and receiving of messages.

For example, when employees listen to a message from the supervisor, several factors come into play. First, the employees evaluate what they hear in relation to their own position, background, and experience, then they also take the sender into account. It is difficult for a receiver to separate what he or she hears from the feelings he or she has about the person who sends the message. Therefore, the receiver often adds nonexistent motives to the sender, which may alter the message received. For example, union members are frequently inclined to interpret a statement coming from administration in a negative manner because they are convinced that management is trying to undermine the union. Often union members consider a hospital's newsletter the administration's propaganda mouthpiece, and its contents are viewed with suspicion. Such mental blocks and attitudes obviously do not promote good communication or understanding.

The supervisor who is trying to be an effective communicator must realize that these status and position differences influence the feelings and prejudices of the employees and thus create barriers to communication. Moreover, not only might the employees evaluate the boss's words differently, but they might also place undue importance on a superior's gestures, silence, smile, or other nonverbal expressions. Simply speaking, the boss's words are not just words—they are words that come from a boss. This is how barriers caused by status work in the downward flow of communication.

Similar obstacles resulting from status and position also arise in the upward flow of communication, as all subordinates are eager to appear favorably in their boss's eyes. Therefore, employees may conveniently and protectively screen the information that is passed up the line. A subordinate, for example, may tell the supervisor what the latter likes to hear and may omit or soften what is unpleasant. Similarly, supervisors anxious to cover up their own weaknesses when speaking to a person in a higher position may fail to pass on important information because they believe that such information would reflect unfavorably on their own supervisory abilities. After two or three selective filterings by different echelons of the administrative hierarchy, you can imagine that the final message may be considerably distorted.

Resistance to Change

Resistance to change can constitute another serious barrier to communication because often a message is meant to convey a new idea to the employees, something that will change either their work assignment, position, daily routine, working environment, or social networks. Most people prefer things as they are and do not welcome changes in their working situation. There are many reasons for resistance to change, but the most common is that many employees feel that keeping the existing environment in its present state is safer. (See Chapter 22 for further discussion of the reasons for resistance to and facilitation of change.)

Ultimately, all of us find our niche in an organization in which we feel comfortable. Our work area—our locker, our desk, our chair—all become part of this small workplace world, even in a large department. Consequently, many employees may be suspicious of a message that threatens to change their niche in the organization or their routine. Their listeners' receiving apparatus works as a filter, rejecting new ideas if they conflict with what listeners already believe. They are likely to receive only the portion that confirms their present beliefs and ignore anything that conflicts with them. Sometimes these filters work so efficiently that the receivers do not listen at all. Even if they hear the entire message, they either reject the part of the message that conflicts with their beliefs as false or they find some way of twisting its meaning to fit their preconceived ideas. In the end, the receivers hear only what they wish to hear. If they are insecure, worried, or fearful in their position, this barrier to receiving communication becomes even more impermeable.

This filtering process can in itself become a barrier to progress. Joel Barker, a well-known speaker and author on this subject, uses the example of the Swiss watchmakers who, in 1970, rejected a digital watch proposal from one of their colleagues because they thought no one would want a nontraditional watch—

one without a face, hands, and gears. Texas Instruments and Seiko then recognized the idea as a breakthrough in technology, and of course, capitalized on the new type of watch. Unfortunately, the Swiss were locked "in gear" and unable to progress past their own watch paradigm.

As a supervisor, you may have been confronted with situations in which your subordinates appeared to only half-listen to what you had to say. Perhaps your employees were so busy and preoccupied with their own thoughts that they only paid attention to the ideas they had hoped to hear. They simply selected those parts of the total communication that they could readily use. The information your employees did not care for, did not apply to their situation at this time, or considered irreconcilable was conveniently brushed aside, not heard at all, or easily explained away. Remember Harry's (Jeff Daniels's) comment in the mid-1990s movie *Dumb and Dumber*?: "Yeah, I called her up. She gave me a bunch of crap about me not listening to her. I don't know; I wasn't really paying attention." The selective perception of information constitutes a serious barrier to a supervisor's communications, particularly when the message was intended to convey a change, a new directive, or anything that could conceivably interfere with the employees' routine or working environment.

Additional Barriers

In addition to the barriers already mentioned, many other roadblocks to communication arise in specific situations. For example, obstacles are caused by emotional reactions such as deeply rooted feelings, biases, and prejudice (recognize that no one is without biases). The subordinate's perception of the sender as not being trustworthy is also likely to cause distortion. Other obstacles result from physical conditions such as inadequate telephone lines, overloaded bulletin boards, lack of a private place to talk, temperature conditions, or noise. Indifference, complacency, or the "they-don't-care" attitude that can be held by supervisors and subordinates also may impede communication.

A supervisor who will not or does not take the time to listen is his or her own worst barrier to communication. In such a case, the message may get through, but it is acted on only halfheartedly or not at all. Unless managers are familiar with all barriers to communication, they are in no position to overcome them. Supervisors should not assume that the messages they send are received as intended; in fact, it may be more realistic, although discouraging, to assume the opposite. Because the effectiveness of the supervisory job depends largely on the accurate transmission of messages and instructions, managers must do everything possible to overcome these barriers to improve their chances for enhancing their communication effectiveness.

OVERCOMING BARRIERS TO IMPROVE COMMUNICATION EFFECTIVENESS

Supervisors can prevent and overcome major communication barriers through adequate preparation, credibility, feedback, direct language, effective listening and sensitivity, appropriate actions, and repetition. Becoming familiar with and using these techniques increases your likelihood for successful communication.

Adequate Preparation and Credibility

Do not initiate communication before you know what you are going to say and what you intend to achieve. According to data from Office Team (1999), employees waste 14 percent of every 40-hour work week as a result of unclear communication; that adds up to seven weeks per year. You must think the idea through until it becomes solid in your mind; do not proceed with imprecise thoughts and desires that you have not bothered to put into final form. Only if you understand your ideas can you be sure that another person will understand your instructions. Therefore, know what you want to communicate and plan the sequence of steps necessary to attain it.

For example, if you want to assign a job, be sure that you have analyzed the job thoroughly so that you can explain it properly. If you are searching for facts, decide in advance what information you need so that you can ask intelligent, pertinent, and precise questions. If your discussion entails disciplinary action, be certain that you have sufficiently investigated the case and have enough information before you reprimand or penalize.

If supervisors are not a reliable source of information, problems of credibility may arise. If, however, communication senders are well prepared and honest, credibility is not a problem. Supervisors must overcome the barriers caused by their managerial position and by the employees' likely interpretation of the message's meaning. Some reactions should be anticipated, and the message should include clarifications of some questions it may cause.

Feedback

Probably the most effective tool for improving communication is feedback. It is the link between receiver and sender that makes certain that effective communication has taken place. Managers must always be alert for some signal or clue indicating that they are being understood. Merely asking the receiver if he or she understands and getting a simple "yes" is not usually enough. Affirmation is required to make sure that the message is received as intended and that understanding is actually taking place. The medium used in the communication affects the type of feedback you may receive.

The simplest way to obtain such reassurance is to observe the receiver and judge the responses by nonverbal clues such as a facial expression of understanding or bewilderment, a raised eyebrow, or a frown. This form of feedback is only possible in face-to-face communication, of course, which is one of the outstanding advantages of speaking to someone in person.

Another way of obtaining feedback in any oral communication is for the senders to ask the receivers to repeat in their own words what the sender has just said. If the receiver can restate the content of the message, the sender knows what the receiver has heard and understood. At the same time, the receiver may ask additional questions that the sender can answer immediately.

Additional feedback can be obtained by observing whether the receivers behave in accordance with the communication. If direct observation is not possible, such as occurs with a written message, the senders must watch for responses, for reports, and, ultimately, for results. If these are as expected, the sender can assume that the message was received correctly.

Direct Language

Another helpful way to overcome blocks in communication is for the manager to use words that are as understandable and simple as possible. Although the supervisor should not "speak down" to the employees, long, technical, complicated words, acronyms, and jargon should be avoided unless both the sender and the receiver are comfortable with them. The sender should also be aware of the possible different meanings that words can have for different receivers, as discussed earlier. Again, the single most important question is not whether the receiver *should have* understood it, but if he or she did understand it.

Effective Listening and Sensitivity

An additional means for overcoming barriers to communication is to carefully and completely listen to the other party. Good listening means more than a mere expression of attention. It means putting aside biases, listening without a fault-finding or correcting attitude, and paying attention to the meaning of the idea rather than to only the words (see Figure 5.3).

The supervisor who pays attention and listens to what the subordinate is saying learns more about the employee's values and relationships to the working environment. Understanding, not agreement, is essential. It may even be advisable for the supervisor to state occasionally what he or she believes has been expressed by asking, "Is this what you mean?" The receiver must patiently listen to what the other person has to say, even though it may seem unimportant. Such listening greatly improves communication because it reduces misunderstandings.

Furthermore, being sensitive to the receiver is necessary for effective communication. This means being aware and respectful of the receiver's perspective and position, and possibly even expressing empathy. Careful listening and sensitivity allow a speaker to adjust the message to fit the responses and world of the receiver. This adjustment opportunity is another advantage of oral communication over written messages.

Appropriate Actions

As discussed earlier, supervisors communicate by actions as much as by words. In fact, actions usually communicate more than words. Consider the accounting

FIGURE 5.3 EFFECTIVE LISTENING GUIDE

1. *Stop talking!* You cannot listen if you are talking. Polonius (*Hamlet*) says, "Give every man thine ear, but few thy voice."

2. *Put the talker at ease.* Help a person feel free to talk. This is often called a permissive environment.

3. *Show a talker that you want to listen.* Look and act interested. Do not read your e-mail while someone talks. Listen to understand, rather than to oppose.

4. *Remove distractions.* Don't doodle, tap, or shuffle papers. Will it be quieter if you shut the door?

5. *Empathize with talkers.* Try to help yourself see the other person's point of view.

6. *Be patient.* Allow plenty of time. Do not interrupt a talker. Don't start for the door or walk away.

7. *Hold your temper.* An angry person takes the wrong meaning from words.

8. *Go easy on argument and criticism.* These put people on the defensive, and they may clam up or become angry. Do not argue; even if you win, you lose.

9. *Ask questions.* This encourages a talker and shows that you are listening. It helps to develop points further.

10. *Stop talking!* This is first and last, because all other guides depend on it. You cannot do an effective listening job while you are talking

    - Nature gave people two ears but only one tongue, which is a gentle hint that they should listen more than they talk.

    - Listening requires two ears, one for meaning and one for feeling.

    - Decision makers who do not listen have less information for making decisions.

Source: K. Davis and J. W. Newstrom. 1985. *Human Behavior at Work: Organizational Behavior, Seventh Edition,* 413. New York: McGraw-Hill Book Company. Reproduced with permission of The McGraw-Hill Companies.

supervisor who preaches that all staff must be at their desks and working by 8:00 a.m. but who arrives routinely somewhere between 8:20 and 8:40. Managers who fail to bolster their talk with action fail in their job as communicators, no matter how capable they are with words. Whether supervisors like it or not, their superior position makes them the center of attention for the employees. The boss communicates through all observable actions, regardless of whether they were intended.

Verbal announcements backed up by appropriate action help the supervisor overcome barriers to communication. If the supervisor says one thing but does another, sooner or later the employees will "listen" primarily to what the boss does. For example, the director of central supply services who says she is always available to see a subordinate undermines the verbal message if her office door is kept closed or if she becomes irritated whenever someone comes in. Regardless of what may or may not be written in your position description, you as a supervisor serve as a role model for your staff, and your staff mirror your actions.

Repetition

At times it is advisable for a supervisor to repeat the message several times, preferably using different words and means of explanation. A certain amount of redundancy is especially advisable when the message is important or when the directives are complicated. As mentioned earlier, adults remember 70 percent of a message that they hear, read, and see. Ideally, a supervisor uses multiple and overlapping tools to communicate a complex instruction for how to use a new computer application, for example: (1) orally discuss the instruction; (2) read aloud written instructions, inserting additional comments or pointing to fields or icons on the screen to reinforce the written instructions; (3) demonstrate how to use the application, referencing the written document; and (4) watch the employee use the application once or twice to ensure the process is understood.

The degree of redundancy depends on both the content of the message and the experience and background of the employee. The sender must be cautioned, however, not to be so repetitious that the message may be ignored because it sounds overly familiar or that the listeners feel patronized by the constant reminder. If in doubt, a degree of repetition is safer than none.

THE GRAPEVINE: THE INFORMAL COMMUNICATIONS NETWORK

Although developing sound formal channels of communication is essential, the dynamics of organizational life tend to create additional channels. This informal communication network among people in an organization is commonly referred to as the *grapevine*. Every organization has its grapevine—a network of spontaneous channels of communication. Informal communication is a logical and normal outgrowth of the informal and casual groupings of people, their social interaction, and their natural desire to communicate with each other. People exchanging news through the grapevine must be looked on as a perfectly natural activity. It fulfills the subordinate's desire to be kept posted on the latest information. The grapevine also gives the members of the organization an outlet for their imagination and an opportunity to relieve their apprehensions in the form of rumors.

Attempts to eliminate the grapevine will be in vain. An efficient manager acknowledges the grapevine's presence and may even put it to good use. For example, by learning who the key sources of information are, the manager can sound out employee reactions to contemplated changes before making a decision. An informal communication network also enables the manager to surreptitiously feed some information into this channel and obtain some valuable information from it. Being attuned to the grapevine gives the supervisor excellent insight into what the subordinates think and feel.

Operation of the Grapevine

Sometimes the grapevine carries factual information and news, but most often it passes on inaccurate information, half-truths, rumors, private interpretations, wishful thinking, suspicions, and other various bits of distorted information. The grapevine is active 24 hours a day and spreads information with amazing speed, often faster than most official channels. The telephone, fax machines, voicemail, e-mail, cell phones, text messaging, and even palm-size personal digital assistants help news to travel even faster via the grapevine and reach more people at the same time. The grapevine has no definite pattern or stable membership, is present at all levels of an organization, and carries information in all directions. The news is carried in a flexible, meandering pattern, ignoring organization charts. Its path and behavior cannot be predicted, and the path it followed yesterday is not necessarily the same today or tomorrow.

Most of the time only a small number of employees are active contributors to the grapevine. Most employees hear information through the grapevine but do not pass it along. Any person within an organization is likely to become active in the grapevine on one occasion or another. However, some individuals tend to be active more regularly than others. They believe that their prestige is enhanced by providing the latest news, and thus they do not hesitate to spread the news or even change it so as to augment its "completeness" and "accuracy." These active participants in the grapevine know that they cannot be held accountable, so it is understandable that they exercise a considerable degree of imagination whenever they pass information along. The resulting rumors give them, as well as other members of the organization, an outlet for discussing their apprehensions.

During periods of insecurity, upheaval, and great anxiety, the grapevine works overtime. In general, it serves as a safety valve for the emotions of all subordinates, providing them with the means to say freely what they please without the danger of being held accountable. Because everyone knows that tracing the origins of a rumor is nearly impossible, employees can feel quite safe in their anonymity as they participate in the grapevine.

Uses of the Grapevine

Because the grapevine often carries a considerable amount of useful information, it can help to clarify and disseminate formal communication. Informal communication often spreads information that could not be disseminated through the official channels of communication. For instance, the COO "resigns" suddenly. Although top administration does not want to say publicly how the resignation came about, it does not want to leave the impression that she was treated unfairly or discriminated against. In such a situation, someone in administration may tell someone in the hospital, who "promises" not to spread it further, what really happened.

Supervisors who deal effectively with the grapevine are attuned to it and learn what it is saying; normal grapevine listening is not unethical behavior by supervisors. They must look for the meaning of the grapevine's communication, not merely for its words. They must learn who the key participants are and who is likely to spread the information. By feeding the grapevine facts, supervisors can counter rumors and half-truths, using the grapevine's energy in the interest of management.

Rumors can be caused by several different factors such as wishful thinking and anticipation, uncertainty and fear, or even malice and dislike. For example, employees who want something badly enough commonly start passing the word that their wish is fact. If they want a raise, they may start a rumor that management will be giving everybody an across-the-board pay increase. No one knows for certain where or how it started, but this story spreads like wildfire. Everyone wants to believe it. Of course, building up hopes in anticipation of something that will not happen is bad for a group's morale. If a story is spread that the supervisor realizes will lead to disappointment, the manager should move vigorously to debunk it by presenting the facts. Toward this end, a straight answer is almost always the best answer. If the supervisor has been able to build a climate of trust, the employees will believe the manager.

The same prescription applies to rumors caused by fear or uncertainty. If, for example, the activities of the institution decline and management is forced to lay off some employees, stories and rumors quickly multiply. In such periods of insecurity and anxiety, the grapevine becomes more active than at other times. Usually the rumors are far worse than what actually happens. Here again, giving the facts is better than concealing them. In many instances, much of the fear and anxiety can be eliminated by maintaining open communication channels. Continuing rumors and uncertainty are likely to be more demoralizing than even the most unpleasant facts. Thus, it is usually best to explain immediately why employees are being laid off. When emergencies occur, when new procedures are introduced, or when policies are changed, explain the reasons. Otherwise, your subordinates make up their own explanations, which are often incorrect.

Other situations may arise, however, in which you as a supervisor do not have the facts either or the facts are so confidential that they cannot be revealed. In such instances, let your superior know what is bothering your employees. Ask your superior for specific instructions on what information you may give, how much you may tell, and when to give it. Next, meet with your assistants and lead employees. Give them the story and guide their thinking. Then they can spread the facts before anyone else can spread the rumors.

Although this procedure may work with rumors caused by fear or uncertainty, it might not be appropriate for rumors that arise out of dislike, anger, or malice. Once again, the best prescription is to try to be objective and impersonal and to come out with the facts, if possible. Sometimes, however, a supervisor finds that the only way to stop a malicious rumor peddler is to expose him or her personally and reveal the untruthfulness of the statement. If employees believe in your fairness and good supervision, they quickly debunk any malicious rumor once you have exposed the person who started it or have given your answer to it. Thus, although there is no way to eliminate the grapevine, even its most threatening rumors can be counteracted to the management's advantage. Every supervisor, therefore, will do well to listen to the informal channels of communication and develop the skill for dealing with them.

SUMMARY

Communication is the process of transmitting information and making oneself understood by another or others. As long as two persons understand one another, they have communicated. Agreement is not necessary for communication to be successful. To perform the managerial functions, a supervisor must realize the crucial importance of good communication.

Throughout every organization are formal and informal channels of communication. These channels carry messages downward, upward, horizontally, and diagonally. The formal channels are established mainly by the organizational structure and authority relationships. The position of the supervisor plays a strategic role in the communication process in all these directions.

Although the spoken word is the most significant medium of communication, one must not overlook the importance of nonverbal language as another meaningful medium. In addition, action is a communication medium that often speaks louder than words. In the healthcare field, the written word is a major medium of communication. Of all media, however, oral, face-to-face communication between supervisors and employees is still the most widely used and the most effective because it provides immediate feedback.

Messages frequently become distorted or are not accurately received for many reasons. The manager must be aware of the major barriers to effective communication and how to overcome them; some barriers can be attributed to the sender, the receiver, the interaction of the two, or the environment.

In addition to the formal channels, an informal network exists, usually referred to as the grapevine. This is the personal network of information among employees fostered by social relationships; it is a natural outgrowth of the informal organization and the social interactions of people. The grapevine serves a useful purpose in every organization. Instead of trying to eliminate it, the supervisor should accept it as a natural outlet and at times participate in it for the benefit of the organization.

New communication technologies such as e-mail, voicemail, and cell phones have affected how business is being done. However, regardless of these new technologies, one must follow the fundamental concepts of successful communication.

REFERENCES

Allen, G. 2000. *Supervision*. [Online information; retrieved 02/08/06.] Denton, TX: RonJon Publishers. http://www.telecollege.dcccd.edu/ mgmt1374/book_contents/3organizing/commun/communic.htm.

Altman, S., E. Valenzi, and R. M. Hodgetts. 1985. *Organizational Behavior: Theory and Practice*. New York: Harcourt Brace Jovanovich, Inc.

Coughlin, C. M. 2000. "Show Your Stuff." *Today's Dietitian* 3 (3): 20.

Kelleghan, K. M. 1999. "Use Memos for Clear, Concise Communication." *Office Hours* 408: 1.

National Right to Read Foundation. 2005. [Online information; retrieved 9/11/05.] http://www.nrrf.org/essay_Illiteracy.html#thegrimstatistics.

OfficeTeam. 1999. "Do You Hear What I Hear? Survey Finds Poor Communication Devours Seven Work Weeks Per Year." Press Release, September 3. Menlo Park, CA: OfficeTeam.

Exhibit 5.1

POORLY WRITTEN MEMO

Memo to: The Boss
From: The Subordinate
Re: Today's Events

Three days ago, Joe Hansen, the BME, noticed some seepage from wall 5E. The seepage continued, so Joe contacted the evening TL to periodically check the seepage and see if it could be repaired. The TL, Tim Walters, determined the water source was from the outside. After some investigation, he found it might involve the Water Company. He sent an e-mail to the Water Company. The Water Company sent out a man to check out the situation, and he determined that they had a water main leak in the ground next to 5E. They came out again today to repair the main, but in doing so, the main burst. This caused flooding in the boiler room, and it destroyed one of our boilers. The Water Company said they would pay the repair bill. We have issued a PO to have an emergency replacement installed. Just thought you ought to know about this.

WELL-WRITTEN MEMO

Memo to: The Boss
From: The Subordinate
Re: Boiler Destroyed

The Water Company's water main, located on our exterior wall, broke today, causing flooding of the boiler room and destruction of one of our boilers. The Water Company is paying for the replacement boiler that we ordered today on an emergency purchase order.

One of our Boiler Maintenance employees noticed the seepage three days ago and advised the Team Leader, Tim Walters. Tim contacted the Water Company to take care of the situation, but, unfortunately, the main was so weak that when they started to work on it, it burst.

Just thought you'd like to know about this. Let me know if you need further information.

Exhibit 5.2

GUIDANCE FOR BETTER COMMUNICATION

by Roger P. Holland, M.D., Ph.D.

LANGUAGE

Language used properly is incredibly compelling. We want to compel them [physicians/readers] to act quickly and in the direction that we think they should go. Let's gaze at some incredibly powerful words.

But

The most consequential word to avoid in any discussion is "but." If I were visiting you at your hospital to provide an educational in-service, what would you think if I began the exit session as follows: "Ms. Smith, you have a well-managed, quiet department, with an extremely friendly staff that gave me every assistance in performing this chart review, but . . . ." Now, quickly, what are you thinking? Did you remember all the nice things I just said about your department and staff? No, you're waiting for the other shoe to drop. You're waiting for what? Bad news! It doesn't really matter what I say next because all you're waiting for is bad news. In fact, you'll actually be uncomfortable or confused if I don't say something bad. What have I accomplished by using the word "but"? First, all my preceding compliments at best will be forgotten and at worst will be now regarded with suspicion. Second, you're bracing yourself for the bad news. I've placed you in a defensive posture. Anything I hope to convey to you after the "but" will be blunted.

Rather than "but," the word I should have employed is "and." Reread my sentence, this time replacing the "but" with "and." Don't you feel better? Now, instead of bad news, you're probably anticipating some good news. Even if I'm going to give you bad news ("and your DRG coders have a problem coding cancer records"), you'll keep smiling because your brain is programmed to receive good news. I recommend that you try this on your spouse and children. Avoid "but" at all costs. (See Table I for a list of other words like "but" that should be avoided. See Table II for a list of words like "and" that should be used.)

Table I: Words to Avoid	Table II: Words to Use
but	and
yet	in addition
however	also
still	plus
except	moreover
	likewise
	further
	as well as

You

Let's say I walk into your office and begin a conversation with, "You. . . ." To some people, this immediately triggers a defensive posture. Perhaps you are querying a physician and your query begins, "You said that this patient was admitted with pneumonia . . . ." Many physicians will feel threatened. Yes . . . it's not a rational response. We are creatures of emotion. Words can trigger, amplify, and blunt any emotion. Now the physician is waiting for you to drop the other shoe. So, let's drop it.

"You said that this patient was admitted with pneumonia, but the x-ray indicates. . . ." Now your physician is subconsciously thinking all sorts of negative things, not only about *him,* but of *you* as well. The lesson here is this: do not use pronouns that center on the physician. It doesn't matter what is going to be said next. He's already thinking of something mean to either say to you or an act of violence toward the piece of paper he's holding in his hand. This time, let's rephrase it: "This patient was admitted with pneumonia and the x-ray indicates . . . ." Isn't that better?

If a pronoun is necessary with the query, try to use plurals such as "we," "us," or "they." Don't use "you."

There are many words that elicit a defensive response. "Always" and "never" are among them. Even if you and Coding Clinics are correct, telling a physician, "According to Coding Clinics, you can never code unstable angina as the principle diagnosis in the setting of an acute myocardial infarction" is worse than waving a red cape in front of an angry bull. You can imagine the response you'll receive from most physicians! Personally, if I used either of these 2 words with my spouse, her immediate response is, "Always?!" or "Never?!"

The Because Clause

Contrary to what you may have been taught as a child, the most powerful word in the English language is not "please." It is "because." Sentences that begin with "because" get answered positively more often than any other kind of sentence. Just as "but" evokes an immediate and strong negative response, "because" evokes a very strong positive response in the mind of the listener or reader. Scientific studies have demonstrated how powerful this word is.

"Because" puts our brain into a state of positive expectancy. When the brain hears the word "but," it immediately ignores everything that came before and braces itself for something different. It's in a state of negative expectancy. When the brain hears "because" it tends to ignore everything that comes after and rushes on to, "Of course, I agree." Therefore, begin every query with "because." Use it early in the query and use it often!

Example

> Dear Dr. Jones:
>
> Did this patient have atrial fibrillation and did you address it during the patient's stay?
>
> Sincerely,
> Susie Smith, DRG Coder

First, what's right with this query? You didn't use the words "but," "always," or "never."

And what's wrong with this query? First, it asks the physician to think. He is going to have to review the medical record. Second, you've worried him. Now he's thinking: "Did this patient have atrial fibrillation? Did I address it? Did I treat him appropriately? Didn't I transfer that patient? Didn't I already see that patient in my office for follow-up? Don't these medical record people have anything better to do than to hound me? I've got better things to do with my time. Here's what I think of their query. Swish. Three points."

Let's try again:

> Dear Dr. Jones:
>
> Because this patient was admitted with an acute myocardial infarction and because the patient's atrial fibrillation, noted on the rhythm strips of 7/17 and 7/18, was successfully addressed with Digoxin, may we include a secondary diagnosis of atrial fibrillation because it more completely characterizes the patient's care?
>
> Sincerely,
> Susie Smith

Though this sentence is long-winded and somewhat unwieldy, it will be far more success-ful than the first example. Why?

1. "Because" is used 3 times.
2. You are not asking the physician to think. You've clearly stated that the patient had atrial fibrillation. You even referenced the dates of the EKG two monitor strips.
3. You give the physician no reason to worry. The patient clearly had atrial fibrillation. The physician clearly treated it appropriately and with a positive outcome. In fact, you have just reminded him of what an excellent job he did.
4. You are doing him a favor by suggesting a way in which he can more completely characterize the patient's care.
5. The word "you" is not present. You have depersonalized this query.
6. It doesn't even sound like a question. As we will discuss, the less a query sounds like a question, the more successful it will be.

Questions

A query by definition is a question, but it doesn't necessarily need to be stated as a question. There are a number of problems with questions.

First they require a person to think, which as we've already mentioned, is something you may wish to promote in your children, but not in physicians.

Life is too short.

Second, questions promote a defensive posture.

Getting to Yes

Most people want to agree with you. When you query to physicians [others], most of the time you know what the answer is that you want. Your mission is getting physicians [others] to answer in the affirmative and making it painful for them to answer in the negative.

I've noticed two things wrong with query sheets that facilities use. First, the query ends with "Yes" and "No." Try changing this to "Agree" and "Disagree." It's hard to say "No" and it's harder still to say, "I disagree." The former has no object toward which the "No" is directed; the latter implies that I—a human being with feelings—disagree with you. Nobody likes to consistently disagree with another human being. Make it hard for the physician [reader] to disagree with you.

Second, the query gives too much space for the physician to answer the query. All that space transmits a not-so-subtle message: "Doctor, I want an explanation from you. I want you to think. Fill up all the empty space!"

Think back to when you were in school and were taking a test. There, all alone on an otherwise blank sheet of paper was this question: explain the reasons that led to the war between the States.

How did you feel? Did you feel threatened with all that blank white paper facing up at you? Would you not have felt better if there were only two inches of paper or half a dozen lines for you to respond within? Doctors are people who also went through decades of schooling and who are called on every day to write essays in the form of History and Physicals and Discharge Summaries. They hate it, but they feel compelled to do it just the same.

Paradoxically, by leaving them only a few lines in which to respond, they will feel more kindly toward the query. Looking at a few lines sends another message: the correct answer to this query is "Agree." "If I disagree, I'm going to have to explain myself and in such little space and all for no remuneration!" What's the easiest (and least painful) thing to do? To simply agree!

Example

To: Dr. Jones

From: Susie Smith, DRG Coder

Because this patient was admitted with an acute myocardial in-farction and because the patient's atrial fibrillation, noted on the rhythm strips of 7/17 and 7/18, which was successfully addressed with Digoxin, we will include a secondary diagnosis of atrial fibrilla-tion because it more completely characterizes the patient's care.

____ Agree   ____ Disagree

_____

Physician's signature: _____

Date: ____ / ____ / ____

By changing "may we include" to "we will include," we changed the form of the query from a question to a statement of fact. We also included "Agree" and "Disagree" instead of the usual "Yes" and "No" and added a single line in the unlikely instance that the physician has something to add. Finally, we deliberately avoided the format of a letter. It has been my experience that physicians generally do not like letters on printed stationery. Letters from lawyers; insurance agencies; and people wanting money, appointments, and favors don't look too different from a query letter. Memorandums, on the other hand, come from colleagues. They usually supply information or announce something. Write your query in a memo format so that the physician doesn't judge it before reading it.

Roger P. Holland, M.D., Ph.D., FAAFP, is president of Utilization PRO, Inc., and provides physician-assisted reimbursement training for health information management, utiliza-tion management, and physician advisor personnel. He can be reached at (918) 649–1100 or rph2750@hotmail.com. This exhibit is excerpted with permission by *For The Record Newsmagazine* (September 6, 1999, Vol. II, No. 18).

CHAPTER SIX

Legal Aspects of the Healthcare Setting

CHAPTER OBJECTIVES

After you have studied this chapter, you should be able to do the following:

1. Understand basic information on legal issues affecting the healthcare environment.

2. Outline the basis of institutional responsibility for healthcare rendered to patients.

3. Recognize key causes for liability.

4. Identify employee litigation issues.

5. Understand the key concepts of major regulations affecting management.

ENORMOUS PRESSURES on the healthcare industry continue to create a legal environment of change and uncertainty. Courts have demonstrated an increasing willingness to adopt new theories of liability for healthcare institutions, both as providers of medical services and as employers. Government agencies continue to issue regulations that constrain hospitals and other healthcare provider activities in an attempt to meet two distinct and possibly conflicting goals: holding down healthcare costs and improving the quality of care.

An unbelievably growing number of federal and national regulatory entities govern healthcare organizations (see Figure 32.3). Healthcare institutions have lost their traditional role as charitable providers of medical care. Instead, hospitals, integrated delivery systems, home health agencies, managed care organizations, and a host of ancillary providers and payers are now recognized

The following individuals have contributed to this chapter: Pamela Marshall, formerly of the American College of Healthcare Executives; Brian L. Andrew, J.D. of TLCVision; and Carolyn A. Haimann, J.D., and Lynne Morgenstern, J.D., formerly of the law firm of Lewis, Rice, and Fingersch.

as business entities that, tax-exempt or not, must maintain a bottom-line profitability to survive. These providers can no longer escape the legal liability that general business has had to cope with for decades. Any advertising and marketing projects developed to address the present competitive climate in the industry must reflect their legal implications.

Furthermore, the development of integrated delivery systems (IDSs) increases the potential for spreading liability over an entire network of healthcare entities and thus compels the need to recognize high-risk activities. These IDSs need to be concerned with liability based on traditional doctrines.

To function effectively in this atmosphere, healthcare managers unquestionably must be aware of the legal considerations that may arise from their activities and decisions. All persons involved with the operation of a healthcare institution should recognize the importance and effect of law in healthcare delivery, as they apply laws and legal principles in their daily routines. This is true of the problems faced not only by the members of the board, administrators, and physicians but also by all supervisors, department heads, and possibly everyone involved in healthcare delivery in a private healthcare setting.[1]

This chapter is intended to provide general and basic information in nonlegal language and should not be used in place of the advice of or consultation with legal counsel. The purpose is to give department heads and supervisors an overall perspective on some of the legal aspects of their positions. The reader should be aware that issues of healthcare liability evolve from state and federal statutes and also from court decisions based on principles of common law and that they can vary between jurisdictions. As with all aspects of law, health law and court decisions applying these principles evolve and change on a continuous basis.

For example, for a long time the courts protected hospitals and other charitable institutions from lawsuits that might infringe on their assets as such institutions. This was generally known as the *doctrine of charitable immunity*. Currently, however, as discussed later in this chapter, nearly every state has established the doctrine that charitable organizations are obliged to compensate for injuries caused by them.

LIABILITY

Liability is a word (and a problem) that has become more and more familiar to administrators, supervisors, and employees in healthcare organizations. This type of liability primarily relates to torts and related actions, as distinguished from liabilities associated with the organizational aspects of a healthcare entity (e.g., antitrust, tax, fraud and abuse, insurance, or regulatory issues). A *tort* is a legal wrong or an act, or omission of acting that results in injury to another. Managers and employees at all levels are constantly being reminded of the potential for liability and its resulting costs to the institution. The need for in-house legal counsel, risk managers, consent forms, incident reports, and numerous requirements for documentation are reminders of the litigious environment within which the healthcare team works. Liability is on everyone's mind, and the growing number of multimillion-dollar judgments against institutions and their staffs has become a hindrance to management and physicians.

Just as charitable institutions were able to avoid liability that was traditionally applied to general business corporations, so too have managed care entities been able to avoid the liability concerns that were pervasive throughout the healthcare industry. However, a growing number of courts have applied traditional vicarious liability doctrines to managed care entities, particularly to HMOs. *Vicarious liability* is a concept that one party may be held responsible for the actions of another even though the original party was not involved in the act. For example, the ambulatory surgery center has vicarious liability for the anesthesiologist who overdoses the patient because the center allows the anesthesiologist to practice there. Vicarious liability, in contrast to a tort, is based on a relationship between two or more individuals or entities rather than on the conduct or actions of the individuals or entities. The relationship is often that of independent contractor–contracting agent rather than employer-employee.

HMOs, a hybrid between health insurers and healthcare providers, are now subject to the same liabilities as a traditional healthcare provider, including negligence and ostensible agency actions. To establish a healthcare organization's liability for an independent contractor's medical malpractice based on ostensible agency, a plaintiff must show that (1) he or she had a reasonable belief that the contractor (physician, therapist, temporary employee) was the agent or employee of the hospital, (2) such belief was generated by the organization holding out the individual as its agent or employee or knowingly permitting the individual to hold himself or herself out as the organization's agent or employee, and (3) he or she justifiably relied on this "appearance" of authority. This includes an HMO being liable for the medical malpractice of a physician if it creates the appearance that the physician is its employee, regardless of his or her actual status or a hospital using a contracted nurse or release-of-information form. Thus, all of the discussion in this chapter of potential legal concerns to healthcare providers and institutions naturally apply to managed care organizations as well. The following section addresses various aspects of liability for the healthcare institution, the supervisor, and the employee.

THE INSTITUTION'S DIRECT RESPONSIBILITY

Although liability is frequently imposed on institutions for negligence resulting in injuries to visitors and employees, most lawsuits filed against healthcare facilities involve patient injuries and allegations of negligent care. Therefore, this discussion focuses on the institution's liability for injuries to its patients and its responsibility for the medical care rendered by its physicians.

The law states that any organization that the public relies on for its safety has a duty to exercise ordinary care to prevent injury. In most jurisdictions a hospital owes a duty of due care to its patients to provide that degree of skill, care, and diligence that would be provided by a similar hospital under the same or similar circumstances. More specifically, a hospital has a legal duty to provide its patients with, among other things, premises kept in a reasonably safe condition, appropriately trained and skilled staff, reasonably adequate equipment, and proper medications. Whether the hospital has breached any of its duties to the patient in a particular situation is usually decided by a jury. If a jury finds that a hospital has failed to meet the various standards of care owed to its patients, thereby breaching its duty, the hospital can be found negligent.

For the purpose of this book, assume that any time one does not follow the healthcare organization's policies and procedures, his or her action(s) or lack of action may cause injury and therefore result in a claim of negligence for which the entity and possibly the employee will be held liable.

What are some examples of torts that could occur and result in a claim of negligence? One obvious example is the environmental services worker who wet-mops the floor and fails to post the stand-up signs notifying visitors or others that the floor is wet. A visitor comes along and slips, cracking a hip and fracturing a wrist. The environmental services employee committed a tort. The facility is responsible for the employee's negligence. Consider the plant engineering department that neglects to change the air filters in the air conditioning units of the pediatric floor. Suddenly a rise in infections occurs in pediatrics. The infection control committee investigates to determine the cause of the infection increase and discovers that the filters were not changed as scheduled. While the patient may choose not to sue the facility, the failure to follow protocol did result in increased cost to the patient or patient's insurer. If the patient's infection was so severe that he or she died, the hospital could face a lawsuit for plant operations' negligence.

RESPONDEAT SUPERIOR

Thus far we have seen that not only is the institution directly responsible for its actions in relation to the patient, but it is also indirectly liable for patient injuries. It is legally responsible for the actions of those persons, employees, and staff over whom it exercises control and supervision. This vicarious liability arises from the doctrine of respondeat superior. Under this doctrine, the institution-employer is legally responsible for the negligent or wrongful acts or omissions of the employee even though the facility itself committed no wrong; the negligence of the employee is imputed to, or placed on, the employer. If an employee commits a negligent act that is the direct cause of injury to a patient, the employer may be liable for the damages awarded to the injured party. The doctrine of respondeat superior applies only to civil actions; thus, an employer is not responsible for the criminal actions of its employees.

For the institution to be liable under respondeat superior, the employer must have the right to control the actions of employees in the performance of their duties (i.e., the method, time, and manner of work performance). If the jury determines that this is the case and that the employee (or agent) was acting within the scope and course of employment, the institution will be found liable. An act is generally considered within the scope of employment when the employee is acting on behalf of (or perceives himself or herself to be acting for) the benefit of the institution.

The doctrine of respondeat superior, however, does not release the employee from liability for his or her wrongful act. The employee as well as the employer may be found liable in damages to an injured third party. Under the law, the employer may pursue indemnification or recovery from financial loss from the employee when his or her actions caused the facility to be responsible for the loss. This occurs infrequently because the adverse effect on employee morale outweighs the benefit of attempting to collect monies from the employee. The following example illustrates the application of respondeat superior.

Assume Joe Smith has been employed by Hospital X for the past five years as a full-time registered nurse on its medical floor. He has a good job record with no incidents of poor performance or poor exercise of nursing judgment. While Joe is on duty during his assigned shift on his assigned floor, he is responsible for passing evening medications to the patients. One day Joe fails to carefully check the order for patients Ms. Jones and Ms. Brown and administers the medication ordered for Ms. Jones to Ms. Brown. As a direct result of the wrong medication being administered to her, Ms. Brown suffers a severe, sudden drop in blood pressure that results in shock. Ms. Brown recovers, but not until after an extended hospital stay in the intensive care unit. She then sues the nurse and the hospital for negligence. The jury finds the nurse liable for negligence and finds the hospital vicariously liable because it was the employer. The jury awards a single sum of money, $50,000, against both the hospital and the nurse jointly, even though the nurse was negligent and the hospital's responsibility was based solely on the theory of respondeat superior. The hospital pays the $50,000 to Ms. Brown and, in accordance with its policy, does not exercise its right of indemnification; that is, it does not ask Joe to pay the hospital $50,000.

In this example, the employer-employee relationship existed; Joe was a salaried employee whose hours of work, type of duties, and procedures for carrying them out were all controlled by his employer. Furthermore, the wrongful act, giving the wrong medication to the wrong patient, occurred while Joe was on his assigned shift performing his assigned duties; thus, the act was "within the scope and course of his employment."

Just as the hospital in this example was found responsible for the acts of its nurses, it is also responsible for the acts of all other employees, professional and nonprofessional. Thus, an institution will be liable for the negligent acts of technicians, orderlies, transporters, housekeepers, dietary personnel, and so forth.

The "borrowed servant" theory and the related "captain of the ship" doctrine are often mentioned in connection with the principle of respondeat superior. The borrowed servant doctrine applies in certain situations in which a private physician has "borrowed" the employee from the hospital to aid him or her, and thus the physician has assumed the right to control and direct the employee in the performance of a duty or task. Here, the physician and not the facility-employer is liable for that employee's negligent acts.

The captain of the ship doctrine, a narrower concept than the borrowed servant theory, applies in the operating room setting. Under this doctrine, the surgeon is considered the "captain of the ship"; that is, he or she has complete and total control and supervision over the personnel assisting him or her. Therefore, the surgeon is responsible for the employee's negligent acts that occur during the procedure. The captain of the ship doctrine does not apply outside the operating room setting. It is important to note that this doctrine has been increasingly rejected by the courts in various jurisdictions. The current trend is to hold the institution, rather than the surgeon, responsible under respondeat superior for the actions of its operating room personnel.

In both the borrowed servant and captain of the ship situations, the key element is the extent and right of control the physician has over the employee whose acts caused the alleged injury. Courts carefully examine and juries decide whether an employee truly has become the borrowed servant of the physician before liability can be imposed on the physician for the employee's negligent acts. Generally speaking, in non-operating-room settings, a physician is not liable for negligence of an institution-employed nurse who carries out the physician's order in the regular course of the nurse's duties. If a physician issues a medically inappropriate order, a court may apportion a measure of the liability to the nurse, and therefore to the institution, if another nurse possessing the same skill and training would have questioned the order rather than carried it out.

The concept of respondeat superior also plays an important role in the question of the institution's responsibility for actions of certain members of its medical staff. The facility is liable under respondeat superior for the actions of those physicians who are employed by the facility or are under its direct control and supervision. Interns and residents in a training program, for example, are considered hospital employees. They are salaried by the hospital to render care to its patients; they do not have private patients; and they are under the control and supervision of the hospital, usually through a chief physician who is a hospital employee. Because of these factors, hospitals are almost always held liable for their actions.

In the past, hospitals (and other healthcare institutions) were not held liable for the actions of their private physicians practicing in the hospital or for other physicians who act as independent contractors and over whom the hospital exercises no direct control. The private physician was considered an independent contractor because he or she has an independent relationship with the patient apart from the hospital. The private physician made independent judgments regarding care of the patient and was not compensated by the hospital for patient care services. He or she was merely making use of the institution's facilities and support staff for the benefit of the patient. The facility exerted no control over the patient's choice of physician and had no right of control over the physicians' actions regarding their patients. However, as the frequency of individuals fraudulently posing as physicians have been admitted to healthcare organization's medical staffs through faulty credentialing practices, liability has increased. This has occurred for a number of reasons, one of which is the perception by the public that the healthcare organization is responsible for using reasonable care in the selection of members of its medical staff to serve the patients treated at the facility. Credentialing failures have been widely publicized since the Swango experience.[2]

OSTENSIBLE AGENCY

A clear trend has emerged in which the hospital has been held vicariously liable for the actions of an independently contracted private practice physician when no employer-employee relationship exists. In these situations, several courts have held that if the hospital caused the patient to believe that the physician rendering care to him or her was a hospital employee or agent and if the patient did not choose the physician, the hospital was responsible for the physician's acts under the theory of ostensible agency.

This principle is most often applied in circumstances in which a group of private physicians has contracted with the hospital to render special services such as anesthesiology, pathology, radiology, or emergency room coverage. These physicians are considered independent contractors, not hospital employees. Some courts have held, however, that patients who come for treatment to the emergency room of a hospital that uses these contracted services do not know, and are not expected to know, that the physicians are not hospital employees and do not choose which physician they want to attend them. In fact, the courts hold that it appears to the patient that the physician is the hospital's employee. The same applies when a hospitalized patient is taken for tests to the radiology department staffed by private physicians who have contracted with the hospital to provide services. In most cases, the patient does not select an individual radiologist to conduct the test; the patient accepts treatment from the radiologist assigned. Although the radiologist is a private physician and an independent contractor, he or she appears to the patient to be a hospital employee who was provided by the hospital to render care. The courts that have adopted this doctrine have made it clear that the patient cannot be expected to know or understand the specific contractual relationship between the hospital and the treating physician.

Because hospitals routinely contract with outside entities to provide services formerly rendered entirely by hospital departments, the risk of this type of exposure is great in those states that have adopted this doctrine. A carefully drawn contract can afford moderate protection for the institution, although a contract's provisions cannot absolutely ensure that a court will not find the institution liable for the acts of an independent contractor.

The courts have found a variety of factors that determine whether vicarious liability or ostensible agency exists. Any combination (although not necessarily all) of the following factors may result in a court determining liability:

- The healthcare entity invites patients to use its services.
- A patient receives treatment at the hospital by a physician provided by the hospital without specific selection by the patient.
- The hospital fails to advise the patient that the emergency room (ER) physician or another hospital-based physician was not an agent or employee of the hospital.
- The hospital arranges for a specific group of physicians to exclusively provide certain types of medical service.
- The hospital directly bills patients for services of the ER or the hospital-based physician.
- The hospital undertakes to collect the accounts receivable of the ER or the hospital-based physician.
- The hospital shares the ER, radiology, anesthesiology, or pathology collections with physicians or guarantees them a minimum compensation level.
- The ER or another hospital-based physician is prevented by a contract with the hospital from conducting a private medical practice or from practicing at any other hospital.
- The hospital owns the equipment and operates the department used by ER or hospital-based physicians.
- The hospital through its employees indicates that the physician is an agent of the hospital (e.g., referring to the physician as "our" doctor).
- The hospital's management controls the appointments of physicians.

Healthcare institutions should take steps to address these factors if their entities are located in a jurisdiction favoring the ostensible agency doctrine.

INSTITUTIONAL RESPONSIBILITY FOR MEDICAL CARE AND TREATMENT

Traditionally, nonprofit, tax-exempt healthcare institutions (most often hospitals) were not considered legally responsible for the negligence of private physicians chosen by the patients themselves and therefore were protected by the doctrine of charitable immunity. The hospital was considered to be merely the provider of the physical premises where physicians carried out their work. The hospital did not "practice medicine," only the physicians did. The hospital's legal responsibility for the quality of care rendered by private physicians in its facility, however, has expanded greatly in recent years and now falls under the category of corporate negligence.

The *corporate negligence* doctrine is primarily the result of case law beginning in 1965 with the Illinois Supreme Court case of *Darling v. Charleston Community Memorial Hospital*.[3] In this case, the plaintiff sustained a fracture in his leg during a football game and was taken to Charleston Community Memorial Hospital for treatment. There the leg was casted, but severe complications arose, resulting in the eventual amputation of the plaintiff's leg. The plaintiff brought suit against the physician and the hospital. The Illinois Supreme Court held the hospital liable for the patient's injuries and held that the hospital owed a direct duty of care to the patient. This was a landmark decision because it imposed on the hospital the duty to monitor the quality of patient care.

The Darling case has been cited, followed, and expanded on by courts in most other states, and the implications of the Darling decision for hospitals have been widely debated. The general trend since the decision, however, has been toward holding the institution directly responsible for the medical care rendered to its patients. The court in this case said:

> The conception that the hospital does not undertake to treat the patient, does not undertake to act through its doctors and nurses, but undertakes instead simply to procure them to act upon their own responsibility, no longer reflects the fact. Present-day hospitals, as their manner of operation plainly demonstrates, do far more than furnish facilities for treatment. They regularly employ on a salary basis a large staff of physicians, nurses, and interns, as well as administrative and manual workers, and they charge patients for medical care and treatment, collecting for such services, if necessary, by legal action. Certainly, the person who avails himself of "hospital facilities" expects that the hospital will attempt to cure him, not that its nurses or other employees [sic] will act on their own responsibility.

Clearly at this point, although the hospital is not legally responsible for the negligent acts of its private physicians acting as independent contractors, a hospital has a legal duty to monitor the quality of patient care and the care given by its private physicians. A hospital is usually held directly liable under the corporate negligence doctrine for failing to (1) select and retain only competent physicians on its medical staff; (2) regularly and routinely review the activities of its physicians; (3) formulate, adopt, and enforce adequate rules and policies to ensure quality care; and (4) take necessary action against those physicians when the hospital has knowledge or reason to know that they are not performing according to set standards, are incompetent, or are endangering patient welfare.

In fact, state and federal legislation (e.g., the Health Care Quality Improvement Act of 1986) imposes peer review responsibilities on hospitals that include reporting disciplinary actions and lawsuits against physicians on the hospital's staff to government agencies (e.g., through the National Practitioner Data Bank). Some states have extended the reporting requirements to include nurses.

Liability exposure has also resulted from changes in reimbursement for healthcare services, primarily as a result of increased managed care products. The principal method used to manage healthcare under a health benefit plan is utilization review; a medical insurance company, for example, designates a specified number of days for hospitalization of a plan enrollee. If complications develop and the patient requires a longer stay, the physician must seek third-party payer approval for the additional time. If that request is denied, the hospital is not paid for the extended stay. These developments have given rise to the perception, whether or not it is true in practice, that patients are being prematurely discharged. Suits for injuries caused by premature discharge may not only be brought against hospitals but against physicians and third-party payers as well.

Thus, in those situations in which hospitals act as the managed care entity, concern is increasing about potential liability for medical treatment decisions that may arise out of adverse payment determinations. The notable California Appellate Court case known as *Wickline v. State of California*[4] held that third-party payers could be held liable to a patient if their prior authorization programs were administered in such an arbitrary or negligent manner so as to injure the plaintiff. However, in this case, the court absolved the payer from liability, ruling that the responsibility for deciding the course of the medically necessary treatment, including when to discharge a patient from the hospital, belonged to the treating physician rather than to the third-party payer. In those situations in which hospitals have significant oversight of physician practices, it is incumbent on the hospital to ensure that the physicians use to the extent possible all appeals and other grievance mechanisms set forth by the payer.

The growth of sophisticated information systems and the increased demand for data mean that more outsiders have access to patient specific information. As maintaining the confidentiality of patient records becomes increasingly difficult for healthcare entities, providers, and payers alike, patients are becoming more concerned with the release of what they consider to be personal information. In turn, as more healthcare entities install electronic health records, information becomes increasingly accessible to providers, payers, employers, and other organizations. Recent federal and state initiatives toward complete healthcare information automation and broad interchange of such information requires greater attention to the confidentiality and security of patient records. Although it is the institution's responsibility to develop security and confidentiality procedures, it is a supervisor's responsibility to make employees aware of these procedures and to monitor compliance.

NEGLIGENCE AND MALPRACTICE

Malpractice is a term often used synonymously with negligence in reference to the actions or wrongful acts of physicians, nurses, and other healthcare professionals. In fact, these terms are not identical but are similar. Negligence is defined in *Black's Law Dictionary* (West Publishing 1979, 930) as follows:

> The omission to do something which a reasonable man, guided by those ordinary considerations which ordinarily regulate human affairs, would do, or the doing of something which a reasonable and prudent man would not do.

Malpractice is the term for negligence of professional persons. Malpractice is defined in *Black's Law Dictionary* (Garner 1999, 959) as follows:

> Professional misconduct or unreasonable lack of skill . . . is usually applied to such conduct by doctors, lawyers, and accountants. Failure of one rendering

professional services to exercise that degree of skill and learning commonly applied under all the circumstances in the community by the average prudent reputable member of the profession with the result of injury, loss, or damage to the recipient of those services or to those entitled to rely upon them. It is any professional misconduct, unreasonable lack of skill or fidelity in professional or fiduciary duties, evil practice, or illegal or immoral conduct.

Any individual can be negligent, such as when one drives carelessly and strikes another vehicle or when a homeowner fails to rope off a hole in his front walk that is not easily visible. Only a professional person such as a physician, however, can commit malpractice.

To determine what constitutes negligence, the law has developed a measuring scale called the *standard of care*. Generally speaking, this is determined by what a "reasonably prudent person" would do under similar circumstances. This reasonably prudent person is, more specifically, a hypothetical person with average skills, training, and judgment and represents the yardstick for measuring what others should do in similar circumstances. If someone's performance fails to meet the standard, negligence has occurred. Also, if it was foreseeable that failure to meet that standard would cause injury and if the negligence was the direct and proximate cause of injury, liability is imposed.

A number of elements are necessary to maintain an action for negligence: (1) there must be an injury to someone, (2) a duty must be owed to the injured person, (3) a breach of that duty must occur, and (4) the breach of this duty must have been the proximate cause of the injury. If any one of these elements is missing, a negligence claim theoretically cannot be maintained successfully. The standards of care that medical professionals must meet are higher than those imposed on laypersons. The following is an example of how these elements of negligence apply in the hospital setting in reference to a professional person.

Assume Jane Doe is a registered nurse in a jurisdiction that permits recovery against nurses for malpractice. Jane is assigned to give medicine to Mr. James, a patient under her care. She misreads the order, which is for 40 milligrams (mg) of the antibiotic gentamicin, and instead gives him 400 mg of gentamicin. This drug is extremely potent, and Jane knows that an excessive dose can cause renal (kidney) problems. Mr. James suffers renal shutdown and has to be hospitalized for several more weeks. Applying the elements as previously outlined, Jane has a duty to the patient to possess that degree of skill and learning ordinarily possessed by nurses. She also has the duty to meet the standard of care for nurses in this same situation—that is, to act as a reasonably prudent nurse would have acted. In this case, to meet that requisite standard of care, she should have given the ordered medication to the right patient, in the ordered dose, at the ordered time, and by the ordered mode of administration. Jane deviates from the standard of care (breaching her duty) by failing to give the correct dosage and is thus negligent. If her negligence is the proximate cause of harm to the patient, she is liable for damages. The burden is on the plaintiff to prove the standard and deviation from it. The jury must then decide whether the negligent act is the cause of the injury.

Despite the perceptions of most plaintiffs, it is important to recognize that not all bad results or unexpected outcomes come from negligence or imply liability for the person committing the act. Assume Jane gives the correct dosage of medication to the patient. Assume further that Mr. James has never taken the medication before and on inquiry has said he has no known allergies to any drugs. Five minutes after he receives the medication, he suffers a severe, unanticipated allergic reaction resulting in a cardiac arrest. In this case, although the medication causes injury to Mr. James, Jane is not liable. She meets her duty of care. She gives the correct dose to the right patient, at the right time, and in the correct manner of administration. She has no reason to anticipate that Mr. James would have an allergic reaction. Because she does not breach her duty, she is not negligent. Therefore, without committing negligence, Jane cannot be found liable.

Often the most difficult element to prove in a negligence action is causation. One may be negligent but not held liable if the negligent act is not the cause of harm to the other party. If Jane gives the wrong dose of medication to Mr. James but he suffers no ill effects, she is still negligent. Because her negligent act causes no harm, however, she probably will not be held liable for damages. Furthermore, as the time between the negligent act and the injury lengthens, the more difficult it becomes to prove causation.

SUPERVISOR'S LIABILITY

The previous sections describe how the healthcare professional can be held personally liable for his or her actions. Can the healthcare professional be held personally liable for his or her negligent actions as a supervisor as well?

The supervisor is not liable for the acts of those supervised on the basis of respondeat superior because the supervisor is not the employer of those he or she supervises. The institution is the employer, and the supervisor has only administrative responsibility for those he or she directs. A supervisor is also not liable just because someone under his or her supervision acts negligently and causes injury to a third party.

Using these guidelines, a supervisor's performance may be measured against the standard of care for a reasonably prudent person in the same or similar supervisory position. If a supervisor fails to meet the standard, he or she as a supervisor may be held liable for the harm caused. If a supervisor permits or directs someone to perform a duty that he or she knows (or reasonably should know) the person is not trained to perform, the supervisor may be held liable for negligent supervision if that person causes harm.

Assume Betty Green is a head nurse in Hospital X. The hospital has a provision stating that no nurse employed less than three months shall be allowed to do endotracheal suctioning without assistance unless the head nurse is familiar with and has reviewed and approved the new employee's performance of that task. Ms. Wanda Burnside, a new employee, has been working under Betty's supervision for one month. Betty has observed Wanda help another nurse suction a patient and concludes that Wanda does not perform the task adequately and needs some additional in-service training. Mr. Kane, a patient, has an order to be suctioned if needed, and Betty tells Wanda to suction him. Wanda does so, but incorrectly, causing injury to the patient's tracheal wall. Betty will probably be held liable for negligent supervision. She has reason to know that Wanda by herself could not yet adequately and skillfully perform suctioning on a patient.

Liability for the nursing supervisors frequently arises as a result of the actions of nursing students under their direct control and supervision. Supervisors need to exercise particular care in not permitting nursing students and others in training to perform tasks and duties for which they are not yet trained or do not have adequate skill, information, or experience.

Remember the example given earlier in which Joe gave the medication intended for Ms. Jones to Ms. Brown? In this case, Joe had worked on his floor for five years with a good record and no incidents of poor performance or faulty nursing judgment. The head nurse, Joe's supervisor, is not liable for Joe's negligent act. Because the head nurse is not Joe's employer, she is not liable under respondeat superior. Also, she is not liable as a supervisor because she has no reason to think Joe is not able to properly perform the task of passing out medications. If, on the other hand, Joe made ten similar mistakes in the past several months and the supervisor is aware of this and takes no action to counsel Joe or make sure he is performing properly, the supervisor may be held liable for negligent supervision.

As a practical matter, legal actions against healthcare supervisors are not as common as those against healthcare professionals, primarily because the potential for injury to plaintiffs is relatively remote.

ADDITIONAL POTENTIAL CAUSES FOR LIABILITY

Many other areas of healthcare activities have potential for liability of the institution, its supervisors, and its employees. These include obtaining informed consent from patients; following proper admission and discharge procedures to avoid charges of false imprisonment, negligent failure to render treatment, or abandonment of care; negligent selection or credentialing of providers; and ensuring a safe work environment for employees. Institutions and personnel must also deal with controversial issues fraught with philosophical, moral, legal, and ethical complexities such as abortion, sterilization, and the right to die with dignity. A discussion of these is beyond the scope of this chapter.

EMPLOYEE LITIGATION

Employees are becoming increasingly aware of their legal rights, resulting in an explosion in the number of legal actions brought by employees against their current or former employers. Often these claims involve a former employee alleging unlawful discharge by the employer. This is a recent phenomenon; historically the law viewed the employment relationship as "at will"; that is, if there was no contract for a specific term, the employee or employer could terminate the employment relationship at any time and for any reason.

The first exceptions to this legal principle originated with statutory and constitutional prohibitions against discrimination based on race. More recently sex, national origin, age, handicap, and pregnancy discrimination have been prohibited by statute and regulation. Consequently, the courts in many states have begun to acknowledge other situations in which an employer cannot rely on the "employment-at-will" doctrine. Courts have recognized claims in which an employee was discharged for refusing to perform an illegal act, for whistleblowing (Qui Tam)[5] against the employer, or for breaching what the employee alleges to be an express or implied contract. In many states, employees have successfully claimed that employee handbooks are essentially valid written contracts or that statements made during job interviews constitute implied contracts.

Employee litigation, however legitimate, places additional burdens on supervisors because part of the responsibility of a supervisor is to treat an employee fairly, to follow institutional policy regarding discipline, and to monitor and document the employee's performance accurately. If a supervisor fails to follow proper procedures and to document incidents and the manner in which employees discharge their duties, the institution is left open to claims that an employee was disciplined for discriminatory or wrongful reasons and not for poor performance.

OTHER AREAS OF CONCERN

An increasing number of new regulations are being passed by Congress to protect employee rights and to protect them from injury. The supervisor is responsible for ensuring his or her department or work area complies with these regulations. Often the human resources department provides supervisors with instructions for these evolving regulations. However, if you have not received policies or procedures, you may need to contact the human resources department for guidance.

Americans with Disabilities Act

The Americans with Disabilities Act (ADA) is a comprehensive federal statute that was enacted to protect those with physical or emotional disabilities. It makes it illegal for most entities to discriminate against individuals with disabilities in such areas as employment and public accommodations. The ADA has spawned a variety of novel claims that could not have been predicted even a short time ago. Therefore, expert healthcare employment relations' legal counsel should be consulted for additional information.

The act identifies a disability as a past, current, or perceived physical or mental impairment of a major life activity. Employers are prohibited under the ADA from doing any of the following:

1. limiting, segregating, or classifying a disabled job applicant or employee in a way that adversely affects job opportunities or status;
2. participating in an arrangement that has the effect of discriminating against a disabled individual;
3. using standards, criteria, or methods that have the effect of discriminating on the basis of disability;
4. denying equal jobs or benefits to individuals based on their relationship or association with an individual known to be disabled; or
5. using standards or tests that screen out disabled individuals unless the standard or test is job related and consistent with business necessity.

The ADA imposes on employers a duty to "reasonably accommodate" a disabled individual's ability to perform essential job functions. The Equal Employment Opportunity Commission defines reasonable accommodation as "any change in the work environment or in the ways things are customarily done that enables an individual with a disability to enjoy equal employment opportunities." Such reasonable accommodation includes the following:

- making facilities accessible to and usable by disabled persons;
- job restructuring;
- modifying work schedules;
- reassigning a disabled person to a vacant position;
- acquiring equipment or devices;
- adjusting or altering tests;
- providing training materials;
- furnishing readers or interpreters; and
- making other similar adjustments to a job.

A reasonable accommodation need not be the best accommodation available, as long as it is effective for the purpose. A disabled individual must request a reasonable accommodation from the employer. A request can be made by a "family member, friend, health professional, or other representative" on behalf of a disabled individual. Once a request is received, management is expected to act promptly. Not all requests are initiated by the disabled person or his or her representative. As the supervisor, you may see the need for a reasonable accommodation and initiate the request. For example, assume you are the radiology supervisor for transcription of radiology reports. You notice that one of your transcriptionists nearly presses her nose to the monitor of her computer. After private questioning, you find that she has a visual deficit. At this point you would initiate the order for a larger monitor with larger fonts. Similarly, a plant engineering foreman may notice that one shop hand has to reach for items hanging on the post board behind the workbench. The foreman may initiate an order to have the workbench height lowered or order a raised platform that the shop hand can use. Although height may not be considered a disability for many, it does cause a "handicap" when doing one's job in this situation.

An employer may not use qualification standards or selection criteria that screen out or tend to screen out an individual with a disability on the basis of his or her disability unless the standard or criterion is job related and consistent with business necessity. (The standard or criterion must be a legitimate measure or qualification for the specific job for which it is being used and must relate to the essential functions of the job.) In screening applicants for positions, however, an employer is not required to lower existing production standards applicable to the quality or quantity of work for a given job in considering the qualifications of an individual with a disability if these standards are applied uniformly to all applicants and employees in that job.

Under the ADA, an employer may not inquire into an applicant's medical condition or disabilities prior to making a conditional offer of employment. An employer, however, may ask a job applicant about his or her ability to perform specific job functions, tasks, or duties, as long as those questions are not phrased in terms of a disability. An employer also may ask an applicant to describe or demonstrate how he or she will perform specific job functions if this is required of everyone applying for a job in this job category, regardless of disability. The ADA regulations have many facets. You will be wise to seek additional guidance from your human resources department.

Sexual Harassment

Organizations must strive to promote a workplace that is free from sexual harassment and should have policies against such harassment. Sexual harassment is considered a form of sex discrimination and is therefore a violation of Title VII of the Civil Rights Act of 1964 and the amendments thereto. In addition, the 1991 Civil Rights Act amended Title VII and provided for compensatory and punitive damages and jury trials.

The Equal Employment Opportunity Commission (EEOC), the federal agency that enforces this law, has issued guidelines regarding sexual harassment. The guidelines define sexual harassment as unwelcome sexual advances, requests for sexual favors, and other verbal or physical conduct of a sexual nature when

1. submission to such conduct is made, either implicitly or explicitly, a term or condition of an individual's employment;
2. submission to or rejection of such conduct by an individual is used as the basis for employment decisions affecting such an individual; or
3. such conduct has a purpose or effect of substantially interfering with an individual's work performance or creating an intimidating, hostile, or offensive working environment.

Sexual harassment can involve individuals of the same or different sex. Examples of sexual harassment include, but are not limited to, unwelcome sexual advances whether or not physical touching is involved; sexual jokes or comments of a sexual nature whether conveyed verbally or in writing (including e-mail or voicemail messages); whistling; leering; unwanted touching; the display of sexual pictures, magazines, or photographs; or other physical or verbal conduct of a sexual nature that interferes with a person's work or that creates a hostile workplace for a person. It also includes instances in which a supervisor or coworker asks for a sexual favor (including kissing) in exchange for any term or condition of the job such as a favorable review, salary increase, or promotion.

Supervisors should pay particular attention to working relationships and conversations among employees. What some employees consider inoffensive, humorous, or harmless flirting could be offensive to others. Supervisors should remember that it is not the intent of the harasser but the impact on the other person that could potentially create a hostile work environment and create a liability for the employer. It is important that employees feel they can discuss such situations with their supervisor or the human resources department.

Any employee who feels that he or she has been subjected to harassment of any type should consider telling the offending party that he or she objects to the conduct. If the employee is uncomfortable confronting the offending party or if the conduct continues, the employee should report the incident to his or her supervisor or the human resources department. Guidance on acts that constitute sexual harassment at your healthcare organization can be obtained from the human resources department.

Family and Medical Leave Act of 1993 (FMLA)

This act provides up to 12 weeks of absence to eligible employees for certain family and medical reasons. Reasons for taking leave include (1) to care for a child after birth or placement for adoption or foster care; (2) to care for a spouse, child, or parent who has a serious health condition; or (3) to care for oneself because of a serious condition that makes one unable to perform one's job.

A serious condition is one that requires inpatient care in a hospital, hospice, or residential medical facility; results in a period of incapacity of more than three consecutive days that involves treatment two or more times by a healthcare provider or one occasion that results in a regimen of continuing treatment under the supervision of a healthcare provider; is a chronic condition requiring periodic treatment by a healthcare provider that continues over an extended period of time; is a permanent, long-term condition requiring supervision; or is a nonchronic condition that requires multiple treatment such as restorative surgery after an accident or cancer or kidney disease.

Guidance on the actions required by management to extend or document conditions qualifying for FMLA leave can be obtained from the human resources department.

OTHER HEALTH ADMINISTRATION REGULATIONS

OSHA Recordkeeping Rule

Employer recording and reporting of occupational injuries and illnesses is one method that OSHA uses to monitor workplace safety. The reporting and recording rules require employer records to include any work-related injury or illness at work and in in-home offices resulting in one or more of the following conditions:

- death,
- days away from work,
- restricted work or transfer to another job,
- medical treatment beyond first aid,
- loss of consciousness, or
- diagnosis of a significant injury or illness by a physician or other licensed healthcare professional.

Supervisors need to review the working conditions in their departments to identify potentially hazardous or other conditions that could cause a work-related injury or illness. Some of the common situations are as follows:

- lifting injuries when moving patients (nursing and therapy),
- wrist and shoulder injuries when filing records (health information),
- falling-object injuries when items are stacked high on shelves (central supply),
- falls when a floor is wet (environmental services), and
- needle sticks when needles are not properly disposed of (environmental services).

Recordkeeping rules require employers to record all needle sticks and sharp-object injuries involving contamination by another person's blood or other bodily fluids. These rules support the need for privacy by prohibiting the recording of an individual's name on certain types of injuries or illnesses (e.g., sexual assaults, HIV infections, mental illnesses).

Because the hospital is open to the public, it, like other businesses, may have workplace violence (e.g., assaults, shootings, hostage situations, domestic disputes, failed coworker love affairs) and may be a target for terrorists. Heightened publicity of deaths resulting from improper administration of medications and other causes encouraged the Joint Commission on Accreditation of Healthcare Organizations (JCAHO) to establish new standards for patient, staff, and public safety. Additionally, the Centers for Disease Control and Prevention has issued recommendations to facilities to be prepared to respond to an act of biological or chemical terrorism. Organizations have implemented educational programs and procedures to safely open mail and expand workplace security;

offered additional opportunities to telecommute; increased criminal and background checks; and established more protective policies regarding layoffs, retention of positions for individuals who are called to military duty, and antidiscrimination practices.

Although Occupational Safety and Health Administration monitors workplace safety, it cannot prevent it. Guidelines to prevent workplace injuries such as back and repetitive motion injuries and needle sticks can usually be obtained from your occupational therapy or employee health departments. Emphasizing these guidelines with your staff contributes to providing a safe environment. You as a supervisor must try to see conditions that could cause injury, sense changes in employee attitudes or personalities that may erupt and result in a hostage situation or shooting, and keep a pulse on illnesses that may flag a work condition cause.

HIPAA

The Health Insurance Portability and Accountability Act of 1996 (HIPAA) has several components that affect day-to-day management activities. One component of the act (healthcare portability) allows employees, after termination by an employer, to remain insured. This component is managed effectively through the payroll and human resources department. Other components address security, privacy, and transaction issues. HIPAA affects all employees working in any healthcare organization or entity.

HIPAA specifically requires healthcare providers to take precautions to protect patient-identifiable information from unauthorized release or access, tampering, or misuse. Inappropriate disclosures may result in fines up to $250,000 and prison time. With these penalties in mind, confidentiality statements are more important than ever.

As a result of HIPAA and other compliance-related concerns, the use of passwords and, in some organizations, biometrics (e.g., fingerprints, cornea scans, palm scans) and other security measures are being used to ensure that the user is (1) authorized to have access to the system or specific application and (2) authorized to have access to the data or data field. Time-outs on computers have been shortened to ensure that when one walks away without logging off, the computer automatically logs off to reduce the possibility of an unauthorized user accessing confidential or proprietary data. JCAHO has monitored this in their on-floor rounds during their surveys.

However, as a supervisor, your role is to ensure that computer access is controlled and that patient-identifiable information is discarded in appropriate containers and not released inappropriately.

Ethics and Qui Tam

In recent years there have been several high-profile corporate misconduct cases, including Enron, HealthSouth, HCA, Tenant, Tyco, Rite-Aid, and Worldcom.

While most of these cases emanated from accounting improprieties, the results had serious negative impacts for the employees, stockholders, and public, destroying some of the world's largest companies, shattering retirement programs, and putting thousands of employees out of work. As a result, Generally Accepted Accounting Principles and corporate ethical behavior have changed. The Sarbanes-Oxley Act of 2002 incorporates harsher penalties for certain crimes, more independent directors, transferring the setting of auditing standards from the private sector to the public sector (the Public Accounting Oversight Board), and so forth. Federal initiatives have set minimum expectations for organizations with regard to ethical practice and compliance with regulations.

Stronger ethics policies have been initiated at healthcare organizations to address accounting, billing, coding, purchasing, and patient care practices. Health-South's ethics statement appears on its web site (see Figure 6.1).

The Department of Justice (DOJ) reports that after violent crime, healthcare fraud is the department's top priority. The number of healthcare fraud investigations pending at the DOJ is in the thousands. The DOJ's primary weapon in prosecuting healthcare fraud is the federal False Claims Act (FCA) of 1863 (31 U.S.C. secs. 3729–3733). The DOJ may entertain lawsuits filed by private individuals on behalf of the federal government as a Qui Tam claim. These claims may include charging organizations with submitting false claims to the government. The FCA rewards qui tam or whistleblowers with a share of any resulting recoveries as a bounty and protects them from discharge for filing false-claims lawsuits against their employers. In 1997, healthcare providers were the targets of 54 percent of the 530 private qui tam lawsuits filed that year (Project Muse 2005).

Supervisors are responsible for reviewing, supporting, and signing code of ethics documents and for educating their subordinates about the organization's ethical policies. At the same time, healthcare organization compliance programs encourage and often require employees at any level to report, at a minimum, inappropriate practices anonymously to the compliance "hotline." Supervisors should encourage a climate of doing what is legally and ethically right and identify any variances to the contrary.

SUMMARY

The healthcare institution's legal responsibility for what occurs on its premises or by its employees and agents is cause for concern by administrators, supervisors, and employees alike. The professional members of the healthcare team also are being held to stricter and higher standards of care and continue to be held liable for their negligent acts.

Those practicing in the healthcare field are well advised to familiarize themselves with the various aspects of their job that could result in liability to themselves or their institution. They must be able to recognize potential legal issues, understand the practical ramifications, and exercise caution and care in the per-

FIGURE 6.1: CORPORATE GOVERNANCE & ETHICS

HealthSouth is fully committed to good corporate governance and the highest standards of business conduct. In today's culture, good corporate governance and adherence to a high ethical standard is simply good business.

We are dedicated to conducting our business with the highest level and integrity while maximizing value for its investors. In October 2003, we implemented our revised Corporate Compliance and Ethics Program to assist HealthSouth directors, officers and employees in making the right choices regarding our business practices. Our revised Corporate Compliance and Ethics Program is described in our Corporate Compliance Handbook, which includes our revised Standards of Business Conduct.

We are also dedicated to effective corporate governance. In January 2004, the Board of Directors approved a number of changes in our corporate governance platform in the interest of transparency and accountability to our stakeholders. Our principles of corporate governance meet or exceed the requirements of the Sarbanes-Oxley Act of 2002 and, although we are not currently listed on the New York Stock Exchange, the revised listing standards of the New York Stock Exchange. HealthSouth's principles of corporate governance are set out in our Corporate Governance Guidelines and the various charters of the standing committees of our Board of Directors.

Source: Courtesy of HealthSouth. 2005. [Online information; retrieved 9/11/05.] http://www. healthsouth.com/medinfo/home/app/frame?cntx=01abouths&1=leftnav.jsp,abouths_nav&2= article.jsp,section_banner,abouths_corpgov.

formance of their duties. A growing number of entities impose regulations on healthcare organizations and their management.

Recent fraudulent activities have resulted in closure of large organizations and imprisonment of corporate officers. These indictments combined with DOJ initiatives in false-claim submissions have encouraged expanded compliance and ethics practices, policies, and procedures at most healthcare organizations. The supervisor is in a pivotal role to set the tone for workplace safety, compliance, and fairness.

NOTES

1. This chapter does not cover situations in facilities operated by the Veterans Administration, Army, Navy, Air Force, Public Health Service, or other federal agencies.

2. Michael Swango had successfully been admitted to several medical staffs across the United States and the world. Faulty credentialing practices failed to reveal a pattern of patient deaths that occurred during his

assignment at different hospitals. He was indicted for murder on numerous accounts. Known as "Dr. Death," it is thought that he may have been responsible for 30 to 60 patient deaths.

3. *Darling v. Charleston Community Memorial Hospital,* 33 Ill. 2d 326, 211 N.E. 2d 253, 14 A.L.R. 3rd 860 (1965), cert. denied, 383 U.S. 946 (1966).

4. *Wickline v. State of California,* 239 Cal. Rptr. 810 (Ct. App. 1986) review granted, 231 Cal. Rptr. 560 (1986), review dismissed, remanded, ordered published 239 Cal. Rptr. 805 (1987).

5. Qui Tam ("who as well for the king as for himself sues in this matter") is a provision of the Federal Civil False Claims Act that allows a private citizen to file a suit in the name of the U.S. government (Garner 1999, 1262).

REFERENCES

Garner, B. D. 1999. *Black's Law Dictionary, Seventh Edition.* St. Paul, MN: West Group Publishing.

Project Muse. 2005. [Online information; retrieved 9/11/05.] http://muse.jhu.edu/cgi-bin/access.cgi?uri=/journals/journal_of_health_politics_policy_and_law/v025/25.2ruhnka.pdf&session=25809279.

West Publishing. 1979. *Black's Law Dictionary, Fifth Edition.* St. Paul, MN: West Publishing.

PART III

Planning

CHAPTER SEVEN

Managerial Planning

CHAPTER OBJECTIVES

After you have studied this chapter, you should be able to do the following:

1. Describe the planning function and its importance as a primary management tool.
2. Discuss the various planning periods and how they are integrated.
3. Relate goals and objectives to organizational planning.
4. Describe how management by objectives can be used to implement plans.

P LANNING IS THE primary managerial function. It is the process of deciding in advance what is to be done in the future. Logically, planning must come before any of the other functions because it determines the framework in which the other management functions—organizing, staffing, influencing, and controlling—are carried out. Planning begins with decision making, the process of selecting from alternatives. Modern healthcare activities operate in an environment that is always changing in ways institutions can neither control nor predict precisely. This increases the need for planning. The only way healthcare organizations can survive is to plan rationally and prepare for change. Although many plans are not carried out exactly as anticipated because of changing circumstances, experience has shown that institutions that plan tend to be more successful than those that do not plan.

In planning, management is concerned with formulating a strategy, establishing the objectives (critical success factors or key performance indicators) to be achieved, and determining how to achieve them. Critical success factors may include patient satisfaction, employee turnover, outcomes, and infection rates. Planning information is assembled, the external and internal environments are studied, planning premises are set out, and decisions to reach organizational goals are made. The decisions made in planning provide the operational units of the organization with their objectives and with the standards against which performance is measured.

Thus, when the manager plans a course of action, he or she attempts to ensure a consistent and coordinated operation aimed at achieving the desired results. Plans alone do not bring about these results; to achieve them, effective operation of the healthcare center by managers knowledgeable of the plan is necessary. Without plans, however, random activities by all managers prevail, resulting in confusion and possibly even chaos. The plan serves as the road map for managers to follow as they chart their path to the goal.

THE NATURE OF PLANNING

How can a manager properly and effectively organize the workings of the department without having a plan in mind? How can the department head effectively staff and supervise the employees without knowing either the objectives or the avenues, policies, procedures, and methods to follow? How could the activities of the employees be controlled? None of these functions could be performed without planning. No substitute exists for the hard thinking that planning demands. Therefore, only after having made the plans can the manager organize, staff, influence, and control.

However, planning does not end abruptly when the manager begins to perform the other functions. It should not be a process used only at occasional intervals or when the manager is not too engrossed in daily tasks. Rather, planning is a continuous process. With day-to-day planning, the supervisor realistically anticipates future problems, analyzes them, determines their probable effect on activities, and decides on the plan of action that will lead to the desired results.

Planning Is a Task of Every Manager

Planning is the job of every manager, whether chair of the board, clinic administrator, information technology director, or materials management supervisor. By definition, all of these people are managers and therefore all of them must plan. The importance and magnitude of the plans depend on the level at which plans are determined. Planning at the top level of administration is more fundamental and more far reaching than at the supervisory levels of management, where the scope and extent of planning become narrower and more detailed.

Thus, the administrator is concerned with the overall aspects of planning for the entire healthcare organization, such as constructing new facilities, adding new services, aligning with other organizations, and enlarging outpatient services. While the chief information officer's (CIO) long-range planning may include setting objectives for achieving a paperless environment for the organization, the information systems supervisor who is knowledgeable about this plan defines priorities (i.e., which areas should be involved, what equipment is needed), writes new procedures, and determines activities to fulfill these objectives. A supervisor is more concerned with departmental plans for getting the job done promptly and effectively each day, or, as some say, "operationalizing" the plan or making "it" happen, while the administrator or senior-level executive is determining what "it" will look like in the future.

Today's long-range planning must make certain that the healthcare facility's services are appropriate, timely, and competitive; that shared services and affiliations with other healthcare providers are considered; and, above all, that quality of care and health outcomes are improved. As reimbursement declines, today's managers must work to plan programs that are cost effective, that are efficient, and that manage health.

Although planning is the manager's function, this does not mean that others should not be called on for advice. Some healthcare institutions have full-time employees known as "planners," usually in a staff position. They are normally employed to help the CEO in his or her long-term strategy and planning decisions. Most supervisors are not likely to need such planners' help. However, at times a manager may require special knowledge as he or she plans, such as human resources (scheduling as a result of nursing shortages), information systems (implementing an electronic medical record), accounting (procedures to record the lease of a Pyxis drug dispensing machine), or other professional and technical aspects. In such instances, the supervisor must feel free to call on specialists within and outside the organization to help with the planning.

Benefits of Planning

Planning is a rigorous process of establishing objectives; deciding on strategies, tactics, and activities to achieve them; and formally documenting expectations. It results in purposeful organization and activities, which in turn minimize costs and reduce waste. Deciding in advance what is to be done—and how, by whom, where, and when—promotes efficient and orderly operations and reduces errors. All efforts are directed toward a desired result so that haphazard approaches are minimized, activities are coordinated, and duplications are avoided. Thus, planning has many benefits that no manager can afford to neglect.

Effective management demands optimum use of the organization's resources. As a manager, you are entrusted with the management of both the employees and physical resources (space, equipment, tools, and materials) of the department. How all these resources are used is your primary responsibility and the basis on which your managerial performance is judged.

Only by planning are you able to make the best possible use of resources and bring out the best in your employees.

THE STRATEGIC PLANNING PROCESS

Planning can occur at any level of an organization. Although this chapter focuses on upper management planning, similar steps are appropriate for the department, section, or team. The development of missions and visions and discussion of other concepts in this chapter are not limited to the interests of boards of trustees. As a supervisor, you will be able to apply the steps discussed to your work team.

Managers may be asked to contribute information for consideration during the strategic planning sessions typically attended by the board of trustees or directors and senior management or administration of the healthcare organization. In addition, the strategic planning facilitator may invite external experts to guide the thinking. Such experts may include the organization's external auditors, professional or trade association leaders, bankers, and community leaders.

Validating the Mission

One of the first steps during any strategic planning process is to validate the organization's mission, a statement that concisely describes what the organization does, what its purpose is, or why it exists. Generally, the mission statement is timeless; a mission statement may be, "We provide long-term, skilled nursing and rehabilitative services for individuals residing in our facility in a cost-effective and high-quality manner." The ideal mission statement is short and concise. Examples appear in Figure 7.1.

With the merger of organizations, the mission of one entity may change when it merges with another, or the mission may change naturally over time as new services are added by the organization. Consider how the first mission cited in Figure 7.1 might change if these organizations begin to offer telemedicine.

Once the organization's mission is established, each department's mission can be developed and should be supportive of the organization's mission. For example, the physical therapy department's mission may be, "We provide quality and effective rehabilitative services for our patient and home care clients."

As mentioned earlier, much information is needed for planning effectively. The review of this information is known as the environmental assessment and is not limited to internal information. To be able to predict the impact of changing or adding services, linking with another organization, and so forth, one must know what is happening outside the walls of the organization specifically and in the healthcare industry in general. Therefore, the environmental assessment includes a comprehensive analysis of information about the following (Purcell 2001, 27):

- the organization's current, past, and potential future customers;
- competitors in the region and those who may invade the region served by the organization;
- societal changes such as demographic shifts in the aged population, movement of the population, or expectations from society in general of health-care providers;
- industry indicators and comparative data (such as Hospital Compare, Leapfrog, Solucient);
- regulatory and accreditation changes; and
- how your own organization is performing (e.g., financially; in terms of patient outcomes and volume; staff and patient satisfaction; licensure issues). Strategic planners have an acronym for these elements of the environmental assessment: *PESTHR analysis*—political, economic, social, technological, human resource, and regulatory forces.

Assume that several organizations in the community have had their accreditation survey and passed accreditation. However, your facility received "conditional accreditation." While the management team is working toward improving their compliance with the accrediting agency's standards, the major concern for administration now is that the managed care companies in the community only extend contracts with those hospitals that passed and had higher Hospital Compare scores. This environmental condition will force all in the organization to focus and coordinate their plans to quickly resolve the issues causing the conditional status.

The last component, the internal organization review, often includes what is known as a *SWOT analysis*. SWOT (strengths, weaknesses, opportunities, and threats) analysis evaluates the internal organization based on its strengths compared to competitors and regional and societal demands, weakness compared to competitors or related to just the internal functions, opportunities for advancing ahead of competitors or serving a patient population not served or well served currently, and threats from external or internal agents that could stymie the organization's success.

Figure 7.2: Vision Statements

Fayette Memorial Hospital, Connersville, Indiana

Our Team will serve the health needs of the residents of the Whitewater Valley by providing compassionate, high quality, cost-effective care. Recognizing our community's needs, we will continue to expand our services and technological base.

Rush University Medical Center, Chicago

Rush University Medical Center will be recognized as the standard for an academic medical center delivering the highest quality care integrated with research and education in health fields.

Sources: Courtesy of Fayette Memorial Hospital, Connersville, IN. Reproduced with permission of Rush–Presbyterian–St. Luke's Medical Center, Chicago.

Creating the Vision

Once the environmental assessment and analysis have been completed, the leadership of the organization (those participating in the strategic planning activities) formulates a vision. The vision of an organization is a statement about where the leadership sees the organization going in a designated period of time; hence, the vision is timebound (Zuckerman 2000). The vision should be clear and concise, and ideally should be a single statement (see Figure 7.2).

The next planning step is to prioritize those actions indicated for the organization to continue to succeed and deliver its mission as it progresses toward its vision. To expand on our earlier example, the vision may read as follows: "Within five years Shady Oaks Nursing Home will be a system of three nursing homes to provide high-quality residential care for those needing skilled nursing and rehabilitative care, as well as one location providing residential housing for those who can care for themselves in a continuing care community located in the suburbs of our community." The strategic plan for the next year may be to open one of the skilled homes. Each department manager will be responsible for developing action plans to ensure the home is efficiently designed and constructed in a timely manner.

Determining the Critical Success Factors or Objectives

Once the vision is determined and the analysis of the environmental data completed, the board of directors and senior administration establish broad strategic thrusts to achieve the vision. (See Nickols [2000] for more definitions of strategy.) Strategic thrusts may also be called strategies, which are approaches to achieve the vision. The thrusts for our example may include (1) a fund-raising program to raise the money needed to build or acquire two additional nursing

FIGURE 7.3: STRATEGIC PLANNING MODEL

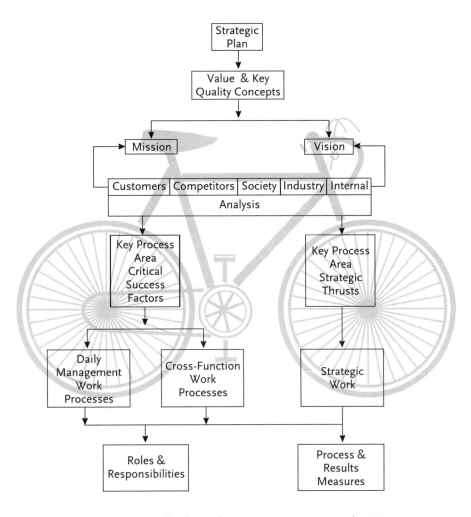

Source: Courtesy of Kevin J. McArdle of McArdle Enterprises, Inc., Minneapolis, MN.

homes and the property and buildings for the residential housing, (2) lobbying the legislature or regulatory agencies to avoid any delays that would prevent the organization from achieving its vision, or (3) proposing a bond issue to support the expansion. The planning group not only sets the vision but also identifies various routes for management to take to achieve the organization's broadest goals. In effect, the strategic planning group could be perceived as sitting on the seat of a bicycle and pedaling it down a path toward the vision (see Figure 7.3).

In addition to the strategic thrusts, the information from the environmental assessment identifies critical success factors. One may be obtaining a state certificate of approval before a competitor obtains one for a given community location or establishing an effective marketing campaign to support the fund-raising program. In some organizations, a critical success factor may be called an organization goal.

With the vision, strategic thrusts (strategies), and critical success factors (goals) defined, senior management and administration identify the objectives that support critical success factors and bring the vision to reality. The burden of the effort to make the organization successful lies with management and staff. The full strength of this group must be marshaled to achieve the vision. As a supervisor, you will meet with your administrative leader and possibly your subordinates to define the objectives for your department, the impact of these objectives on your daily work processes, and the interdepartmental relationships that must be established or strengthened for total organizational success (see Figure 7.4).

Other Planning Considerations

The length of time for which the manager should plan is called the *planning horizon*. The planning horizon is usually distinguished as long term, interme-diate, or short term. The exact definitions of long-term and short-term planning depend on the manager's level in the hierarchy, the type of institution, and the kind of activity in which it is engaged.

Generally, *short-term planning* covers a period up to one year, and planning of activities to be carried out over a period of one to five years is known as inter-mediate planning. This planning horizon contains fewer uncertainties than the long-range planning, which has to contend with highly uncertain conditions of several decades hence. Thus, *long-term planning* usually involves a considerably longer horizon—generally, any plan that extends beyond five years. Because of this industry's dynamics, administrators, such as board members and CEOs, find it difficult to plan beyond a decade. So much regulatory change is dependent on the political party controlling Congress and the potential for congressional and presidential changes every four years.

The supervisor's planning period is probably short range—that is, for one year at the most or perhaps for six months, one month, one week, or even one day. A supervisor can definitely plan some activities in certain departments three, six, nine, or twelve months in advance, such as the preventive mainte-nance planning. On the other hand, with other activities in a healthcare facility, supervisory planning is for a shorter time—a week, a day, or only a shift. Such short-range planning is frequently needed in patient care services and in other departments that have difficulty recruiting talented staff, such as for engineer-ing and coding.

It is more desirable if the supervisor is able to make longer-range plans, but for practical purposes, proper attention must be given to seeing that the work of each day is accomplished. This short-range planning requires the supervisor to take the time to consider the nature and amount of work that is to be done each day by the department, the person(s) responsible for doing the work, and when

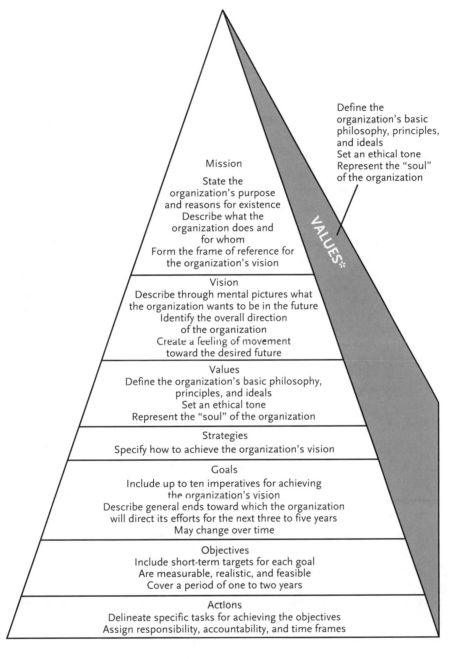

Define the organization's basic philosophy, principles, and ideals
Set an ethical tone
Represent the "soul" of the organization

VALUES*

Mission
State the organization's purpose and reasons for existence
Describe what the organization does and for whom
Form the frame of reference for the organization's vision

Vision
Describe through mental pictures what the organization wants to be in the future
Identify the overall direction of the organization
Create a feeling of movement toward the desired future

Values
Define the organization's basic philosophy, principles, and ideals
Set an ethical tone
Represent the "soul" of the organization

Strategies
Specify how to achieve the organization's vision

Goals
Include up to ten imperatives for achieving the organization's vision
Describe general ends toward which the organization will direct its efforts for the next three to five years
May change over time

Objectives
Include short-term targets for each goal
Are measurable, realistic, and feasible
Cover a period of one to two years

Actions
Delineate specific tasks for achieving the objectives
Assign responsibility, accountability, and time frames

* The values support each step equally.
Source: Zuckerman (1998).

the work has to be done. Furthermore, this daily planning, by definition, must be done ahead of time; many supervisors prefer to do it at the end of the day or shift, when they can size up what has been accomplished already to formulate plans for the following day or shift.

Occasionally, a supervisor is also involved in intermediate and long-term plans. For example, the boss may want to discuss planning for new activities for the institution. A supervisor may be informed of a contemplated expansion or the addition of new facilities, for instance a nursing home, and is then asked to propose what the department can contribute or what is needed. If a hospital plans for an enlarged outpatient surgical center, the director of nursing as well as the operating room supervisors are asked to be deeply involved. These supervisors are assigned to develop short-term measurable targets, or objectives, and then delineate the specific tasks or actions for achieving the targets. Action plans are the result of this delineation process.

From time to time the administrator might request that the supervisor look into the future and project the long-term trend of a particular activity, especially if it is apparent that such activity will be affected by major breakthroughs in medical science and technology or by regulatory change. Certainly the reimbursement manager was involved in the planning for the many prospective payment systems introduced during the last ten years, and the IT management team was involved in preparations for HIPAA compliance. It is important for supervisors to participate in such long-range planning because the plans may require some employees to be reassigned or others to acquire additional skills. Some planning suggestions are offered by The Economics Press, Inc. (1999):

> Start your planning by asking questions about the new project: "How does the upcoming job differ from the one my team is working on now?" Even a small change, such as a tighter deadline or a change of location, could lead to big problems if you and your team are not prepared for it. Once you've decided what makes the upcoming job different from the last one, ask yourself: "What problems and mistakes are likely to occur? And what's the best way to avoid them?" If you have to coordinate your efforts with another department or team, you will have to work out a joint, detailed schedule with them. If needed, materials must be obtained before the project can begin. Another question: "Will anyone need additional training?"

The long-range plans also may indicate that subordinates with completely new skills and education are needed and that a search for them must start immediately. Learning new procedures and techniques might be necessary as a result of new and different ways of diagnosing and treating medical conditions. For instance, consider the transition from a film library in the radiology department to a picture-archiving communications system with web access for telemedicine. Even though these technologies are readily available, their implementation date is often placed in the long-range term because of the high cost and the time it takes to acquire the equipment (a capital expenditure). In these situations, the supervisors must participate in long-range planning to ensure adequate space, staff and user training, and so forth.

The Integration and Communication of Plans

Integrating, coordinating, and balancing the long-range, intermediate, and short-range plans are essential. Therefore, the supervisor's short-range plans must support intermediate plans, which in turn should support long-range plans. Long-range planning should not be viewed as an activity separate from or contrary to short-range planning. All too often, however, there is a gap between the knowledge of top management and that of lower-level management concerning planning. This gap is often justified by the claim that many of the plans are confidential and cannot be divulged for security or proprietary reasons. Most employees know that very little can be kept secret in any organization. On the other hand, supervisors should realize that some limitations to what they are allowed to know exist, and top-level administration may not wish to disclose all their plans for competitive reasons.

To the extent necessary, plans should be communicated and fully explained to subordinate managers so that they are in a better position to formulate derivative plans for their departments. Along the same line, supervisors should always bear in mind that their own employees are affected by the plans they make. Not only supervisors but their staff must clearly understand the objectives of their own department as well as how their goals support the goals and objectives of the entire institution. Because employees are needed to execute whatever has been planned, the supervisor should explain in advance the plans for the department. The manager may even want to consult his or her subordinate supervisors, team leaders, and line employees for suggestions because some may be in a position to make helpful contributions. The supervisor must bear in mind that the successful completion of a task depends on the full understanding of its purpose by those who have to carry it out. The supervisor should also remember that well-informed employees always are better employees. Such employees appreciate that they have not been kept in the dark. It is therefore good management to make certain that all employees at all levels are thoroughly informed about the objectives to be achieved.

THE USE OF OBJECTIVES IN PLANNING

I am from the school that never used the terms goals and objectives interchangeably. However, today's literature often does; thus, this chapter has done so as well. Therefore, let me distinguish between the two:

Goals support the vision and define results; for example, our medication error rate will be lower than the regional average as defined by our liability carrier. *Objectives* set targets and describe how our goals will be achieved. One such objective may be to eliminate and/or reduce the acceptance of handwritten orders by securing 90 percent of all orders through computerized physician order entry by the end of the first quarter.

All planning has the purpose of achieving organizational goals and objectives. In this sense, objective has a broader meaning. For example, it was George W. Bush's objective to win the 2000 presidential election. In this context, objective and goal are synonymous. Therefore, the first step in planning is to develop a statement of the goals and objectives[1] for the institution that becomes the target or the end results that the institution seeks to attain through organized efforts and toward which all activities are directed. These goals and objectives must be expressed clearly and communicated fully so that all managers have a common understanding around which to coordinate their activities. The objectives largely determine how the managers go about their organizing, staffing, and influencing functions. Also, the controlling function would be meaningless without a set of objectives as guidelines.

Effective management is always management by objectives. This holds true for the CEO of a hospital, for the supervisor on the "firing line," and for all managers on the levels in between. Formulating objectives should therefore be foremost in every manager's mind. Once the goals have been established, additional plans, such as policies, standard procedures, methods, rules, programs, projects, and budgets, are then designed to achieve the objectives.

Primary Objectives or Goals

In general, many healthcare centers have such primary objectives as providing primary, secondary, or tertiary care[2] to the sick and injured; providing healthcare at a reasonable cost; doing research; helping in the maintenance of health and in the prevention of sickness; recruiting outstanding interns, physicians, and employees; providing education; and training employees in all the professional and nonprofessional activities customarily associated with a healthcare institution. In addition to these goals, a healthcare facility can have many other objectives such as implementing process improvements, maintaining a fine reputation among hospitals, achieving excellent outcomes, establishing a good and caring image in the community, discharging numerous social and charitable responsibilities, and maintaining fiscal viability. For healthcare entities organized as a for-profit undertaking, profit certainly is also one of the major objectives.

A healthcare institution also strives toward many other, less tangible objectives. In relation to its employees, for instance, its goal is to be a good and fair employer. The objective in this case is to establish the reputation of being a good place for people to work. These objectives may actually speak to the organization's values. According to Zuckerman (1998), "values define the organization's basic philosophy, principles, and ideals." A *value statement* answers the question, "what is important to this organization?" and cites the beliefs and behavioral standards that are fundamental to the organization. It should express the entity's moral and ethical basis (Purcell 2001, 27). An example of a stated set of hospital values appears in Figure 7.5.

FIGURE 7.5: EXAMPLE OF VALUE STATEMENT

Catholic Healthcare West, San Francisco

OUR VALUES

Catholic Healthcare West is committed to providing high-quality, affordable health care to the communities we serve. Above all else we value:

- Dignity—Respecting the inherent value and worth of each person.
- Collaboration—Working together with people who support common values and vision to achieve shared goals.
- Justice—Advocating for social change and acting in ways that promote respect for all persons and demonstrate compassion for our sisters and brothers who are powerless.
- Stewardship—Cultivating the resources entrusted to us to promote healing and wholeness.
- Excellence—Exceeding expectations through teamwork and innovation.

Source: Courtesy of Catholic Healthcare West.

Any organization has many primary objectives, and the real difficulty lies in ranking and balancing them. This is especially true for healthcare facilities. If the CEO chose a single objective and excluded all the others, the effectiveness of the institution's overall performance could be jeopardized. Because healthcare activities must function in a constantly changing and increasingly challenging environment, it is necessary to continually reevaluate past objectives and to add new ones.

Secondary or Departmental Objectives or Goals

The primary objectives of an institution are its goals. In turn, goals specific to departments can be called secondary, operative, supportive, or derivative objectives. Because each department or division has a specific task to perform, each must have its own clearly defined goals. These secondary goals and objectives of the departments must stay within and contribute to the overall framework of the organization's primary goals.

Because they are concerned with only one department, however, secondary objectives are necessarily narrower in scope. They enable departmental managers to operate at their own discretion, although, again, always within the limits of the overall institutional (primary) goals. For instance, if the stated organizational goal is, "to support research so that our clinicians are able to deliver state-of-the-art healthcare," the stated mission of the facility's decision-support department may be, "to systematically collect and maintain all patient demographic and medical data and to facilitate analysis of the data so that the resulting information benefits the user." Therefore, the departmental objectives or goals for the decision-support department may be to (1) work closely with patient financial services, health information, and accounting to obtain timely data; (2) collect, analyze, and publish various hospital and clinical comparative statistics; and (3) review and assess concurrently and retrospectively the outcomes and utilization of services.

Obviously these departmental objectives are specific, but their fulfillment contributes significantly to the achievement of overall institutional goals. In fact, the primary objectives could not be achieved if these and all other departmental objectives were not fulfilled.

Developing Objectives

Planning is a dynamic process. Because all healthcare activities operate in an increasingly complex and dynamic environment, new situations and new information necessitate revising and updating the established long-range and intermediate plans. This, in turn, creates the need for changing the objectives. Objectives must be flexible and adaptable to changes in the internal and external environments. Therefore, reviewing, revising, or updating objectives on an increasingly frequent basis is a managerial duty on all levels.

As noted above, objectives represent measurable targets that we develop to achieve a given goal. The acronym SMART indicates the steps to writing strong objectives—specific, measurable, attainable, result-oriented, time-limited (Allen 2000)[3]. Objectives must be established for each critical success factor or goal. An example of an organizational goal may be, "to expand community access to primary healthcare services." A corresponding objective may be, "to open three off-site ambulatory care clinics in the coming fiscal year at a cost not to exceed $1.5 million." For objectives to be achievable, senior management must ensure that the resources are available. The clinic manager cannot open additional facilities if the board does not allocate funding to do so.

MONITORING THE EFFECTIVENESS OF THE STRATEGIC PLAN

Once management has created the strategic plan, the plan must be implemented through the efforts of all departments and staffs of the healthcare entity. Top down or bottom up, an organization's workforce implements any changes; if the staff do not respect or understand the undertaking, the plan is doomed at inception (Purcell 2001). As with any plan, knowing whether the decisions were right or wrong requires monitoring the implementation and effectiveness of the plan. This monitoring effort is known as *performance management* (PM). PM uses the critical success factors (CSFs) and their respective measures, collects data, and monitors the results of the CSFs, making necessary revisions to the plan or operations to achieve corporate goals. Involving all employees in the development of CSF measurements defines what management is interested in and the results it expects. Sometimes, this process is carried out through a management by objectives approach.

Management by Objectives

To achieve specific results from setting these departmental objectives, organizations use a process called *management by objectives* (MBO). The term and concepts were first introduced by management expert Peter Drucker in the early 1950s and have become very popular.

MBO is an integrative management concept, containing elements of the planning function together with participative management, collaboration, motivation, and controlling. It is the process of collaborative goal setting by the manager and subordinate. The degree to which goals are accomplished plays a major role in evaluating and rewarding the subordinate's performance. MBO demonstrates the interrelationships of the managerial functions and the systems approach to management. Therefore, MBO is also discussed in other chapters of this book. This section, however, is primarily concerned with the meaning of MBO in connection with setting and achieving objectives.

When a facility begins an MBO program, top administration must communicate the reason that MBO has been adopted, must indicate that the program starts at the top of the organization, and must project the results the program is expected to produce. All managers and employees also need to be educated and informed about their role in the program. Often organizations create "dashboards" to monitor their progress.

As stated, MBO is concerned with goal setting for individual managers. In this process, a manager at any level and his or her immediate subordinate jointly develop departmental goals in accordance with organizational goals. Once institutional goals are clarified, the manager and the subordinate, on a one-to-one basis, should develop and agree on the subordinate's goals during a stated period. The subordinate then defines the objectives to achieve the goals. To be operational, these performance objectives must be specific, measurable (quantifiable), and challenging, but they should also be realistically attainable within the time frame established. This means that each objective must provide a plan showing what work is to be done, in what time frame it is to be done, which individual is to do it, and what resources the individual can use to get it done. Quantitative indicators must also be established to measure what work is achieved.

To be realistic, it should be possible to carry out the activity within the time frame set—a period long enough to meet the objective, but short enough to provide timely feedback and still permit intervention if necessary. In general, the goals should meet the three criteria of specificity, conciseness, and time frame. The degree to which these goals are achieved is a major factor in evaluating and rewarding the subordinate's performance.

Goal	Expected Date
Reduce by 50% the denials for inappropriate admissions.	4th Quarter
Capture data (by physician and payer) on inappropriate admissions	1st Quarter
In cooperation with the VP Medical Affairs, develop an educational program for the Medical Staff	2nd Quarter
Present education program for each clinical service	2nd Quarter
Present one-on-one educational program for those physicians with the majority of admission denials	2nd Quarter

It is important that these goals be jointly established and agreed on ahead of time. At the end of the period, both the supervisor and the subordinate participate in the review of the subordinate's performance to see how results for the period compare with the objectives he or she set out to accomplish. If the goals were achieved, new goals are set for the next period. If a discrepancy exists, efforts are made to find solutions to overcome these problems and the manager and subordinate agree on new goals for the next period. MBO clearly is a powerful tool in achieving involvement and commitment of subordinates (see Figure 7.6).

The next four chapters explore other tools that are necessary to planning success.

SUMMARY

Planning is the managerial function that determines in advance what is to be done in the future. It is the function of every manager, from the top-level administrator to the supervisor of each department. Planning is important because it ensures the best utilization of resources and economy of performance. The planning period at the supervisory level is usually much shorter than the period at the top administrator's level. Nevertheless, the short-range plans of the supervisor must coincide with the long-range plans of the enterprise.

Establishing the vision is an essential step in planning. The vision guides managers to set goals and objectives. Although the overriding or primary objectives are determined by top-level administration, many secondary objectives or department goals must be clarified by the supervisor and must be in accordance with the primary objectives of the overall undertaking. The work of "operationalizing," or making the vision become reality, is in the hands of the managers and their staff who develop measurable objectives and action plans to accomplish the goals.

One useful technique for implementing plans is management by objectives, a process of collaborative goal setting that leads to evaluation. To be successful, this approach must establish realistic time frames and expectations that are mutually agreed on.

NOTES

1. The terms goals and objectives are used interchangeably in this chapter. Some experts point out that the terms differ in meaning—objectives mostly describe short-term results on the operational level, whereas goals describe the major results the organization seeks to accomplish.

2. Primary care means ambulatory, emergency, and initial physician contact. Secondary care refers to high-morbidity, low-mortality, inpatient care provided by specialists. Tertiary care means high-mortality, low-morbidity, highly sophisticated and specialized inpatient care.

3. As viewed on Internet on 2/11/06 at http://ollie.dcccd.edu/mgmt1374/book_contents/2planning/perf_objectives/perf_obj.htm.

REFERENCES

Allen, G. 2000. *Supervision, Second edition*. Denton, TX: RonJon Publishers.

Nickols, F. 2000. "Strategy Is . . . a Lot of Things." [Online article.] http://home.att.net~nickols/articles.htm.

Purcell, T. 2001. "Strategic Planners Lead the Pack." *Journal of Accountancy* 192 (December): 27.

The Economics Press, Inc. 1999. "Plan for Success." *Better Supervision* 738: 3–4.

Zuckerman, A. M. 2000. "Creating a Vision for the Twenty-First Century Healthcare Organization." *Journal of Healthcare Management* 45 (5): 298.

———. 1998. *Healthcare Strategic Planning: Approaches for the 21st Century*, 37. Chicago: Health Administration Press.

CHAPTER EIGHT

Forecasting

CHAPTER OBJECTIVES

After you have studied this chapter, you should be able to do the following:

1. Discuss the need for and extent of forecasting, which provides the background for managerial planning.
2. See the value of projections and population changes in planning for the healthcare industry.
3. Identify skill needs and potential generational diversity issues.

ALTHOUGH THE FUTURE is fraught with uncertainties, managers must make certain assumptions about it to be able to plan. These assumptions are based on forecasts that provide information essential to the planning process. Forecasting is done by scanning the external and internal environments for useful information. Because the appraisal of future prospects is inherent in all planning, the success of an enterprise greatly depends on the skill of management, first in forecasting and second in preparing for future conditions.

FORECASTS AS THE BASIS OF PLANNING

Management typically confines its forecasting effort to factors that experience suggests are important to its own planning. Thus, chief administrators of the healthcare facility select those forecasts that have a direct material bearing on the healthcare field in the broadest sense.

In trying to make predictions, administrators consider the general economic, political, labor, and social climates in which the healthcare institution must operate during the next few years. This information comes from reviewing forecasts on government policies, legislation and regulation, government spending, merger and consolidation activities, and insurer penetration to determine how these might ultimately affect the activities of healthcare providers.

Thus, top-level administrators do not actually perform the research and statistical analysis for all their forecasts. They frequently use data published in government and trade publications or made available by hospital or healthcare organizations, healthcare system research staffs, and other experts in various fields. Administrators then try to predict the general trends for the delivery of healthcare as it affects the various providers and users in relation to cost effectiveness and other considerations.

With the recent turn of the century, top-level management has been vitally interested in forecasts of changes in the U.S. population. The population is growing, graying, and diversifying. In Census 2000, 281.4 million people were counted in the United States. The U.S. Census Bureau (2000; 2004) estimates the population count will be 419.9 million for 2050 and approximately 498 million people for 2080. The breakdown of population figures by age and sex provides even more meaningful data, depending on whether administrators are planning for a general short-term hospital, long-term healthcare facility, women's services, and so forth. Figure 8.1 shows us that the babies born during the baby boom that occurred after World War II will be reaching Medicare age shortly after the turn of the twenty-first century. The boom creates a surge of 60-year-olds starting in 2010 that will continue to ride the timeline horizon through 2030+/— and will place demands on the healthcare system for treatment and care. These demands are similar to the ones that occurred in the early 1950s for schools and teachers to accommodate the school-aged children created by the baby boom.

As can be seen in Figure 8.1, starting with 2010, there will be more people eligible for Medicare (65 and older) than people contributing to the Medicare fund. A report released on February 29, 2000 by the White House, "America's Seniors and Medicare: Challenges for Today and Tomorrow," predicts that the nation's 65+ population will grow from 34.71 million in 2000 to 61.95 million in 2025. This growth not only affects healthcare service utilization but also tax expense for employers to fund Medicare benefits. As a supervisor, you will likely be asked to identify processes to deliver high-quality service while using less labor to stem the growth of compensation expenses for your organization.

Growth in the diversity of our population will continue as well. The U.S. Census Bureau (2004) predicts a decline in the white population as a percentage of total population, from 81 percent in 2000 to 72.1 percent in 2050. This means that our healthcare organizations and our management styles need to change to address alternative medicine preferences, language barriers, family values of different cultures, signage needs, food preferences, cultural superstitions/beliefs, holy day recognition, and religious beliefs.

SUPERVISORY FORECASTS

Scientific and Technological Developments

When supervisors make departmental forecasts, their assumptions about the future cover a much narrower field than those of administrators. A supervisor should forecast mostly those factors that may have some bearing on the future

FIGURE 8.1: BABY BOOMER BULGE

Change in Workforce & Retired Age Groups

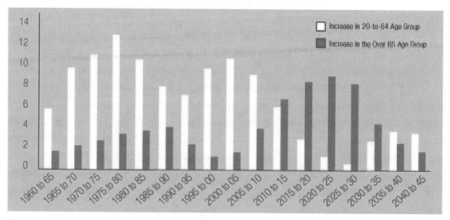

Originally published in *Chief Learning Officer* magazine, www.clomedia.com. Used with permission.

of his or her department. For example, supervisors should determine whether a trend is growing for more sophistication or more simplification of the function they oversee or whether this function seems to be of increasing or decreasing significance to the healthcare institution. It is important to keep abreast of the rapid and often revolutionary developments in the medical field, in technology, and in automation. Of course, supervisors also have to contend with some broader assumptions such as cost containment, government involvement, staff recruitment, skill requirements, and other concerns in the healthcare field.

Based on past events, the supervisor should make some assumptions on what the future holds. In making such assumptions, he or she can look to the sources of supplies, available technology, and equipment used for assistance. Supervisors can also learn by attending lectures, national meetings, and exhibitions and by joining professional organizations and reading their journals. Advances in the medical sciences and technology are progressing so rapidly that in several years a department's functions and staff's responsibilities may be significantly different from what they had been or are today. Consider, for instance, the impact of further computerization and automation in laboratories, where automated analyzers have become more sophisticated, smaller, and less expensive such that the technology can easily be installed at physician offices, thus reducing the demand for testing at the hospital laboratory. Such projections are essential for the planning done by supervisors in clinical laboratories: Will more, less, or about the same number of employees be needed with the same, different, or additional education or training? Should the equipment be bought or leased? The supervisor must consider these and similar questions.

Employees and Skills

Supervisors also have to make forecasts about the types of employees that will be working in the department in the future. When Bill Gates proposed in a college paper that every household would have a personal computer, his professor rejected the paper. We know now that the Industrial Age has given way to the Information Age. According to the U.S. Department of Labor, at least 44 percent of all workers performed data services—for example, gathering, processing, retrieving, or analyzing information at the beginning of this century (Pritchett 1999). The explosion in computing power geometrically increases the amount of data available for decision making. However, the key to quality decision making is the conversion of data to information. Some experts indicate that data supplies double every five years. Pritchett (1999) states that more information has been produced in the last 30 years than during the previous 5,000 years. Given this explosion, data collection, screening, management, manipulation, and display skills are a premium asset for employees to possess.

Changes in healthcare technology will probably create a need for some employees who have been educated and trained in completely new and advanced scientific fields and are capable of coping with state-of-the-art technology and areas such as robotics, genetics, electronics, use of artificial intelligence, and neural networks.

At the same time, the nation is experiencing serious shortages of nurses, transcriptionists, information systems professionals, coding specialists, secretaries, and even clerical staff. These positions are no longer glamorous to young people joining the workforce. Similarly, conventional full-time jobs are perceived to limit time available for family or personal activities and are going unfilled. Supervisors should be aware of the noneconomic demands that young people expect to fulfill on their jobs and the potential for generational clashes at the work site. Cultural and generational diversity will be a challenge for staff and leaders alike, as Generation Y 20-year-olds, raised with computers in every aspect of their lives, work side by side with 50- and 60-year-olds. Planning for the team-building efforts that may be required will be imperative for supervisors. Meeting all types of demands, such as material, psychological, and professional, will be particularly important if supervisors must find people who possess skills that up to now may not have been required in the department.

In addition, supervisors may find that reduced reimbursement from third-party payers could force downsizing or elimination of some clinical services and their associated staff. Alternatively, department reorganization could result in the need for fewer supervisors and employees, but retention of those who have skills in a variety of areas. In 1995, one of the Reports of the Pew Health Professions Commission was published. This report, and its subsequent studies, represent the thinking of participants from all healthcare professions. One theme that permeates the report is that "Schools must develop strategies that will create an environment conducive to the education of a generalist practitioner." The report goes on to say, "It [the education system] will require the alteration of some organizational structures and the development of new and different relationships with affiliated institutions and community-based practitioners. In part, these needs will be met by working across professional lines in clinical settings and by courses aimed at instilling the value of primary care, providing the skills necessary to maintain primary care, and promoting the team work skills vital to participation in primary care" (Pew Health Professions Commission 1995). The supervisor's role as a coordinator and collaborator will be paramount.

At the supervisory level, you will be expected to select new employees who have certain basic skills that can be built on with internal educational programs to enable them to perform multiskilled tasks. Further, you will be asked to develop educational programs to teach these individuals the many skills they will be required to master. You will need to plan both time and effort to bring existing staff up to par with a varied skill set as well as plan the educational curriculum to teach new employees. Lastly, you will need to create monitoring tools to ensure the employees have learned the skills, maintain their skills, and are performing according to your expectations. Your planning spectrum in this type of environment will be quite vast.

SUMMARY

All planning must be done with forecasts of the future in mind. Forecasting is an art, not a science. As of yet, no infallible way of predicting the future exists; however, forecasting accuracy increases with experience. One should always remember that at the base of all forecasts lie certain assumptions, approximations, opinions, and judgments. Entitywide forecasts or assumptions are made by top-level administration, and the supervisor narrows these down to forecasts for the departmental activity.

Over time, making assumptions about the future should become a normal activity for all managers. They should exchange ideas, help each other, and supply information whenever it is available. They most likely will act as a check on each other, and their analysis of what the future holds will probably be quite reliable. Even if some of the events that have been anticipated do not materialize or do not occur exactly as forecasted, it is better to have foreseen them than to be suddenly confronted with them. Having foreseen these events, supervisors have prepared themselves and the state of the organization's affairs to be able to incorporate changes whenever they are needed. Although this task may sound formidable for supervisors, it is their job to be alert to all possible changes and trends. Based on these assumptions and forecasts, the supervisor then makes plans for the department. This is the only way supervisors can prevent their own and their employees' obsolescence.

REFERENCES

Pew Health Professions Commission. 1995. "Critical Challenge: Revitalizing the Health Professions for the Twenty-First Century." Commission Report, 25–26. San Francisco: UCSF Center for Health Professions.

Pritchett, P. 1999. *New Work Habits for a Radically Changing World*. Plano, TX: Pritchett Rummler-Brache.

U.S. Census Bureau. 2000. "NP-D1-A Projections of the Resident Population by Age, Sex, Race, and Hispanic Origin: 1999 to 2010." [Online article; retrieved 9/13/05.] www.census.gov/population/projections/nation/detail/ d2071_80.pdf.

———. 2004. "US Interim Projections by Age, Sex, Race, and Hispanic Origin." [Online article; retrieved 9/13/05.] http://www.census.gov/IPC/ wwww/USinterimproj/.

CHAPTER NINE

Tactical Considerations in Planning

CHAPTER OBJECTIVES

After you have studied this chapter, you should be able to do the following:

1. Define and discuss different strategies for resource planning.
2. Recognize that planning requires attention to other elements, including timing, resource utilization, financial considerations, and safety.
3. Identify approaches to planning for the proper utilization of materials, machinery, and manpower.

WHILE PLANNING, SUPERVISORS must keep in mind how these plans affect others. Peers and subordinates assess the impact that plans or changes to their environment have on them or their departments first. Any perceived negative impact may result in resistance or lack of support for the initiatives. Success or failure of planning depends largely on the reaction of those involved in the plans, whether they are employees, supervisors of other departments, top-level administration, the medical staff, patients, or visitors. Several tactical or political strategies are at the supervisor's disposal to help minimize negative reactions and to facilitate the success of the plans.

Tactical approaches are short term. They are a means to get to the desired end. A combination of these approaches may be used, depending on the situation at hand. For example, a plan to outsource the environmental and food services functions of an organization requires tactical considerations by the current departmental managers and the administrator for these functions. Administration may involve managers, supervisors, and possibly some of the line staff such as lead cooks and housekeepers to help develop some of the criteria that will be used in selecting a firm. In addition, these same individuals may be part of the interview team. The goal is that by involving staff in parts of the decision, administration will gain their buy-in to the change.

PLANNING STRATEGIES

Because timing is a critical factor in all planning, the manager may choose the strategy that tells him or her to strike while the iron is hot. This strategy advocates prompt action when the situation and time for action are favorable. On the other hand, the supervisor may prefer to use the wait-and-see strategy, which takes the approach that time is the great moderator. This is not an endorsement of procrastination but of moving more slowly and seeing if factors take care of themselves after a short period of time.

When significant changes are involved in planning, the supervisor may use the strategy known as *concentrated mass offensive*. This strategy advocates a quick pulling together of all resources and taking radical action all at once to get immediate results. The creation of quasi-immediate service "hospitals" during Hurricane Katrina may be one example. Another approach may be team involvement. This strategy involves employees using various techniques such as brainstorming to solve what-if questions. This approach may be used if the organization has set a goal to improve patient satisfaction during the next year. Team involvement takes time but also provides for buy-in on plans by the employees. It also allows management to use the input of the employees as an information resource. On the other hand, the supervisor may prefer to just get a foot in the door. This approach may be used to initially introduce a pending change such as "we will need to expand coverage of our department to seven days a week. However, we will not be able to add staff. Be thinking about this, and we'll discuss it further at next week's department meeting." This tactic implies that proposing merely a portion of the plan in the beginning may lead to gradual acceptance, especially if the program is of such magnitude that its total acceptance is doubtful.

Sometimes one supervisor's plan may involve changes that could come about more easily if supervisors of other departments participate. It may therefore be advisable to seek allies to promote the change—that is, to adopt the strategy that promotes strength in unity. For example, if a supervisor plans to propose to increase the salaries of the employees, it may be wise to get other supervisors to join the effort in presenting a general request for higher compensation to the management. This may involve the you-scratch-my-back-and-I'll-scratch-yours strategy. This tactic, known as *reciprocity*, is practiced in business, in political circles, and by colleagues who wish to present joint action on a particular issue.

The choice and application of these political tactics depend on the people involved, the magnitude and urgency of the objective, timing, means available, and various other factors. Mentioning these tactical considerations, however, should not be construed to mean that they are always recommended. Properly applied, however, they can minimize difficulties and increase the effectiveness of the supervisor's planning.

PLANNING THE UTILIZATION OF RESOURCES

Every supervisor is entrusted with a large number of valuable resources to accomplish the job. These resources are grouped into three categories—materials, machinery, and manpower (the 3 Ms). The supervisor has a duty to specifically plan how to use the resources available so that the work of the unit can be managed efficiently and cost effectively. This means that detailed plans must be made for the proper use of equipment, instruments, space, materials and supplies, and supervisor's and employees' time.

Patient Care Equipment and Other Machinery

Because the institution has made a substantial investment in the equipment, plans for its efficient use must be made to protect that investment. In many departments, much of the equipment's usage depends on the orders of the physicians and surgeons. However, it is the supervisor's job to ensure that employees use the equipment with care.

Furthermore, the supervisor must ensure that the department is properly maintained. Equipment that is poorly maintained and does not function properly could lead to an incident resulting in a patient's lawsuit for damages. When the supervisor discovers that a piece of equipment is malfunctioning, he or she should immediately determine if it is being operated properly or if a maintenance problem exists. The proper steps to remedy the malfunction should be taken at once. Supervisors should work closely with the maintenance department or biomedical services and plan for periodic maintenance checkups.

Most facilities have an established program to check equipment at regular intervals in accordance with the manufacturers' guidelines. Records of these checks should be maintained. If a piece of equipment becomes worn, these records provide the supervisor with evidence to support replacement. In addition, such records of maintenance, repair, and corrective action are often reviewed by regulatory and accrediting agencies at the time of facility inspections.

Also, it is the supervisor's job to determine if the equipment serves its purpose and if better options are available for doing the work. This does not mean that a supervisor must always have the very latest model available; however, the supervisor should plan to replace inefficient equipment. The medical staff working in this area should be actively involved in deciding to update the equipment and recommending the replacement models or manufacturers as well. If the enterprise uses an outside biomedical service, supervisors would be wise to obtain its advice on replacement brands because the service may have encountered a more reliable model or brand elsewhere.

Once supervisors decide to replace old equipment or introduce new equipment, they must plan such replacements very carefully. In addition to consulting with the medical staff, they must read professional journals and literature circulated by hospitals and related associations, listen to sales presentations of equipment and instruments, and keep themselves abreast of current developments within their fields. Only with this type of background can the supervisor submit to his or her boss intelligent plans and alternatives for the replacement of the equipment. The recommended changes should be well substantiated. The proposal should include such items as projections of better patient care, utilization, cost effectiveness, community need, collaboration required, payback or return expected, customer sensitivity, and the important considerations of leasing versus buying.

Financial Considerations When Proposing the Purchase of New Equipment

Every year department managers submit requests for new equipment. The requests are often evaluated by an administrative or board committee, generally known as the capital expenditures committee. Funds for the equipment, or capital, are derived from an accounting process that sets aside a portion of monies each month or year in a fund called accrued depreciation.

Competition for the accrued depreciation is usually high. All managers want to update their facilities, equipment, and furnishings. Furthermore, new technologies for patient care purposes may be requested by members of the medical staff.

The final decision, however, remains with higher management. Even if the request is turned down, the supervisor has demonstrated that he or she is on top of the job, planning for the future. Eventually the plans for replacing equipment probably will be accepted, and the administrator will realize that the supervisor planned for the department's equipment with foresight (see Figure 9.1).

PLANNING A SAFE ENVIRONMENT

Traditionally healthcare providers have been very aware of the need for safety for their patients, employees, and visitors; after all, many accident victims end up in hospitals and, unfortunately, some hospital deaths are caused by unsafe conditions within the healthcare facility. Furthermore, the emphasis by accrediting agencies, the push for computerized physician order entry, and the federal government's support of an electronic health record for every individual by 2014 make every healthcare employee doubly aware of the importance of safety.

Although most healthcare facilities have a safety committee or safety department, its existence alone cannot fulfill the institution's obligation to plan, create, and maintain a safe environment for clients, visitors, and employees. As part of their responsibilities, managers and supervisors must diligently watch their areas and attempt to eliminate safety hazards. The recent flood of liability suits against hospitals and the publicity on medication errors have put additional emphasis on the need for safety.

When preparing a capital expenditure request, a manager should consider the following points recommended by Sweeny and Rachlin (1987):

1. Is the request supportive of, and consistent with, the organization's strategic plan?
2. Is the request responsive to the needs of the customers served as described by the marketing department?
3. Is the request responsive to the needs of the operating department? Will it solve an operational problem?
4. Has the request been fully justified by analysis of the benefits it will offer the organization/department?
5. Is the proposal supported by firm price quotations by vendors and contractors?
6. Is the request financially fundable?

Source: H. W. A. Sweeny and R. Rachlin. 1987. *Handbook of Budgeting, Second Edition*, 103. New York: John Wiley & Sons, Inc.

A patient is entitled to expect that the healthcare facility staff follow proven protocols and that the premises are reasonably safe. Care must be taken regarding equipment, instruments, and appliances so that they are adequate for use in the diagnosis or treatment of patients. If defective equipment causes injury to a patient, the hospital may be liable. Patients have brought lawsuits against healthcare facilities and their professional staffs because of defective beds, medication errors, broken thermometers, inoperative patient call systems, improperly calibrated x-ray equipment, and improperly prepared food. These examples indicate why JCAHO stresses the patient safety performance improvement activities and the Life Safety Code in its surveys.

Exposure to potentially dangerous materials or chemicals is common in healthcare facilities. For example, the food service and environmental staffs are exposed to cleansing agents and disinfectants, and the pathology staff is exposed to various media used to assist in evaluating tissues and bodily fluids. It is the supervisor's duty to keep his or her staff informed of chemical agents with which they may come in contact. When chemical agents of any type, such as detergents, correction fluid, printer toner, or laboratory chemicals, are used in the work setting, a Material Safety and Data Sheet (MSDS) should be prominently posted in the work area. These MSDSs provide staff with information such as how to treat the employee if the chemical is ingested or gets in the eyes. This OSHA and JCAHO requirement helps ensure staff safety from and knowledge of the chemicals and materials to which they may be exposed.

Another concern supervisors must take into account today is the rise in workplace violence. Consider the following five events:

- In June 2000, a resident physician who was fired from a medical center in Washington allegedly shot and killed a high-ranking doctor at the center before turning the gun on himself. Apparently, the resident physician was told that his contract would not be renewed, harming his prospects for future employment (Opus Communications 2001).
- In 2003, a woman fatally shot a doctor with whom she worked and then killed herself in an office at Massachusetts General Hospital (Business and Legal Reports 2003).
- A nurse at Long Island College Hospital in Brooklyn was held captive for 30 minutes by a patient who held scissors to her throat on November 19. (New York State Nurses Association 11/24/2003).[1]
- A drunken, 50-year-old Salem man was brought to Beverly Hospital for treatment. As a nurse helped him get ready to leave, he lunged at her, grabbed her crotch and tore through her hospital scrubs. He refused to let go. (Massachusetts Nursing Association April 2005)[2]
- "A female physician was accosted and sexually assaulted in an elevator at Bridgeport Hospital." "Police sources said Stanford may have posed as a hospital employee." "She managed to grab the elevator telephone but no one answered." (Connecticut *Post* May 2005).[3]

In 1999, the Bureau of Labor Statistics reported a rate of 8.3 assaults per 10,000 workers in the healthcare industry. This rate compares to 2 nonfatal assaults per 10,000 workers in the private sector.

No place or individual is immune from violence today. Taking training courses and reviewing publications such as the Centers for Disease Control and Prevention's NIOSH report[4] can help you identify precursors to violence, such as marital discord or depression, and prepare you to take appropriate measures if violence erupts in your workplace. Your organization's safety officer and the local police department are two excellent resources for prevention and safety advice.

The final safety concern discussed here is workplace injuries. Overall, the number of fatal work injuries recorded by the U.S. Department of Labor has declined. Today, however, much emphasis is placed on reducing or eliminating injuries caused by repetitive hand and finger motions, often linked to the increased use of computers and keyboards in the workplace. The Bureau of Labor Statistics (2001) reported that the median number of days away from work for 27,922 job-related cases of carpal tunnel syndrome in 1999 was 27 days or more. Therefore, it is to your advantage to reduce or eliminate such causes of injuries among your staff. Safety evaluations are not limited to at-facility work sites. Some staff, such as transcriptionists and billing employees, now telecommute or work at home. Working at home does raise job site safety issues, however. You may need to inspect home offices, offer ergonomic furniture, and hold safety classes. The occupational therapy department will be able to assist you in having your staff's workspace evaluated for appropriate ergonomics.

The true responsibility for safety lies with every manager, from the CEO down to the supervisors. The supervisor, being the person on the spot, must stress safety more than anyone else and must enforce safety procedures. Safety must be foremost in the supervisors' and employees' thoughts and must be a constant consideration in all supervisory planning. It must be integrated in all policies, procedures, methods, practices, and directives so that accidents and incidents do not occur or at least are significantly reduced.

PLANNING SPACE

Supervisors must also plan for the best utilization of space. First, they should determine whether the space assigned to the department is being used effectively. Some industrial engineering help, if available, may be requested to make this determination. If such help is not available, the supervisor should make a layout chart showing the square footage of the department, the location of equipment and supplies, and the work paths of the employees. Such a chart can then be studied to determine whether the allocated space has been laid out appropriately or whether areas need to be rearranged so that the department's work can be done more efficiently.

For example, say the chief laboratory scientist of the clinical laboratories shows that their annual workload has been increasing by approximately 10 percent annually, which would nearly double the workload in approximately nine years, from 40,000 to 70,000 tests. She also points out that the increased volume requires additional instrumentation that requires more square feet of room. She may also show how long the laboratories have occupied the same space. The chief technologist then draws up a typical laboratory space plan, showing a layout for separate work units or technical sections—hematology, urinalysis, biochemistry, histology, serology, bacteriology, immunology, blood bank, and the support areas. At the same time, the supervisor points out that laboratory facilities should preferably be on the first floor near the emergency room and patient registration areas and should be easily accessible to surgery, rather than on the present upper-floor location. The supervisor also discusses the feasibility of moving the labs to an off-site location. She then presents these materials during a discussion with the administrator and the medical director of the laboratory.

Layout planning may show the need for additional space, a different location, or both. If such a request, based on thorough planning of the space currently allotted, is made to the administrator, the likelihood that it will be granted is greater. In this case, the chief laboratory scientist most likely will be competing with many other managers who probably also requested more space and another location. Even if the request is denied, these plans will not have been drawn up in vain. They most likely will alert the chief laboratory scientist to some of the conditions under which the employees are working, and perhaps that information can be used to plan more efficient work methods according to the existing conditions.

Exhibit 9.1 shows sample forms and floor plans and discusses some of the intricate details you may be asked to address when planning new or expanded space.

PLANNING UTILIZATION OF MATERIALS AND SUPPLIES

The supervisor must plan for the appropriate use, security, and conservation of the materials and supplies entrusted and charged to the department. Every department has some supplies that are ideal for the household and therefore, lend themselves to pilferage. Items such as thermometers, file folders, trash bags, and even scrubs are examples of such supplies. (It is not uncommon to experience increased supply usage—specifically, for pencils, pens, and tablets—in September, which coincides with the start of school.) In most departments, the quantity of materials and supplies used is substantial. While a single item may represent only a small value, the aggregate of these items adds up to sizeable amounts in the budget of a healthcare facility. Controlling access to these items through the use of locked storage cabinets, using RFID (radio-frequency identification) tags to monitor whereabouts of small equipment (such as IV stands), periodic inventorying, and minimizing the quantity on hand help to limit loss. Not all loss is intentional, as there is "pocket loss"—supplies that leave the facility (innocently) in the pockets of lab coats or uniforms. Proper planning ensures that materials and supplies are used as conservatively as possible without compromising sterility, asepsis, and sanitary requirements. Although proper planning for the control and use of materials and supplies helps budgetary constraints, it does not prevent all waste.

PLANNING UTILIZATION OF THE WORKFORCE

The employees in a department are the most valuable resource. Therefore, planning for their full utilization must be foremost in every manager's mind.

Planning for the best utilization of the workforce also entails developing methods for recruiting good employees, enhancing employee satisfaction, searching for all available sources of qualified employees, and working for their retention. Furthermore, proper utilization means conducting an ongoing search for the best ways to group employee activities and to train, supervise, and motivate employees.

Finally, effective use of workers means the continual appraisal of their performance, appropriate promotions, adequate plans for compensation and rewards, and, at the same time, fair disciplinary measures.

All these considerations play an important role when the supervisor plans for the best utilization of the department's workforce. Only through such human resource planning can a situation be created in which workers willingly contribute their utmost to achieve both personal satisfaction on the job and the department's objectives. Employees, in turn, amply reward a supervisor who considers their personal satisfaction important. Planning for the best utilization of employees is at the heart of expert supervision.

SUMMARY

Plans must be made for the full utilization of all the resources at the supervisor's disposal. More specifically, he or she must plan for proper use of equipment and instruments, work methods, and processes. The supervisor should plan to effectively use the space available and to maintain control of materials and supplies under his or her supervision. The efficient use of time also must be planned. Most importantly, the supervisor must plan for the best overall utilization of the employees in the unit. This means, among other things, seeing that employees are able to find satisfaction in their work.

Throughout all planning, the supervisor should be concerned with the effects of these plans on other members of the organization. At times, the manager may need to resort to various tactical considerations that are helpful in getting the department's plans accepted and effectively implemented.

NOTES

1. Viewed 2/11/06: http://www.nysna.org/news/press/pr2003/112403.htm.

2. Viewed 2/11/06: http://www.massnurses.org/News/2005/04/massnurse7.htm.

3. Viewed 2/11/06: http://www1.va.gov/vasafety/page.cfm?pg=13.

4. Viewed 4/21/06: http://www.cdc.gov/niosh/pdfs/2002-101.pdf.

REFERENCES

Bureau of Labor Statistics. 1999. "Workplace Violence in Healthcare Settings." [Online report; retrieved 4/21/06.] www.lni.wa.gov/safety/topics/AtoZ/wpv/wpvhealthcare.asp.

Business and Legal Reports. 2003. "Security at Hospitals in Focus after Fatal Workplace Violence." [Online library; retrieved 4/14/03.] http://hr.blr.com/display.cfm?id=8366.

Opus Communications. 2001. "Workplace Violence Happens." Safety Update for Briefings on Hospital Safety. [Online newsletter; retrieved 02/11/06.] http://www.hcmarketplace.com.

U.S. Bureau of Labor Statistics. 2001. "Days Away from Work Highest for Carpal Tunnel Syndrome." Table 9: Selected (Sprains, Strains, Tears; Carpal Tunnel; Tendonitis) Natures by Worker and Case Characteristics. [Online report; retrieval 12/17/01.] http://www.bls.gov/opub/ted/2001/apr/wk1/art01.htm.

Exhibit 9.1: Space Planning Tools

It is said that a manager needs no desk nor for that matter an office because he or she should be observing what is happening among the staff in their work sites. Immediate feedback should occur when something is done right and observed firsthand. Managers cannot do this in an office. Often the size of an office is proportional to the rank of an individual in an organization. Office size, therefore, may help explain positions that appear on an organizational chart. However, offices do not exist in all organizations.

The chairman of Aluminum Company of America (ALCOA) moved out of his lush executive suite into a Spartan cubicle in the mid-1990s. The chairman and other executives decided they should spend their workdays in a cluster of cubicle offices that allowed them to lean over a makeshift wall to confer rather than wait for formal meetings. Changes such as these occurred at IBM, Nickelodeon, and the American Health Information Management Association (AHIMA). Open office arrangements increase communication and possibly increase production, as individuals cannot hide inside an office to read a book or have long telephone conversations. These open office arrangements are usually less expensive and provide design flexibility, as cubicles can be easily rearranged. For departments that have staff who telecommute for part of the week, open office and cubicle arrangements allow telecommuters to use available cubicles.

At some time during your career, you will be asked to work with a design specialist to lay out new or renovated workspace. To do so, it is important for you to know fundamental office design practices. A typical design worksheet appears in Exhibit A. Workspace areas typically vary by position level. Directors may have enclosed offices or cubicles with higher walls to provide additional privacy for meetings and conversations. Their space may be 155 square feet to 175 square feet and include a desk, credenza, bookcase, and round meeting table. Managers may be assigned space that ranges from 110 to 144 square feet. The larger work area allows space for a small round conference table for the manager and two or three staff members to meet spontaneously in the manager's office (Exhibit B). Supervisory positions may have space allocations, ranging from 64 to 100 square feet. Typically, this area includes sufficient desk and filing space for the supervisor and an extra chair for a staff member or visitor (Exhibit B). Staff members who require desk space, such as data analysts, transcriptionists, billing and collections staff, and dietitians may be allocated 40 to 90 square feet (Exhibit B).

Some areas require extensive filing space, such as radiology, information systems tape library, pharmacy, and medical staff library. In these areas, the manager needs to determine whether stationary open shelving or moveable shelving (Exhibit C) meet their needs. Using moveable, condensed filing systems may reduce the floor space requirement by as much as 50 percent. To use this type of filing system one must consider (1) whether the weight-bearing load of the floor accommodates the weight of condensed shelving, (2) the number of access aisles required, and (3) reasonable reaching height. When selecting shelving units, the items to be stored on the shelves must be measured. Patient records require a 9" to 10" opening (height) between shelves. Depth of shelving also is a factor:

Farnsworth GROUP
ENGINEERS
ARCHITECTS
SURVEYORS
SCIENTISTS

DESIGN CRITERIA WORKSHEET

Date: _____

Project: _____

Project No.: _____

Department:	Room Name:	Room No.

General Requirements:

A. Floor:
- ☐ Vinyl Composition Tile
- ☐ Rubber Tile
- ☐ Sheet Vinyl
- ☐ Sheet Tile
- ☐ Seamless Flooring
- ☐ Ceramic Tile
- ☐ Quarry Tile
- ☐ Terrazzo
- ☐ Carpet Tile
- ☐ Carpet Broadloom
- ☐ Unfinished
- ☐ Sealed
- ☐ Conductive
- ☐ Patch
- ☐ Existing
- ☐ _____
- ☐ _____
- ☐ _____
- ☐ _____
- ☐ _____

B. Walls:

N	S	E	W	
☐	☐	☐	☐	Plaster
☐	☐	☐	☐	Cement Plaster
☐	☐	☐	☐	Gypsum Board
☐	☐	☐	☐	Concrete Block
☐	☐	☐	☐	Brick
☐	☐	☐	☐	Paint
☐	☐	☐	☐	Vinyl Wallcovering
☐	☐	☐	☐	Epoxy Coating
☐	☐	☐	☐	Ceramic Tile
☐	☐	☐	☐	Structural Glazed Tile
☐	☐	☐	☐	Unfinished
☐	☐	☐	☐	Borrow Lite
☐	☐	☐	☐	Folding Partition
☐	☐	☐	☐	Demountable Partition
☐	☐	☐	☐	Patch
☐	☐	☐	☐	Existing
☐	☐	☐	☐	Fire Rated
☐	☐	☐	☐	Sound Wall
☐	☐	☐	☐	_____
☐	☐	☐	☐	

E. Doors:
- ☐ Width
- ☐ Operation
- ☐ Label
- ☐ Solid
- ☐ Hollow
- ☐ Vision Panel
- ☐ _____
- ☐ _____

F. Casework:
- ☐ Steel
- ☐ Plastic Laminate
- ☐ Wood
- ☐ Corrosion Resistant Top
- ☐ Plastic Laminate Top
- ☐ Solid Surface Top
- ☐ Stainless Steel Top
- ☐ _____
- ☐ _____

C. Base:
- ☐ Vinyl
- ☐ Rubber
- ☐ Ceramic Tile
- ☐ Quarry Tile
- ☐ Terrazzo
- ☐ Structural Glazed Tile
- ☐ Seamless Integral
- ☐ Patch
- ☐ Existing
- ☐ Wood
- ☐ _____
- ☐ _____
- ☐ _____
- ☐ _____

D. Ceiling:
- ☐ Acoustical
  - ☐ Lay-in
  - ☐ Concealed
  - ☐ Adhesive
- ☐ Plaster
- ☐ Cement Plaster
- ☐ Gypsum Board
- ☐ Unfinished
- ☐ Existing
- ☐ Patch
- ☐ Paint
- ☐ Fire Rated
- ☐ _____
- ☐ _____

G. Special Construction
- ☐ Prefabricated Construction
- ☐ X-ray Shielding
- ☐ R-F Shielding
- ☐ Neg./Pos. Pressure Room
- ☐ Isolation Room
- ☐ ICU Doors
- ☐ _____
- ☐ _____
- ☐ _____
- ☐ _____
- ☐ _____
- ☐ _____
- ☐ _____

H. Notes and Comments:

_____

_____

_____

_____

_____

_____

_____

_____

_____

_____

_____

_____

_____

_____

_____

_____

(continued on following page)

Farnsworth GROUP
ENGINEERS
ARCHITECTS
SURVEYORS
SCIENTISTS

DESIGN CRITERIA WORKSHEET

Electrical Systems:	Mechanical Systems:

Electrical Systems:

A. Utilities and Services:
- ☐ 110V duplex Outlets
- ☐ 220V duplex Outlets
- ☐ Wire Mould
- ☐ X-ray Outlet
- ☐ Special Outlet
- ☐ 110V Emergency Power
- ☐ 220V Emergency Power

B. Lighting:
- ☐ Fluorescent
- ☐ Compact Fluorescent
- ☐ Incandescent
- ☐ Halogen
- ☐ Mercury Vapor/Halide
- ☐ Emergency Lighting
- ☐ Surgical Lighting
- ☐ Dimmable
- ☐ Ballast
- ☐ _____
- ☐ _____

C. Communications:

Rough-in
  Wiring
    Equipment
      Special Outlet

☐	☐	☐	☐	Telephone
☐	☐	☐	☐	Intercom
☐	☐	☐	☐	Public Address
☐	☐	☐	☐	Paging
☐	☐	☐	☐	Music
☐	☐	☐	☐	Nurse Call
☐	☐	☐	☐	Central Dictation
☐	☐	☐	☐	Physiological Monitoring
☐	☐	☐	☐	Charting
☐	☐	☐	☐	CCTV
☐	☐	☐	☐	Cable TV
☐	☐	☐	☐	Data Processing
☐	☐	☐	☐	Internet
☐	☐	☐	☐	Emtek
☐	☐	☐	☐	_____
☐	☐	☐	☐	_____

D. Notes and Comments:

_____
_____
_____
_____
_____
_____
_____
_____
_____
_____
_____
_____
_____
_____
_____
_____

Mechanical Systems:

A. HVAC:
- ☐ Air Conditioned
- ☐ Special Environment
- ☐ Temperature
- ☐ Humidity
- ☐ 100% Exhaust
- ☐ _____
- ☐ _____

B. Utility and Services:
- ☐ Hot Water
- ☐ Cold Water
- ☐ Deionized Water
- ☐ Chilled Water
- ☐ Natural Gas
- ☐ Steam
- ☐ Sprinklers

C. Medical Gases:

Wall
  Ceiling
    Column

☐	☐	☐	Air
☐	☐	☐	Oxygen
☐	☐	☐	Vacuum
☐	☐	☐	Nitrogen
☐	☐	☐	Nitrous Oxide

D. Plumbing:

Handicapped
  Conventional
    Knee
      Foot
        Wrist Blade
          Goose Neck
            Divertor Valve
              Aerator Valve
                Vacuum Breaker
                  Hose Spray

☐	☐	☐	☐	☐	☐	☐	☐	Lavatory
☐	☐	☐	☐	☐	☐	☐	☐	Counter Sink
☐	☐	☐	☐	☐	☐	☐	☐	Scrub Sink
☐	☐	☐	☐	☐	☐	☐	☐	Clinic Sink (Flushing Room)
☐	☐	☐	☐	☐	☐	☐	☐	Mop Receptor
☐	☐	☐	☐	☐	☐	☐	☐	Water Closet
☐	☐	☐	☐	☐	☐	☐	☐	Urinal
☐	☐	☐	☐	☐	☐	☐	☐	Shower
☐	☐	☐	☐	☐	☐	☐	☐	Floor Drain
☐	☐	☐	☐	☐	☐	☐	☐	Drinking Fountain
☐	☐	☐	☐	☐	☐	☐	☐	Cup Sink
☐	☐	☐	☐	☐	☐	☐	☐	Tub
☐	☐	☐	☐	☐	☐	☐	☐	Emergency Eyewash
☐	☐	☐	☐	☐	☐	☐	☐	Emergency Shower

E. Notes and Comments:

_____
_____
_____
_____

Source: Courtesy of Farnsworth Group, Inc., St. Louis, MO.

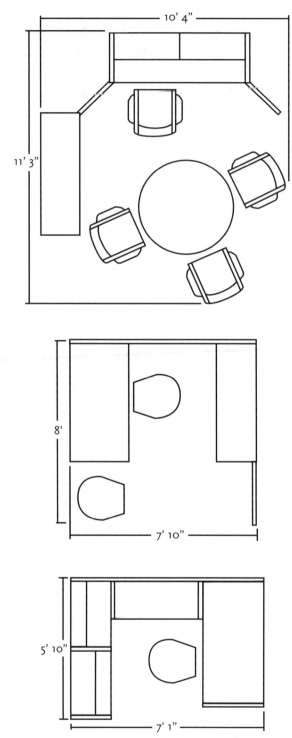

Exhibit C

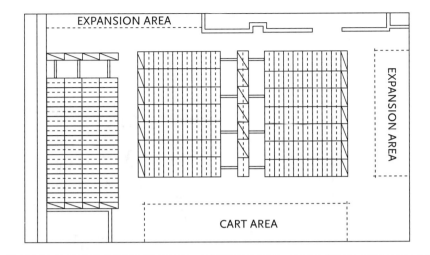

EXPANSION AREA

EXPANSION AREA

CART AREA

Exhibit D

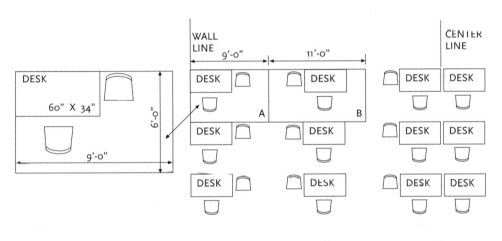

WALL LINE

CENTER LINE

9'-0"   11'-0"

DESK

60" X 34"

6'-0"

9'-0"

DESK | DESK | DESK | DESK

A   B

DESK | DESK | DESK | DESK

DESK | DESK | DESK | DESK

WORK STATION 3-A - 54 SQ. FT.
            3-B - 66 SQ. FT.

books may require 10"; radiology films may require 18". When using moveable shelving, ensure the shelves are deep enough for the item to be pushed in all the way on the shelf. If it sticks out, it may trigger a safety switch that does not allow the shelving units to move. Shelves typically have widths of 36", 42", and 48". Other filing options are vertical and lateral files. A typical five-drawer vertical file cabinet provides 125 linear inches of file space and consumes 6 square feet of floor space. Lateral file cabinets that are 36" wide provide

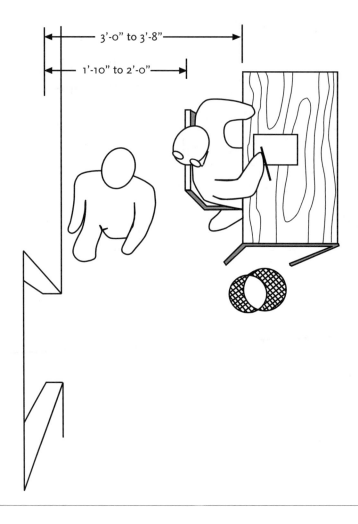

204 linear inches of filing space and consume 3 square feet of floor space. Generally, lateral file cabinets are more expensive than vertical file cabinets.

Aisles between desks should be no less than 24" to 26" (Exhibit E). The same holds true for work areas that have file cabinets (Exhibit F).

This overview emphasizes the value of utilizing space planners from the organization's construction and design department or from a local architect to ensure that you do not shortchange your needs. These professionals also are able to suggest alternative arrangements and space-saving features such as overhead storage units, worklights, and hanging storage pedestals that help your staff work more efficiently.

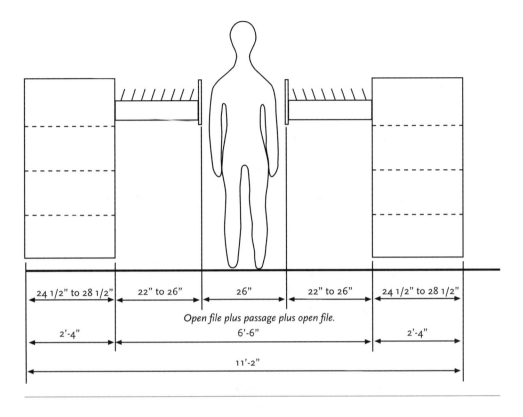

24 1/2" to 28 1/2"	22" to 26"	26"	22" to 26"	24 1/2" to 28 1/2"

Open file plus passage plus open file.

2'-4"	6'-6"	2'-4"

11'-2"

CHAPTER TEN

Planning Tools

CHAPTER OBJECTIVES

After you have studied this chapter, you should be able to do the following:

1. Describe the types of and distinguish between standing plans, repeat-use plans, and single-use plans.

2. Discuss the various types of standing plans and their effect on managerial decision making.

3. Differentiate policies from procedures, procedures from methods, and policies from rules.

4. Discuss the value of organizational manuals.

O NCE THE ENTITYWIDE goals are established and the objectives are determined, managers must design numerous plans necessary to achieve fulfillment of the goals. Several different types of plans are devised to implement objectives: policies, procedures, methods, rules, programs, projects, and budgets. All these plans must be designed to reinforce one another; that is, they must be internally consistent, integrated, and coordinated. Because every manager probably has to devise or at least use each type of plan at some time, he or she should be familiar with the meaning of all of them. The major plans are formulated by top administration, but department supervisors have to formulate their own departmental plans accordingly. The purpose of all these plans is to ensure that the thinking and actions taken on different levels and in different departments of the institution are consistent with and contribute to the overall objectives.

These different types of plans can be divided into two major groups: repeat-use plans and single-use plans. Policies, procedures, methods, and rules are commonly known as repeat-use or standing plans. They are used for problems that occur regularly. *Repeat-use plans* are applicable whenever a problem situation presents itself that is similar to the one for which the standing plan was originally devised. *Single-use plans* are used for nonrecurring situations. These plans are no longer needed once their objective is accomplished. Within this single-use plan category are programs, projects, and budgets.

POLICIES

Policies are probably the most important and frequently invoked repeat-use plans among the various plans a manager must depend on. Generally, they are issued and set by the top management of the organization. Policies provide managers with a general guideline for decision making, such as "all staff should wear clothing that is appropriate for a business environment and for meeting with the public." They are general statements that channel the thinking of all personnel charged with decision making. Because they are broad, policies do not have definite limitations and boundaries. Policies reflect constraints, and as long as a supervisor stays within these limitations, he or she will make an appropriate decision—one that conforms to the policy.

In this way, policies facilitate the job of both managers and subordinates. They ensure uniformity of decision making throughout the organization. Policies are standing plans that express the organization's general response to a problem or situation. Thus, top management directs decisions toward the achievement of the organizational goals, expressing values and ideas it deems important. Policies help to coordinate activities, and as the organization grows larger and more complex, the need for policies increases.

Policies as an Aid in Delegation

Policies cover the various areas of the organization's activities: some relate to the managerial functions (e.g., a promotion-from-within policy), others relate to operational functions (e.g., patient care policies, public relations, marketing), and still others cover the safety and health of the employees. By issuing these policies, top-level administration sanctions or supports in advance the decisions made by subordinate managers, as long as they stay within the broad policy guidelines. After having set policies, a higher-level manager should feel reasonably confident that whatever decisions subordinates make fall within policy limits. In fact, subordinates probably come up with decisions comparable to those the manager would have made. Thus, policies make it easier for the higher-level manager to delegate authority to subordinates.

Policies are a great help to the subordinate managers as well. They provide guidelines that help subordinates make decisions and at the same time ensure uniformity of decisions throughout the enterprise. Therefore, the clearer and more comprehensive the policy guidelines are, the easier and more effective they are for the higher-level managers to delegate authority and for the subordinate managers to exercise authority.

The Origin of Policies

Policies are determined by management, particularly by the higher administrative levels. Formulating policies is one of the most important functions of top-level management. These managers are in the best position to establish the various types of policies that help achieve the enterprise's objectives. Once the corporate policies have been set by the top-level administrator, they in turn become the guidelines for various policies covering divisions and departments, such as patient care policies. Such divisional and departmental policies are created or developed by the various managers lower in the managerial hierarchy. This type of policy formulation, originated at the top administrative level and pursued by the lower managerial levels, is the most important source of policies.

Occasionally, however, a supervisor may have a problem situation not covered by an existing policy. Here the supervisor has two choices: (1) confer with the boss or human resources to determine if any existing policies may be applicable or (2) jointly agree on the appropriate action until a policy is issued to cover such situations if it is likely that the current problem will recur.

For instance, suppose that one of your employees asks for a leave of absence to care for a neighbor. To make the appropriate decision, you would prefer to be guided by policy so that your decision is in accordance with all other decisions regarding leaves of absence. You may find, however, that the administrative and FMLA (Family Medical Leave Act) policies do not apply to this situation and therefore you are in a quandary on granting or denying the leave of absence. Instead of making an ad hoc decision (a decision that pertains to this case only), you ask your department's human resources liaison to issue a policy, which you can refer to whenever leaves of absence for similar reasons are requested in the future. You probably do not have to make such a request very often because a good administrator and his or her human resources advisor usually foresee most of the areas in which policies are needed. On occasion, however, you may have to appeal to your own boss, stimulating the formulation of what is known as an *appealed policy*.

In addition to originated and appealed policies, some policies are externally imposed on an organization by outside factors such as the government, accrediting agencies, trade unions, and trade associations. The word "imposed" indicates having to comply with compulsory rules. For instance, to be accredited, hospitals and other healthcare facilities must comply with certain regulations issued by the accrediting agency—JCAHO. These regulations must be translated into institutional policy, and all employees must abide by them.

JCAHO requires hospitals to have formal written policies on patient care matters. Another body that imposes policies externally is the EEOC. Unless the healthcare center was an equal opportunity employer before federal and state fair employment codes were legislated, such a policy statement can be regarded as one that was externally imposed on the institution.

Clarity of Policies

Because policies are such a vital guide for thinking and thus for decision making, it is essential that they be stated simply and clearly. Policies must be communicated so that those in the organization who are to apply them understand their meaning. This is no easy task. It is difficult to find words that can be understood by all people in the same way because different meanings can be attached to the same word. Although there is no guarantee that even the written word can be properly understood, still it seems more desirable to put all policies in writing. This at least will prevent the added ambiguity of trying to remember someone's spoken words. An example of policy that guides vital thinking is a "Code Policy," which is common to many healthcare organizations (see Figure 10.1).

In addition to better comprehension, other benefits are derived from written policies:

1. The process of writing policies requires the top-level administrator to think them out clearly and consistently.
2. Written policies are easily accessible; the subordinate managers can read them as often as they wish.
3. The wording of a written policy cannot be changed by word of mouth because it can always be consulted.
4. Written policies are especially helpful for new managers who need immediate help in solving a problem.
5. Written policies can be made available electronically on the organization's intranet to enhance access by all staff.

Although these advantages are significant, one disadvantage is connected with written policies. Once policies are in writing, management may be reluctant to change them. Thus, some enterprises prefer to have their policies communicated by word of mouth because they believe that this is more flexible, allowing the verbal policies to be adjusted to different circumstances with greater ease than is possible with written policies. The exact meaning of a verbal policy may become scrambled, however, making it difficult to apply the policy properly. For this reason, written policy statements are generally considered far more desirable and necessary.

The Flexibility of Policies

Although policies must be consistent to successfully coordinate the activities of each day, they must also be flexible. Some policies even explicitly state this flexibility using such words as "whenever possible," "whenever feasible," or "under usual circumstances." For instance, one of the most widely practiced policies today is, "Our enterprise believes in and practices promotion from within whenever possible." If these qualifying clauses are built in, the manner in which the supervisor applies the policy determines its degree of flexibility. The supervisor must intelligently adapt the policy to the existing set of circumstances. Such flexibility, however, must not lead to inconsistency; policies must be administered by supervisors with regularity and continuity.

The Supervisor and Policies

Although supervisors seldom have to issue policies, they must frequently use them. Supervisors primarily apply existing policies in making their daily decisions, but they must also interpret and explain the meaning of policies to employees of their departments. Therefore, it is essential that they clearly understand the policies and learn how to apply them appropriately.

A manager who heads a major department, such as the director of patient care services, or a department that normally comprises half of the institution's employees and has many subdivisions within it may find it necessary to issue and write policies for the department. In fact, JCAHO examines such patient care policies for compliance with its regulations. All of them must reinforce and be in accordance with the overall policies of the healthcare organization. Included among these policies probably is a patient care policy stating that the welfare of the patient is the foremost concern of the patient care service and that it takes precedence over all other considerations. In all likelihood, the institution's overall policy of fairness and nondiscrimination also shows up in a patient care policy. The policy may state that patients shall be accorded impartial access to treatments or accommodations to the extent that these are available and medically indicated, regardless of the patient's race, color, creed, or national origin. The policy also may state that the patient's right to privacy shall be respected, consistent with medical needs, and so forth.

Periodic Review of Policies

Changes in the healthcare environment, accompanied by changes in an institution's own goals, require older policies to be periodically reviewed, revised, or removed, regardless of how well-thought-out the policies were when originated. Such a review may uncover policies that contradict other policies or policies that have become so outdated that no one follows them. In such cases, top-level administration must either rewrite or abandon the questionable policies because an institution certainly cannot afford to let its various subordinate managers decide which policies are still current or whether they should still be observed.

PROCEDURES

Procedures are repeat-use plans for achieving the institution's objectives. They are derived from policies, but are much more specific. Procedures are guides to action, not guides to thinking. Procedures specify a set of actions to be followed step by step. They outline a chronological order for the acts that are to be performed. In brief, procedures prescribe a path toward the objectives; they describe in detail how a recurring activity is to be performed and are commonly used in the daily operations. For example, recall the policy that stated, "Our institution promotes from within whenever possible." The purpose and objectives of this policy are clear. The procedure designs the steps to be taken in

FIGURE 10.1: CODE ORDER POLICY STATEMENT

BARNES-JEWISH HOSPITAL
Nursing Policy and Procedure

Document: <u>C15</u>
Reviewed: <u>7/99</u>
Revised: <u>2/00</u>

CODE 7

I. POLICY

    A. Upon recognition of an unconscious patient, visitor or staff member, the first responder must call for help to ensure immediate overhead code is called and delivery of the nearest defibrillator and crash cart.

    B. Any BLS (Basic Life Support) trained employee can initiate CPR. It is of utmost importance that the first BLS responder begin CPR immediately and that delays in CPR till code team arrival are unacceptable. RN's, LPN's, PCT's are to be BLS certified every two years utilizing the American Heart Association/Red Cross course.

    C. Cardiopulmonary resuscitation must be initiated on all patients unless there is a written order not to resuscitate.

    D. Designated BLS instructors for each area are responsible for providing BLS classes each year for on-going staff certification.

    E. Each RN, LPN and PCT is responsible for maintaining a current BLS certification.

    F. Nurse managers or their designees are responsible for maintaining records of the employees' BLS certification and to provide a method to keep staff familiar with the crash cart contents.

    G. For patient safety, transport of the post-arrest patient from north to south campus of BJH must be minimized. Communications between the nursing supervisor or code team member and the ICU attending MD or charge nurse must first be made to acquire an ICU bed on the north campus for that patient (i.e., lowest acuity patient moved out to allow for post-arrest patient's ICU admission). In the event that all north campus ICU beds are completely filled with high acuity patients, transport via the link to the south campus must be arranged via the nursing supervisor. The transport of any post-arrest patient to an ICU, either between campuses or intra-hospital, must include the following: A physician and nurse familiar with the patient must physically stay with that patient until the patient is transported to an ICU and report of events is given to the accepting physician and nurse. Other personnel needed for transport may include dispatch (2-3), RT's, other RN's or physicians.

Source: Courtesy of Barnes-Jewish Hospital, St. Louis, MO.

a chronological sequence to fulfill the meaning of the policy. These steps might be stated as follows:

1. Every opening in the institution must be posted on the employees' bulletin board in the employees' cafeteria for two weeks.
2. The potential candidates should obtain a job description from the manager in whose department the job is open.
3. Potential candidates must inform their present boss before arranging for an interview.
4. An interview between the applicant and the manager in the department with the opening will be arranged with the assistance of the human resources department.

There are literally hundreds, if not thousands, of procedures in a healthcare center. Just think of the number in nursing services alone, such as the procedures for administering medications, turning techniques, examining critically ill patients, initiating protocols without a physician order, and discharging patients.

Although supervisors do not have much opportunity to issue policies, they have many opportunities for devising and issuing procedures. Because supervisors are the managers of the department, they determine how the work is to be done. The difficulty is that many supervisors work under considerable pressure and find little time for this type of planning. Moreover, the supervisor is often so close to the jobs performed in the department that he or she believes the prevailing work methods are satisfactory and that not much can be done about them. The level of detail in written procedures may differ, depending on the skill, educational level, or both of the staff. As educational levels increase, more freedom to act based on tested and demonstrated experience is permitted.

Some employees already have been thoroughly trained in standard practices and procedures before being hired for the position. For example, nurses, therapists, radiology technologists, laboratory technicians, and database administrators receive many years of schooling and training, during which great emphasis is placed on the proper procedures and methods for performing certain tasks. In managing a department in which such highly skilled employees are at work, the supervisor's job is simplified. One of the main concerns is to ensure that good, generally approved procedures and methods are performed in a professionally accepted way.

However, even with that training, most healthcare institutions "do things differently from everyone else." Even after many years of good schooling and experience in other healthcare settings, new employees have to become familiar with the procedures, methods, and idiosyncrasies of the new facilities. This is the reason each healthcare organization requires employees and others to participate in new employee orientation, which may take several days to complete. In addition to a facilitywide organization, often the department that the employee is joining provides an orientation to the department-specific policies, procedures, schedules, and job-related activities. Therefore, new employees probably go through an orientation program that lasts for many weeks to familiarize them with the procedures and methods of the institution and the department. This is often done by matching them with a coworker who can serve as a mentor and resource in the early weeks and months.

Effective work procedures designed by the supervisors for the institution result in definite advantages. One of these is that the process of preparing a procedure requires analyzing the work to be done. To maintain a high level of efficiency and the best possible patient care, occasionally the supervisor must study the operations performed to be able to plan improvements. If the department begins doing something new, the supervisor has to write a complete set of new procedures and methods for this new activity. For example, if the hospital staff begins using new laser techniques, the manager of that unit has to develop new procedures for this operation. The manager does so with the help, information, and support of medical specialists, technologists, and possibly the manufacturer of the equipment.

Moreover, once a supervisor establishes a procedure, its existence helps ensure consistent and uniform action and a predictable outcome. In addition to these benefits, procedures provide the supervisor with a standard for appraising the work of the employees. Because a procedure specifies the sequence of actions, it also decreases the need for further decision making. This makes the supervisor's job, as well as that of the employees, easier. The supervisor is also more likely to assign work fairly and to distribute it evenly among the employees.

A good supervisor spends considerable time and effort in devising efficient procedures for the department. From time to time, of course, the supervisor needs to review and revise departmental procedures because some are likely to become outdated. The supervisor should try to look at all of the department's operations from the point of view of a newcomer. In other words, he or she should look at the current operations objectively. The supervisor should ask the following questions: Is each operation really necessary? What is the reason for it? Could the procedure be combined with another operation? Are the various steps necessary? Are they performed in the best possible sequence? Are there any avoidable delays? The supervisor should also seek ideas from employees who are doing the job because they often can make valuable suggestions for improved methods and procedures. The use of employee teams can also be very useful in developing new procedures and identifying external barriers to performing their jobs effectively. These barriers may require the supervisor to work with peer supervisors outside of his or her department to improve the flow of work inside.

METHODS

A *method* also is a standing plan for action, but it is even more detailed than a procedure. A method may also be called a practice. Whereas a procedure shows a series of steps to be taken, a method is concerned only with a single operation, or with one particular step. The method tells exactly how this particular step is to be performed. For instance, one typical patient care procedure guides nurses step by step in how to account for controlled substances at the beginning of each shift by both the nurse going on duty and the nurse going off duty. For each step in this procedure, there exists a method. For example, one method explains exactly what is to be done in case of unavoidable spilling or accidental destruction of narcotics: the nurse involved must record what happened; the remnants are to be returned to the pharmacy, if possible, or discarded altogether; and another professional nurse must verify the spill and witness the report form.

For most work done by the employees of a department, there exists a "best method"—that is, a best way for doing the job, and it is the supervisor's responsibility to specify to employees what that is. Indeed, a large amount of the supervisor's time is spent in devising methods. Once a method has been devised, it carries with it all the advantages of a procedure already stated such as uniformity of action, predictability of outcome, and standard for appraisal.

Using established methods, supervisors also may be asked to establish productivity standards for their staff. Doing so takes time, because production history, methods of improving production, equipment used, and industry norms must be assessed. Supervisors must be able to define not only the quantity expected but also the quality of the activities expected. The definitions form the framework within which management establishes the standards of performance. Once the standards are established, a simple and timely reporting mechanism must be developed as a control system. (Control is discussed in chapters 27 through 29.) It is outside the realm of this book to discuss in depth the various techniques to gauge production and establish productivity standards. Supervisors are encouraged to obtain more information on these techniques before embarking on a program of establishing standards.

In determining the best method as well as establishing standards, a supervisor may occasionally need to enlist the help of another professional such as a physician, human resources specialist, or a management engineer (a specialist in motion and time study), if such a person is available in the organization. Most often, however, the supervisor's own experience and the input of his or her team members are probably broad enough to allow him or her to design the best work methods.

RULES

A *rule*, probably the most explicit kind of a standing plan, is a statement that either forbids or requires a certain action or inaction without variation. A rule does not provide a guide to thinking; it does not leave any discretion to the party involved. A rule is related to a procedure insofar as it is a guide to action and states what must or must not be done. A rule, however, is not the same as a procedure because it does not specify a time sequence for the particular action.

Rules pertain whenever and wherever they are in effect. A no-smoking rule, for instance, is one issued by management and is probably just one of a long list of safety rules. This rule is a guide to action, or more precisely a guide to inaction. No order of steps is involved, however; it simply requires "no smoking" wherever and whenever it is in effect.

Rules develop from policy; they are not part of it. For example, the institution's safety policy is to make the facility a safe place for the patients, employees, and visitors. Safety considerations play an important role in all procedures and methods, and the no-smoking rule is just an outgrowth of the original safety policy. The same applies to the rule issued by the supervisor of the clinical laboratories that all employees are to wear gloves and impervious gowns at all times.

It is the supervisor's duty to apply and enforce the rules and regulations of the healthcare institution uniformly, whether they are defined by higher management or set by the supervisor. There are many occasions when supervisors have to set their own departmental rules. For example, the dress code may state that employees must come to work "appropriately attired" for their job. This general rule gives each director the right to devise a more detailed dress code to meet the needs of the department, including requiring uniforms for the food service and security staffs. The pediatric patient care manager may have a more lax dress code to allow staff to wear costumes and other paraphernalia to raise the spirits of their young patients. Because supervisors have the obligation to see that rules are observed, they should be involved in the formation of these rules. Again, these rules are developed from overall organizational policies and must reinforce and support them.

WORK SIMPLIFICATION

This chapter points out that the supervisor is deeply involved in designing, developing, and writing procedures and methods. The supervisor should continually review and, if necessary, revise procedures and make plans concerning improved work methods and processes in the department.

Much has been written on *work simplification* or methods improvement, which is "an organized approach to determine how to accomplish a task with less effort in less time or at a lower cost while maintaining or improving the quality of the outcome" (Abdelhak et al. 1996). The efforts of the Gilbreths, discussed in Chapter 2, focused on methods improvement. Ben B. Graham (2001) offers a summary of work simplification in Exhibit 10.1.

According to Abdelhak and colleagues (1996), "The fundamental objectives of work simplification are (1) simplify, (2) eliminate, (3) combine, and (4) improve." For more information on work simplification process charts, the reader is encouraged to review the recommended readings noted in Ben Graham's article (see Reference list at the end of this chapter). Additionally, we explore this process and other approaches that focus on process improvement in Part VII.

ORGANIZATIONAL MANUALS

The *organizational manual* is another helpful tool for communicating the organization's practices effectively. It provides in comprehensive written form the decisions that have been made with regard to the institution's structure. It defines the institution's major policies and objectives, contains organizational charts of the institution and of specific departments (see Chapter 13), and provides job descriptions. Moreover, the organizational manual is a readily available reference defining the scopes of authority, responsibilities of managerial positions, and channels to be used in obtaining decisions or approval of proposals.

One of the chief advantages of a manual is the analysis and thinking necessary before it can be written. Another advantage is that the manual is also of great assistance in the indoctrination and development of managerial personnel. The manual should clearly specify for each manager what the responsibilities of the job are and how they are related to other positions within the organization. In addition, it reiterates for the individual manager the objectives of the enterprise and of the department, and it provides a means of explaining the complex relationships within the organization. Supervisors should familiarize themselves with the contents of the institution's manual, especially those parts affecting their own department. Often, managers create department manuals to serve as communication tools for their staff.

Organizational manuals are valuable tools only if they are up-to-date. Because the manual is in written form, it is more difficult to change. Unless manuals are kept current and incorporate changes, they are more of a hindrance than a valuable aid. As stated before, another difficulty with a manual is the initial effort it takes to compile one.

Content

Although the content of both the organizational and departmental manuals varies from one healthcare institution to another, almost all include statements of goals and objectives, overall policies, department procedures, job descriptions, organizational charts of the institution and specific departments, and possibly an explanation of titles.

Objectives and Policies

In the organization manual, top-level management states the major objectives and goals of the institution. For a hospital the manual would state the institution's mission, vision, values, and broad policies in regard to code of conduct and ethics, compliance, patient care, the quality of medicine practiced, social responsibility, and other areas that cross over many departments. The manual would mention, for example, the organizational objectives concerning the education of medical and other professionals, investigative studies, and possibly care of the indigent. It may state an objective, "to be alert and responsive to the changing needs of the community and the environment." The manual should be comprehensive enough to guide departmental managers on overall organizational issues and is often supplemented with a departmental manual that includes more detailed policies and procedures.

PROGRAMS AND PROJECTS

A *program* is a single-use plan with a complex set of activities to reach a specific major objective. The program may have its own guidelines, such as policies, procedures, and budgets, and may extend over several years. For instance, building a new extended care facility within a healthcare system is a major one-time undertaking. Such a program involves many derivative plans, each of which can be considered a project. Such plans would include selecting the architects and contractors for the new construction, arranging public information for the local community, providing information for the local medical society, and recruiting the needed personnel. Arranging the financing itself is a project. At the department level the program may be designing the new laundry department for the extended care facility. One project for the laundry department includes evaluating and selecting new laundry equipment. The laundry manager is also expected to develop a staffing plan and budget for the new department.

A project, therefore, is similar to a program but is smaller in scope. It is an undertaking that can be planned and executed as a distinct entity within the overall program; all projects must be coordinated and synchronized so that the major program can become a reality. Programs and projects are single-use plans; once they are achieved, they are filed away. Planning a program is usually a concern for top-level administration, whereas department heads and supervisors are often involved in one of its many projects. It is also possible for a project to be initiated without a connection to a major program.

For instance, assume the new extended care facility is located in a rather affluent community and the economy is such that unemployment in the area is extremely low. As such, it may be difficult to recruit laundry workers. Therefore, the manager may need to work with the human resources department to develop both a transportation plan and compensation structure that attract individuals to commute to this community to do the job. As such, it is not the program—the extended care facility—that caused the shortage of staff, but rather the combination of the location of the facility and the economy.

Some projects may be quite complex. To manage these endeavors, the project manager may use Gantt or PERT charts.

The *Gantt chart* was introduced by Henry Gantt (see Chapter 2). The project is displayed as a bar chart that shows the planned and actual activities. Once the manager decides which activities need to happen and the amount of time that is allotted to each of them, the manager plots them on the chart. The chart becomes a control device that allows managers to see when activities are falling behind and/or taking more time than anticipated to accomplish. This type of planning tool is useful when there are a few activities to manage and when

FIGURE 10.2 GANTT CHART EXAMPLE

Activity	Month 1						Month 2				Month 3		
Revise policy manual	███	██	██	██	██								
Obtain executive approval							██						
Make revisions requested								██	██				
Obtain final executive approval										██			
Print sufficient quantity for department heads											██		
Distribute													██

PERT CHART EXAMPLE

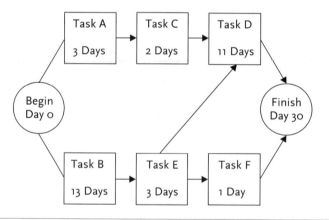

they are independent of each other. Figure 10.2 provides an example of a Gantt chart.

PERT is a planning tool developed by the U.S. Department of Defense, originally used to ensure that complex military projects remained on schedule. In its sophisticated form, PERT uses probabilities and three time estimates for each task involved in the project. PERT is an effective tool for scheduling complex projects and when activities are dependent on one another. The visual display allows the manager to compare what effect alternative actions have on the completion of the project or subset of activities. The steps involved in PERT planning are (1) identify each task involved in the project; (2) estimate the time required to complete each task; (3) determine the relationships among tasks— which must occur first, second; which is dependent on another; and which ones may occur simultaneously with or independently from others; and (4) determine when the project must be completed. Once these factors are known, a graphical representation or chart is drawn depicting one or more paths for the various tasks, linking those tasks dependent on one another's completion before the next task can occur. The time estimates are entered along the linking lines between tasks. The cumulative times for a given path represents the total time required to complete that path. If the cumulative time exceeds the "due date" for the project's completion, the project will be delayed. PERT helps managers to identify when resources have to be shifted to keep on schedule.

In the above PERT diagram, Task C is dependent on Task A. Task D is dependent on Task C and Task E. Task E is dependent on Task B. Therefore, before Task D can begin, 16 days will elapse (Task B + Task E). Tasks A and C will have been completed before Task B is completed. Because Task D requires 11 days, the project should be completed within the 30-day timetable required.

BUDGETS

Budgets are usually thought of only in connection with the controlling function, but this is too narrow a view. In this context, we look at budgets as plans that express the anticipated activities and results in numerical terms. Such terms may be dollars and cents. However, most items start out in other measurable terms such as nursing hours, hours per patient day, or kilowatt hours; tests to be run; output; materials; computer time; inventory levels; or any other unit used to perform work or to measure specific results. Because the overall budgets for the entire institution are ultimately expressed in the one common denominator of dollars and cents, and because most values are convertible to monetary terms, all budgets are eventually translated and expressed in monetary terms. Although budgets are an important tool for controlling, developing a budget is also part of the planning function. As we know, planning is the duty of every manager. Using the budget and working within it is part of the manager's controlling function, which is in Chapter 29.

Because a budget is a plan expressed in numerical units, it has the distinct advantage of being stated in exact and specific terms instead of in generalities. The figures put into a budget represent actual plans that are seen as goals and standards to be achieved. These plans are not mere projections or general forecasts; they are considered a basis for daily operations, cost effectiveness, and the bottom line. They are guidelines about the institution's expectations.

Because budgets are so important for the daily operations of every department, supervisors who have to use them should participate in their preparation. It is only natural that people resent arbitrary orders, and this applies to having to abide by budgets they see as arbitrary. Thus, it is necessary that all budget objectives and allowances be determined with the full input of those who are responsible for executing them. All supervisors should actively participate in the budget-making process for their units, and this should not be mere "pseudo-participation." They should participate in what is commonly known as "grassroots budgeting," and supervisors also should be allowed to submit their own budgets.

Each supervisor has to substantiate the budget proposals in a discussion with the boss and possibly with top-level administration, where the budgets are finalized. This is what is meant by active participation in budget making, and it ensures the effectiveness of the process. Such participation, however, should not be construed to mean that the suggestion of the supervisor will prevail. The supervisor's budget should not be accepted if the higher-level manager believes it is based on plans that are inadequate, overstated, or incorrect.

Differences among budget estimates should be carefully discussed by the supervisor and higher-level manager, but the final decision rests with higher management. Nevertheless, if a budget is arrived at with the participation of the supervisors, the likelihood that the supervisors will live up to it is higher than if the budget had been simply handed down to the supervisors by their boss.

In conclusion, it is important to remember that the budget is a single-use plan. When the period is over, the budget is no longer valid. A new budget will have to be drawn up, and a new planning period will have to be established.

SUMMARY

To reach all the objectives, different types of plans must be devised. The broad range of plans can be grouped into repeat-use and single-use plans. The first group is designed for a course of action that is likely to be repeated several times, whereas the latter is designed for a course of action that is not likely to be repeated in the future.

Policies, the major type of repeat-use plans, are guides to thinking, and most originate with the chief administrator. In most cases, the supervisor's concern with policies is primarily in interpreting them, applying them, and staying within them whenever decisions are made for the department. Although supervisors do not usually originate policies, they are often called on to design procedures, methods, and rules, which are other repeat-use plans. These plans are guides for action, not guides for thinking. Supervisors also participate in the establishment of budgets, which are single-use plans expressed in numerical terms. Occasionally supervisors are involved with programs and projects, which are two more examples of single-use plans.

It is a supervisor's duty to simplify work processes. Continual, periodic assessment of job descriptions, procedures, and methods is key to ensuring departmental efficiency.

REFERENCES

Abdelhak, M., S. Grostick, M. A. Hanken, and E. Jacobs. 1996. *Health Information: Management of a Strategic Resource*, 550. Philadelphia, PA: Saunders.

Graham, B. B. 2001. "Rediscover Work Simplification." [Online article; retrieved 9/17/05.] http://www.worksimp.com/articles/rediscover%20work%20simplification.htm.

Exhibit 10.1

WORK SIMPLIFICATION

Work Simplification has generated billions of dollars through effectiveness and efficiency for organizations that focused on their people and gave them tools for continuous improvement. Over the past two decades, the glamour of electronics has seduced many organizations into treating their people as expenses rather than resources. For those organizations whose leaders truly believe that their people are their most valuable resource, the tools of work simplification are still available, and better than ever.

In 1946, the American Society of Mechanical Engineers (ASME) did something that was even then a long time in the making. They established a set of symbols as the ASME Standard for Operation and Flow Process Charts. Twenty-five years earlier, in 1921, Frank and Lillian Gilbreth had presented "Process Charts—First Steps in Finding the One Best Way" at the Annual Meeting of ASME. By the time the symbols were standardized, they had evolved into a solid set of five symbols that covered every aspect of work, in any work environment, that can be used with very little confusion. The first process charts appeared as a series of symbols strung down a page in sequential order. This was (and still is) a simple and effective way to track the flow of a person or a piece of material through a work process.

In 1932, Allan Mogensen (1989) founded work simplification, which is defined as the organized application of common sense. Mogensen used the process chart (among other tools) to organize and study work, and he drew on the common sense of the people who did the work for improvement ideas. Mogensen defended participative improvement with these words, "The person doing the job knows far more than anyone else as to the best way of doing that job, and therefore is the one person best fitted to improve it." It is this human element of work simplification that distinguishes it from most other improvement techniques. It is predicated on people who do the work being involved in improving that work. It does not treat people, products, and information as inputs and outputs, using accounting terminology. It regards people as a treasured resource, the safekeepers of the corporate (or organizational) memory, which is the most vital factor in successful continuous improvement! Mogensen described the process chart as follows: "In order to achieve measurement, tools are needed and the most important of these is the process chart. . . . The process chart is the lifeblood of work simplification. It is an irreplaceable tool. It is a guide and stimulant. It takes time to properly utilize but there is absolutely no doubt that it works" (Mogensen 1989, 44–46).

Mogensen began conducting work simplification conferences at Lake Placid in 1937 and continued them for nearly 50 years. (Lillian Gilbreth was part of the original staff returning each year until the mid-1960s.) Ben S. Graham was a student at Mogensen's 1944 Conference. He was unique in his class in that he did not come from a manufacturing environment. He learned the methods of work simplification and adapted them from the machine shop into the office while directing the paperwork simplification effort at The Standard Register Company. There he developed the horizontal process flow chart to accommodate multiple information flows. He also embraced an employee team approach to process improvement, which is summarized in this statement he made in 1958: "Participation by the worker in developing the method eliminates many causes of resistance and assures enthusiastic acceptance. This is more important than all the techniques put together." Graham subsequently joined Mogensen's staff as the resident expert in paperwork simplification.

A few of the organizations that have embraced work simplification in the past include the following (Mogensen 1989):

- *Texas Instruments*. Its former CEO Pat Haggerty described work simplification as "TI's most effective program for fostering personal involvement at all levels of the organization while yielding tangible benefits to the company."
- *Maytag*. Its former CEO Daniel J. Krumm stated, "Work simplification plays an integral part in Maytag's total cost-reduction efforts and makes a significant contribution year after year."
- *Procter & Gamble*. In 1983, P&G realized nearly $1 billion in first year savings as a result of work simplification.
- *Ford*. Ford-Connersville's annual first year savings increased from $400,000 to $10 million during 11 years of applying work simplification. Savings in administrative processes grew from $820,000 to $1.5 million in three years.
- *Standard Register*. The company introduced work simplification to the office environment, and it was the first to offer business process improvement to clients to support the sales of new information systems.
- *The US Navy*. Over a period of 14 years, about 250 projects produced a typical annual return for the Navy of over $150,000 per project.

These days, processes change so fast that many organizations have failed to keep up. Their work is undocumented and as changes are made the complexity mounts. The simple and effective approach of work simplification has more to offer than it ever had. However, its use is not widespread. It appears that many organizations are focusing their attention on purchasing solutions for their business rather than mastering their work themselves. Where the purchased solutions lead to downsizing, the corporate memory is discarded, leaving the organization dependent on those from whom it purchased its processes.

The work simplification approach utilizes the corporate memory rather than discards it. It counters increasing complexity with continuous improvement and enables the workforce to be the masters of their processes. It is on the program at many universities, and it is being applied in increasing numbers of organizations across the United States and

Canada and in South America, Europe, and Australia, as these companies seek to regain control of their operations.

New methods for studying work are introduced on a regular basis. Usually they focus effectively on one or another aspect of improvement, but they often fail because they do not deal rigorously with the work itself. This is a good time to look back and discover again a simple tool that visually displays processes in a universal language that can be readily understood by anyone who wants to understand.

Today, if you are pursuing Six Sigma or lean manufacturing, using kaisan or value stream mapping, managing your supply chain, developing a business-to-business strategy, establishing an electronic commerce presence, managing day-to-day internal operations, or documenting your processes for certification or audit, understanding the fundamental steps in your work processes will help you get those things done. Work simplification helps you get there . . . faster, cheaper, and better!

Mogensen, A . H., with R. Rausa. 1989. *Mogy: An Autobiography*. Chesapeake, VA: Idea Associates.

Source: Adapted from Ben B. Graham, "Rediscover Work Simplification." Ben Graham Corporation website, 2001.

CHAPTER ELEVEN

Time Management Techniques

CHAPTER OBJECTIVES

After you have studied this chapter, you should be able to do the following:

1. Classify how time is spent.
2. Identify tools for managing one's time.
3. Define the benefits of a time-use chart.
4. Distinguish how one may need to manage staff and plan staff's time depending on the management theory followed.
5. Describe the pros and cons of flexible work alternatives.

T O WASTE YOUR time is to waste your life, but to master your time is to master your life (Lakein 1972; Carnahan et al. 1987; Kiechel 1984). If supervisors want more time, they have to "make" it themselves. The supervisor's own time is one of the resources for which he or she is responsible. Every supervisor has probably experienced days that were so full of pressures and demands that he or she began to feel as though all the matters that needed attention could never be resolved. (See Figure 11.1.) The only way to keep such days at a minimum is for the supervisor to plan for the most effective use of time. Technologies that had promised huge time savings have actually consumed more of a manager's time. The individual who received 10 to 20 letters and memos a day in the past may now receive dozens, even hundreds of calls, faxes, and e-mail messages (The Economic Press 1999).

Unfortunately, problems at work come up constantly but without any order of importance or priority. Thus, the first thing the supervisor must do is to determine which problems must be attended to personally and which can be assigned to someone else. The supervisor cannot delegate some matters, but most can be assigned to staff members. Every time the supervisor assigns one of his or her duties to an employee, time is gained to take care of matters that represent a more effective use of his or her time. This delegation of tasks is worthwhile even if some valuable time must be spent training one of the employees in a particular task. When in doubt, the supervisor should delegate. Remaining matters have to be classified according to their urgency.

USE OF TIME

Stephen R. Covey (1989), in his popular book, *The Seven Habits of Highly Effective People*, identifies four ways in which we spend time. If managers follow Covey's advice, they will work to concentrate their time preparing for the future rather than being driven by the future when it arrives, thus causing a crisis. In addition, Covey provides guidance in setting priorities. Two factors that define an activity are the terms "urgent" and "important." Urgent items require immediate attention because they act on us. For example, a ringing phone is urgent. Important items have to do with results, and those important actions contribute to the manager's mission, values, or goals (Covey 1989).

Unless supervisors distinguish between those matters that must be done (urgent items) and those that ought to be done (important items), they are inclined to pay equal attention to all matters before them. Consequently, planning and other more important tasks may not receive the attention they truly deserve. By distinguishing between the two, supervisors are giving priority to matters that need immediate attention. A supervisor should therefore plan his or her time so that the most important things appear at the top of the schedule. The supervisor must make certain, however, that free time is scheduled to attend to new urgent items. Some emergencies occur that a supervisor must deal with when they arise. The flexibility makes it possible to take care of these situations without significantly disrupting the other activities planned on the time schedule.

Many techniques have been devised to help supervisors control their time schedules. One of the simplest methods is to use a desk calendar or computer scheduling system to schedule or make a to-do list of those items that need attention such as appointments, meetings, reports, and discussions. The supervisor should schedule these events far in advance, so they will automatically come up for attention when they are due. Electronic calendars and reminder lists on your computer or personal digital assistant (PDA) can help you organize your time as long as you do not become a slave to entering items on the lists rather than completing them.

Another effective way of planning each week's work, as well as knowing what is being accomplished as the week progresses, is to keep a planning sheet. This sheet is prepared at the end of one week for the week to follow. It shows the days of the week divided into morning and afternoon columns and a list of all items to be accomplished. Then a time for accomplishment is assigned to each task by placing it in the morning or the afternoon blocks of the assigned day. As a task is accomplished, its box is circled. This approach can be accomplished using a PDA or your computer's software in lieu of paper.

Those tasks that have been delayed during the day must be rescheduled for another time by placing them in an appropriate block on a subsequent day. Those tasks that are planned but have not been accomplished during the week

Figure 11.1

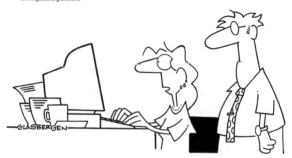

"Is there a file compression program that will help me
squeeze 12 hours of work into an 8 hour schedule?"

(the ones that remain uncircled) must be rescheduled for the following week. Such a record shows how much of the original plan has been carried out at the end of the week and provides a good answer to the question of how the supervisor's time was spent. Based on this record, the supervisor is then able to plan the next week, and so on. Over time, the supervisor can become better at forecasting the time required to accomplish tasks and at planning his or her own workload. Furthermore, the accounting of time spent allows assessment of which activities were time wasters and serves as a reminder to eliminate those activities.

Regardless of whether this particular system or another is used, the supervisor must schedule the time each week and must have some method of reporting the tasks that are planned and those that have been accomplished (see Figure 11.2). Remember, build into your schedule time for unplanned and urgent events; these consume time that you may have set aside to do something else. By incorporating time in your schedule for these unexpected events, your other projects do not fall behind.

Many short, easy-reading booklets on time management are available. Reading one or two of these provides you with ample ideas for making the most of your time.

Time-Use Chart

A manager needs to assess how his or her time is being used to eliminate time wasters. He or she can figure out how time is spent by keeping a time-use chart or a time log. Midway through and at the end of the day, or every half-hour if the supervisor chooses, he or she should list, on a half-hour basis, all of his or her activities that occurred. This log should be kept during a typical work cycle for at least two weeks. At the end of the week, a review of this log will tell the supervisor

FIGURE 11.2: SAMPLE METHOD FOR RECORDING TASKS

MONDAY 10/23	TUESDAY 10/24	WEDNESDAY 10/25	THURSDAY 10/26	FRIDAY 10/27
AM	AM	AM	AM	AM
	Work on job descriptions	See Personnel Director about Helen	Arrange dates for evaluation interviews.	Work on dress code revisions
		Talk to maintenance about new ff outlets.		
PM Check leave of absence policy	PM	PM Read minutes, last meeting of infection con.	PM Start on work on new budget.	PM Attend Management Seminar

how much time he or she spent in counseling and instructing employees, on the phone, answering emails, in meetings, on personal chores, socializing, or having lunch. Then the supervisor should create some broad classifications for daily activities such as routine duties, regular supervisory duties, special duties, emergencies, and innovative thinking.

The supervisor may find that 20 percent of the time was spent on routine work, which could and should be assigned to some of the subordinates. A large percentage of time was devoted to regular supervisory duties such as checking performance, giving directives and instructions, evaluating and counseling employees, and promoting and maintaining discipline. These are supervisory duties that the manager alone should do. Then the supervisor should find out how much time he or she spent on special duties such as serving on committees, attending professional meetings, planning next year's budget, changing the dress code, and reviewing procedures. Again, all this time is probably spent wisely.

A certain amount of time also will be spent on emergencies—that is, unpredictable events that demand some of the supervisor's attention. In addition, some time should be open for creative and innovative thinking, which is essential for planning advances or changes for the department and the progress of the institution. The boss evaluates the supervisor on how well the department's job gets done, which includes his or her implementation of innovative changes and development of suggestions.

Studying the time-use chart illustrates how the time was spent and in which areas a supervisor can make more time. Unless the supervisor has a clear picture of this, routine tasks can creep in and reduce the time available for real supervisory duties.

This raises the question, "Who controls the supervisor's time?" Throughout our discussion, the fact that only the supervisor can control time has been emphasized, and that it is his or her responsibility for what is done with this time. However, another interesting approach to managing time is suggested by Oncken and Wass (1974). They examine three kinds of managerial time:

1. *Boss-imposed time* is time used by an individual to accomplish those activities that the boss requires and the supervisor cannot disregard.
2. *System-imposed time* is time used by an individual to give support to peers and to cooperate with and coordinate activities of the organization.
3. *Self-imposed time* is time used by an individual to accomplish the items the supervisor originates and agrees to do himself or herself.

The supervisor cannot do much about the boss- and system-imposed time. The self-imposed time, however, is where you can make changes. During the self-imposed time, some of the supervisor's time is taken up by the subordinates or by subordinates "passing the monkey" to the supervisor, which can be called subordinate-imposed time. Subordinate-imposed time can be consumed by such things as counseling, idle chitchat, providing direction, evaluating situations or dilemmas posed by subordinates, and settling disputes. The latter has become a significant time consumer (see Figure 11.3). The remaining time is called discretionary time. To increase discretionary time, the supervisor must reduce the subordinate-imposed time by counseling employees on their issues but sending the employees back to their office to resolve the issues rather than doing the problem solving work for them.

In summary, effective time management increases the manager's discretionary time for managerial tasks and innovative thinking. Another important benefit of time management is that stress can be controlled and reduced if the individual does a good job of managing time.

MANAGING THE EMPLOYEES' TIME

When planning for the effective use of the subordinates' time, much will depend on the supervisor's basic managerial strategy and assumptions about human na-

FIGURE 11.3: PLAYING PEACEMAKER

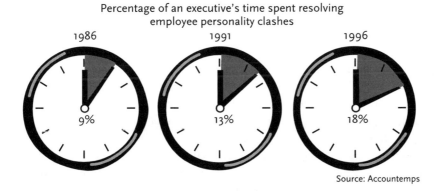

Percentage of an executive's time spent resolving
employee personality clashes

1986   1991   1996

9%   13%   18%

Source: Accountemps

Source: Reprinted with permission from *The Journal of Accountancy,* © 1996 by the American Institute of Certified Public Accountants (AICPA). Opinions of the authors are their own and do not necessarily reflect policies of AICPA.

ture. Recalling what we learned about human nature in Chapter 2, the human resources school provides some guidance. Douglas McGregor (1985) states that most managers base their thinking on one of two sets of assumptions about human nature, which he calls Theory X and Theory Y. The Theory X manager believes that the average employee dislikes work, avoids work, and tries to get by with doing as little as possible. The employee has little ambition and has to be forced and closely controlled in each and every job. In these cases, the manager may require the use of specialized software, such as project management software. The manager estimates the time required for the project and expects the employee to explain any variances from that time allocation.

The Theory Y manager operates with a drastically different set of assumptions regarding human nature. He or she believes that most employees consider work natural and that most are eager to do the right thing, seek responsibility under the proper conditions, exercise self-control, and do not need to be constantly reminded to do their work.

If a supervisor is a Theory Y manager, he or she expects employees to do the right thing and to turn in a fair day's work. Because one cannot expect employees to work indefinitely at top speed, however, the plans for their time are based on a fair output instead of a maximum output. Allowances are made for fatigue, personal needs, unavoidable delays, and a certain amount of unproductive time during the workday.

In planning employees' time, as in other aspects of planning, the supervisor may be able to get assistance from a specialist employed by the facility, preferably a motion and time specialist. However, most supervisors usually can figure out what can be expected of their employees. Managers are generally capable of planning reasonable performance requirements that their employees accept as fair. Such requirements are based on average conditions and not on emergencies. These reasonable estimates of employees' time are necessary because the supervisor must depend on the completion of certain tasks at certain times. The supervisors themselves may have been given deadlines, and to meet them, they must have a reasonable estimate of how fast the job can be done.

In some situations, the subordinate's time is paced and is set by someone or something other than the supervisor because of the nature of the activity performed. For instance, the time an operating room nurse or technician spends on a case is determined by the type of surgery and the speed and skill of the surgeon. In the clinical laboratories and even in the food service dish room, the time required is set by the speed of the equipment used. Unexpected complications may add to the time normally necessary to complete the job. In these cases, average time estimates can still be made, but the time allotted must allow for the various contingencies that can arise.

Because employees are a high-cost commodity, supervisors must coordinate the use of this valuable resource. In some healthcare departments, such as information systems and engineering, project management software can be used to help team leaders and team members organize tasks, track costs, and meet deadlines. However, the supervisor may need to write an action plan that captures the important steps of the process and due dates. This type of plan forces the supervisor to consider the issues that affect the process and gives staff expectations in terms of timeliness. Gantt charts may be used to display the impact of various steps in the process. Work simplification efforts help management find wasted time as a result of redundant or outdated efforts. Knowing how the time is spent helps to identify time that can be captured to do things that must be done by eliminating things that are no longer necessary.

In addition to planning for the normal employee time, it may be necessary to plan for overtime. Overtime should be considered only as an emergency measure. If the supervisor finds that overtime or working a double shift is regularly required, plans need to be changed by altering work methods, obtaining better or more equipment, or hiring more part-time or full-time employees. The supervisor must also plan for employee absences. One cannot plan for those instances in which employees are absent without notice, but one can plan for holidays, vacations, leaves of absence, or layoffs for overhaul. Plans for these absences should be worked out in advance to ensure smooth functioning of the department thereafter.

Flexible Work Schedules and Alternatives

Work schedules for many employees in different organizations have become more flexible. The idea behind this is that employees should have some autonomy to adjust their work schedules to fit their lifestyles and to choose the hours they would prefer to work while ensuring that a core workforce is available to attend to the department's operations. One such alternative is flextime. *Flextime* enables employees to choose a schedule that fits into their off-the-job activities. It enables working parents or others with responsibilities at home the opportunity to combine work with family life. Another work-scheduling option that is popular is the 4–10 or 3–12 arrangement. Employees choosing to work these schedules work either four 10-hour days or three 12-hour days. Often, organizations offering the 3–12 arrangement pay the employee for 40 hours, even though only 36 hours are worked. One concern with these extended day schedules is that they can potentially cause fatigue and an increase in errors. Regardless, flexible work schedules tend to improve employee satisfaction and should contribute positively to productivity and time utilization.

Another work arrangement option, *telecommuting*, has gained popularity in many industries and is penetrating the healthcare industry as well. Telemedicine advances and computer and telecommunication technologies allow radiologists to work from their home offices and other specialists to serve rural and unserved area through remote television. Faced with tight labor markets in a number of areas in a hospital, managers continue their efforts to attract and retain professionals by establishing an environment in which professionals can achieve work-life balance and reduce the stress of commuting and distractions of the office. Global Telematics offers a checklist that management can use to assess telecommuting options. This checklist appears in Exhibit 11.1.

Baldiga and Doucet's (2001) study indicates that the percentage of women returning to work full-time after childbirth declined from 73 percent to 61 percent between 1994 and 2000. Because a hospital's workforce is predominantly composed of women, supervisors must consider alternative work schedules for their staff.

Flexible working schedules and remote working arrangements undoubtedly create some additional scheduling and planning challenges for supervisors. Managers must consider how to supervise staff working on different shifts and how to coordinate activities with other departments.

The concerns noted above and others are additional challenges for supervisors. However, as long as flexible working schedules and arrangements produce good results (e.g., easier staff recruitment, better staff retention, higher morale, fewer absences, less tardiness, less dissatisfaction, and better patient care), supervisors make every effort to overcome these problems by better planning and supervision.

Some departments must plan for variable workloads. Consider the central supply room as one such department that at year-end must take a physical inventory of all supplies both in stock and throughout the organization. This is no easy task. Using overtime may be an option, but it will be a costly one. Therefore, it may be necessary for supervisors to hire temporary or part-time employees to work hours during inventory. Alternatively, by recruiting staff who are willing to adjust their schedules at different times of the year PRN (on an as-needed basis), the supervisor is able to manage labor expenses and fulfill the work requirements.

SUMMARY

Of the many resources a supervisor is responsible for, probably the most valuable one is time, both the supervisor's and his or her employees'. Identifying time wasters and eliminating them, whether through delegation, reassignment, or discontinuance, is necessary to accomplish one's work. The supervisor must set priorities for the unscheduled events of the day and distinguish between those items that must be done.

Several techniques and tools are available to supervisors today, including scheduling software, desk calendars, planning sheets, and time-use charts. Understanding what is consuming one's time is the first step in organizing and prioritizing it to accomplish more tasks more effectively.

To recruit talented staff, flexible work alternatives may be required. Modifying the schedule to meet the needs of those staff members who are hard to recruit and understanding what motivates the staff working in the department create a more satisfying environment for them and still allow the department to continue to be productive. In cooperation with the human resources department, today's supervisor can find a variety of work schedules and technology-driven alternatives from which to choose.

REFERENCES

Baldiga, N. R., and M. S. Doucet. 2001. "Special Report. Having It All: How a Shift Toward Balance Affected CPAs and Firms." [Online article; retrieved 2/13/02.] www.aicpa.org/pubs/JOFA/may2001/news_sr.htm.

Carnahan, G. R., B. G. Gnauk, D. B. Hoffman, and B. C. Sherony. 1987. *To Improve Management Effectiveness.* Cincinnati, OH: South-Western Publishing Co.

Covey, S. R. 1989. *The Seven Habits of Highly Effective People.* New York: Simon & Schuster.

Kiechel, W., III. 1984. "Beat the Clock." *Fortune* (June 15): 147–48.

Lakein, A. 1972. *How to Get Control of Your Time and Your Life.* New York: Peter H. Wyden, McGraw-Hill Book Co.

McGregor, D. 1985. *The Human Side of Enterprise,* 25th Anniversary Printing, chapters 3 and 4. New York: McGraw-Hill Book Co.

Oncken, W., Jr., and D. L. Wass. 1974. "Management Time: Who's Got the Monkey?" *Harvard Business Review* (November–December): 75–80.

The Economic Press. 1999. "Managing Your Time: Think Quality, Not Quantity." *Office Hours* 405: 1.

Exhibit 11.1

TELEWORK SOLUTIONS CHECKLIST
FROM GLOBAL TELEMATICS

Telework means using telecommunications and computers to let employees do their work in novel locations such as new remote offices or their own homes.

Here are the main considerations in deciding to establish additional office work locations:

1. Be on the lookout for business problems that telework helps to solve.
   - Difficulty filling jobs because appropriate workers do not live close to the office
   - Employees who would be happier working closer to their homes
   - Need for headquarters expansion or relocation
   - Location- or facility-related operational problems
2. Consider both of the telework location options.
   - In additional company facilities
   - In employees' own homes
3. Take a comprehensive approach to telework.
   - Recognize that installing the right technology is only one piece of the telework solution
   - A bigger issue is maintaining the effectiveness of staff interactions when people are less frequently in the office for face-to-face interactions
   - Involve business planning, personnel management, facilities planning, and operations management in setting up telework
   - Don't count on telework as an easy "off-the-shelf" purchase
4. Encourage employees to submit proposals on work site location.
   - Let individual employees propose working at home (telecommuting)
   - See if any managers propose relocating their work groups
   - Evaluate these proposals for energy and ideas to drive improvement
5. Look for opportunities to improve customer focus.
   - Survey customer attitudes toward present location
   - Consider advantages of a second company location closer to the airport, a business center, an important customer, or a cluster of customers
   - Examine if a second location would provide better facilities for meeting customers
   - Evaluate if splitting certain units away from sales and service would yield more customer focus
6. Seek retention and recruitment improvements.
   - Survey employee attitudes toward present and potential locations
   - Map out where employees live to see a better location for certain offices
   - Respond to individual employee needs by offering work-at-home opportunities

7. Evaluate the facility cost reductions from split operations.
   - Back office operations—functions not requiring customer contact in the office—can be placed in lower-cost space
   - Mobile personnel who meet customers in the field instead of at the office can be placed in lower-cost space
8. Find potential operational improvements from telework.
   - Moving a work group to a new location may support more creativity and single-minded focus
   - Logistical factors—moving people or materials in and out—may be eased for some work groups in a new site
9. Use telework for additional flexibility to handle change.
   - Set up new work sites for temporary task forces, special projects, and seasonal hires
   - Multiply flexibility by using portable office equipment and modular furniture
10. Check out the many telecommunications options for linking worksites.
    - Define what you want in functionality and keep looking until you find it; technology is improving and costs are dropping
    - Seek long-term relationships with sources of expert technical support
    - Remote access to your company network (local area network or intranet) is important and feasible
    - Remote access to the company voice network is also important and feasible
    - Still, occasional remote telework can sometimes be set up for tasks that don't require full connections to the office network
11. Address the teamwork and company culture issues arising from dispersed work sites.
    - Make extra effort to maintain company teamwork and culture when employees formerly working together start to work apart
    - Schedule additional inter-facility meetings and social gatherings as telework replaces some face-to-face interaction
12. Move forward on telework only on finding a "killer" advantage.
    - Telework is complex and risky enough to be justified only when the advantages are projected to be very important and near certain
    - Start on the easy parts
    - Try telework confidently, but leave room for modifications as experience builds
    - Recognize that office environments continue to have some advantages over a network of dispersed workers

Source: Prepared by Global Telematics, http://www.globaltelematics.com. Used with permission. © 2001, Global Telematics. All rights reserved.

PART IV

Organizing

CHAPTER TWELVE

Fundamental Concepts of Organizing

CHAPTER OBJECTIVES

After you have studied this chapter, you should be able to do the following:

1. Discuss why organizing is an important managerial function.

2. Identify the organizing function as the process of designing the structural framework and establishing authority relationships based on major principles.

3. Enumerate and discuss two fundamental organizational underpinnings—namely, authority and span of management.

4. Describe the meaning and major sources of formal, positional authority.

5. Explain the importance of the span of management and the relationships of span to levels leading to a shallow or tall organization.

6. Discuss the major factors that influence the width of the span.

7. Review the concept of team management as an approach to expanding the span of management.

P LANNING DEFINES THE goals and objectives of the institution; the function of organizing is closely related to that process. It defines and arranges the activities needed to accomplish these objectives and es- tablishes the relationships among various functions. *Organizing* is the process of deciding how best to group and relate organizational activities and resources. These activities and functions form subsystems that are synchronized and co- ordinated into a larger system, called the *formal organization.*

How this structure looks and works depends on the organization's overall objectives, its size, geographic span, space constraints, technology, culture, and many other factors. One such factor is change. The healthcare environment is constantly changing. Management must have an organizational strategy that can be adapted to a competitive and changing environment. The structure of the organization will follow that strategy and will require restructuring from time to time to accommodate demands for new services, technologies, and expertise.

The managerial function of organizing is an impersonal function, which means that the organization is designed with the activities in mind and not around the individual personalities in place to perform them. Of course, the organization must be a structure that can be inhabited by people, the most valuable asset of any organization. It must be a structure in which people can function and thrive. The human element obviously is important, and we discuss all these considerations in the staffing and influencing functions. When the manager designs the structure, however, it is done without thinking of specific persons.

Formal organizational theory rests on several major principles:

1. Authority is the lifeblood of the managerial position, and the delegation or distributing of authority makes the organization come alive. Authority may be line or staff in nature, a subject discussed in Chapter 15.
2. The span of management sets outside limits on the number of subordinates a manager can effectively supervise.
3. The division of work is essential for efficiency. This may require designing jobs (job or work specialization).
4. The formal structure is the main network for organizing and managing the various activities of the enterprise. Often this is done through departmentalization.
5. Unity of command must prevail; that is, each person should take orders from and report to only one boss.
6. Coordinating activities and resources is a primary responsibility of management and is fulfilled by performing the managerial functions properly.

These major principles of organization are a primary concern of the senior executives of the organization, the CEO and the COO. He or she must translate these principles into a formal organizational structure so that the institution operates smoothly and accomplishes its objectives.

Organizational structure is the formal arrangement of jobs in the organization. The structure is displayed in the organizational chart or table of organization (TOO). An organizational chart typically includes the title of each manager's position and, by means of broken or solid connecting lines, who is accountable to whom, who has authority for each department, and what type of authority is held.

Because the application of these formal organizational principles involves all levels of management, it is also necessary for you as a supervisor to understand them and know how they are used. This knowledge helps you organize your own department and coordinate its activities with those of the rest of the institution. As a supervisor, you will certainly be asked to carry out (and may even be asked to help make) such decisions involving reorganization, departmentalization or the division of work, the span of supervision, and the delegation of authority.

As you move up the managerial hierarchy, you will probably be called on to participate in more and more organizational decisions. Some of these deal with organizational design to respond to the changing environment. *Organizational design* is a process involving decisions about such things as work or job specialization, departmentalization, chain of command, span of control, and centralization or decentralization. Thus, although the COO initially applies the formal principles to establish the overall organizational structure and activities, the department heads, supervisors, and other middle- and lower-level managers must make these principles and the resulting structure work. This is why a discussion here of the organizing process on an overall, or institutional, basis is essential before discussing it on the departmental, or supervisory, level.

The many contingencies facing management are a constant challenge, and the dynamic nature of organizing enables the manager to bring about change and to absorb and accommodate change as the need arises. This enables the enterprise to pursue and achieve its objectives continuously.

Although organizing is a dynamic process, it rests on two fundamental concepts, authority and span of management (also known as span of control), which this chapter examines. *Authority*, the right to direct others and to act and give orders, is one of the bases through which the manager gets the job done. It is the underpinning of the organization. *Span of management* deals with another dimension: the scope of supervision, or the number of people who report to a particular manager.

AUTHORITY

In chapters 1 and 2, we referred to the importance of authority to the managerial position. That discussion of authority merely stated that it is the lifeblood of the supervisory position and one of the characteristics of a manager. In addition, we mentioned that delegating authority breathes life into an organization; without it, an organization cannot and does not exist. Therefore, we must first examine and understand the concept of authority.

Authority is the key to the managerial job; at the same time, it carries many interpretations. In a general sense, authority refers to the formal or official power of a manager to influence decisions and to obtain the compliance of the subordinate by using directives, communications, policies, and objectives. Such authority is associated with the manager's function in the organization; it is vested in organizational roles or positions, and it is legitimized by the organization. As long as an individual holds the position, he or she has the privilege of exercising the authority that is inherent in it.

Positions are meaningless unless they are occupied by someone. Therefore, we generally speak of the authority of the manager, the authority that is delegated to the manager, and so forth. Although it would be more precise to speak of the authority of the managerial position itself or the authority delegated to that position rather than to the person who occupies it, the difference is generally regarded as semantic. As long as we understand that authority in this sense resides in the position, we may speak rather loosely of the authority of the manager, supervisor, and so on.

Source of Nature of Authority

Max Weber (1974) first expressed authority as "legitimate power" to give orders. The subordinates' compliance rests on the belief that it is legitimate for managers to give orders and illegitimate for subordinates not to obey them. This kind of authority is vested in organizational roles and positions, not in the individuals who occupy these positions. As long as an individual holds the position, he or she has the privilege of exercising the authority that is inherent in it. Once a manager leaves an organizational position, he or she loses the authority inherent in it, and the authority goes to the successor.

While examining the foundation for this organizational authority, Weber identified three bases of authority: tradition, rules and regulations, and charisma. *Traditional authority* "rests on the belief in the sacredness of the social order" (Weber 1985). For instance, in a patriarchal society, the father receives legitimacy as an authority through custom. Rules and regulations form a second basis.

Subordinates comply with orders because, in a bureaucratic organization, superior-subordinate authority relationships are defined by rules and regulations. While today's managers may have had concerns about Generation X employees refusing to comply, the same does not appear to be true of "Millennials" (Generation Y—those born in the 1980s and now entering the workforce). These individuals experienced the Cold War, 911 and terrorism, and dramatic advances in technology. They seem to want to make a positive impact in their jobs and communities and willingly work within the structure to effect this change.

Other explanations of the meaning and sources of authority are presented by Barnard (1989). The formal authority theory and the acceptance authority theory are two contradictory theories of the source of authority. In *formal authority theory*, authority originates at the top of the organizational hierarchy and is delegated downward from superiors to subordinates. In *acceptance authority theory*, a leader's authority originates at the bottom of the organizational pyramid and is determined by his or her subordinates' willingness to comply with it. Each of these theories is discussed below to provide further insight.

Formal Authority Theory

Formal authority is the top-down theory. It traces the flow of authority downward from top-level management to subordinate managers. You can trace your authority directly from your boss, who has delegated it to you. He or she in turn receives authority, for example, from an associate administrator, who receives authority from the chief administrator, who traces authority directly back to the board of directors, who receive their authority from the owners or the stockholders. In private corporations, therefore, one may say that the actual source of authority lies in the stockholders, who are, loosely speaking, the owners of the corporation. These owners delegate their power to administer the affairs of the corporation to those they have put into managerial positions. That power flows down from the top administrator through the chain of command until it reaches the supervisor.

Limitations of Authority

The authority that a manager has by virtue of his or her position in an organization is limited, either explicitly or implicitly. Moreover, some limitations stem from internal sources while others are from external sources. *External limitations on authority* include such factors as our mores, folkways (community practices), and lifestyle, along with the many legal, political, ethical, moral, social, and economic considerations that make up our society. For example, laws referring to collective bargaining and resulting contractual obligations and fair employment practices are specific examples of external limitations on authority.

In contrast, *internal limitations on authority* are set mainly by the organization's articles of incorporation and bylaws. In addition to these overall internal restrictions, each manager is subject to the specific limitations spelled out by the administrator when duties are assigned and authority is delegated. Generally, there are more internal limitations on the scope of authority the further down one goes in the managerial hierarchy. In other words, the lower the rung on the administrative ladder, the narrower is the area in which authority can be exercised. This is known as the *tapering concept of authority*, as shown in Figure 12.1.

All these limitations are explicit, fairly obvious restrictions on authority. In addition to these, a number of more implicit limitations, such as biological restraints, exist simply because human beings do not have the capacity to do certain things. No subordinate should be expected to do the impossible. Thus, physical and psychological restrictions on authority must be recognized and accepted. In today's society, such considerations significantly limit the scope of authority of every manager.

Thus far, the discussion has centered on the formal way of looking at the origin of authority as a power that results from our recognition of private property. According to this theory, then, the ultimate source of all managerial authority in the United States is the constitutional guarantee of the institution of private property. Because the U.S. Constitution was created by the people and is subject to amendment and modification by the will of the people, it follows that society is the source from which authority flows (Peterson et al. 1962).

This theory is in agreement with Weber's definition of formal authority, as management's right to give orders is legitimate and the employees are obliged to carry out these orders because the orders are legitimate. A problem could arise, however, when such an order seems unethical to the employee or outside the limits of the job. This raises the question of whether the subordinate has some say in this matter, thus leading to the acceptance theory.

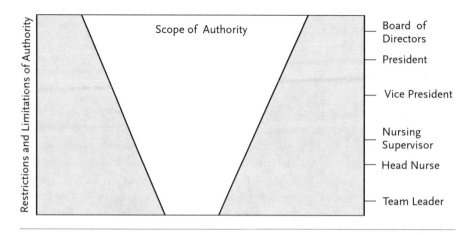

Acceptance Authority Theory

The acceptance authority theory addresses the role of subordinates in managerial authority. It is a bottom-up approach in which employees give managers their authority. In addition to Chester Barnard (1886–1961), other experts do not agree with the formal theory and maintain that management has no meaningful authority unless and until subordinates confer it; that is, formal organizational authority is effective only to the extent that subordinates accept it. In reality, subordinates often do not have a real choice between accepting or not accepting authority. The only choice they have is to leave the job. Nevertheless, this is a worrisome consideration, indicating that there is considerable merit in looking at authority as something that must be accepted by your employees.

Advocates of the acceptance theory state that in most cases a manager does not have a real problem; an employee, on accepting a job, knows that the boss of the department has the authority to give orders, take disciplinary action, and take whatever appropriate action that comes with the managerial position. Whenever an employee decides to work for a healthcare institution, he or she agrees, within the limits of the job, to accept orders given by the organization. The decision of whether an order carries authority, however, lies with the person to whom it is addressed and does not reside in "persons of authority" or those who issue those orders (Barnard 1956). Furthermore, Barnard emphasizes that employees cannot accept a manager's orders if they do not understand what the manager wants them to do or if they do not have the ability or resources to comply with the manager's directive.

Those who support Barnard's theory encourage supervisors to heed the following management recommendations: (1) establish and maintain an ongoing and effective communication system, (2) hire and retain effective staff, and

(3) motivate those hired. Communication has already been discussed in Chapter 5; the other topics are discussed in Parts V and VI of the book.

Formal Authority Theory Versus Acceptance Authority Theory

Differences between the formal authority theory and the acceptance authority theory significantly influence the practice of supervision, or the manner and the attitudes with which supervision is approached. This becomes more obvious with the realization that adhering to the acceptance theory does not necessarily rule out the downward delegation of authority from upper to lower levels of management. The acceptance theory can be thought of as merely another dimension to the formal concept of organizational authority. That is, in addition to having formal authority delegated from above, managers must also have such authority accepted from below. All managers must be aware that they possess formal authority and, if need be, can resort to it as a final recourse.

Today no one wants to rely exclusively on the weight of this formal authority to motivate workers to perform their jobs. At times, however, every manager has to make full use of this authority and power, but with hope that these occasions are the exceptions and not the rule. Even when the manager must invoke this authority, the manner in which it is done makes a difference in whether it is resented or accepted fully. If such actions are accepted graciously most of the time, the manager will know that the subordinates have chosen to recognize and respect the authority that superiors have formally delegated to him or her.

Types of Authority

Authority carries attributes that allow us to categorize it into various types. The following examines the various types of organizational authority: positional, functional, and personal.

Positional authority is based on organizational position and rests on the legitimacy of the manager's position as the agent of a socially valid organization. This authority is vested in the position and in the organization and is impersonal. Positional authority exists in all types of organizations, including healthcare, educational, business, military, religious, and fraternal. We may not like or care for a particular individual, but we recognize and accept the legitimacy of that person's position and authority.

Functional authority is based on expertise and knowledge. We accept expert advice and recognize that this person is an "authority" in a particular specialty. Functional authority exists in all branches of learning and crafts and comes from specialization. Healthcare institutions provide an example of the role and importance of functional authority. The specialist's statements and directives are accepted because he or she is recognized as the authority in the field and carries the weight and power of functional authority.

Whereas positional authority is impersonal, functional authority in this sense is highly personal. It is association with the individual whose knowledge and expertise make him or her the authority. Whereas positional authority can and must be delegated, functional authority cannot be delegated; it remains with the individual wherever he or she may be and work. Although it is highly personalized, functional authority has some aspects of positional authority because some organizations, especially healthcare centers, demand that certain positions can only be filled by individuals with special skills and expertise. Many examples and applications of functional authority may be found in a hospital, probably more than in any other organized activity. Functional authority rests on acceptance, but it stems from an individual's knowledge and not from society.

Personal authority is based on an individual's characteristics, magnetism, and charisma. Some call this charismatic authority. In *charismatic authority*, the compelling personal characteristics and charisma of the leader inspire the subordinates and followers to carry out the orders. Subordinates and followers accept personal authority because their needs are consistent with the leader's goals. Personal authority motivates the subordinates to work willingly and enthusiastically toward the achievement of the objectives. This concept of personal authority can be equated with leadership, which is discussed in Chapter 23.

French and Raven (1960) defined several types of power (outside of legitimate power or power based on one's position we have discussed), including coercive (based in fear), reward (based on the ability to distribute something of value), and referent (based on another person liking you or wanting to be like you).

Integrated Approach to Authority

To be an effective manager in any industry, it is not enough to depend on the weight of positional authority based on legitimacy, although occasionally this may be the last resort. It is much more desirable if the manager relies on a combination of all three types of authority—positional, functional, and personal—to manage effectively. This is even more important in the healthcare field because of the occupational and professional characteristics of the people involved.

New fields of scientific advances and new technologies make greater expertise a necessity, leading to more and more functional authority. For instance, the lead coding professional should not rely on only positional authority as the "lead" of the coding team; he or she should also use personal expertise and knowledge in this field as well as leadership ability and charisma. Reliance on all three types of authority creates a highly desirable and motivating organizational climate.

SPAN OF MANAGEMENT

Another important element of an organization's foundation is the number of people who report to a particular manager. This defines the *span of management*, also known as span of control.[1] This concept deals with the number of people any one person can supervise effectively. Thus, several factors that influence the span of one's control include the following:

1. competence/skills of the supervisor and his/her employees,
2. physical proximity of employees to each other and their supervisor,
3. extent of time spent by the manager performing nonsupervisory duties,
4. frequency of required interaction between employees and the employees and their supervisor,
5. extent of standardized procedures,
6. similarity and complexity of tasks being supervised, and
7. frequency of changes in process.

Each of these factors must be considered when pondering span of control. Should it be relatively narrow, with few subordinates per manager, or reasonably wide, with many subordinates per manager?

To make these reporting relationships as effective as possible, depending on the diversity of tasks and activities involved, organizations must create divisions, departments, sections, or teams and place someone in charge of each. In doing so, the resulting organization may be *tall* or *flat*. In Figure 12.2, we see the organization starting as flat and eventually becoming tall—that is, with more layers. *Tall organizations* may be more expensive because more managers are required and communication may be challenged because there are additional channels through which it must pass. *Flat organizations* tend to have higher employee morale and productivity. Both morale and productivity can be hindered by having too many direct reports causing the supervisor to be spread too thin to adequately respond to employee or customer concerns.

The establishment of departments in an organization is not an end in itself. It is not desirable per se because departments are expensive; they must be headed by someone and staffed by additional employees, all of which costs large sums of money. Furthermore, creating departments is not intrinsically desirable because the more there are, the more difficulties are encountered in communication and coordination. However, as discussed earlier, departments do make the division of work possible. Some departments are too large and require further compartmentalization into sections or teams. Equally important, this compartmentalization allows an organization to incorporate the principle of the span of management, or the span of supervision. This principle states that there is an upper limit to the number of subordinates a manager can effectively supervise. This is a very crucial factor in structuring organizations.

The Relationships of Span to Levels

Many types of superior-subordinate interactions are possible, including (1) direct relationships between the superior and the immediate subordinates, (2) direct group interactions between the superior and different groupings of the subordinates, and (3) cross-relationships among the subordinates themselves.

However, the number of superior-subordinate interactions that can be effectively handled is limited.

Because no one can manage an infinite number of subordinates, the administrator must create departments, or distinct areas of activities, over which a manager is placed in charge. The administrator delegates authority to this manager. The manager in turn re-delegates authority to some subordinates, who in turn supervise only a limited number of employees. In this manner, not only are departments and subsections of the department created, but the span of supervision is established. The number of managerial levels in the organization is determined as well.

To examine this relationship between the span of supervision and the levels of an organization, imagine a hypothetical organization in which 81 subordinates report to one chief executive, thus representing an organizational level (see Figure 12.2). Few will disagree that 81 subordinates are too many people for the executive to manage. However, everyone tends to want to report directly to the boss. To ease his or her burden, the executive is given three associates. Under each of these three associate administrators there would now be 27 employees. By creating associate administrators, however, we have established two levels of organization and have a total of four executives. Now, assuming that 27 subordinates are still too many and that this number is reduced to nine, the organization will require a third managerial level, increasing the total number of managers to 13. Each of the four executives on the upper two levels will have three subordinates, and each of the nine supervisors on the lowest level will have nine subordinates. The span of supervision has thus been reduced drastically from the original 81 to a maximum of nine.

This example shows what occurs when one begins to narrow the span of supervision. The narrower the span becomes, the more levels of management have to be introduced into the organizational setup. As with departments, this is not desirable either because it is expensive and may interfere with communication and coordination. Every manager costs money, not only in salaries, but in supporting expenses (offices, furnishings, educational allowances, and possibly support staff salaries). More levels will complicate communication, even distort it with omissions and misinterpretation of the messages. Finally, adding levels to an organization creates problems with morale because it increases the distance between employees and upper administration. Therefore, a constant conflict exists between the width of the span and the number of levels: the narrower the span, the more managerial levels. The problem is whether to have a broader span of supervision or more levels, or vice versa, and it is a problem that all managers face throughout their careers and one for which a clear solution is still not evident.

All of the issues discussed thus far were confirmed in two studies. The first study, conducted by Doran et. al (2004), sought to determine if the cost-cutting and restructuring in healthcare had an impact on nursing employee retention, patient satisfaction, outcomes, and other factors. The key findings indicate a correlation between the width of the span of control and turnover

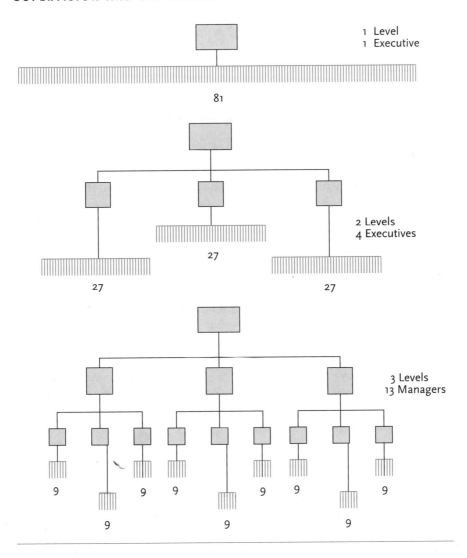

and employee and patient dissatisfaction. The second study, conducted by the College of American Pathologists on hospital clinical laboratories, does not define the ideal span of control but shows a correlation between smaller span of management and increases in productity (Valenstein, Souers, and Wilkinson 2004).

However, attempts to quantify an optimum span of control appear in the works of Graicunas (1937), Urwick (1956), Davis (1951), and Hamilton (1921). While Graicunas developed a formula that accounted for interactions between the supervisor and subordinates and subordinates to their peers, he, Urwick, and Hamilton all gravitated to a number of five to six direct reports at least at the executive level. Davis stretched the number to 30 at the manager level, depending on the type of work being performed by the subordinates and the level of the supervisor. Thus, no definitive answer exists to the question, "How many subordinates should report to a given manager?" One can only say that there is an upper limit to this figure.

Although we do not know exactly what the upper limit should be, it is interesting that in many enterprises the top-level administrator has only five to eight subordinate managers reporting directly to him or her. Descending down the managerial hierarchy, the span of supervision generally increases. It is not unusual to have 15 to 20 people reporting to the supervisor. On closer inspection, the number of subordinates who can be effectively supervised by one manager actually depends on numerous different contingency factors. These factors determine not only the actual number of relationships but also their frequency and intensity. Therefore, before deciding the proper span of supervision in a particular organization, it is necessary to examine the more important contingencies that influence the magnitude of the span.

Factors Determining the Span of Supervision

As mentioned earlier, one of the factors that influences the magnitude of the span is the competence of supervisors—that is, quality of management, experience, and expertise. Some supervisors are capable of handling more subordinates than are others. Some are better acquainted with good management practices; others have had more experience and are simply better all-around managers. A person who is a "good manager" probably can supervise more employees. Limitations still exist, however, on the human capacity and the amount of time available during the workday.

What the manager does with this time is of utmost importance in determining the span. For example, a supervisor needs more time to make an individual decision for every problem that arises than to make initial policy decisions that anticipate problems that might arise later. Clear and complete policy statements reduce the volume of, or at least simplify, the personal decision making required of a manager and thus can increase the span of supervision. The same applies to other managerial processes that determine in advance definitions of responsibility and authority, procedures, methods, and performance standards. Predeterminations such as these reduce the number of decisions the manager has to make and likewise increase the potential span of management.

Another factor that determines how broad a span a manager can handle is the competence and makeup of the subordinates. The greater the capacities and self-direction of the employees, the broader the manager's span can be. The education, experience, and training possessed by the subordinates are also important. The more experienced they are at their jobs, the less they need their supervisor, thus freeing the manager to increase the span.

Another contingency on the manager's span is the amount and availability of help from staff specialists within the organization. If a healthcare organization has a range of experts who provide various kinds of advice, support, and service, the manager's span can be wider.

The number of subordinates who can be supervised also depends on the nature and importance of the activities the subordinates perform. If these activities are complicated, are highly important, carry critical consequences, or change frequently, the span of supervision has to be small. The simpler, less complicated, or more uniform the work, the greater can be the number of persons supervised by one supervisor.

Closely related factors that have a bearing on the span of supervision are the dynamics and complexity of a particular activity. In those departments engaged in dynamic, critical, and unpredictable activities, such as the emergency room, the span is very narrow. In those departments concerned with more or less stable activities, such as food production in the dietary department, the span of supervision can be broader.

Another factor that determines the span of supervision is the degree to which a fairly comprehensive set of standard procedures and objective standards can be applied. If enough procedures and standards exist and are available for subordinates to gauge their own progress, subordinates do not need to report to and contact their boss constantly. Objective standards and standard procedures result in less frequent interactions, freeing the manager for a broader span.

Finally, organizations have had success expanding the span of control through the use of self-directed teams. These teams further compartmentalize a department. Each team has a leader who is formally appointed or selected by the team. The team assumes some of the traditional supervisory duties and authority, such as assigning workloads to team members, scheduling vacations or weekend duty, checking each other's work, and even preparing performance reviews, thus relieving the supervisor of those duties (see Figure 12.3). Team management allows authority to be shared, broadens the span of control, and encourages staff to work together rather than compete with one another. With broader spans of control, the organization also functions with fewer supervisors.

Teams are often assembled on an ad hoc or temporary basis to study a process or a complex issue. These ad hoc teams usually include individuals with expertise or knowledge of the issue and who have an interest in improving the process. Team members typically serve on these teams because they wish to encourage cooperation between departments, divisions, or other teams. Often teams are provided training to help them in their team activities. Such training may include meeting facilitation, problem identification, problem solving, and interpersonal skill building.

Regardless of the factors considered, management must keep in mind that the economic benefits of a broad span of control are rapidly diluted if communication is compromised. Urwick (1956, 43) states it succinctly: "There is nothing which rots morale more quickly and more completely than poor communication

FIGURE 12.3: TEAM AUTHORITY

Authority Template   Date: _____

You will need to obtain authority from your team members to successfully get your team's work accomplished. At the beginning of your project, together you should negotiate with your team members and your team leader as to who has responsibility for each of the following authorities. Sometimes you will need to share these authorities with your team leader or other leaders. Therefore, these other team leaders may need to be involved in the negotiation too. All agreeing with the delegated duties are to enter their initials in the initial column.

This worksheet can be used as a negotiation tool, to make sure that all relevant authorities are clear, have been discussed, and are agreed to by all participating parties.

1. Which team members were involved in the granting of authorities?

    a. _____

    b. _____

    c. _____

2. Were any team leaders or non-team members not involved in this decision?

    Yes: _____   No: _____

3. Who were the team leaders or non-team members who were not involved in this decision? _____

4. As a team, discuss and decide which the of the following authorities are required in order to accomplish the project or work assigned. Also discuss which authorities should remain with the team leader or with others outside of the team in order to successfully accomplish this project. Make notes in the blocks below or on additional paper as necessary and make sure everyone involved receives a copy of this document.

Delegated Authorities for Meeting Project Needs

Authorities	Team Leader	Comments	Team Members	Initials
Assigning tasks or duties to team members.*				
Identify products or services.				
Select products or services.				
Select vendors, suppliers, or contractors.				

(continued on following page)

Authorities	Team Leader	Comments	Team Members	Initials
Eliminate or terminate the services or products of vendors, suppliers, or contractors selected.				
Identify team members or others who would work well on this project.				
Select team members or others.				
Eliminate or reassign team members or others.				
Recommend how/how much supplier, contractors, or vendors are paid.				
Authorize payments to suppliers, contractors, or vendors.				
Recommend how much team members are paid or if bonuses are to be issued.				
Authorize pay and/or bonuses for team members.				
Define work that is to be accomplished.				
Establish timetable for work to be accomplished.				
Offer alternatives to achieving goals.				
Approve or disapprove alternatives offered by team members or others.				
Monitor the timeliness and report of progress.				
Prepare budget.				
Approve budget.				
Approve variances to budget.				
Summarize "lessons learned" and success or failure.				

* Will this authority differ if more than one team leader is involved?

and indecisiveness . . . And there is no condition which more quickly produces a sense of indecision among subordinates or more effectively hampers communication than being responsible to a superior who has too wide a span of control."

SUMMARY

Organizing defines and arranges the activities needed to accomplish the objectives of the organization. To do so, one must assess the organization's overall objectives, its size, geographic span, space constraints, and changing environment. If an organization exists in a rapidly changing environment it may need to restructure itself often.

On establishing the structure, positions within the organization are granted authority to manage resources and activities assigned to them.

Authority and span of management are two basic elements of the organizing function. Authority is the right to give orders and directives and to expect that they be carried out. Much has been said and written about the source of authority. The formal authority theory is top down; it views authority as coming from the U.S. Constitution, the recognition of private property, social institutions, owners, stockholders, boards of directors, higher management, and so on down the line to the supervisor.

The opposite view, the acceptance authority theory, views authority as coming from the bottom up. This theory states that managers have no authority unless and until the subordinates accept their authority, and subordinates normally accept only those directives they perceive to be legitimate.

Tradition, rules, and charisma are the bases of authority, which lead to three major types of organizational authority. Positional authority is based on the position in the organization; functional authority is based on knowledge and expertise; and personal, or charismatic, authority comes from the subordinates' needs being consistent with the leader's goals.

Many factors must be considered when defining the structure of an organization and the span of control assigned to each of the managerial and supervisory positions. Too broad a span may result in lackluster performance of the staff and the supervisor, poor morale, and customer as well as employee dissatisfaction; too narrow a span may result in too many supervisors—a costly endeavor for the organization. While a definitive size for the ideal span of control has not been discovered, there has been research done in this area that indicates a consensus of 5–6 direct reports, at least at the executive level, and possibly up to 30 at the manager level.

Determining the span of supervision at each level and the number of managerial levels is important. The span of supervision states that there is an upper limit to the number of managerial levels. The actual width of this span is determined by such factors as the competence of the supervisor as well as the competence and experience of the subordinates to be supervised by one manager. The manager knows, however, that when the span of supervision is decreased, an additional supervisor has to be introduced to supervise the excess employees.

In other words, the smaller the span of supervision, the more levels of supervisory personnel are needed. This shapes the organization into either a tall, narrow pyramid or, in the case of a broad span of supervision, a shallow, wide pyramid. On the other hand, broadening the span of control or increasing the use of team management enhances the shallow pyramid or flat structure and allows employees to manage their own activities without consuming a manager's time to do so.

NOTE

1. Span of management may also be called span of authority, span of supervision, or scope of supervision.

REFERENCES

Barnard, C. I. 1989. *Management, Fourth Edition*, edited by R. Krietner, 281. Boston: Houghton Mifflin Co.

———. 1956. *The Functions of the Executive*, 163. Cambridge, MA: Harvard University Press.

Davis, R. 1951. [Online article; retrieved 9/19/05.] www.aviation.sosu.edu/salluisi/avia3133/chapter-6-notes.pdf.

Doran, D., A. S. McCutcheon, M. G. Evans, K. MacMillan, L. McGillis, D. Pringle, S. Smith, and A. Valente. 2004. "Impact of the Manager's Span of Control on Leadership and Performance." [Online article; retrieved 9/18/05.] http://www.chsrf.ca/final_research/ogc/doran2_e.php.

French, J. P., Jr., and B. Raven. 1960. "The Bases of Social Power." In *Group Dynamics*, edited by D. Cartwright and A. Zander, 607–23. New York: Harper and Row.

Graicunas, V. A. 1937. "Relationship in Organization." In *Papers on the Science of Administration*, edited by L. Gulick and L. F. Urwick, 183–87. New York: Columbia University's Institute of Public Administration.

Hamilton, I. 1921. *The Soul and Body of an Army*, 229. Arnold, London: Hamilton.

Peterson, E., E. G. Plowman, and J. M. Trickett. 1962. *Business Organization and Management, Fifth Edition*, 83. Homewood, IL: Richard D. Irwin, Inc.

Urwick, L. F. 1956. "The Manager's Span of Control." *Harvard Business Review* (May–June): 39–47.

Valenstein, P. N., R. Souers, and D. S. Wilkinson. 2004. "Staffing Benchmarks for Clinical Laboratories: A College of American Pathologists Q-Probes Study of Staffing at 151 Institutions." *Archives of Pathology and Laboratory Medicine* 129 (4): 467–73. [Online article; retrieved 9/18/05.] http://arpa.allenpress.com/arpaonline/?request=get-document&doi= 10.1043%2F1543-2165(2005)129%3C467:SBFCLA%3E2.0.CO%3B2.

Weber, M. 1985. "The Three Types of Legitimate Rule." *Berkeley Journal of Sociology* 4: 3–10.

———. 1974. *The Theory of Social and Economic Organizations*, edited by T. Parsons, 324–63. New York: Oxford University Press.

CHAPTER THIRTEEN

Division of Work and Departmentalization

CHAPTER OBJECTIVES

After you have studied this chapter, you should be able to do the following:

1. Describe the importance and benefits of division of work—that is, job specialization.

2. Describe the advantages and disadvantages of departmentalization and departmentalization methods.

3. Explain the supervisor's goal when designing the "ideal" department.

4. Consider alternative models for displaying the organization chart.

AS STATED IN the previous chapter, organizing means deciding how best to group the activities and resources of the organization. Formal organization theory, also as stated earlier, rests on several major principles or premises. Two of these are division of work and departmentalization. Division of work, or job specialization, means the degree to which each task of the organization is broken down into component parts. This is essential for efficiency and for the achievement of objectives.

Departmentalization, or compartmentalization, is the process of grouping many activities into distinct units according to logical arrangements. Departmentalization creates the building blocks for the formal structure, the main network for managing the various activities of the enterprise.

These two major premises of organization are a primary concern of the CEO in a smaller organization or the COO in a larger one. He or she must translate these principles into a formal organizational structure for the institution. Because the application of these formal organizational principles involves all levels of management, it is also necessary for you as a supervisor to understand them and know how they are used. This knowledge helps you in organizing your department and in coordinating its activities with those of the rest of the

MAKING A PIN (NAIL) INVOLVES 18 TASKS

Without Specialization
1 worker doing all 18 tasks yields approximately 20 nails day.
20 workers make 400 nails a day.

With Specialization
20 workers make 100,000 pins (nails) a day.
1 worker makes approximately 5,000 pins (nails) a day.

Source: Smith, A. (1776, 1967). *The Wealth of Nations.* Chicago: Henry Regnery. As viewed on Internet at http://www.fordham.edu/halsall/mod/adamsmith-summary.html.

institution. You will certainly be asked to carry out, and maybe even help make, decisions involving departmentalization and division of work. As you move up in the managerial hierarchy, you will probably be called on to participate in many more such organizational decisions.

DIVISION OF WORK: JOB SPECIALIZATION

Division of work is an age-old practice. Consider the division of work in many tribal societies: women plant and maintain the gardens and wash clothes, while men hunt for food and protect the tribe. *Job specialization* is the degree to which the overall task is broken down and divided into smaller parts. Each part or step of the task may be performed by a different individual. Thousands of years ago, human beings divided work in this manner because they realized a group of people, each performing a small specialized part of the overall job, could accomplish more than the same-size group in which each individual was trying to do the whole job alone. Adam Smith's oft-cited example from 1776 of job specialization in a pin (nail) factory confirms this advantage (see box).

Furthermore, with specialization, each individual learns how to do his or her task exceptionally well, decreases transfer time between tasks, and allows high-skilled workers to concentrate on highly skilled tasks while lesser-skilled workers perform lower-skilled tasks. Additionally, teaching an individual a single task makes employee replacement easier. In other words, the division of work results in greater efficiency and higher production. This explains the mass production capabilities owed to specialization achieved in industrial settings in the United States in the twentieth century. However, excessive specialization can lead to employee boredom. Adam Smith, known as the Father of Economics, stated, "The man whose life is spent in performing simple operations . . . has no occasion to exert his understanding. He generally becomes as stupid and ignorant it is possible for a human creature to become" (Box et al. 1999).

Healthcare organizations, in particular, function under this acceptance of specialization and division of work theory. Continuous advances in medical sciences and technology resulted in greater specialization of professionals, facilities, and equipment and increased fragmentation of the delivery of care. Both healthcare professionals and healthcare organizations continue to attain a high degree of specialization in extremely challenging occupations and service foci. For example, ophthalmologists have attained the same basic specialty training in ophthalmology, some specialize in retinal conditions while others specialize in surgical techniques such as Lasik surgery. One home care agency may specialize in serving newborns, while another agency specializes in serving the geriatric population. Because of the proliferation and specialization of medical sciences and technologies, healthcare centers have become very large and complex organizational structures.

This proliferation of specialties provides clear advantages for patients in terms of their receiving state-of-the-art care. However, this specialization creates problems in administrating healthcare institutions, because of the need for various organizational structures to coordinate the specialties. It also causes problems for the patients who can no longer go to one physician for everything that ails them.

In essence, as the healthcare industry becomes more sophisticated, higher degrees of expertise are required, thus forcing specialization of its professionals and staff. In light of Adam Smith's concern, the impact specialization may have on motivating your workforce is discussed in Part VI of the book.

DEPARTMENTALIZATION

When organizational or specialization growth is such that a single person can no longer personally supervise all personnel in the organization, additional managers are employed and assigned specific employees to supervise. Almost every organization must departmentalize because healthcare organizations are diverse in their workforces and the division of work into such specialized tasks produces a much more efficient operation. As stated, *departmentalization* is the process of grouping various activities into natural units by logical arrangements. A department, by definition, is such a unit; it is a distinct area of activities over which a manager or supervisor has been given authority and for which he or she has accepted responsibility. The terminology may vary and a department may be called a division, service, section, unit, office, bureau, or similar term, but it still represents a closely related set of activities. Departmentalization relies on specialization, which is the core determinant. By departmentalizing the organization, a horizontal grouping of specialized activities is attained.

The major departments in an organization are established by the CEO or COO. The top-level executive is the one that groups the various activities into departments. Some departments established this way are small and require no further subdivision; others are so large that managers have to subdivide their departmental staffs into smaller units, sections, or teams to create an effective span of control. For this reason, every manager must become acquainted with the various alternatives available for grouping activities.

The process of departmentalization can be done on the basis of (1) functions, (2) process and equipment, (3) territory (location), (4) customer (patient), (5) time, or (6) product.

Functions

The most widely accepted practice of departmentalizing is to group activities according to functions[1], or common tasks. All activities that are alike or similar and involve a particular function are placed together into one department under a single chain of command (see Figure 13.1). For instance, all patient care services are placed under the chief nurse executive or all information-generating departments (i.e., health information management, information systems, registration, utilization review, risk management, and patient financial services) may be organized under the chief information officer.

As the institution grows and undertakes additional work, often these new duties are added to the already existing departments. For instance, an addition of an outpatient surgical center, in which surgery is performed with reasonably low risk on patients who do not stay overnight, may logically be assigned to the operating rooms department and its director. However, when we study product- or customer-oriented organizations, this function may be more appropriately placed with ambulatory services. Regardless, such increased activities require adding more employees and levels of supervision within the functional departments, a topic that was discussed in Chapter 12. Occasionally, however, new services may require adding a new department; for example, a rural hospital that purchases several physician practices and a rural health center may need to establish a physician practice management department.

To departmentalize by function is a natural, logical way of arranging various activities. This kind of departmentalization takes advantage of specialization by combining the functions that belong together and that are performed by experts in that functional field with the same type of education, background, equipment, and facilities. The experts for each function are brought together under a supervisor for the area where they can share their common expertise and participate in technical problem solving. Each functional supervisor is concerned with only one type of work and concentrates all of his or her energy on it. This leads to an efficient use of resources and reduces duplication of resources.

Functional departmentalization also facilitates and enhances coordination because one manager is in charge of one type of activity throughout the entire organization. Coordination is easier to achieve in this way than it would be in an organization in which the same function is performed in several different divisions. Another advantage of functional departmentalization is that it makes the outstanding abilities of one or a few individuals available to the enterprise as a whole.

Functional design also facilitates in-depth skill development and allows for clear career paths. For example, an employee may start out at the Technician I level and after a year move up to the Technician II level. If the technician

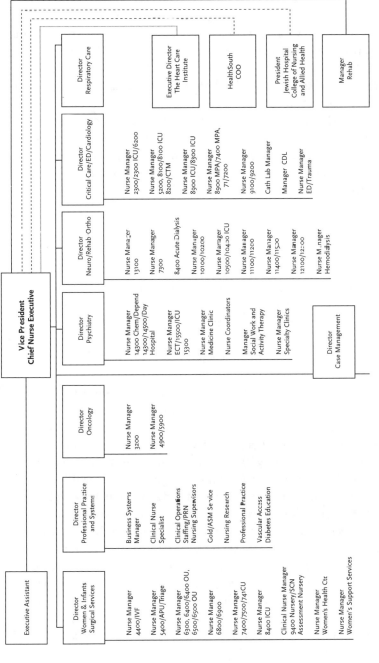

Source: Courtesy of Barnes-Jewish Hospital, St. Louis, MO.

has three or more years of experience, he or she may qualify for the team leader position; after five years, the day supervisor position; and so forth. Eventually, the individual becomes an expert in each of the tasks performed by the department. Because functional departmentalization is a simple and logical method and has all these advantages, it is the most widely used way of setting up departments.

Some disadvantages to functional departmentalization have arisen in large organizations, especially when the undertaking grows in size. It may limit staff's seeing the full picture of the complete process, emphasize routine tasks, and increase boredom. Interdepartmental communication may break down and turf battles may ensue over new services offered. The expertise gained from working in a single department leaves an individual with a narrow perspective or focus on the big picture. If technology advances to such a point that the specialized expertise is no longer needed, the individuals who are very specialized in one area only will be laid off or may require extensive retraining to be used elsewhere in the organization. Finally, department managers may become so protective of their own goals that the organizational goals may be compromised. In a healthcare setting, however, these disadvantages can be minimized by supervisory awareness and therefore should not prevent management from opting for functional departmentalization.

Process and Equipment

Activities can also be grouped around the equipment, process, customer flow, and technology involved. This way of departmentalizing is often found in hospitals because they usually operate sophisticated equipment and handle certain processes that require special installations, training, and expertise. Every task involving the use of certain equipment and technology is then referred to the particular specialized department that is equipped to do the task. This type of organizational structure is similar to functional departmentalization, the major difference being the emphasis on person-machine relationships or a process that supports mass production. For instance, in imaging and nuclear medicine departments, specific equipment is used but only certain functions are performed. Another area in which organizing occurs around equipment is in large laboratories, where the laboratory has discrete sections, each focusing on one high-volume type of testing. Here staff may be assigned to work with the microbiology equipment or the chemistry equipment and remain in this area for their entire career. Organizing by equipment, process, and technology results in the staff becoming very specialized in the defined area, but this is beneficial during disaster situations when patient care services are triaged in large numbers.

Therefore, departmentalization by function and by equipment frequently become closely allied. In fact, within a functional department, one may organize staff by process or equipment. However, it does create disadvantages for management and staff. Because employees are specialized, they may not be able to be used to fill vacancies in other areas or positions because they lack the additional skill sets. Conversely, the employee is limited on positions into which he or she may advance because his or her skill set is technically limited or narrow.

Territory (Location)

An alternative way to departmentalize is according to location (see Figures 13.2 and 13.5). This means setting up departments based on defined geographic areas or sites. The extent of the area may range from the entire hemisphere to a number of cities, a few blocks of a large city, or different floors in the same building. Again, this type of departmentalization is common in national and regional healthcare systems. For example, a hospital or nursing home in a large city may have several physically dispersed units, such as St. Mary's East on one side of town and St. Mary's West on the other. If the same functions are performed in different locations and different buildings, geographic departmentalization is necessary. This type of departmentalization is also common for county health departments and home health agencies. As staff members join the agency, depending on their residence or client load, they are assigned to the agency's office that serves that region. The same considerations are applicable even if all activities are performed in one building but on different floors and wings, such as a medical-surgical nursing unit, third floor, west wing and another on the fourth floor, south wing.

One of the advantages of territorial departmentalization is placing decision making close to where the work is done; managers develop expertise solving problems unique to the location, and managers are familiar with their customers and their problems. This departmentalization has the possible disadvantages of duplications of effort and resources, diverting attention to a given location's goals rather than the organization's, and may require extensive rules or procedures to enable managers to coordinate and ensure uniformity of quality of care between locations. On the other hand, territorial departmentalization provides opportunities for the development of more managerial talent.

Customer (Patient)

At times, management may find it advisable to group activities based on customer (patient) needs and characteristics, hence the term customer (or customer-focused) departmentalization. Two examples of organizations that have departmentalized along customer lines are universities and hospitals. In some universities, night programs and day programs comply with the requests and special needs of the "customers"—namely, part-time and full-time students. With hospitals, certain services and activities are grouped for outpatients and inpatients, such as outpatient surgery. Some healthcare organizations have built entire facilities to specifically serve a patient type, such as women's centers, cancer centers, and children's hospitals. In so doing, the healthcare center delivers its services to more people because the services are less diverse and allow the staff to specialize in treating a certain customer or patient type.

Healthcare services delivered by this approach are on the rise. It is most apparent in the outpatient arena, which has grown rapidly since inpatient prospective payment was implemented and with the advent of new technology. Outpatient services are a significant factor in a hospital's revenue picture and ultimately result in fewer overnight patients.

The customer departmentalization approach offers several advantages, including facilitating the attention to patient (customer) needs by centralizing specialists' focus on a specific patient or condition type and developing managers to become customer advocates. It also has disadvantages such as fostering conflicts over resource allocation, restricting problem-solving skills to a single patient type, possibly contributing to coordination problems between specialties or departments, duplicating resources, and resulting in decisions that please the customer but hurt the company.

Time

Some organizations find it helpful and necessary to group activities according to the period during which they are performed. An enterprise such as a hospital or public utility, which operates around the clock, must departmentalize activities on the basis of time, at least to a certain extent. In other words, the institution must set up different time shifts—usually day, afternoon, and night or only day and night. The many work-time arrangements currently practiced by healthcare personnel may necessitate different time-shift demarcations. Activities typically are grouped first on some other basis, such as by function, and then are organized into shifts. The activities to be performed on the other shifts are largely the same as those performed during the regular day shift. Thus, such groupings often create serious organizational questions of how self-contained each shift should be and what relationships should exist between the regular day-shift supervisors and the off-shift supervisors.

Product

This departmentalization approach is similar to customer departmentalization and has gained acceptance in healthcare institutions often through the establishment of centers of excellence within the organization. To departmentalize on a product basis in industry means that a division is responsible for a single product or group of closely related products so that the emphasis is shifted from the function to the output, or product. For example, a hospital supply company may have a separate department for furniture, another for surgical supplies, and a third for uniforms.

Product departmentalization in a healthcare facility involves the division into departments based on the "product" turned out—for example, maternity, surgery, oncology, cardiology, or psychiatry. Hospitals that have adopted this departmentalization approach often call it a product-line organization. Each such department has its own nursing, dietary, housekeeping, maintenance staffs, and so forth, and each such product department has its own boss—the director of oncology services, the director of maternity, and so on. These directors are in charge of all functions within their product departments, including nursing activities, therapy, food services, laundry, and maintenance. Often decision making is faster in this structure. Having total control over all or most factors allows economic and outcome performance of these individual products to be assessed.

As you can see, such product departmentalization can result in duplication of effort within the organization. Instead of a single director of nursing, there are as many as the number of existing departments. Moreover, coordinating all nursing services and ensuring that the same level of care is rendered throughout the entire organization are difficult because each supervisor reports to a different boss. The same difficulties are found in every department. However, if, for example, a manager is experiencing difficulty recruiting an individual who has a broad set of skills, such as those required to care for babies and the aged, this approach may be helpful but may limit career mobility for these personnel outside their product line.

Additionally, as hospitals have had to compete for market share, they have had to enhance, and to some extent exploit, those areas that are in demand by the population served. Some hospitals have created geographically separate facilities dedicated to one product, such as women's services or mental health services. Furthermore, the increased technology and advances in medicine in some product areas have forced healthcare enterprises to organize by product to permit the manager or product leader to focus on the product, the technology serving it, and the impact of medical advances on its future. Thus, product departmentalization, as practiced in healthcare institutions, also has encouraged specialization, can easily be aligned with customer departmentalization, and presents the same advantages and disadvantages.

MIXED DEPARTMENTALIZATION (COMPOSITE, HYBRID STRUCTURE)

Departmentalization is not an end in itself. In grouping activities, management should not attempt to merely draw a balanced organizational chart. Its prime concern should be to set up departments that help bring about the institution's objectives and coordinate its functions. There are advantages and disadvantages to each method of departmentalization. Choosing a method is a question of balance and deciding which works most effectively. In so doing, management probably has to use multiple departmentalization options and end up with a hybrid structure—that is, a mixed departmentalization; for example, a nursing supervisor (functional) on the surgical unit (subfunction), west wing, third floor (location), during the night (time), in the women's center (customer). In practice, almost all hospitals have this composite type of departmental structure, combining function, location, time, and many other considerations (see Figure 13.2). Any mixture is acceptable, as long as it works and is consistent with the overall objectives of the institution.

ORGANIZING AT THE SUPERVISORY LEVEL

Thus far, we have discussed the organizing process from an overall institutional point of view. We have explored how the chief executive establishes the formal organizational structure and makes it come alive by selecting the right supervisors to whom organizational authority is delegated.

Most department heads and supervisors are not likely to be involved in the major decisions concerning the overall organizational structure of their healthcare institution. However, they are likely to be concerned with the structure of their own department, including departmental goals and objectives, daily operations and activities, and existing personnel and resources.

It should not be surprising to find that the organizing process is basically the same, whether it is performed by the CEO, COO, or first-line supervisor. Organizing involves grouping activities for purposes of departmentalization or subdepartmentalization on the supervisory level; assigning specific tasks and duties; and, most importantly, delegating authority. In essence, this means that the basic organizational principles must be understood and applied by supervisors when they are setting up their own departments, just as they were by the chief administrator when the overall institution was structured. How might a supervisor go about applying these principles, using them on a day-to-day basis so that they are not just abstractions but parts of a healthy departmental body?

Ideal Organization of the Department

Most supervisors are placed in charge of an existing department; only a few have the opportunity to design a structure for a completely new department. When designing or rearranging the organizational structure of the department, the supervisor should conceptualize and plan for the ideal organization. The word "ideal" in this instance is not intended to mean perfect; rather, it is used to mean the most desirable organization for achieving stated objectives. It is the supervisor's job to design an organizational setup that is best for his or her particular department. In so doing, the principles and guides of organizing must be observed. Following these, of course, gives no guarantee that the department will not have any problems. A significant number of problems can be avoided, however, because the organizational network has been designed based on sound and proven principles and is likely to function smoothly in most cases.

The manager must bear in mind that certain organizational concepts and arrangements that work well in a very large organization may not be applicable to a smaller organization as, for example, in a 50-bed hospital, where a supervisor may be supervising two different activities such as purchasing and environmental services. In other words, supervisors must not blindly follow the idea that what is good for one enterprise is also good for another. Moreover, it is not essential that the manager's organizational plans for the department look pretty on paper or that the organizational chart appears symmetrical and well balanced. Rather, this ideal design should represent the most appropriate arrangement for reaching the departmental objectives. It should be uniquely tailored to suit the conditions under which the manager works, instead of some abstract image of what a "perfect" department should look like.

In planning this ideal, but realistic, organization, the supervisor must consider it as something of a standard with which the present organizational setup can be compared. The ideal structure should be looked on as a guide to the short- and long-range plans of the department. Although the supervisor should carefully plan for the ideal structure when becoming the department's manager, this does not mean that the existing organization should be forced to conform to the ideal immediately. Each change in the prevailing organization, however, should bring the existing structure closer to the ideal. In other words, the ideal organization of the department represents the direction in which the supervisor moves as time passes.

Internal Departmental Structure

You may wonder exactly how supervisors would go about designing the ideal departmental structure. In most cases, they are being asked to subdepartmentalize—to establish subdivisions or subunits within their department—just as the chief administrator established the overall divisions or units for the whole organization. Some examples of how a director might subdepartmentalize or set up the internal departmental structure are shown in the organizational charts in Figures 13.1 through 13.3. Organization charts from colleagues at other facilities or from professional journals serve as sources of departmental organizational structures.

More specifically, what supervisors are being asked to do is to consider the groupings of activities in the department, the various existing positions, and the assignment of tasks and duties to these positions. Is this the best possible arrangement for achieving departmental and institutional objectives? Are all the present positions necessary, or could some be eliminated or combined with others? Does each position have a fair assignment of tasks and duties, commensurate with its status and salary? Are the positions related so that there is no duplication of effort and that coordination and cooperation are facilitated? Are there any changes at all that the supervisor would like to see in the internal organizational structure of the department?

Any such changes become the basis for the ideal organization of the department. They become the organizational goals toward which the department head strives when structuring the department.

DEPARTMENTAL ORGANIZATIONAL STRUCTURE

A department can be organized by function, process and equipment, territory, and so on. A department may have sections, divisions, teams, or areas. Your organization may have additional names for these subunits. Each subunit may have a lead employee, team leader, supervisor, or manager, or several subunits

FIGURE 13.2: CAMPUS DEPARTMENTAL STRUCTURE

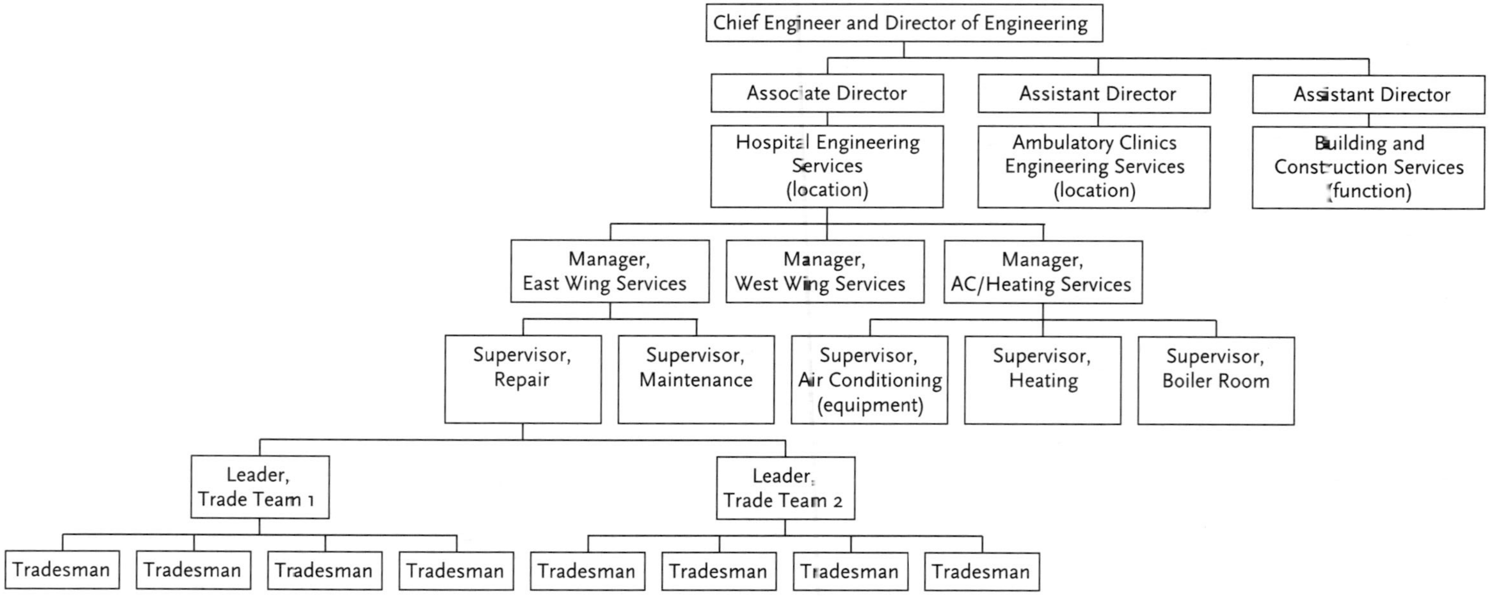

Chief Engineer and Director of Engineering

Associate Director

Assistant Director

Assistant Director

Hospital Engineering Services (location)

Ambulatory Clinics Engineering Services (location)

Building and Construction Services (function)

Manager, East Wing Services

Manager, West Wing Services

Manager, AC/Heating Services

Supervisor, Repair

Supervisor, Maintenance

Supervisor, Air Conditioning (equipment)

Supervisor, Heating

Supervisor, Boiler Room

Leader, Trade Team 1

Leader, Trade Team 2

Tradesman

Tradesman

Tradesman

Tradesman

Tradesman

Tradesman

Tradesman

Tradesman

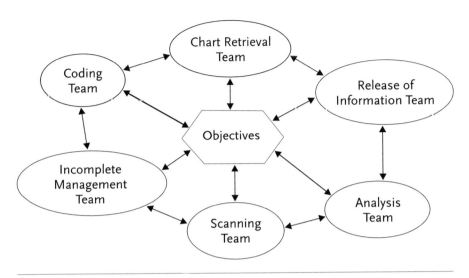

may report to one of these titled individuals. Regardless, the objective of the manager in creating the organizational structure is to ensure that the department's goals are achieved through the proper organization of staff and coordination of duties or work flow. Examples of different departmental structures are given in the following section.

Figure 13.2 displays a departmental structure when the engineering services are centralized under one executive, the chief engineer. He has responsibility for services across a healthcare campus that includes a hospital and several ambulatory clinics. This structure depicts an organizational structure that includes location, equipment, and function models and uses the relatively common titles of director, associate director, assistant director, manager, supervisor, and team leader.

Figure 13.3 depicts a health information management department that has chosen the self-directed team model. Here the manager establishes the objectives but has delegated authority to the teams to achieve the objectives. The manager may use an authority template as explained in Chapter 12, or he or she may have met with each team one-on-one and discussed his or her expectations. To have fully decentralized authority, this manager may even allow each team to select its leader or to choose not to have a leader.

Figure 13.4 is an organizational chart depicting product-line organization. All staff involved in the delivery of surgical services are aligned under the vice president for these services. Note that practitioners with expertise in nutrition, financial management, pharmacy, and so forth are included in this product-line organization.

FIGURE 13.4: PRODUCT-LINE ORGANIZATION

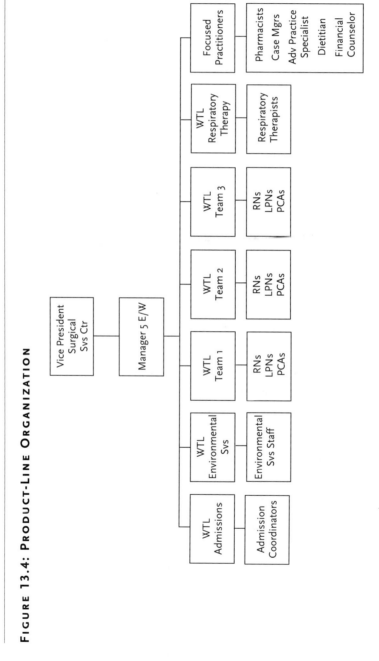

Source: Adapted courtesy of Lakeland Regional Medical Center, Lakeland, FL.

If a supervisor is setting up a new department or working in a newly established institution, much of the ideal structure can probably be implemented in the beginning. This is the most desirable situation, but it is not usually the case. In fact, often the structure that is established at the beginning of a new organization is rapidly changed.

Example of a New Department in a New Organization

Consider the case of a new 80-bed hospital in southwest Florida. The hospital expected to have 25 beds in operation on Day 1 and to be at the 80-bed level within six months. Clearly, the staffing level required for 25 beds was not the same as that required for 80 beds. Furthermore, it was inappropriate to hire staff for 80 beds only to have them be idle for up to six months until the census increased. To manage these staffing challenges, the activities of registration, billing, and health information were initially combined; the positions were titled personal account managers (PAM) (see Figure 13.5). Staff were cross-trained to perform all registration, billing, and health information duties with the exception of coding and transcription. In fact, the staff even obtained the first meal selection from the patient and escorted the patient to the patient care area.

The staff worked 12-hour shifts three days per week and a four-hour shift on any day of their choosing. During peak registration hours the staff performed registration functions; during slow periods or between registrations the staff obtained precertifications or certifications from insurers. Also during slower hours, the staff assembled and analyzed discharged patient records for documentation deficiencies and completed the various billing functions for the day. In the early evening, these same individuals followed up on patient balances for collection purposes. Because they met the patients at the time of admission, staff developed rapport with patients and could check on their at-home recovery progress and report the same to performance improvement.

Generally, the supervisor implements organizational goals gradually while working within the existing departmental structure and with personnel. In this instance, the goals were to ensure the functions were adequately staffed with well-cross-trained individuals who eventually migrated to one specialized function or another as the hospital grew in size and complexity.

ORGANIZATION AND PERSONNEL

The supervisor should design the ideal organization based on sound organizational principles, regardless of the people with whom he or she works. This does not mean that departments can exist without people to staff their various positions. Without people, of course, there can be no organization. The problems of organization should be handled in the right order, however; the sound structure comes first, then the people are asked to fulfill this structure.

FIGURE 13.5: NEW DEPARTMENT

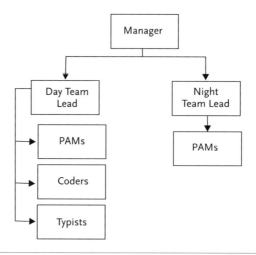

If the department setup is planned first around existing personnel, existing shortcomings are perpetuated. Because of incumbent personalities, too much emphasis may be given to certain activities and not enough to others. Moreover, if a department is structured around personalities, it carries an inherent flaw, which is revealed if a particular employee is promoted or resigns. If, on the other hand, the departmental organization is structured impersonally on the general need for personnel rather than on the incumbent personalities, it should not be difficult to find an appropriate successor for a particular position. Therefore, an organization should be designed first to serve the objectives of the department, then the various employees should be selected and fitted into departmental positions. This, however, is easier said than done.

In most instances, the supervisor has been put into a managerial position in an existing and fully staffed department without having had the chance to decide on the present structure or personnel of the department. Frequently, some of the available employees do not fit well into the ideal structure, but they cannot all be overlooked or dismissed. In such cases, the best the supervisor can do for the time being is to adjust the organization to use the capacities of the employees he or she has. This is an accommodation of the ideal plan to fit present personalities and should be regarded as temporary. Such personnel adjustments are sometimes necessary, but fewer of them are required if the supervisor has already made a plan of the organization he or she would like to have if the ideal human resources were available. Then, as time goes on and attrition naturally occurs, the supervisor can strive to come closer and closer to the ideal departmental setup.

ORGANIZATIONAL DESIGN

So far the discussion of organizational structure has centered around what is often called traditional structure. *Traditional structure* is the most often used in all types of organized activities. It is the most studied and researched form of organization and has a long history of successful performance. Traditional structure is a contemporary design and is not inflexible or rigid. This structure functions successfully under most prevailing conditions and is capable of producing and accommodating change and adapting to contingencies as they arise.

Of course, even the best-designed organization cannot be left without change forever. Changes in technology, care delivery systems, the environment, human and social processes, organizational size, the workforce, economic trends, regulatory activities, and so forth have to be accommodated. The institution must design a structure that works best under these contingencies. The organization is an open system, which means that every change in one part of it affects the activity in another part. The organizational concepts discussed thus far are applicable even under those new contingencies. An example of this flexibility is the recent matrix design of organization, as discussed in the next section.

Matrix Organization (Matrix Design)

One of the newer organizational structures building on traditional concepts is the *matrix organization*. This is an organization structure in which employees have two bosses—one at the department to which they are permanently assigned and one that is directing a service or product over several geographic areas or a special project. Matrix organization, also known as project or grid organization, does not do away with the traditional organization; it simply builds on it and, under certain contingencies, improves on it. It is superimposed on functional organization, creating a grid, or a matrix. Thus, it provides horizontal dimensions to the traditional vertical orientation of the functional organization. It is an organizational design that typically combines technical expertise found in one of the other departmentalization models and product model simultaneously.

Figure 13.6 is the organizational chart of a national managed care organization (MCO). This example shows us a matrix organization for the utilization review function of the MCO. The structure violates unity of command, however; for this organization it is imperative that utilization review policies are consistently applied nationwide. Therefore, the corporate utilization review's vice president's responsibility is to ensure this occurs, and he or she must have some authority to impose standard rules and procedures on the regional operations. Day-to-day oversight and control of these functions rests with the regional vice president. This structure can be used in a diversified healthcare provider as well. For example, consider the JCAHO expectation for consistent nursing practice throughout a healthcare organization that has multiple outlying clinics, an

FIGURE 13.6: UTILIZATION REVIEW MATRIX

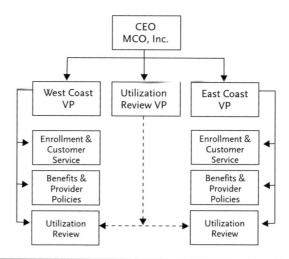

ambulatory surgery center, home health agency, community urgent care centers, and a hospital. The chief nurse executive must have authority to mandate certain nursing practices to ensure compliance with JCAHO's standard. In this scenario, a matrix organization may be best to meet this objective.

During recent years, high-technology industries found a need to create project organizations to focus resources and special talents for a given time on a specific project. For example, if the organization were emphasizing oncology (cancer) care, the oncology division brought in the dietitian, radiation therapy technicians, pharmacists, nurses, pastors, lab technicians, and physicians who specialized in cancer care together from their base departments. These members defined the services to offer to cancer patients. They then developed the plans, recruited the staff needed, organized the functions needed to serve the patients, and delivered the care. Management and the customer became increasingly interested in the end result—cancer care (the product).

The essence of matrix management is a compromise between functional and product departmentalization in the same organizational structure. Figure 13.7 shows a matrix arrangement in a healthcare institution in which the functional managers are in charge of their professional function, with an overlay of two project managers (A and B) who are responsible for the end product—a specific project.

The concept of matrix organization gives an enterprise the potential capacity to conduct several projects simultaneously. For example, the president of the hospital sees the need for three projects to be phased into the institution within the next two years, such as a unit-dose pharmaceutical system, an electronic record system that supports the clinics and the hospital, and preparation for the hospital's accreditation. These three projects could be assigned to three different

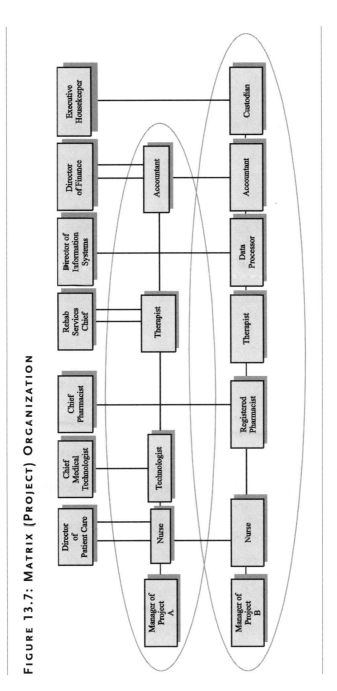

project managers, and matrix organizations could be established for obtaining these objectives.

By establishing a project organization, better coordination can be achieved than would be possible in a traditional organizational structure. As the project proceeds, it is assigned to a project manager from the beginning to its completion, and people from the functional areas needed for this project are assigned either on a full- or part-time basis. The matrix is an overlay on conventional structure; it draws on traditional structure for the various skills required for the project. When the project is finished, the project manager and specialized personnel return to their functional departments or are reassigned to a new project.

The advantages of matrix organization are that it

1. provides an effective way to focus on new products and customers and phase new projects in and out of operation;
2. improves coordination and establishes lateral relationships;
3. offers greater flexibility to consider and implement innovative ideas;
4. creates teams of experts quickly to cope with a sudden change or need;
5. dissolves teams without too much repercussion on the overall structure;
6. exposes members of a project to interaction with experts from other areas, thus offering an opportunity for personal development;
7. identifies individuals who may be selected to serve in future leadership positions; and
8. affords top-level management an additional way to delegate and decentralize.

Matrix design also creates a number of problems. Most result from the team members finding that during the project, their roles have not been clearly defined. Matrix organization is a system in which employees are supervised by two bosses, namely their functional director and the project manager. This structure clearly violates one of the major principles listed in Chapter 12—unity of command. The professional, when assigned to a project, may be faced with duality of command because conflicting directives may come from the two bosses. Additionally, the employees on the project may not be certain to whom they are supposed to report and whose assignments take priority, or worse there may be power struggles between the individual's two bosses. More confusion can arise when one person is assigned part-time to two or more projects.

Further sources of frustration for the professional are that while assigned to the project, he or she may also feel isolated from the mainstream of his or her expertise or home department and penalized by the assignment because evaluations and possible promotion opportunities are usually vested in the functional department head and not in the project manager.

Most of these problems are caused by poor coordination, project preparation, and a lack of concise and clear statements of authority relationships. Well-prepared projects should have the following attributes:

- At the start of the project, the enterprise executive should try to clarify these relationships. He or she should clarify the authority and responsibility of the functional directors.
- The project manager should have full authority and responsibility over the integrity of the design and over the budget. He or she must act as decision maker and coordinator for the duration of the project.
- There must be clear statements about the project manager's frequency of reporting and the scope of the project.
- The project manager must decide on schedules and work out priorities with the functional managers.
- The functional managers should be responsible for the integrity of the service or products that their departments supply to the project.
- Statements concerning these decisions and responsibilities are necessary to guide the project manager and the functional managers whose departments are involved in the project.

Despite the best preparations and clarifications, misunderstandings may still arise. Provisions to resolve such a dilemma should probably be made by referring the misunderstanding or dispute to higher management. Thorough preparation and clarifying authority and responsibility when the project is established minimize many of these problems. Some borderline cases involving problems of dual command may still arise. Remember that all organizational structures can create some problems occasionally. Matrix organization provides a system with a contemporary proven method of implementing a complex new task that has relatively short duration.

Contemporary Approaches to Organizational Structure

Two additional and contemporary organizational approaches appear in the literature: mechanistic and organic (Burns and Stalker 1961). While classified as *organization structures*, they speak more to the *culture* or *atmosphere* established within any of the structures discussed in this chapter. Setting the tone for an organization starts at the top. Recognizing that labels have been created to define these tones is an important lesson for supervisors to learn, as these labels may affect recruitment and retention of talented staff.

A *mechanistic organization* is a structure that is characterized by high specialization, extensive departmentalization, narrow spans of control, many rigid rules and regulations, limited information network, and authority vested in a few higher-level executives. Those who have seen Charlie Chaplin's *Modern Times* know what this type of organization feels like for employees and managers alike. Whereas the organic structure, occasionally called the thinking structure, is one in which jobs tend to be very general; few rules and regulations exist; communication is vertical, diagonal, and horizontal; and the organization is highly adaptive and flexible and encourages decentralized decision making by the employees.

No one culture or structure works for any organization. Common sense helps the manager design the best one and create a culture that encourages productivity and employee satisfaction.

ORGANIZATIONAL CHARTS

Many conflicts in organizations are often caused by the employees not understanding their assignments and those of their coworkers. Proper use of organizational charts, manuals, and job descriptions defining authority and informational relationships helps to substantially reduce misunderstandings and to clarify doubts. The healthcare institution's structure is formalized graphically in charts and in words in the manual. To be helpful, these tools must be available all the time and be up-to-date, which means changes must be incorporated promptly.

Organizational charts are a means of illustrating the organizational structure at a given time—as a snapshot. The chart shows the skeleton of the structure, depicting the basic formal relationships and groupings of positions and functions; that is, it maps the lines of decision-making authority. Most of the time, the chart starts out with the individual position as the basic unit, which is shown as a rectangular box. Each box represents one function. The various boxes are interconnected horizontally to show the groupings of activities that make up a department, division, or whatever part of the organization is under consideration. They are connected vertically to show scalar relationships. Thus, one can readily determine who reports to whom merely by studying the position of the boxes in their scalar relationships.

Advantages

As the organizational chart is prepared, the organization must be carefully analyzed. Such analysis might uncover structural faults and duplications of effort, complexities, or other inconsistencies. Cases of dual-reporting relationships (one person reporting to two superiors) or overlapping positions might also be uncovered. Moreover, charts might indicate whether the span of supervision is too wide or too narrow, and an unbalanced organization can also be readily revealed.

Charts offer a simple way to acquaint new members with the organizational makeup and with their fit into the entire structure. Most employees have a keen interest in knowing where they stand, in what relation their supervisor stands to the higher echelons, and so on. Charts are also helpful in human resources administration; they can indicate possible routes of promotions for managers as well as for other employees.

Another advantage of charts is they assist in developing better communications and relations. Charts can also be valuable for future planning purposes. A supervisor may want to have two charts for his or her department, one showing the existing arrangements and the other depicting the ideal organization. The latter may be used so that all the gradual changes planned fall within the design of the ideal, representing the ultimate organizational goal of the department in the future. Charting shows what is changing and how that change affects the members of the organization.

Limitations

Charts also pose some limitations, especially if they are not constantly kept up-to-date. It is imperative that organizational changes be recorded speedily, or they are of little practical use. Another shortcoming of charts is that the information they give is limited. A chart is a snapshot, not a CT scan; it shows only what is on the surface, not the inner workings of the structure. It shows only formal authority relationships, not the many informal relationships that exist (see Chapter 18). The chart also does not show the amount of authority and responsibility inherent in each position.

Another problem with charts is that individuals confuse authority relationships with status. Sometimes people read into charts and come up with interpretations that are not intended. For example, a person may interpret an employee's degree of power and status by checking how distant that person's position is on the chart from the box of the CEO, or on which level it is shown. Despite these shortcomings, charts are very useful tools for every member of the organization.

Finally, some charts are so complex that they end up confusing the employees. To determine if your organization chart is too complex, ask your employees to identify their position and then work their way up to the individual to whom you report. If they cannot, then reevaluate the chart.

Types of Charts

Three main types of charts commonly used are vertical, horizontal, and circular. Of these, the vertical chart is used most often in organized activities.

A *vertical chart* shows the different levels of the organization in a step arrangement in the form of a pyramid. The CEO is placed at the top of the chart, and the successive levels of administration are depicted vertically in the pyramid shape. One of the main advantages of the vertical chart is that it can be easily read and understood. It also shows clearly the downward flow of delegation of authority, chain of command, functional relationships, and the relationships of those activities. Many of the general shortcomings of charts apply to vertical charts as well.

In addition to the vertical chart, some healthcare institutions may occasionally prefer a *horizontal chart*, which reads from left to right (see Figure 13.8). The advantage of a horizontal chart is that it stresses functional relationships and minimizes hierarchical levels. The left-to-right chart of a matrix or project organization is a combination of these two arrangements. Horizontal relationships are superimposed on the vertical chart.

A *circular chart* can also be used. It depicts the various levels in concentric circles rotating around the top-level administrator, who is at the hub of the wheel (see Figure 13.9). Positions of equal importance are on the same concentric circle. This graphic portrayal eliminates the need to place positions at the bottom of the chart.

A few organizations might prefer an inverted pyramid chart, showing the chief administrator at the bottom and the associate administrators farther up. This type tries to express the idea of the "support" given to each manager by the "superior" (see Figure 13.10).

SUMMARY

Management's overall organizing function is to design a formal structural framework that enables the institution to achieve its objectives. The CEO or COO establishes this framework initially, using the basic principles of formal organizational theory as guidelines. He or she begins with the principle that specialization is necessary for efficiency. This means grouping the various activities into distinct departments or divisions, assigning specific duties to each which, in turn, then assigns the tasks to multiple workers to work on simultaneously. The administrator can approach this departmentalizing effort in several ways. The most widely used concept of departmentalization is grouping activities according to functions—that is, placing all those who perform the same functions into the same department. Besides departmentalization by functions, it is possible to departmentalize by process and equipment, geographical (territorial) lines, customers (patients), time (shift), or product. However, a composite or hybrid structure made up of several of these alternatives is most often used.

Organizing on the departmental level involves the same general steps as organizing the overall institution—that is, grouping activities or subdepartmentalizing, assigning specific tasks and duties, and delegating authority. The supervisor should supplement these steps, however, by designing an ideal organizational structure specifically for his or her particular department. Such a structure represents the way the supervisor would organize the unit if starting from scratch and given ideal resources and personnel. In most cases, however, the supervisor comes into an existing department and cannot immediately implement an ideal organizational design. One reason may be that the available personnel do not fit into this model. What must be done instead is to plan changes or completely reorganize the department to make it come closer to the ideal. Such reorganization is a normal and important part of managerial life; however, it should not be done so frequently that it undermines the security and morale of employees. Organizational changes can be implemented either all at once or gradually, depending on the imminence of the need for them.

One of the newer developments in organizational design is the matrix organization. This stresses horizontal relationships and combines functional and product departmentalization. Matrix design is employed for achieving a special project with a definite result by superimposing a matrix over the traditional

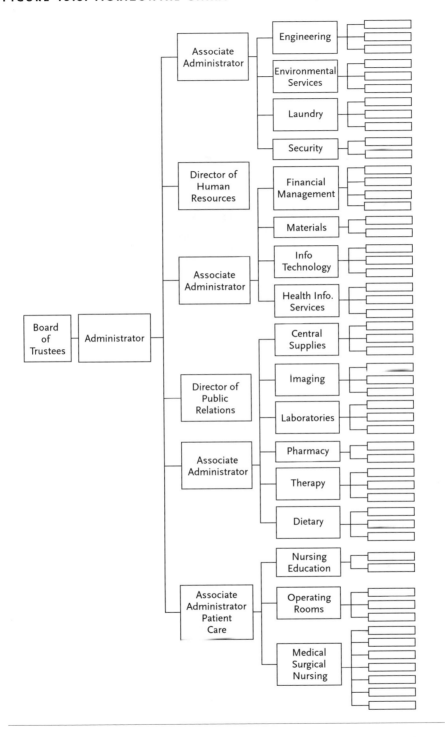

Chapter 13: Division of Work and Departmentalization 231

FIGURE 13.9: CIRCULAR CHART

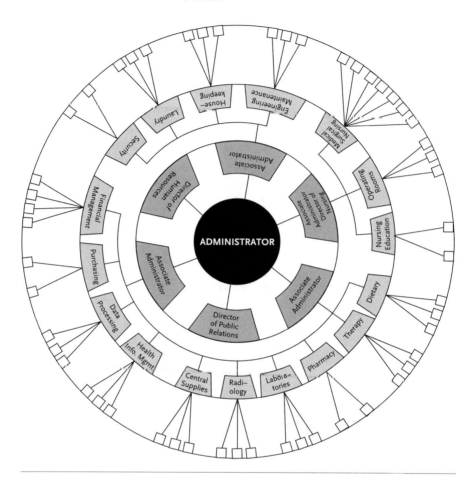

FIGURE 13.10: INVERTED PYRAMID CHART

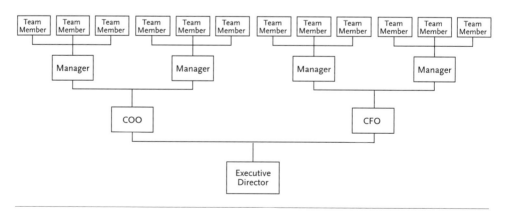

organizational structure. At the project's inception, the CEO or COO must state the authority relationships to the project manager in charge, the functional personnel assigned to the project for the duration, and their functional department heads. This is necessary to minimize possible problems of dual command, dual allegiance, and other conflicts.

Two additional and contemporary organizational approaches—mechanistic and organic—while classified as organization structures, speak more to the culture or atmosphere established within any of the structures discussed in this chapter.

NOTE

1. The term function in this context is used to connote organizational activities such as nursing, pharmacy, laboratories, dietetics, therapy, and environmental services rather than the basic managerial functions of planning, organizing, etc.

REFERENCES

Box, T. A., T. A. West, L. R. Watts, and M. L. Whisman. 1999. "Learning Organizations: Panacea or Partial Answer?" *Academy of Strategic and Organizational Leadership Journal* 3 (2): 57–58.

Burns, T., and G. M. Stalker. 1961. *The Management of Innovation.* London: Tavistock.

CHAPTER FOURTEEN

Delegation of Organizational Authority

CHAPTER OBJECTIVES

After you have studied this chapter, you should be able to do the following:

1. Discuss authority as the lifeblood of the managerial position, and describe how the flow of authority throughout the organizational structure makes it operative.

2. Explain how delegating authority is key to creating an organization.

3. Define delegation of authority.

4. Describe the concepts of the scalar chain and unity of command.

5. Distinguish between authority and responsibility.

6. Describe the spectrum of delegation with centralization on one end and decentralization at the other end.

7. Identify some barriers to delegation.

THE FORMAL ORGANIZATIONAL structure, as stated in the previous chapter, is based on the division of labor and departmentalization. Once this has been accomplished, the second essential step for creating an organization is delegation of authority. *Delegation* is the conferring or granting of authority from superior to subordinate to act as a representative of the superior. Authority is the lifeblood of the managerial position; without authority the manager's job is meaningless. In turn, the process of delegating authority breathes life into the organizational structure: the same process of delegation that brings authority to the manager is used to delegate it farther down the line of command. As managerial responsibilities are divided, additional levels in the chain of command are created. The degree to which authority is delegated throughout the institution indicates the extent of decentralization.

THE MEANING OF DELEGATION

Delegation of authority makes the organization operative. Although the formal structure of an organization may have been meticulously designed by the administrator and carefully explained in manuals and charts, the organization still does not have life until and unless authority is delegated throughout its entire structure. Through this process of delegation, the subordinate manager receives authority from the superior. In other words, if authority was not delegated, there would be no subordinate managers and thus no one to occupy the various levels, departments, and positions that make up the organizational structure. Only in delegating authority to subordinate managers is the organization actually created. Only with such delegation can the administration vest a subordinate with a portion of its own authority, thereby setting in motion the entire managerial process and life of the organization.

Delegation of authority, however, does not mean that the boss surrenders all of his or her authority. The delegating manager always retains the overall authority to perform his or her functions. If necessary, all or part of the authority granted to a subordinate manager can be revoked and reallocated. A good comparison can be made between delegating authority and imparting knowledge in school: a schoolteacher shares knowledge with the students, who then possess this knowledge as well, but the teacher still retains the knowledge.

The Scalar Chain (Chain of Command)

The line of vertical authority relationships from superior to subordinate is the *scalar chain*, or the chain of command. Through the process of delegation formal authority is distributed throughout the organization. It flows downward from the authority at the top, through the various levels of management, to the supervisor, and from there possibly to lower line supervisors. The broad authority necessary to run a private healthcare organization is usually delegated by the board of directors or trustees to the president (administrator or CEO), who in turn must delegate authority to subordinate managers (vice presidents), who then delegate authority to department directors, who then delegate to section managers, and so forth.

An entity's organization chart should pictorially display the scalar chain for all employees to see to whom a person reports and from where their authority and assignments come. Solid lines typically represent line authority, while dashed or dotted lines may represent staff or matrix authority. Line and staff authority relationships are discussed in Chapter 15.

The chain of command must be clearly understood by every subordinate and must be closely adhered to, or the risk exists of undermining authority. By the time this flow of authority reaches the supervisory level, it probably has narrowed considerably, thus focusing the supervisor's range of authority on the function for which he or she is responsible (see Figure 12.1). Nevertheless, it can

FIGURE 14.1: CHAIN OF COMMAND

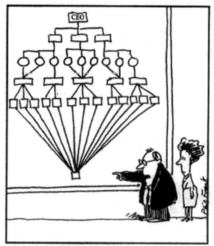

"On the hospital's organizational chart, you're right there, Mrs. Finkle. You report to everyone."

Source: Reprinted from *Hospitals & Health Networks,* Vol. 73, No. 10, by permission, October 1999, © 1999, by Health Forum, Inc.

be traced directly upward to the top executive where authority is at its broadest scope.

Consider the following example. Most organizations have a finance division headed by the chief financial officer (CFO). This individual may have authority to sign contracts and authorize expenditures up to $500,000. The division may have several departments, including accounting, patient billing, accounts payable, cashiering, and auditing. Each department leader (manager or director) also may have contract signing privileges and expenditure authorization limits, generally at a substantially lower level, perhaps to $50,000. Amounts above $50,000 to $500,000 must be approved by the CFO, and amounts above $500,000 must be approved by his or her superior, the CEO. Farther down the chain of command, the accounts payable clerk has no contract signing privileges nor expenditure authorization rights. Everything he or she processes has been authorized by someone more superior in rank.

These scalar relationships are based on positional authority, as discussed in Chapter 12. They are also based on another important managerial principle—unity of command.

Unity of Command

Delegation of authority flows from a single superior to a single subordinate. Each subordinate reports and is accountable to only one superior—namely, that person from whom he or she receives authority. This is known as *unity of command*. A superior manager can have a number of subordinates reporting to him or her (span of control), but for each of these subordinates, the one-to-one relationship (unity of command) still prevails.

The scalar chain provides the major route along which the process of delegation moves. Unity of command is a critical organizational concept; it enables the administration to coordinate activities, pinpoint responsibility and accountability, and define and clarify superior-subordinate relationships. Whenever the principle of unity of command is violated or compromised, management must anticipate complications; we discussed some of these in the matrix model in Chapter 13. Some complications appear as employee frustration because of conflicting directives, others in staff turnover; poor employee morale may surface as well.

THE PROCESS OF DELEGATION[1]

Every manager must be thoroughly familiar with the process of delegation. It consists of three components, all of which must be present. These three components are inseparably related, so that a change in one of them requires an adjustment of the other two. The three essential parts of the delegating process are as follows:

1. the assignment of duties and the defining of the results expected by a manager to the immediate subordinates;
2. the granting of permission (authority) to the subordinates to make decisions and commitments, use resources, and take all the actions normally necessary to perform their assigned duties; and
3. the creation of an obligation (responsibility) on the part of each subordinate to the delegating superior to perform the assigned duties satisfactorily (accountability).

Unless all three of these steps are taken, the success of the delegating process cannot be ensured. This is true no matter which level of management is doing the delegating. The chief administrator does the initial delegation when he or she groups activities, sets up departments, and assigns staff their duties. All managers, from the chief administrator down to the line supervisors, must do their part in delegating authority throughout the entire organization. The managers of each department or division must subdivide and reassign these duties within their own section and at the same time delegate the appropriate amount of authority and exact responsibility to carry them out. In addition, whether it is the chief administrator who delegates authority to the associate administrators and directors, or the line supervisor who delegates authority to a team of nonmanagerial subordinates, the steps in the process of delegation are the same.

Delegation of Authority on the Supervisory Level

Once a supervisor has organized or reorganized the department's structure, or at least planned the changes that are needed and recorded them in an ideal organizational design or position description, he or she is ready to delegate or redelegate authority in accordance with the organizational structure. We assume that the supervisor has been given sufficient authority and that he or she is in charge of all the activities within this section. Just as other managers, supervisors must delegate some of their authority. If this is not done, an organization has not been created. Specifically, the supervisor must assign tasks, grant authority, and create responsibility within each of the subunits and for each of the positions in the department.

Assigning Duties

In assigning duties, the supervisor determines how the work in the department is to be divided among the subordinates and the supervisor. All the tasks that must be accomplished in the department are considered; the supervisor decides which ones he or she can assign to a subordinate and which he or she must do.

First, the supervisor should assign routine duties that can be done by any subordinate. Second, he or she should assign duties that require special knowledge to those subordinates who are particularly qualified for the tasks. Third, the supervisor must decide which functions he or she only should perform. Hence, delegation is the process by which managers assign a portion of their duties and resources to perform these duties to others.

It is better that the assignments be justified and explained on the basis of logical guidelines, rather than on personal likes and dislikes or hunch and intuition. Ensman (1999) suggests delegating by task (e.g., picking up reports), by process (e.g., reconciling inventory), and by absence (tasks individuals can do in your absence). Assigning duties logically is important because the supervisor needs to explain his or her delegations. Some subordinates want to do more work, whereas others believe that they should not be burdened with certain duties. Thus, despite the guidelines, the supervisor should anticipate some difficulty deciding who should do a certain task.

By considering such factors, the supervisor should be able to assign work so that everybody gets a fair share and can do his or her part satisfactorily. One way of doing this is to assign the activity to employees who are involved with the duties most of the time. To achieve this fair distribution of work, the supervisor must clearly understand the nature and the content of the work to be accomplished. Furthermore, one must be thoroughly acquainted with the capabilities of the employees. All this is not as simple as it might appear at first. The supervisor is often inclined to assign an activity or more challenging tasks to those employees who have the skills and interest and are more capable because they are the ones who best carry out the activity and doing so is the easiest solution. In the long run, however, it is far more advantageous to train the less-capable employees so that they also can perform the more difficult jobs. If the manager relies heavily on one person or a few persons, the department is bound to be in a bad situation in the manager's absence. By building up the strength and experience (cross training) of all the employees, the supervisor's problems of assigning various duties become simpler.

The manner and extent to which the supervisor assigns duties to the employees significantly affect the degree to which the employees respect and accept the supervisor's authority (see acceptance authority theory in Chapter 12). Much of the manager's success depends on his or her skill in making assignments and defining expectations. Recall Barnard's communication recommendation from Chapter 2, which includes four conditions that must be met for an individual to accept a directive as authoritative. First, the person must understand the communication. Second, that person must believe that what is to be done is consistent with the organization's purpose. Third, the work is something that the person has a personal interest in. Fourth, the person is mentally and physically able to comply with the communication. However, the first step in delegating authority is to assign certain tasks or duties to each subordinate.

Granting Authority

The second essential part in the process of delegation is granting authority—that is, granting permission to make decisions and commitments, use resources, and take all actions necessary to get the job done. As pointed out earlier, duties are assigned and authority is delegated to positions within the institution rather than to people. Because these positions are staffed by people, however, one typically refers to delegating authority to subordinates instead of to subordinate positions.

To be more specific, granting authority means that a supervisor confers on the subordinates the right and power to act and make decisions within a predetermined and limited area. The manager always must determine in advance the scope of authority that is to be delegated. The range of delegated authority is usually specific when a task is routine and more general when the task is less formalized.

How much authority can be delegated depends on the amount of authority that the delegating manager possesses and on the type of job to be done. Generally, enough authority must be granted to the subordinate to perform what is expected adequately and successfully. There is no need for the degree of authority to be greater than necessary, but it must be sufficient to get the job done. If employees are expected to fulfill the tasks assigned to them and make reasonable decisions for themselves within this area, they must have enough authority to perform.

The degree of authority delegated is intrinsically related not only to the duties assigned but also to the results expected. Whenever management delegates authority, it is necessary to inform the subordinate of the expected results. For example, the employee should know what you expect, when you expect it, how much is expected, in what condition or format, and what resources may be available for him or her to complete the project. Do not expect perfection on the first project. Your subordinate learns from his or her mistakes, as do we all. Delegation is a process that facilitates grooming. Grooming also takes time.

If a supervisor is taking over an existing department consisting of a large and substantial number of employees, broad delegation of authority probably is in effect. It still is necessary, however, to check carefully whether the level of authority latitude is consistent with the ideal organizational plans. The supervisor should check the amount and type of authority delegated to each position and whether the three essential steps in the process of delegation were followed.

At this point, it is sufficient to say that you as a supervisor must be specific in telling each employee just what authority he or she has and what results are expected while exercising that authority. If this is not stated clearly, the subordinate has to guess how far the authority extends, probably by trial and error. As a supervisor, you may have experienced this confusion when your own boss was not explicit about how much authority you really had. To avoid this from happening to your subordinates, you should explain the scope of authority and results you expect and then trust that the employee will do a good job. These assignments are opportunities for you to groom or develop a subordinate into a member of the management team. As time goes on, less explanation will be necessary.

On the other hand, consider the situation in which the number of employees in the supervisor's department is rather small. Such a department consists merely of a supervisor and a few (three to six) employees. The supervisor may wonder if in these circumstances it is necessary to delegate authority. The answer is yes. Even in a small department, the supervisor needs someone who can be depended on to take over if the supervisor should have to leave either temporarily or for any length of time. Even in the smallest department, there should be someone who can work as the supervisor's backup.

It is a sign of poor supervision when no one in a department can take over when the supervisor is sick or has to be away from the job. The supervisor also may miss a promotion because there is nobody to take charge of the unit. Thus, sooner or later every supervisor needs a backup, understudy, next-in-command, or assistant. The supervisor needs to identify potential candidates in the workforce and begin their training. As with any other new initiative, the department manager should always discuss this intention with his or her immediate boss as well. In addition, because of compensation and job description changes that may be necessary down the road, it is beneficial to involve a human resources staff person for guidance. These staff experts may be able to provide guides for your selection process and may have evaluation tools you can use in your assessment of subordinates' strengths for this important role.

Remember that when authority is delegated you remain accountable for the outcome. Therefore, it is advisable for you and helpful to your subordinates to have checkpoints to see how the project is progressing and for them to recognize that you are holding them accountable for completing the assignment as agreed. Furthermore, remember that if you change an employee's job assignment, you must check to see that the degree of authority you have given is still appropriate. If it is more than needed, you may have to revoke some of the delegated authority. Whenever conditions and circumstances of an employee's job change, he or she needs additional clarification of the scope of authority.

The Exception Principle   Although the scope of authority clearly delineates the area of decision making, the supervisor may be confronted by a problem beyond and outside of this area. Then the *exception principle* comes into play. These problems are exceptions and must be referred to the supervisor's delegating manager for decision making. The latter must make certain that this is truly an exception because a danger exists that some subordinate managers may refer too many decisions upward when their own authority is sufficient. In those situations, the superior should refrain from deciding and refer the problem back to the subordinate manager. If it is truly an exception, however, and is beyond the scope of the subordinate's authority, the superior manager must make the decision.

Only One Boss   In granting authority, the principle of unity of command must be followed. Employees must be reassured that all orders and all positional authority can come only from the immediate supervisor, the only boss they have. This principle should be stressed, as situations do occur in which two superiors issue directives and delegate authority to one subordinate. Dual command is bound to lead to unsatisfactory performance by the employee, and it definitely results in confusion about lines of formal authority. The subordinate does not know which of the two "bosses" has the authority that can contribute most to his or her success and progress within the organization. Eventually, such a situation results in conflicts and organizational difficulties.

Revoking Delegated Authority   As stated before, delegating authority does not mean that management has divested itself of its authority. The delegating manager still retains authority and the right to revoke whatever part of the authority he or she delegated to a subordinate. Occasionally, as activities change, a need arises to take a fresh look at the organization and to realign authority relationships. Managers frequently speak of reorganizing, realigning, reshuffling, and so forth. What is meant by these terms is the revoking of authority and reassignment of it elsewhere. Naturally, such realignments of authority should not take place too often because frequent changes create uncertainty, which affects morale. However, periodic reviews of authority delegations are advisable and are necessary in any organization. This applies to top-level administration as well as to the lowest-level manager.

If recentralization of authority is called for, authority must be revoked or realigned. This is a form of reorganization that presents a difficult task for the supervisor because feelings of suspicion, hurt, discouragement, and insecurity on the part of the subordinate are likely to surface. To mitigate these tensions, the supervisor must explain the reasons for this action. Such an unpleasant situation can be lessened by taking great care when choosing a subordinate to whom to delegate authority in the first place.

Because organizing is a dynamic process, it should be emphasized that regardless of the difficulties and unpleasant aspects involved, a supervisor must make organizational adjustments occasionally to keep the department as viable as possible.

Creating Responsibility

The third major aspect of delegating authority is creating an obligation on the part of the subordinate toward the boss to perform the assigned duties satisfactorily. The *acceptance* of this obligation creates responsibility. Without responsibility, the process of delegation is not complete.

The terms responsibility and authority are closely related. Both terms are often misused and misunderstood. Although you may hear phrases such as "keeping subordinates responsible," and "delegating responsibility," these phrases do not describe the actual situation because they imply that responsibility is handed down from above, whereas it really is accepted from below.

Responsibility is the obligation accepted or agreed to by the subordinate to perform the duty as required by the superior. By accepting a job and accepting the obligation to perform the assigned tasks, an employee implies acceptance of responsibility. This responsibility cannot be arbitrarily imposed on a person; rather, it results from a mutual agreement in which the employee agrees to accomplish the duties in return for rewards. Thus, although the authority to perform duties flows from management to subordinate, the responsibility to accomplish these duties clearly flows in the opposite direction, from the subordinate to management. Once an assignment and resources are delegated to a subordinate, allow the employee to establish his or her own plan of action. This allows you to judge planning and decision-making skills.

It is essential to bear in mind, however, that responsibility, unlike authority, cannot be delegated. Responsibility cannot be shifted. Your subordinate accepts responsibility, but you still have it as well. The supervisor can assign a task and delegate the authority to perform a specific job to a subordinate. However, the supervisor does not delegate responsibility in the sense that once the duties are assigned, the supervisor is relieved of the responsibility for these tasks. A supervisor can delegate authority to a subordinate, but not responsibility. See Figure 14.2.

The healthcare administrator must delegate a great deal of authority to the associate administrators for them to oversee the performance of various tasks

FIGURE 14.2

EXAMPLE OF DELEGATION OF AUTHORITY VERSUS RESPONSIBILITY

The Board approves funding for the renovation of an area of the hospital for a new medical staff lounge and library. The chief of the medical staff is notified of the approval. Additionally, the chairman of the board tells the CEO to proceed. The CEO accepts the authority to spend the funds authorized for this purpose.

The CEO asks the VP of Construction and Design for the hospital to design the lounge and library. The VP and CEO agree on a date when the preliminary drawing and cost estimates must be completed and presented to the medical staff.

The VP needs the square footage and current layout of the vacated gift shop, which will be used for the new medical staff lounge and library. He asks his draftsman to measure and provide a perimeter drawing of the area. The draftsman agrees to do so, but with all the holiday activities going on around the hospital, he forgets to do it.

The VP is unable to complete the drawings and cost estimates in time for the meeting with the medical staff. The chief of the medical staff complains to the chairman of the board.

In each step, authority has been granted and accepted. Ultimate responsibility for doing the project rests with the board, but one can be certain that others in the chain of command will be reminded of their failure to meet their obligations.

and services. These associate administrators, in turn and of necessity, have to delegate a large portion of their authority to the managers below them, but none of them delegates any responsibility. Each still accepts all the responsibility for the tasks originally assigned. Similarly, when you as a supervisor are called on by your boss to explain the performance within your department, you cannot plead as a defense that you have delegated the responsibility for such activity to some employee. You may have delegated the authority, but you have remained responsible and must answer to your boss.

Every supervisor should clearly understand this vital difference between authority and responsibility. When managers delegate the authority to do a specific job, they reduce the number of duties that they have to perform. They also conditionally divest themselves of a certain amount of authority, which can be taken back at any time if conditions are not fulfilled. In this process, however, managers do not reduce the overall amount of responsibility originally accepted. Although subordinates also accept a certain amount of responsibility for duties assigned to them, this does not in any way diminish the manager's responsibility. It does add another layer or level to the overall responsibility, thereby creating overlapping obligations. Such overlapping obligations provide double or triple insurance that a job gets done correctly and responsibly. The supervisor however is held responsible for what his subordinate fails to do.

Thus, even though responsibility is something you accept, you cannot rid yourself of it. This thought should not make you overly anxious. After all, delegations and redelegations are necessary to get the job done. Although you try to follow the best managerial practices, you cannot be certain that each of your subordinates uses his or her best judgment all the time. Therefore, allowances must be made for mistakes. In evaluating your performance as a supervisor, your boss should notice how much you depend on your subordinates to get the work of your department accomplished. Although the responsibility has remained with you, your boss understands that you cannot do everything yourself.

In appraising your skill as a manager, your boss considers how much care you have shown in the following areas: selecting your employees, training them, providing constant supervision, and checking their activities. All these matters are taken into consideration in evaluating your ability as a supervisor.

AVAILABILITY OF TRAINED SUBORDINATES

The process of delegation assumes that there is someone available who is willing to accept authority. As a supervisor, you may have wanted to delegate more and more authority to some of your subordinates and to make one of them your assistant, but you have no one within your department who is willing to accept this arrangement and to take charge of an area of activities. You may not have anyone working for you who is capable of handling more authority. In such a case, authority, for the moment at least, cannot be delegated and must be withheld.

On the other hand, you may find yourself in a vicious circle, complaining that without better trained subordinates you cannot delegate. Without delegating additional authority, however, your subordinates have no opportunity to obtain the necessary exposure. With additional experience and training, their judgment may improve and they could become more capable subordinates. Although this lack of trained subordinates is often used by supervisors as an excuse for not delegating authority, they must always bear in mind that unless they begin to delegate authority, no subordinate capable of being a backup and of taking over the department (if necessary) will ever be available.

It is the supervisor's duty to develop and train such a person, and in the process delegate more authority not only to the individual selected as a backup but to other employees as well. Moreover, this process of training for increased delegation gives the supervisor a much clearer view of his or her own duties, the workings of the department, and the various jobs to be performed. Bringing subordinates to the point at which they can be given considerable authority is a slow and tedious process, but it is worth the effort. In the early stages the degree of authority granted will be small, but as subordinates grow in their capacities, more and more authority can be delegated to them.

Selecting a Backup

As mentioned, the process of delegation of authority should include making one particular subordinate into an assistant for the supervisor. The role of this assistant or backup is to serve as a reserve person who is ready to support the supervisor and serve in the supervisor's absence. The first step is to select the right person for the job. The supervisor undoubtedly knows which employees are more competent and capable. These would be the ones to whom the other employees turn in case of questions and who are looked on as leaders.

Outstanding employees, moreover, know how to do their job very well, seem to be able to handle problems as they arise, and do not get into arguments. They should also have shown good judgment in the way they organize and go about their job, should be open minded, and should be interested in further development and moving into better positions. Outstanding employees must have shown a willingness to accept responsibility and must have proven dependability. Sometimes a worker may not have had the opportunity to show all these qualities. Whatever qualities have remained latent, however, show up rather quickly during the actual training process.

If the supervisor has two or three equally good employees in the department, training all of them for greater delegations of authority on an equal basis should begin. Sooner or later it becomes obvious which one has the superior ability, and this individual then becomes the major trainee for the backup position. Once the selection of a single person is made (or in a large department there could be several), it is not necessary to come out with general formal announcements in this respect. Of course, the supervisor should discuss and explain the intentions fully to the employee chosen. More importantly, the supervisor must follow through by laying a thorough groundwork for good training so that the one who has been chosen will work out as an understudy.

Training a Backup

Although the phrase training a subordinate is frequently used, the term training is really not appropriate. It would be more fitting to speak of developing, mentoring, or grooming the backup, or even self-development on the subordinate's part. Understudies must be eager to improve themselves and show the initiative to be self-starters.

The supervisor should gradually let understudies in on the workings of the department, explain some of the reports to them, and show them how needed information is obtained. The supervisor should tell them what is done with these reports and why it is done. The supervisor should also introduce an understudy to other supervisors and other people in the organization with whom they must associate; eventually the understudy should contact them himself or herself. It is advisable to take the understudy along to some of the institution's meetings after this person has had a chance to learn the major aspects of the supervisor's job.

On such occasions, the supervisor should show how the work of the department is related to that of the other departments in the healthcare facility.

As daily problems arise, the supervisor should let understudies participate in them and even try to solve some of them. By letting understudies come up with solutions to problems, the supervisor is given a chance to see how well they analyze and how much they know about making decisions. In time, the supervisor should give the understudy some areas of activity for which he or she will be entirely responsible. In other words, gradually more duties and authority should be assigned.

This whole process requires an atmosphere of confidence and trust. The boss must be looked on by the understudy as a coach and friend, not as a domineering superior and know-it-all. Supervisors should caution themselves that in their eagerness to develop their understudies as rapidly as possible they do not overload them or pass on problems that are beyond their capabilities. The supervisor must never lose sight of the fact that it takes time and experience to be able to handle problems of any magnitude.

All of this requires much effort and patience on the supervisor's part. With increased responsibilities, there should also be commensurate positive incentives for the backup. These may be in the form of pay increases, bonuses, a fancier title, recognized status within the organization, or other rewards of a tangible and intangible nature. Such rewards include the self-satisfaction that the subordinate feels when he or she is able to handle increased responsibility and is moving up in the organizational ranks. Conceivably, just about the time the understudy comes to the point of being truly helpful, he or she may be transferred to another job outside of the supervisor's department. This may be discouraging for the moment, but the supervisor may rest assured that he or she has been recognized and given credit for developing a good new leader and for a training job well done.

RECOGNITION

We have discussed how and why we delegate authority, who may be chosen to receive authority (an individual, a team, etc.), and the importance of clearly communicating expectations and periodically checking on the progress of the tasks assigned. The often forgotten step in delegation is recognizing individuals or the team for the job done and reviewing with them the work completed, including how it or the process might be improved the next time. Grooming subordinates to take on greater responsibility is a duty of every supervisor. The subordinate you assign a task to today may be your right hand tomorrow or may be able to cover for you during an emergency or a much deserved vacation. Just as you appreciate feedback, so do your staff members. Employees want to improve. Like you, they want to feel appreciated for their efforts. A small amount of recognition goes a long way the next time you make an assignment.

EQUALITY OF THE THREE ESSENTIAL PARTS

Always bear in mind that these three components—duties, authority, and responsibility—must blend together to make delegation of authority a success. There must be enough authority (but not more than necessary) granted to your subordinates to do the job, and the responsibility you expect them to accept cannot be greater than the area of authority you have delineated. Subordinates cannot be expected to accept responsibility for activities if they have not been handed any authority. In other words, do not try to keep your subordinates responsible for something that you have not actually delegated to them.

Inconsistencies between delegated authority, responsibility, and assigned tasks generally result in difficult and undesirable outcomes. You may have worked in organizations in which some of the managers had much authority delegated to them but had no particular jobs to perform; this creates misuses of authority and conflicts. You also may have been in positions in which responsibility was exacted from you when you did not have the authority to fulfill an obligation. When responsibility exceeds authority, it is nearly impossible to do the job. For example, assume you are the pharmacy director and have been granted authority to install a Pyxis system within three months. However, the chief nurse executive, chief information officer, and plant engineering director want nothing to do with the project because "their plates are full." You do not have the authority to order them to assist you because they are peers reporting to other administrators. This, too, is a most embarrassing and frustrating situation. Therefore, you must make certain that the three essential elements for successful delegation are of equal magnitude and that whenever one is changed, the other two are changed simultaneously.

Some rare occasions occur when responsibility and authority are not equal and staff take action regardless. For example, in emergencies managers are often inclined and even forced to exceed their authority. One hopes this is the exception and not the normal state of affairs.

CENTRALIZATION-DECENTRALIZATION CONTINUUM

As discussed earlier, delegation of authority is the key to the creation of an organization. If no authority has been delegated, one can hardly say an organization exists. Thus, from an organizational point of view, the problem is not whether to delegate or not delegate authority, but rather how much authority is delegated to middle- and lower-level managers. The question involves the degree of authority to be delegated. Centralization and decentralization represent opposite ends of this delegation continuum.

This question about the degree of delegation is extremely important because it determines the answer to another highly significant organizational question, To what extent is the organization decentralized? How much of what authority should be given to whom and for what purpose?

Variations in the extent of decentralization are innumerable, ranging from a highly centralized structure, in which the concept of an organization barely exists (such as the mechanistic model discussed in Chapter 12), to a completely decentralized organization, in which authority has been delegated to the lowest possible levels of management (as in the organic model). In the first instance, the chief executive is in close touch with all operations, makes all decisions, and gives almost all instructions. Hardly any authority has been delegated, and, strictly speaking, it cannot be said that an organization has been created. Many small enterprises regularly operate along these lines. Some small business owners or executives believe employees can never do anything as well as they can. They fear that something will go wrong or a customer will be lost if someone else takes over a job. Often, these same executives lack time for long-range planning because they are doing the work rather than delegating the work. Often such one-man shows collapse if the chief executive becomes incapacitated, dies, or for some other reason leaves the enterprise. Moreover, although this analogy applies to an entire organization, the same can be said for a large or physically dispersed department. A supervisor cannot single-handedly do all the work of a department, meet department goals, and focus on the objectives and action plans.

A much less extreme situation is found in organizations in which authority has been delegated to a limited degree. In such organizations, the major policies and programs are decided by the top-level manager of the enterprise, and the task of applying these policies and programs to daily operations and daily planning is delegated to the first level of supervision. Few or no other levels exist between the top-level manager and the supervisors. This relatively flat organizational arrangement is often found in medium-sized enterprises. It is advantageous because it limits the number of managers that the general manager must hire, thus keeping expenses down. Furthermore, the particular knowledge and good judgment the general manager possesses can be applied directly. A considerable number of enterprises in the United States have this type of organization with a limited degree of delegation of authority.

At the other end of the centralization-decentralization continuum, we find those organizations in which authority is delegated as far down the chain of command as possible. To find out if an organization is this decentralized, one must determine the type of authority that has been delegated, how far down in the organization it has been delegated, and how consistent the delegations are. The more important the decisions made farther down in the hierarchy are, the more decentralization is prevalent. The number of such decisions and the functions affected by them also serves as a barometer of decentralization. Finally, the less checking that is done by upper-level management, the greater the degree of decentralization.

The answers to all these questions indicate whether you are dealing with an organization that has delegated authority to the greatest extent possible (decentralization). Most healthcare institutions probably find broad delegation of authority and decentralization advisable and necessary because of the nature of the activities involved and the skills, expertise, and expectations of the personnel. Today's better educated and more sophisticated healthcare workforce wants to use individual judgment and expects more authority and responsibility.

ACHIEVING DELEGATION OF AUTHORITY

Broader delegations of authority are not always easily put into practice. To be effective, a sincere desire and willingness to delegate must permeate the entire organization. Top-level management must set the mood by not only preaching but also by practicing broad delegation of authority. Although top management's intentions may be the best, at times the desired degree of decentralization of authority may not be achieved. For instance, top management may find that authority has not been delegated as far down as it intended because somewhere along the line there is an "authority hoarder," a person who simply does not delegate authority any further. This person grasps all the authority delegated to him or her without redelegating any of it.

The Supervisor's Hesitancy to Delegate

Managers may resist further decentralization of authority in this manner for several reasons. To some, the delegation of authority may mean a loss of status (their subordinates "show them up") or a loss of power and control. Others may think that by having centralized power they are in closer contact with top-level administration. Still other managers may believe that their subordinates are already too busy to take on additional duties or are truly concerned with the expenses involved in delegating authority.

Occasionally, supervisors do not like the idea of creating a backup; they may be reluctant to delegate authority because they know that they cannot delegate responsibility. Because the responsibility remains with the supervisors, they may think it is best to make all decisions themselves. Thus, out of fear of their subordinates' mistakes, many supervisors are not willing to delegate authority and, as a result, continue to overburden themselves. Their indecision and delay may often be costlier than the mistakes they hoped to avoid by retaining their authority. Always remember the likelihood exists that the supervisor may make mistakes as well. Moreover, if employees are permitted to learn from some of their own mistakes, they will be more willing to accept greater authority.

The supervisors' reluctance in delegating such authority is understandable in view of their continued accountability for the results. The traditional picture of a good supervisor was one who rolled up his or her sleeves and worked right alongside the employees, thus setting an example by his or her efforts. Such a description is particularly true of a supervisor who has come up through the ranks and for whom the supervisory position is a reward for hard work and professional or technical competence. This person has been placed in a managerial position without having been equipped to be a manager and is faced with new problems that are difficult to cope with. This person therefore retreats to a pattern in which he or she feels secure and works right alongside the employees. Occasionally such participation is needed, for example, when the job to be performed is particularly difficult or when an emergency has arisen. Under these conditions, the good supervisor is always right on the job to help. Aside from such emergencies and unusual situations, however, most of the supervisor's time should be spent carrying out the supervisory job, and the employees should be doing their assigned tasks. It is the supervisor's job not to do but to see that others get tasks done.

Frequently, however, supervisors do not trust their subordinates. They still think that if they want something done right, they have to do it themselves. Often they believe that it is easier to do the job than to correct the subordinate's mistake. Even if the supervisor lets the subordinate do it, the supervisor may feel a strong temptation to correct any mistakes rather than explain to the subordinate what should have been done. It is frequently more difficult to teach than to do a job oneself. Moreover, supervisors often believe that they can do the job better than any of their subordinates, and they are probably right. Sooner or later, however, they have to get used to the idea that someone else can do the job almost as well as they can, and at that point they should delegate the necessary authority.

There are several ways to cope with this problem and to achieve the degree of decentralization that is desired by top-level administration. As stated before, the entire managerial group must be indoctrinated with the philosophy of decentralization of authority. They must understand that by carefully delegating authority they do not lose status, nor do they absolve themselves of their responsibilities. One way of putting this understanding into practice is to request that each manager have a fairly large number of subordinate managers reporting to him or her. By stretching the span of management, the subordinate manager has no choice but to delegate authority. By delegating, they can save their own time for more important managerial jobs, for thinking and planning. If supervisors are willing to see to it that employees become more competent with each job, their own belief and confidence in their employees' work will also grow. This mutually advantageous relationship permits the supervisor to carry out the basic underlying policy of delegating more and more authority as the employees demonstrate their capability in handling it.

Finally, another way to achieve broader delegation of authority is for the enterprise to adopt the policy of not promoting a manager until a subordinate manager has been developed who can take over the vacated position. By doing this, the manager is encouraged to delegate as much authority as possible at an early stage. Moreover, this process creates an ideal organizational climate in which the subordinates can find maximum satisfaction for many of their most important needs.

Despite the fact that a certain amount of authority must be delegated to create an organization, some supervisory duties cannot be delegated. The supervisor should always apply and interpret policies, give general directions for the department, take necessary disciplinary action, and appraise and promote employees. Aside from these duties, however, their subordinates should perform most tasks by themselves.

The Reluctant Subordinate

The delegation of authority and especially the development of an understudy are two-sided relationships. Although the supervisor may be ready and willing to turn over authority, the subordinates may sometimes be reluctant to accept it. Frequently subordinates may feel unsure that they can handle the job assigned to them. They may be reluctant to leave the security of their job and their coworkers. They may have failed in the past or were excessively criticized about how they approached an assignment. Some may refuse because they see no reward for taking on the additional responsibility. Still others just prefer to avoid any additional workload, risk, or confrontation with peers. Merely telling them to have more self-confidence has little effect. When these situations arise, the supervisor should spend time with the subordinate to determine the reason for their resistance and determine if any accommodations can be made to reduce the individual's concerns. The supervisor, as we have said, must engender this self-confidence by carefully coaching and training the subordinate to undertake more and more difficult assignments. Only then will the subordinate be able to accept the increased responsibility that goes along with harder tasks and greater authority.

Organizational Maturity

Timing also plays a role in solving the degree of delegation problem. Although centralized authority may be the most logical organizational form to use in the early stages of an enterprise, later stages usually require the CEO to face the problem of delegating more authority and decentralizing the organization to a greater extent. Such decentralization of authority becomes necessary when centralized management finds itself so burdened with decision making that the top executives do not have enough time to perform their planning function adequately or to maintain a long-range point of view. This type of situation usually occurs when an organization expands. This lack of time to plan should indicate to top-level management that they should delegate authority to lower echelons. In other words, there should be a gradual development toward decentralization of authority commensurate with the growth of the enterprise.

DELEGATION AND GENERAL SUPERVISION

Delegation ends, in the strict sense of the word, when the level of employees who are actually doing the work is reached. When no more authority can be delegated, the question now arises as to how a supervisor can effectively reap the benefits of delegation—that is, how he or she can take advantage of the motivating factors of delegation in the daily working situation. The answer to this question can be found at the point in the philosophy of delegation that is commonly referred to as loose, or general, supervision. General supervision is closely tied to decentralization of authority.

General supervision means merely giving orders in broad, general terms. The supervisor, instead of watching every detail of the employee's activities, is primarily interested in the results achieved. He or she permits the subordinates to decide how to achieve these results within accepted professional standards and organizational requirements and sets the goals and tells the subordinates what is to be accomplished. Thus, the supervisor is setting the limits within which the work has to be done, but the employees are to decide how to accomplish these goals. This is referred to as team management, and it gives each employee maximum freedom within the constraints of organizational and professional standards.

Employees' Reaction to General Supervision

Most employees accept work as a part of normal, healthy life. Accordingly, most managers display the underlying managerial attitude of McGregor's Theory Y (see Chapter 24) toward their employees. Such managers understand that in their daily jobs employees seek satisfaction that wages alone cannot provide. Most employees also enjoy being their own bosses. They like a degree of freedom that allows them to make their own decisions pertaining to their work. The question arises as to whether this is possible if one works for someone else, whether such a degree of freedom can be granted to employees if they are to contribute their share toward the achievement of the enterprise's objectives. This is where the ideas of delegation of authority and general supervision can help.

The desire for freedom, for being one's own boss, can be enhanced and fulfilled by delegation of authority, which in a working situation means general supervision. In the daily work environment, this broad, general type of supervision on the employee level has the same motivating results as the delegation of formal authority throughout the managerial hierarchy.

Advantages of General Supervision

Significant advantages result from this approach to supervision and are similar to those cited in our discussion of the process of delegation. The supervisor who learns the art of general supervision benefits by having more time to be a manager and being less mentally and physically drained. The supervisor is freed from many of the details of the work and thus has time to think, plan, organize, and control. In so doing, the supervisor is positioned to receive and handle more authority and responsibility.

Moreover, the decisions that general supervision allows employees to make probably are superior to those made by a harried manager trying to practice detailed supervision. We have already pointed out that the employee on the job is closest to the problem and therefore is in the best position to solve it. Furthermore, opportunities to make decisions give the employees a chance to develop their own talents and abilities and become more competent. It is always difficult for a supervisor to instruct employees on how to make decisions without letting them make them. They can really learn only by practice.

This leads us to the third advantage of general supervision: it enables employees to take great pride in the results of their decisions. As stated before, employees enjoy being independent. Surveys reveal that the one quality employees most admire in a supervisor is the ability to allow them to be independent by delegating authority. Employees want a boss who shows them how to do a job and then trusts them enough to let them do it on their own. In this way the supervisor provides on-the-job training for them as well as a chance for better positions.

The last advantage discussed here is that general supervision creates an environment for teamwork to thrive. By allowing employees to work together to achieve a goal, they learn that two heads are better than one. But the greater benefit is the camaraderie that develops. In addition, individuals who may not have been recognized by their peers in the past may surface as knowledge leaders and display leadership skills that previously would not have been apparent to the department manager. Thus, we can see that general supervision allows for the progress not only of supervisors themselves but also of the employees, the department, and the enterprise as a whole.

Much more is said about general supervision in the discussion of the managerial function of influencing. Briefly, practicing the general approach to supervision, instead of an autocratic, dictatorial, detailed approach, provides much of the satisfaction employees seek on the job, which money alone does not cover. Because this approach fulfills many of their needs, employees are motivated to put forth their best efforts in achieving the enterprise's objectives.

ADVANTAGES AND DISADVANTAGES OF DELEGATION

Delegating and decentralizing authority provides numerous advantages, which become even more important as the enterprise grows in size. By delegating authority, the senior manager is relieved of much time-consuming detail work and subordinates can make decisions without waiting for approval. This increases flexibility and permits more prompt action. In addition, such delegation of decision-making authority may actually produce better decisions because the team leader on the job usually knows more pertinent factors than the higher-up manager. Delegation to the lower levels also increases morale, interest, and enthusiasm for the work. It provides a good training ground and helps identify up-and-coming leaders. As Andrew Carnegie once said, "The secret of success is not in doing your own work but in recognizing the right man to do it" (Allen 2000). All these advantages serve to make the organization more democratic and more responsive to the needs and ideas of its employees, which ultimately results in delivery of better patient care.

Some disadvantages to extensive delegation also may arise. For example, the supervisor of a department may believe that he or she no longer needs the help of upper-level managers and can develop his or her own supporting services, known as "building an empire." This could easily lead to duplication of effort. Another disadvantage could be a possible loss of control, although if monitoring is occurring, the delegating manager can take steps to see that this does not happen. In most situations, however, the advantages of broad delegation far outweigh the disadvantages.

As stated before, the environment and contingencies of healthcare institutions are such that to deliver the best possible patient care, authority must be delegated broadly. It is a question of balance, of finding the degree of decentralization that works. Remember, no two departments are alike. Each has its own tradition, history, problems, challenges, workforce, and environment to integrate into an organizational structure that works. This is an ongoing process. One must constantly monitor and adjust the degrees of delegation and decentralization as the environment and the institution change.

SUMMARY

In earlier chapters we defined authority as the power that makes the managerial job a reality. Authority is the lifeblood of the managerial position, and the process of delegation of authority breathes life into the organizational structure. Good managers must know how to use formal authority and how to delegate it to their subordinates. Through the process of delegating authority, management actually creates the organization. This process of delegation is made up of three essential parts: allocating or assigning a job or duty, granting authority, and creating responsibility. All three are inseparably related, and a change in one necessitates a change in the other two.

Managers can delegate authority, but they cannot delegate responsibility. Delegation does not relieve the manager from ensuring the work or task is being accomplished. Thus, the manager must clarify the expectations, define the subordinate's range of discretion, monitor its progress, hold the individual accountable for results, and recognize the subordinate for his or her performance. At all times, authority should equal responsibility. An imbalance may result in the task being left undone. When positions and position holders change, authority may need to be realigned or withdrawn. Finally, as mentioned in Chapter 13, avoid making decisions for the subordinate to whom you have delegated authority. The subordinate needs to plan and execute the assignments he or she accepted.

This process of delegation is the only way to create an operative organization. Thus, the question is not whether top-level management delegates authority, but rather how much or how little authority it does delegate. An authority centralization-decentralization continuum exists in all organizations. If authority is delegated freely to the lowest levels of supervision, the organization is highly decentralized. If most authority is in the hands of higher-level managers, the organization is highly centralized. Although centralization might be appropriate when an enterprise is just getting started, far greater advantages arise from decentralization, or broad delegation of authority.

In a large or medium department, the process of delegation is similar to the one outlined in this chapter—assigning duties, granting the authority to carry them out, and encouraging employees to accept responsibility for them. In a small department, the delegation of authority takes the form of developing an understudy who can take over when the supervisor is not there. This is a long and tedious process because it involves careful development and progressively increasing delegations of authority. It is well worth the effort, as it contributes to high motivation and morale among employees. Moreover, unless the supervisor trains someone to be the backup and grants authority to that person, the department is bound to collapse if the supervisor is absent for any length of time or leaves the organization.

This decentralization of authority is not as easily achieved as it might seem. Management frequently runs into obstacles that must be overcome to achieve broad delegation. These obstacles may be caused by an authority hoarder somewhere down the line, a subordinate's reluctance to shoulder authority and responsibility, or the unavailability of suitable subordinates to whom authority can be delegated. Encouraging general supervision fosters an environment of decentralized authority.

At some point in the organization, further delegation of authority is not possible. This is at the interface between the supervisor and nonmanagerial employees as they go about performing their daily tasks. At this level, delegation of authority expresses itself in the practice of general supervision that involves giving employees a great amount of freedom in making decisions and determining how to do their jobs. Such general supervision is probably the best way to motivate employees, whereas dependence on the sheer weight of authority normally brings about the least desirable results. Occasionally the manager must fall back on formal authority, but with the newer attitudes and expectations of our society, the general trend is toward more freedom and self-determination in management as well as in other aspects of life.

NOTE

1. A terminology change is occurring in the United States. Rather than using the term delegation, some organizations have adopted the term empowerment. The meaning is the same—you are empowering your subordinates to make decisions and to act.

REFERENCES

Allen, G. 2000. *Supervision*. Denton, TX: RonJon Publishers. Viewed 2/12/06 at http://ollie.dcccd.edu/mgmt1374/book_contents/3organizing/deleg/ delegate.htm.

Ensman, R. G. 1999. "Delegation: Pick the Strategy that's Right for You." *Advance for Health Information Professionals—Online Edition* July 1999. [Online information; viewed 2/12/06.] http://health-information.advanceweb.com/common/editorialsearch/ searchresult.aspx?FN=p32.html&AD=7/19/1999 &CR=true.

CHAPTER FIFTEEN

Line and Staff Authority Relationships

CHAPTER OBJECTIVES

After you have studied this chapter, you should be able to do the following:

1. Discuss the need to add staff specialists to the organization as an additional consequence of specialization.

2. Describe the typical line and staff organization.

3. Describe the primary chain of line command to achieve unity of command.

4. Discuss and contrast line and staff departments, and explain their positions in the organizational hierarchy.

5. Discuss the typical relationships between line and staff.

6. Define functional authority and explain how it is an exception to the typical relationship between line and staff.

7. State the benefits and shortcomings of functional authority.

A LL OF THE chapters in Part IV of this book are concerned with building an effective organization. We first discussed horizontal organization—how to divide the work into departments—and then we looked at dividing the work vertically by delegating authority. Now, as another consequence of specialization, we have to add staff to the organization. We are creating lateral and diagonal relationships by adding line and staff relationships, another essential building block of the organization.

In healthcare facilities, one usually speaks of different staffs such as the nursing staff, medical staff, plant engineering staff, and administrative staff. In this context, the word staff applies to a group of people who perform similar jobs, such as nurses, physicians, and maintenance engineers. In the general field of management and administration, however, the meaning of the term staff is very different. "Staff" is spoken in connection with "line," and both these terms refer to authority relationships. In the following discussion, any reference to staff means line staff, not the meaning that most people working in healthcare organizations usually associate with staff such as medical staff.

Because no one, not even the CEO, could possibly have all the knowledge, expertise, skills, and information necessary to manage a modern organization, staff becomes an essential and critical part of the institution. Line managers retain the administrative and authoritative parts of the activities, whereas staff representatives supply expert advice and support—the scientific, technological, technical, and informational aspects. Without these aspects, the institution can not function properly.

ORIGIN OF STAFF

The informal meaning of staff is the grouping of individuals together who perform a similar task. In management theory, however, the term has another meaning, one that has developed since the days of ancient Athens and Rome. The technical definition refers to an individual or individuals who serve in an advisory capacity to the manager(s) of an organization. Consider the president of the United States. He has many issues he must keep abreast of and does so through the use of a team of staff advisors. These staff positions may also serve in an *extender role*—that is, they may perform portions of a task or prepare pieces of a project or study for the manager when the manager cannot do everything himself or herself. The previous paragraphs as well as Part I of this book referred to this extender role for the manager who could no longer supervise any more supervisors.

As organizations grow in size and complexity, and as the environment changes and impinges more and more on them, the duties of managers increase. Then managers add subordinate managers by creating more departments and delegating authority. Sooner or later, however, the manager's span of management is so large that no more additional supervisors can be added because the manager cannot pay proper attention to them. At this point, they add personal staff, which means one or more assistants to do the work that cannot be delegated (see Figure 15.1).

Again, sooner or later the assistant's knowledge becomes too general and not sufficiently qualified. Furthermore, other members of the organization also require the help of experts in many difficult areas such as fair employment practices and healthcare law. This is where organizational staffs are added to advise and support any member of the institution who needs this kind of help and support. Today staff activities are increasing, as is the number of people working in them.

LINE AND STAFF ORGANIZATION

At this point, it is important to distinguish between line and staff. Staff personnel are advisory in their duties, whereas line personnel have direct responsibility to ensure goals are achieved through their subordinates. Whereas a line

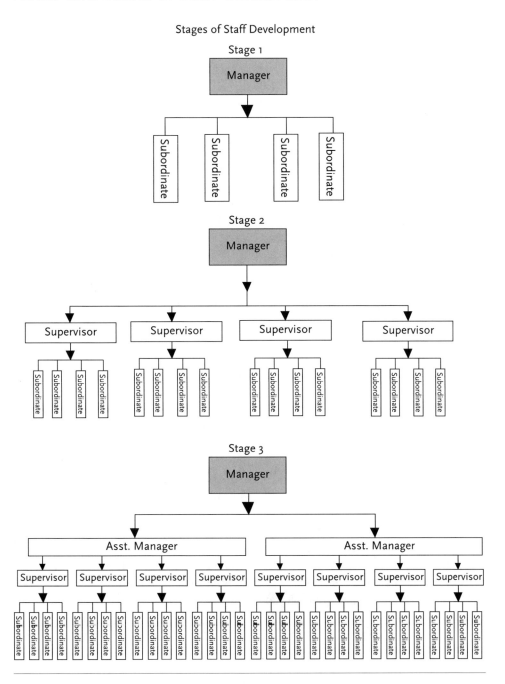

Stages of Staff Development

manager or supervisor may seek advice from a staff advisor, the line supervisor determines the action that must be taken next and then directs the subordinates to carry it out. Recall our discussion about organizational planning in Chapter 7: the guidance of planning staff may be needed. In that situation, staff developed planning premises and may have coordinated the planning activities. They probably collected data or conducted studies for management to use as the basis for decision making. But it was the line managers who made all the decisions involved in preparing the plan. The line managers define the objectives, allocate the resources, establish the timetable in which goals must be accomplished, and so forth.

One staff department commonly found in organizations is the human resources department. The director of human resources serves the management of the organization in a staff capacity. If the director has subordinates (i.e., supervisors of recruitment, benefits, employee relations, and so forth), he or she also has line duties for the ongoing activities of the department. Much has been written and said about the concepts of line and staff, and probably no other area in the field of management has evoked as much discussion as these concepts. Many of the difficulties and sources of friction encountered in the daily life of an organization probably result from line and staff problems. Misconceptions and lack of understanding as to what line and staff really are can cause bitter feelings and conflicts of personalities, disunity, duplication of effort, waste, and lost momentum.

As a supervisor of a department, you should know whether you are attached to your organization in a line capacity or a staff capacity. You might be able to find this out by reading the job description or, if that does not clarify it, by asking your superior manager. Line and staff are not characteristics of certain functions; rather, they are characteristics of authority relationships. Therefore, to ultimately determine whether a department is related to the organizational structure as line or staff is to examine the intentions of the CEO. The CEO confers line authority on certain departments, usually to generate products and services, and he or she places others into the organizational structure as staff to serve in advisory or supportive roles for the line management. Staff are not inferior to line personnel in terms of authority, or vice versa; they are simply completely different in nature. As these differences are discussed, keep in mind that the objectives of the staff elements are ultimately the same as those of the line organization—namely, achievement of the institution's overall goals of delivering the best possible care.

Line Organization

The simplest of all organizational structures is the *line organization*, which depicts the primary chain of command and is inseparable from the concept of authority. Thus, when we refer to line authority, we mean a superior and a subordinate with a direct line of command running between them. In every organization, this straight, direct line of superior-subordinate relationships runs

FIGURE 15.2: A DIRECT LINE OF AUTHORITY

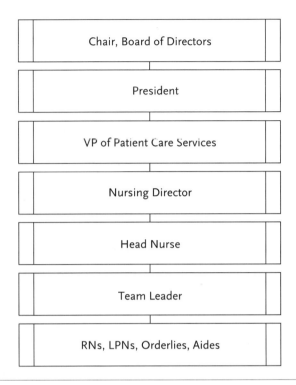

| Chair, Board of Directors |
| President |
| VP of Patient Care Services |
| Nursing Director |
| Head Nurse |
| Team Leader |
| RNs, LPNs, Orderlies, Aides |

from the top of the organization down to the lowest level of supervision. Figure 15.2 depicts one direct line of authority running from the board of directors to the president of the institution through the vice president of patient care services, a nursing director, a head nurse, and a team leader and finally to the other nursing employees.

Unity of Command

The uninterrupted line of authority from the chairperson of the board to the team leader in Figure 15.2 ensures that each superior exercises direct command over the subordinate and that each subordinate has only one superior to whom he or she is accountable. This is known as the principle of unity of command, as discussed in Chapter 14. Unity of command means that one person in each organizational unit has the authority to make the decisions appropriate to his or her position. Each employee has a single immediate supervisor, who in turn is responsible to his or her immediate superior, and so on along the chain of command. Thus, everyone in the line organization knows precisely who the boss is and who the subordinates are. The individual knows exactly where he or she stands, to whom orders can be given, and whose orders have to be fulfilled.

It is easy to see that line authority can be defined as the authority to give orders—that is, to command. It is the authority to direct others and require them to conform to decisions, plans, policies, and objectives. The primary purpose of this line authority is to make the organization work by evoking appropriate action from subordinates. Direction and unity of command have the great advantage of ensuring that results can be achieved precisely and quickly.

This type of direct line structure, however, does not answer all the needs of the modern organization. This structure was adequate when organizations and their environments were not as complex as they are today. In most enterprises now, activities have become so specialized and sophisticated that an executive needs assistance to direct all of his or her subordinates properly and expertly in all phases of their activities. Line management today definitely needs the help of others to make the right decisions.

Staff Organization

Staff is auxiliary in nature; it helps the line executive in many ways. Staff provides information, counsel, advice, and guidance in any number of specialized areas to all members of the organization whenever and wherever a need may exist. However, staff cannot issue orders or command line executives to take their advice. Staff can only make recommendations to the line. That advice can be accepted, ignored, rejected, or altered by the line. Because staff is expert in its specialty, the advice is usually heeded, but it does not have to be. When the line accepts the staff's suggestion, this suggestion becomes a line order. Line authority is based on superior-subordinate relationships; it is positional and managerial. Staff's authority is based on expertise; it is advisory and not managerial. Obviously, staff is not inferior to line and line is not inferior to staff. They are just different, and both are needed to complement each other to achieve objectives.

The right to command is not part of staff authority, with two exceptions. First, within each staff department there exists a line of command with superior-subordinate relationships just as in any other department. Staff's own chain of command, however, does not extend over to the line organization. Rather, it exists alongside the line organization as shown in Figure 15.3. The second exception arises when staff has been given functional authority by the CEO. This very important concept is discussed later in the chapter.

You can probably see more clearly why all supervisors must know whether their position is attached to the organization in a line or a staff capacity. They must know to understand their function and relation to the other members of the organization. If it is a staff capacity, the function is to provide information, guidance, counsel, advice, and service in their specialized area to whomever may ask for it. As far as the supervisor's own department is concerned, however, it will not matter whether the position is line or staff. Within every department the supervisor is the line manager. He or she is the only boss, regardless of whether the department is attached to the organization in a staff or a line capacity.

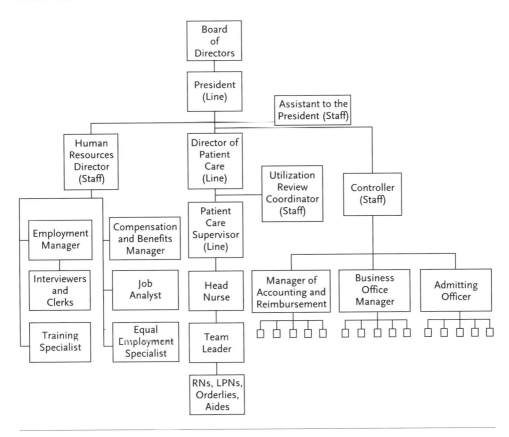

At this point, we must distinguish between personal staff, briefly mentioned already, and specialized staff. When executives find themselves in a position in which they need a personal aide (sometimes referred to as an "administrative assistant," or "assistant to" such as "assistant to the president") to help them in performing duties that they cannot delegate, a personal staff position may be created. The person in this position is a staff aide to the particular executive rather than to the organization at large; the placement of the assistant to the president in Figure 15.3 shows this relationship.

This person performs a variety of tasks for the executive such as gathering information, conducting research, and relieving the executive of detail work. This position is also often used to train and develop junior managers to acquaint them with how higher-level executives function. The assistant-to position has no line authority. This individual, however, often plays a role in the channels of informal communications and in the workings of the informal organization.

Eventually, however, a personal staff member may be inadequate because this person may not be sufficiently qualified and specialized in the many areas that challenge the executive; furthermore, many other members in the organization also need expert advice and guidance. At this juncture specialized staffs and possibly staff departments are introduced into the institution to provide counsel and advice in various special fields to any member of the organization who needs it. The discussion in this chapter refers to these specialized staff positions.

The Relationship Between Staff and Line

Conflict over organizational and operational problems may occasionally arise between line and staff, regardless of how well the relationships were defined. This is because of the two types of authorities at work: positional and formal on one side, with the weight of expertise and knowledge on the other. In most organizations, line and staff work together harmoniously. Harmonious cooperation between line and staff is especially important in a healthcare institution because the input of so many specialists is necessary for the delivery of good healthcare. Much depends on the sensitivity and tact of the staff people and the clarity of organizational arrangements.

It is common practice for certain activities in each organization to be undertaken as staff activities. This does not mean, however, that one can assume these are always staff activities. Line and staff, as stated before, are characteristics of authority relationships and not of functions. Thus, even a title does not offer any clue in recognizing line or staff. In many enterprises, one typically finds a vice president of engineering, a vice president of human resources, and a vice president of operations. None of these titles, however, indicates whether the position is line or staff. The little square box on the organizational chart also does not offer any help in this dilemma.

The function of a staff human resources department is to provide advice and service on personnel matters to all the other departments of the institution. The human resources department is there to recruit, screen, and test applicants; keep personnel records; help provide reasonable wage and salary administration; and advise line managers when difficult problems of fair employment practices or discipline arise. Whenever a line manager has a personnel problem, therefore, the specialized services of this staff department should be requested. Someone in the department of human resources certainly is best qualified to supply the current advice and information.

All that the human resources manager can do, however, is submit suggestions to the line manager, who in turn can accept, alter, ignore, or reject them. In essence, the human resources manager serves in the role of consultant to the line manager. If the line manager believes that the suggestions (consultant's advice) of the human resources department are not feasible, he or she is at liberty to make a different decision. Because the reason for establishing a staff in most instances is to obtain the best current advice, however, it is usually in the interest of the line manager to follow staff suggestions. For all practical purposes, the authority of the staff lies in their expertise in dealing with problems in their field. They will sell their ideas based on their authority of knowledge, not on their power to command. A person who acts in a staff relationship must know that his or her task is to advise, counsel, and guide, not to give orders, except within his or her own department. If any of the suggestions of the staff are to be carried out, they are carried out under the name and authority of the line officer, not that of the staff person.

Functional Authority

As stated before, in most instances staff provides advice and counsel to line managers, but staff lacks the right to command them. One important exception to this concept exists: a particular staff office may be given functional authority. *Functional authority* is authority restricted to a narrow area; it is a special right given to someone who normally would not have authority and therefore could not command. Although functional authority is limited to this area, it is full authority and gives the staff member the right and power to give orders outside of normal authority lines in this limited area. This right is based on expertise in the specialized field.

For example, an executive director decides that the human resources director's office should have the final word in cases of employee dismissal. In recent years, the laws, regulations, court decisions, and interpretations referring to fair employment practices have become an important area of managerial concern and a specialty that requires daily attention by someone in the organization. The department of human resources probably is best suited to keep up-to-date in this area. To avoid and minimize problems of this nature for the health-care center, the administrator decides to confer final operations decisions on the human resources department. In this instance, the administrator has conferred functional authority on staff in the special area of dismissals. Now the human resources director, rather than the line supervisors, has the authority to discharge employees. Other departments with functional authority commonly found in healthcare organizations are the compliance and materials management departments.

Functional authority undoubtedly violates the principle of unity of command. This principle, as you recall, states that the subordinate is subject to orders from only one superior regarding all the functions. Functional authority, however, introduces a second superior for one particular function such as the discharging of employees in our example above. Functional staff orders have to be carried out by the line supervisor to whom they are directed. If the line supervisor should disagree strongly, he or she can appeal to the superior manager up the line. However, unless these orders are changed, which is unlikely, the supervisor has to comply with them.

Functional authority is advantageous because it allows the maximum effective use of a staff specialist, leading to improved operations. It enables staff to intervene in line operations in situations designated by top-level management. Assigning functional authority is an effective way to use staff because, while still maintaining the overall chain of command, we make use of the specialized staff expertise. There is a price for this intervention-violating unity of command, and this may cause friction in some organizations. It is up to the administrator to weigh the advantages and disadvantages before functional authority is assigned.

THE AUTHORITY OF ATTENDING PHYSICIANS AND SURGEONS

At this point, another line of internal authority, found only in a healthcare setting such as a hospital, HMO, clinic, or the like, must be discussed—the authority exercised by physicians and surgeons. Here we are referring to those physicians who are members of the medical staff group. They are full-time chiefs of a medical specialty, physicians under contract by the hospital or HMO to serve in various "director" roles, and other "private," "community," or "part-time" physicians and surgeons who are members of the medical staff.

With the many changes that have been taking place during the last decade, some or all of these physicians may be compensated by the hospital. In the past, the chiefs usually received some compensation from the hospital, whereas the other physicians did not. The part-time or private physicians were compensated through their own efforts on a fee-for-service or some other clinic compensation arrangement. The growth of managed care organizations and the acquisition of physician practices by healthcare systems have resulted in a variety of compensation arrangements as well as changes in the roles physicians hold in these new healthcare enterprises.

The potential exists for tensions and misunderstandings between administration and members of the medical staff; this is understandable. The administration must consider the entire healthcare entity or system as an organized activity—that is, its relationships with all its employees, financial viability, and its role in the community. The physician's interests, however, are likely to be focused on the patient and at times on the physician's own economic well-being. Members of the medical staff often wonder whether the administrative staff really understands their problems, and vice versa.

There may also be conflicts between the full-time and part-time members of the medical staff. These may relate to policies established by the full-time members that adversely affect the part-time members. Examples of this may be control over the care plan of the patient or teaching obligations that may be imposed on part-time physicians whose compensation is directly related to the amount of time they have to serve patients in their offices. In recent years, the addition of *hospitalists*, who have demonstrated positive outcomes (Dichter 2003), are being inserted between the attending and his or her patient as well as between the attending physician and the patient's nurse. In these cases the nurse or other patient care professional may find himself or herself in a triad of command—taking orders from the immediate functional supervisor, the attending physician, and the hospitalist.

In most hospitals, clinics, and HMOs, these frictions and violations of unity of command are minimal because both groups strive toward the best results for the healthcare center. In most situations, a natural partnership exists between administration and the medical staff, the first providing the necessary facilities and personnel and the latter, regardless of their staff status, providing the medical expertise.

There is little doubt that the physicians direct the care of the patients they admit to the healthcare facility or serve in their offices. In this connection they have clinical-therapeutic-professional authority and exercise substantial influence throughout the healthcare entity at many organizational levels and in many functions. These physicians allowed to practice at the hospital, surgical center, or clinic, usually referred to as the medical staff, are not shown on the hospital organizational chart in any direct line or staff relationship under the CEO unless they are employees of the hospital or clinic. They are usually placed in a vague relationship to the board of directors on the chart. They practice medicine at the hospital, but they are outside of the administrative line of authority. They are "guests" who are granted practice privileges to perform certain services, but they have much authority over various people in the hospital. Their authority is exercised over the patient and especially over the nursing and patient care staff regarding medical issues. They also give orders to and expect compliance from many other employees of the hospital—for example, personnel in the respiratory therapy department, laboratories, and cardiac diagnostic services.

As a second line of authority, such orders from the physician or surgeon clearly violate the principle of unity of command. In fact, while in the operating room, the surgeon is known as the "captain of the ship," a concept discussed in Chapter 6. This may lead to a situation in which operating room personnel in particular are accountable to two bosses; that is, they must take orders from and are responsible to their supervisor and to the physician on the case at the same time. This can cause difficulties when orders from the administrative source of authority and the medical professional source of authority are not consistent. Nevertheless, the physician constitutes an outside source of authority who can marshal the resources of the facility without being in the chain of command. The physician also is not responsible to the administrator, except for his or her professional medical responsibility to the medical world and to the hospital policies, rules, and regulations governing the medical staff.

This dual command obviously creates administrative and operational problems, as well as difficulties in communication, discipline, and organizational coordination. Moreover, dual command can cause considerable confusion in cases in which it is not clear where authority and responsibility truly reside. This may lead to the attending physicians trying to circumvent administrative channels. Additionally, the administration may think that the physicians, through their power and authority, are interfering with administrative responsibilities. There probably will need to be some clarifications concerning this situation as hospitals' overall legal responsibilities are defined more clearly in the future. Regardless of all the complications inherent in this duality of command, it is an integral part of every healthcare organization.

SUMMARY

Management's organizing function is to design a structural framework that enables the institution to achieve its objectives. Work is divided horizontally into departments, then divided vertically by delegating authority. Another result of specialization is adding of staff to the organization. No manager could possibly possess all the knowledge, expertise, and information necessary to manage a modern healthcare institution, or any other organized activity, without the expertise and knowledge of specialists.

The CEO must decide whether a department is attached to the organization in a line or in a staff capacity. Because line and staff are quite different, it is essential for every supervisor to know in which capacity he or she serves. The supervisor in a straight, direct chain of command that can be traced all the way to the top-level administrator is part of the line organization. The line organization generally follows the principle of unity of command, which means that each member of the organization has a single immediate superior.

The person who is not within this line of command is attached to the organization as a staff person to provide expert counsel and service in a specialized field to whomever in the organization needs it. Staff people are not inferior to line staff, or vice versa; rather, they represent different types of authority relationships. The line manager has the authority to give orders, whereas the staff manager usually only has the authority to make recommendations. The advice can be accepted, ignored, rejected, or altered by the line manager who requested it. Because staff represents expertise in a specialty, however, the advice is usually accepted. Staff's authority is based on expertise; it is advisory, not managerial authority.

This situation changes in the case of functional authority. Sometimes the CEO may decide to confer functional authority on a staff office—that is, the right to give orders in a narrow area based on the staff person's expertise in a specific area. Although functional authority is limited to this area, it is full authority and the right and power to command outside of normal lines. Such functional authority violates the principle of unity of command. A similar difficult situation of duality of command is created by an attending physician's clinical-therapeutic authority. These additional channels of command result from the nature of healthcare delivery. Many areas of functional authority exist in most healthcare centers.

REFERENCE

Dichter, J. R. 2003. "Teamwork and Hospital Medicine: A Vision for the Future." *Critical Care Nurse* 23: 8–11.

CHAPTER SIXTEEN

Reorganization

CHAPTER OBJECTIVES

After you have studied this chapter, you should be able to do the following:

1. Discuss why organizations must reorganize.
2. Define reorganization and reengineering.
3. Review the various approaches available for organizing and reorganizing.
4. Distinguish between job design, job redesign, job rotation, job enrichment, and job enlargement.
5. Define quality.
6. Discuss approaches to quality improvement.
7. Describe how Six Sigma can be applied in the healthcare environment.

ALFRED CHANDLER (1962), did the original work on the strategy-structure relationship. His finding that *structure followed strategy* demonstrated that as organizations change their strategies, they must change their structure to support that strategy. Throughout Part IV of the book we discuss the executive's and the supervisor's roles in organizing staff, equipment, supplies, and other resources to achieve the goals of the entity. One must keep in mind that organizational structure is not static, and just like humans, its shape and needs change. The organization is a living institution and therefore needs a certain amount of adjustment as time goes on and as the organization's priorities or goals change. For this reason, the manager's organizing function is constant; checking, questioning, and appraising the soundness and feasibility of the departmental structure are ongoing processes. Organization is not an end in itself, but rather a means to an end—the accomplishment of the objectives of the department. A manager must be on the lookout for new developments,

Special thanks for their contributions to this chapter to Robert Sutter, R.N., M.B.A., M.H.A., Six Sigma Master Black Belt, of Six Sigma Academy, Arizona, and Michael Troncone, M.P.H., CHE, administrator, Calvary Hospital, New York, and principal, Michael T. Troncone & Associates, New Jersey.

practices, and thinking in the field of organizing. The supervisor must be willing to reorganize the department if developments warrant it, if it is indicated that the existing structure does not permit effective and efficient functioning, or if it is apparent that the services or products being produced are defective.

The term *reorganization* has many connotations. In this discussion, the term refers to changes in the organizational structure, departmentalization, the assignment of activities, or authority relationships. From time to time, a manager makes such changes because of scientific and technological advances, the dynamic and changing nature of the department's activities, financial needs, or a change in supervisors. As noted previously, reorganization also may be necessary to overcome existing deficiencies. When supervisors study those deficiencies, they use a variety of tools to improve the processes of the department and organization. Often reorganization is closely aligned with reengineering and process improvement activities such as Six Sigma. Occasionally, it is confused with downsizing and rightsizing, driven by cost reduction.

In an effort to prepare for the future, healthcare organizations have concluded that the trend toward more sophisticated specialization and computer literacy will continue and that employees with higher levels of technical skills will replace lower-skilled employees because higher levels of technical skill will be needed to treat future acute care patients. More technology that permits services to be performed remotely, the transition to an electronic health record, PACS, robotics, virtual private networks, smart toilets[1], remote heart monitoring, and more healthcare workers and physicians working remotely or telecommuting require many healthcare organizations to reorganize or restructure to accommodate the services and staff that remain onsite at the bedside of the patient versus those who serve the organization and patients from a distance. In addition, these technologies will affect the levels of staffing and skills required. Electronic health records will eliminate the need for clerical staff who now file items in or courier the record, laboratory staff who processed samples may find their jobs changing as more technology like smart toilets and glucose monitoring units are managed by the patient, and specialists will use robots to visit their patients so that they can "see" more patients in a given day. There are many tools available to organizations and their management team to orchestrate the restructuring caused by these changes.

REORGANIZATION CONCEPTS AND TOOLS

Two closely associated terms are reengineering and Six Sigma. For people new to healthcare management, reengineering can be difficult to distinguish from traditional cost-cutting approaches to organizing. *Reengineering* is an organizational approach introduced in the 1990s. According to Michael Hammer, "the simplest way to define reengineering is to say it means taking a 'clean sheet' approach to forget how you've done things in the past and to ask what's the very best way to get your work done. It's about rethinking how you do your work, working backwards from what customers need and then determining what's required to deliver it." Hammer contends that the concept has nothing to do with profit and loss, and it is not about buying and selling, merging, or divesting: "It's about serving customers' needs" (Deloitte & Touche 1996a).

The increased awareness about medical treatment errors and deaths as a result of medication errors has caused healthcare organizations to look more closely at their services, structure, and processes with a single goal in mind—to eliminate errors. When we couple the reengineering principles with quality improvement approaches that focus on delivering defect-free services and products, we introduce Six Sigma. *Six Sigma* was developed by Motorola in the 1980s and subsequently has been used at healthcare systems like Providence Health System and Baptist Health Care System. "Six Sigma is a management method that addresses error prevention, problem solving, problem detection, and managed change. Six Sigma uses a collection of management practices to achieve its specified goal to achieve defect-free processes and decrease variation in services offered. Some of these practices are based on" failure mode and effects analysis and "statistics, but many are not" (Barry, Murcko, and Brubaker 2002; Woodard 2005).

In Chapter 2, we discussed the early theorists who focused on production improvement techniques during the scientific management era from 1890 through 1940. Additionally, we have said that supervisors should seek the input of their staffs for ideas to improve processes and the environment in which they work. Encouraging supervisors to involve their staffs started as early as the 1950s with the human resources school of management. Quality improvement approaches have attempted to merge these two distinctively focused schools together.

Quality improvement programs are also known as total quality management, total quality control (Feigenbaum's term)[2], continuous quality improvement, companywide quality control (Ishikawa's term), Little Q and Big Q (Juran's terms), performance improvement, zero defects (Crosby's term)[3], quality circles, and multiple variations of these terms. Quality improvement is the practice of monitoring activities, identifying variations from expected outcomes, establishing corrective actions, and assessing whether the actions have corrected the variation. There is interdependence and overlap in the three concepts of reengineering, Six Sigma, and quality improvement. The reader can find a thorough discussion of quality improvement models in the July/August 2005 issue of the *Journal of Healthcare Management*.

To help you through the reorganization effort, the following are some terms that describe activities and components of the reorganization process.

- *Job design* is the process managers complete to define the specific tasks, methods, and relationship of a given job or position to others in the organization. When a supervisor is first setting up a department or planning for a new function, job design is essential.

- *Job redesign* is the process by which the manager reviews the various tasks assigned to a job or position and alters the assignments to improve productivity, enhance quality, or enrich the employee's work experience. This is one reorganizing approach.
- *Job rotation* is an enlargement technique whereby employees periodically move from one job to another, thus expanding their skills and comprehension of the entire process.
- *Job enlargement* is a method used in redesigning the job by adding variety to it through more tasks of a similar nature.
- *Job enrichment* is similar to job enlargement in that it is a method used to redesign jobs. However, in the process of doing so, the employee is allowed more participation in decision making by increasing the depth of the employee's authority and adding a variety of tasks to the job.
- *Work redesign* focuses on the work itself—what is being done and how it is being done. The idea is to identify and eliminate duplication, waste, and process steps that do not add value. Organizations may be able to combine functions, merge units, redesign jobs, streamline processes, and/or eliminate organizational layers (bureaucracy) as a result of such efforts (Thomas 2002).

Each of the above tools evaluates jobs. Do not allow the redesign activity to become too complex or it will overwhelm you.

However, recognize that every job does contributes to a process. For the reorganization process to effectively and efficiently use the resources (manpower, money, equipment, and materials) allocated, the supervisor must continuously monitor the process changes to ensure that services and products being produced are at a quality level acceptable to the organization and the customer and, when necessary, to tweak the processes or organizational structure to achieve the goals of the organization. This is the supervisor's role in process or quality improvement.

THE SUPERVISOR'S ROLE IN QUALITY MANAGEMENT[4]

All managers are responsible for ensuring the quality of the product or service they oversee. The manager must continuously assess the performance of the operation within his or her span of control and maintain or improve its outcome. This is accomplished through others. The manager must continuously monitor, motivate, and communicate with subordinates, peers, and superiors—team members who participate in the quality management process.

The customers, persons, or departments dependent on the manager's unit for their own satisfaction define quality by assisting the manager to set the performance expectations necessary to achieve satisfactory results. Customers may be internal—other units of the organization the department interacts with—or external—the patients, families, and public the organization serves.

FIGURE 16.1

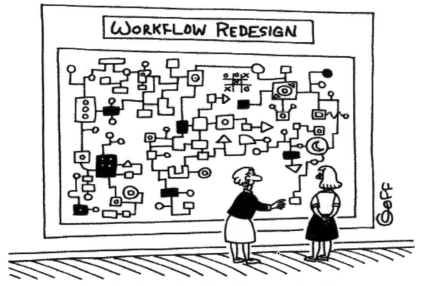

"And this is where our ED workflow redesign team went insane."

Source: Reprinted from *Hospitals & Health Networks*, with permission, September 2004, © 2004, by Health Forum, Inc.

What Is Quality?

Many experts have attempted to define *quality*. While definitions vary, there are three standard levels of quality that are accepted today. At the most basic level is *conformance quality*. For the supervisor, this means ensuring that the outcomes of the work they oversee meet the minimum standard set by the organization. For instance, the new medical records supervisor may be responsible for ensuring that a given number of charts are coded each day or that the records are filed correctly. Conformance is the act of doing the right thing.

The second level of quality is often called *requirements quality*. At this level, the supervisor is responsible for meeting customer expectations. Every supervisor has a number of customers—their employees, the departments they interact with, and so forth. When a supervisor ensures requirements quality, they are perceived as running a good department.

The highest level of quality is *quality of kind*.

This means providing a service that exceeds customer expectations or that delights the customer. This is the quality that Deming alludes to when he defines quality as "pride of workmanship" (Deming 1986)—but this is relatively common information if one had studied Deming.

Approaches to Quality

To achieve quality of kind, the supervisor must be familiar with and practice ongoing performance improvement techniques, both to motivate employees and to continuously improve the work product. Many of today's organizational approaches to quality are based on *DMAIR—Design, Measure, Assess, Improve, Redesign.* This process defines the continuous cycle of quality improvement. Its elements are as follows:

1. *Design.* The first step in improving any process is to understand its design. Questions to ask are
   - What is the purpose of the process? What is its objective?
   - Who is involved in the process?
   - What are the steps of the process? (These should be defined at the most basic level. Flow charts are an excellent method to identify redundancies or inefficiencies in the process.)
2. *Measure.* "You can't manage what you don't measure" is an oft-quoted phrase. To obtain baseline measurement, questions to ask are
   - What parts of the process are being measured?
   - What parts of the process should be measured based on its design and the desired outcome?
   - Are the results satisfactory, or is there a need for improvement?
3. *Assess.* When the design of the process is understood and measurement results have been obtained, it is necessary to ask
   - Is the process efficient? Are there redundancies, extra or duplicate steps, inefficiencies, or unnecessary steps?
   - Can the results be improved?
4. *Improve.* Based on the assessment, changes to the process can be identified to improve the end result.
5. *Redesign.* As the improvements are implemented, two important steps must be taken:
   - Define the redesigned process and communicate it to all parties involved.
   - Establish measures to ensure that the improvements accomplish what was intended.

The Six Sigma approach to quality is quite similar to the DMAIR approach. Its steps are *DMAIC—Define, Measure, Analyze, Improve, and Control.* While the methodology calls for a rigorous, scientific approach to statistical analysis, the fundamental cycle of quality is quite similar. (Read more discussion of Six Sigma later in this chapter.)

Quality Improvement Teams

In the Word Web on-line dictionary,[5] the primary definition of a team is a "cooperative unit." The second definition is "two or more draft animals that work together to pull something." The new manager leading or participating in a process improvement team may sometimes appreciate the second definition.

Each member of the quality improvement team has a defined role in the performance improvement process. The manager may be called on to serve in any one of these roles:

- *Team leader.* The team leader is the owner of the performance improvement project under study and leads the team through the DMAIR or DMAIC process. The leader works closely with the facilitator to plan the work of the team. He or she must start meetings on time, assign roles and responsibilities, ensure that work is evenly distributed, ensure that everyone has an opportunity to participate, ensure accurate record keeping, and ensure that all tasks are accomplished.
- *Facilitator.* The facilitator is responsible for keeping the team on track by keeping time and ensuring that each topic is covered as laid out in the work plan.
- *Team member.* Team members are chosen because they are associated with the process under study, either as participants or customers, or because of their knowledge of the process. They must support the work of the team and support its recommendations throughout the organization.
- *Recorder.* The recorder is often a rotating role and is responsible for keeping an accurate record of the team's proceedings.
- *Consultant.* A consultant is an invited guest. He or she does not need to attend every meeting of the team but may be called on when his or her particular expertise is needed.
- *Team champion.* The team champion is a senior leader who has the authority to support the work of the team and ensure that the team receives resources and support needed.

Additional Methods for Involving Employees in Quality Efforts

While the contributing author, Michael Troncone, has outlined the benefit of quality improvement teams, there are other methods to gain employee participation.

The *quality circle*, sometimes called the quality control circle (QCC) or do-it group (DIG) (see Figure 16.2), is a method of increasing employee participation in the daily work routine. The underlying ideas of this approach are derived from the work of McGregor, Maslow, Herzberg, Deming, Drucker, Sherman[6], and others; the first practical applications of the quality circle were made in Japanese industries. The resulting Japanese management technique claims much credit for high levels of productivity, quality, and worker satisfaction. Now as continuous quality improvement (CQI) and performance improvement (PI) are becoming more prevalent in healthcare institutions, the quality improvement or quality management task force is being used to accomplish the goals of PI and CQI.

FIGURE 16.2: DO-IT-GROUP ESTABLISHMENT FORM

This DIG is __ intradepartmental (within 1 department) or __ interdepartmental (more than 1 department).

_____   _____ __   _____
Employee's Name   Department   Extension

We are looking for ways to improve what we do. We do that by offering suggestions and establishing DIGs to make our ideas work. A DIG idea may be started by anyone. If you have an idea or have identified a problem and would like to have a DIG created, complete this form. Discuss the idea or problem with your supervisor. Drop this completed form in the DIG Box next to the ATM machine.

Is this an idea? ____ , or is this a problem ____?

(1) If this is an idea, please tell us more about it: _____

_____

_____

If this is a problem, tell us more: What is the problem? _____

_____ __   __

(2) Where is it located? _____

(3) When does it occur? _____

(4) Who does it affect? _____

(5) How big is the problem? _____

(6) What do you think causes the problem? _____

Have you had DIG training? _____ Have you participated in a DIG before? _____ Have you ever been a DIG Chairman? _____ Will you join this DIG committee? _____ Will you Chair this DIG? _____

If this problem is fixed or idea is implemented it will improve:
Customer Satisfaction _____ Quality _____ Productivity _____ Organization _____
Finances _____ People Skills _____ Other: _____

Supervisor's Initials: _____ Date: _____

Source: Adapted from DIG Creation Form from Fayette Memorial Hospital, Connersville, IN.

In some settings, employees may recommend the establishment of a quality improvement task force. These members volunteer to meet regularly, during regular working hours, after hours, or both to discuss work, work processes, and quantity- and quality-related problems and to stimulate innovation. The task force is either assigned a project to assess or is asked to identify problems, isolate the causes, and develop practical solutions or more effective methods to ensure that the work is accomplished error free the first time. The supervisor may act as the facilitator of this group, but often a worker or individual from outside the work team serves in this capacity or in the role of team leader.

Usually the improvement team leader is first exposed to some basic training course in group dynamics, problem solving, and similar techniques. The members are often given some training in problem-solving techniques, establishing priorities, brainstorming, and so forth. Because there may be many problems to solve or ideas to explore, the team may apply the Pareto Principle to determine what problems to solve and in what order (Spath 2001). The *Pareto Principle*, also known as the 80/20 rule, states that 80 percent of the results are caused by 20 percent of the causes. In everyday terms, the principle could be any of the following:

- 80 percent of the ICU days are consumed by 20 percent of the patients treated in the hospital.
- 80 percent of the tardiness in a department is caused by 20 percent of the department employees.
- 80 percent of the needle sticks occur in 20 percent of the areas.

The thought underlying the use of any improvement team is to tap the minds of an organization's own workforce, realizing that the employees doing the job often know best why productivity may be hindered and why product quality is poor. Often they have excellent ideas and answers. These ideas surface through such team sessions as brainstorming. Successful *brainstorming* sessions follow certain ground rules: (1) ignore the hierarchy (rank does not count); (2) suspend judgment (make it clear that ideas are being gathered); (3) encourage quantity, not quality (get as many ideas on the table as possible); (4) nurture a no-limits session (ask questions such as, "what would our competitor do in this case?"); and (5) don't rush (do not set a fixed time, serve refreshments, and so on) (*Journal of Accountancy* 2000). These brainstorming ideas and solutions are then presented to management or a PI steering committee.

The QCC or DIG idea fits into the existing organizational structures, following the existing channels of communication and authority. Because improvement teams are an application of participative management, the concept can be introduced with success into any organization in which administration's philosophy has been democratic, open, and participative. It is unlikely that these teams would produce results in an environment that practices autocratic and highly centralized management. Many organizations have found the adoption of improvement teams to be successful, whereas others have found them disappointing (Rice 1984.)

The improvement team or task force may be empowered to implement their recommendations without a presentation to management (recall our discussion of decentralized authority in Chapter 14). In a quality-driven environment, much like that found in the culture of Japanese industries, total trust exists between management and employees. Employees are encouraged to make changes and test their hypotheses of improving processes and output without fear of management repercussion. The employees are empowered to make decisions about their work environments and are rewarded for taking the initiative. Management serves as coach and facilitator of the brainstorming effort. This type of managerial attitude develops over time and creates a culture of mutual trust and freedom of communication in a facility. This cultural style is more closely identified with the Theory Z philosophy. *Theory Z* is fairly new in healthcare, and the management culture it requires is different than in most businesses in the United States; it may be several years before we see Theory Z in our healthcare organizations.

One approach to help staff deal with redesigning a process is demonstrated in the chart developed by SSM Healthcare System (see Figure 16.3). This approach is used when a process or procedure for doing something, such as obtaining the information to register and the activities involved in registering a patient for treatment, becomes so cumbersome or error prone that it needs streamlining.

Preparation of staff to participate in performance improvement teams may consume some productive time, but it must occur to make the process successful. All team members, whether they serve on the steering committee or the team assessing an opportunity to improve, must have a common vocabulary and use tools to transform data into meaningful information. Some of the tools often used are shown in Figures 16.4 and 16.5.

The success of any process that places subordinates and supervisors together requires communication. To encourage communication without fear of reprisal, the *nominal group technique* is practiced. This technique tries to provide a way to give everyone in the group an equal voice in problem or process identification.

According to Witt (1996), the key questions that should guide the team or group are as follows:

- Who is the customer in the process?
- What is the desired outcome?
- What would the process look like under ideal conditions?
- What are key points where problems have been observed in the past?
- How can we design quality into the process, rather than inspect for it after the fact?

For the healthcare supervisor, the most challenging part of any quality improvement process is the implementation of the improvement. Six Sigma has gained momentum as an approach that speaks to each of Witt's questions.

FIGURE 16.3: CQI MODEL: PROCESS (RE-)DESIGN APPROACH

Team Information

A PLACE TO:

- Post Team Project Planning Work Sheet.
- Display team meeting minutes.
- Solicit comments using self-stick notes.
- Recognize individuals who provided support to team.

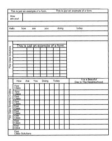

① Identify Opportunity

OBJECTIVE:
Identify an opportunity for improvement and the reason for working on it.

KEY ACTIVITIES:
- Research the opportunity:
  —Review indicators.
  —Survey patients and other customers and suppliers.
  —Interview individuals involved in the process.
- Consider patient and other customers' and supplier' needs to help select the opportunity.
- Schedule the CQI Model activities.

CHECKPOINTS:
1. The criteria for selection were customer oriented.
2. A schedule for completing the CQI Model steps was developed.

OUTPUTS:
- Mission Statement Form.
- Team Project Planning Work Sheet.

② Conceptual Design

OBJECTIVE:
Develop ideal process flows.

KEY ACTIVITIES:
- Design the ideal process flows.
- Perform customer needs analysis to define requirements at the hand-off and interfaces in the process.
- Write a clear outcome statement.
- Document mutually agreed upon requirements between customers and suppliers.

CHECKPOINTS:
3. The sequence of activities in the new process was documented.
4. The potential benefits of the new process were clearly identified.
5. Customers' valid requirements were identified.

OUTPUTS:
- Clear outcome statement of the process.
- Flowchart of the ideal process.
- Valid requirements of each customer/supplier relationship in the process.

③ Analysis

OBJECTIVE:
Design the control system for the process to prevent problems from occurring.

KEY ACTIVITIES:
- Consider potential problems.
- Consider potential causes.
- Develop methods for preventing potential problems.
- Design a measurement system.

CHECKPOINTS:
6. Potential causes of problems were identified and prioritized.
7. Appropriate actions were taken on major potential causes.
8. The measurement and control system is specific enough to pinpoint future problems.

OUTPUTS:
- Control system with measurable indicators.

(continued on following page)

④ Implement New Process

OBJECTIVE:
Put the new process in place.

KEY ACTIVITIES:
- Develop an action plan that:
  —Identifies who, what, when, where, and how.
  —Reflects the barriers and aids needed for success.
- Obtain cooperation and approvals.
- Implement the process.
- Develop performance targets for the process.

CHECKPOINTS:
9. Action plan addressed who, what, when, where, and how.
10. Action plan reflected the barriers and aids necessary for successful implementation.
11. Cooperation of relevant managers in impacted organizations was obtained.
12. Performance goals/targets were identified.

OUTPUTS:
- Action Plan.
- Targets for measurable indicators.
- Implementation of new process.

⑤ Measure Results

OBJECTIVE:
Confirm that the process is working well and that the performance targets for the process have been met.

KEY ACTIVITIES:
- Compare results obtained to the target.
- Change the process, as necessary, if results are not satisfactory.

CHECKPOINTS:
13. Data was collected to measure performance relative to targets.
14. Results met or exceeded targets. (If not, specific follow-up as planned.)

OUTPUTS:
- Compare the results obtained to the target.
- Change the process, as necessary, if results are not satisfactory.

⑥ Standardization

OBJECTIVE:
Ensure that the process is still working and is incorporated into daily work.

KEY ACTIVITIES:
- Ensure that solutions become part of daily work:
  —Create/revise standards.
- Educate employees/medical staff on the process and/or standards and explain need.
- Establish periodic checks with assigned responsibilities to monitor the new process.

CHECKPOINTS:
15. Method to ensure process becomes part of daily work was developed.
16. All impacted personnel were trained (include explanation of need).
17. Periodic checks were put in place with assigned responsibility to monitor the proposed solutions.
18. Specific areas for replication were considered.

OUTPUTS:
- Education of people.
- Incorporation into standard operating procedures.
- Replication.

⑦ Future Plans

OBJECTIVE:
Plan what to do about any remaining problems and evaluate the team's effectiveness.

KEY ACTIVITIES:
- Analyze and evaluate any remaining problems.
- Plan further actions if necessary.
- Review lessons learned related to problem-solving skills and group dynamics:
  —What was done well.
  —What could be improved.
  —What could be done differently.

CHECKPOINTS:
19. Plan for any remaining problems was developed.
20. Applied P-D-C-A to lessons learned.

OUTPUTS:
- Plan for the future of the team.
- Evaluation of the team and its work.

Source: © SSM Health Care CQI Manual, St. Louis, MO, SSM Health Care System 1990 (pp 279–80). Reprinted with permission.

FIGURE 16.4: PERFORMANCE IMPROVEMENT CQI MODEL: PROBLEM-SOLVING APPROACH

CQI Data Tools	Purpose/Description of Tool

Brainstorming

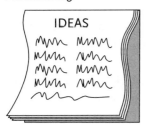

A discussion forum used to get a group of people to quickly generate, clarify, and evaluate a number of ideas that are listed regardless of their viability to support a solution to the problem.

Cause-and-Effect Diagram (also known as the "fishbone" and Ishikawa Diagram)

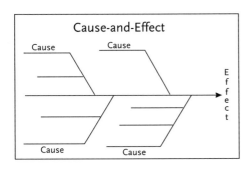

A diagram that depicts causes of a problem and attempts to narrow the problem down to the most likely, or root, cause. Contributing issues to the problem are grouped together such as people, materials, machinery (equipment), and methods.

Flow Charts or Process Diagram

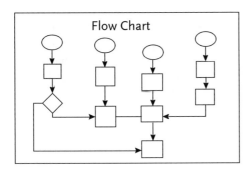

Pictorial description of the flow or steps in a process to allow visualization of the tasks. Flow charts are used to "document" a process or procedure.

◯ — Start and stop symbol

☐ — Process step symbol

◇ — Decision symbol

(continued on following page)

CQI Data Tools	Purpose/Description of Tool

Pareto Charts (also known as 80-20 rule)

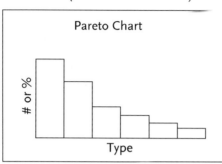

These charts are used to display data in the order of its relative importance or weight. It identifies the "few major causes" of variation from the "trivial" to many. It comes from the 80–20 theory that 80% of the problem is directly related to 20% of the causes. For example, 80% of the delinquent medical records are for 20% of the physicians on the medical staff.

Run Charts (Trend or Line graphs)

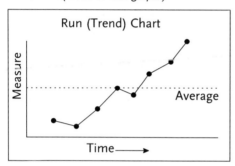

This graph shows with a single line data or results occurring at different times for a time period.

Histograms

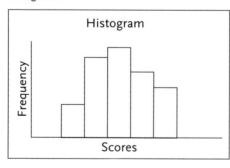

This graph, usually in bar format, displays the frequency with which something occurs. It shows a distribution that may or may not be bell shaped. It may illustrate the stability of a process.

(continued)

FIGURE 16.4: *(continued)*

CQI Data Tools   *Purpose/Description of Tool*

Scatter Diagram

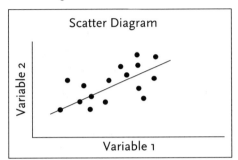

This diagram is used to demonstrate the relationship between two variables such as processing time and volume of specimens received.

Control Chart

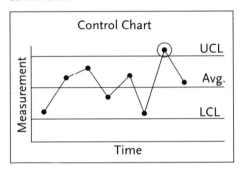

This chart reflects the tolerances of something happening within limits. Normal limits are established and concern should rise when the number of occurrences outside of the limits increases.
UCL — Upper Control Limit
LCL — Lower Control Limit

Affinity Diagram (also known as KJ Diagram and named for its founder Kawakita Jiro)

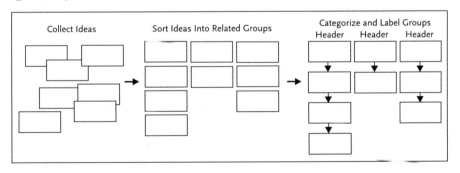

A tool used to sort large amounts of ideas or opinions gathered through brainstorming into groupings of similar ideas and then relationally into categories.

Source: Adapted from *The Memory Jogger II*™ © 1994, GOAL/QPC, Salem, NH, www.goal/qpc.com. Used with permission.

FIGURE 16.5: WHEN TO USE WHICH TOOL

Step	Who	QI Tool
1. List and Prioritize Opportunities	Steering Committee	Data Collection, Pareto Analysis, Brainstorming, Affinity Diagrams, Flow Charts, Graphs and Charts
2. Identify Customer(s) and Expectations	Steering Committee and Team	Brainstorming, Affinity Diagrams, Flow Charts, and Data Collection
3. Define Project and Team	Steering Committee	Flow Charts and Graphs and Charts
4. Formulate Theories	Steering Committee and Team	Brainstorming, Affinity Diagrams, Cause-and-Effect Diagrams, and Flow Charts
5. Test Theories	Team	Flow Charts, Data Collection, Graphs and Charts, Pareto Analysis, Histograms
6. Identify Root Cause	Team	Flow Charts, Data Collection, Graphs and Charts, Pareto Analysis, Histograms, Cause-and-Effect Diagrams
7. Identify Solutions and Control Systems	Team	Brainstorming, Affinity Diagrams, Flow Charts, Data Collection, Graphs and Charts, Cause-and-Effect Diagrams
8. Address Resistance to Change	Team	Brainstorming, Affinity Diagrams, Flow Charts, Cause-and-Effect Diagrams
9. Implement Solutions and Control Systems	Steering Committee and Team, and Others	Flow Charts, Graphs and Charts, Pareto Analysis, Histograms
10. Evaluate Performance	Steering Committee and Team	Data Collection, Graphs and Charts, Pareto Analysis, Histograms, Flow Charts
11. Standardize Process	Team, Steering Committee, Senior Management	Data Collection, Graphs and Charts, Pareto Analysis, and Histograms
12. Monitor Control Systems	Steering Committee, Senior Management	Data Collection, Graphs and Charts, Flow Charts, Pareto Analysis, Histograms

AN EXAMPLE OF SIX SIGMA[7]

Six Sigma is permeating healthcare at an increasing rate. This is a favorable trend because it is a perfect fit for healthcare organizations: the methodology follows the medical model, and the healthcare industry is wrought with defects and process variation. Defects such as billing errors, postoperative infections, and unplanned readmissions are quite common in healthcare today. Also contributing to the adoption of Six Sigma is evidence that healthcare organizations have realized substantial improvements by deploying Six Sigma (Dlugaz 2004; Frankel et al. 2005; Lenaz 2004; Torres and Guo 2004; Yound 2004).

Six Sigma is a systematic process improvement method that is focused on reducing process defects and variation. There are five phases associated with Six Sigma: define, measure, analyze, improve, control (DMAIC). These phases are collectively referred to as DMAIC, and as Figure 16.5 depicts, these five phases correspond to the medical model of diagnosis, treatment, and follow-up. In other words, dysfunctional processes are treated methodologically just like physicians treat sick patients. The only difference is that Six Sigma uses a set of tools and methods appropriate for process improvement.

Diagnosis: Define, Measure, Analyze

In the diagnosis phase, physicians conduct a history and physical as well as various diagnostic tests to determine the root cause of an illness. The define, measure, and analyze phases of Six Sigma are focused on diagnosing the root cause of process defects and variation. The define phase establishes what process is to be treated and the process boundaries. Subsequently, the measure phase involves collecting data and establishing baseline performance measurements. The analyze phase identifies the root causes of dysfunctional processes through the use of various statistical methods. This rigorous use of data and statistical analysis is the hallmark of Six Sigma, compared to other process improvement methods.

Treatment: Improve

Once a diagnosis of a patient's illness is confirmed, a physician then prescribes a treatment—medication, surgery, and so on—to eradicate the cause of illness. During the improve phase, methods such as reengineering and design of experiments are employed to remove or fix the root causes identified in the analyze phase.

Follow Up: Control

Once a physician institutes treatment a comparison of the patient's condition after treatment to before treatment is made to ensure that the treatment is effective and remains effective. The control phase is designed to accomplish the

FIGURE 16.5: FIVE PHASES OF SIX SIGMA

Medical Model		Six Sigma
• Diagnosis	⟶	• Define
— H&P		— Project Charter
— Laboratory		• Measure
— Imaging		— Process Maps
— Stress Testing		• Analyze
— Microbiology		— Regression
• Treatment	⟶	• Improve
— Medication		— Re-engineer
— Surgery		— Design of Experiments
— Rehabilitate		
• Follow Up	⟶	• Control
— Laboratory		— Control Plan
— Imaging		

same goal: to ensure that the process has improved and that the improvement is sustained. Six Sigma uses the control plan to achieve this objective. The control plan is a document that specifies what components of the process are measured, how they are measured, what constitutes acceptable measurements, and who is responsible for monitoring the measurements and taking action if the measurements are unacceptable.

The DMAIC methodology can be used to improve many processes in a healthcare organization just as the medical model—diagnose, treat and follow up—is used to treat virtually any illness..

Six Sigma Case Study: Thrombolytic Administration

To demonstrate the use of Six Sigma in a healthcare organization, the following is a brief description of a Six Sigma project to improve the timeliness of thrombolytic administration in patients with acute myocardial infarction in a community hospital. At the time of this project, the American College of Cardiology practice guidelines called for a thrombolytic to be administered within 30 minutes of a patient's arrival.

Define

An initial meeting with the hospital's CEO, COO, and chief of the emergency department (ED) was held to garner the support of senior management and medical staff to the project. Subsequently, the problem was defined as excessive cycle time and variability associated with thrombolytic administration in the ED. The boundaries of the process were established as beginning with patient arrival to the ED and ending with thrombolytic administration in the ED. Project objectives and a multidisciplinary team of ED personnel were established.

Measure

Baseline data were collected to establish baseline performance measurements of door-to-needle time:

- Average (minutes): 44.3
- Standard deviation (minutes): 33.9
- Defect rate (proportion of patients with door-to-needle time = 30 minutes): 68.75 percent

The data were then analyzed with a control chart, which revealed the process to be fairly stable. Subsequently, process mapping was conducted to document the process steps and flow as the current process is executed. Finally, a cause-and-effect diagram as well as failure mode and effects analysis were conducted to identify factors that affected door-to-needle time.

Analyze

The process map, cause-and-effect diagram, and failure mode and effects analysis were reviewed to determine what data elements to include in the data collection plan. A data collection form and definitions were derived, and personnel from the medical records department were trained to collect the data. Variables, including age, EKG results, and the presence of chest pain, were analyzed using linear regression to ascertain which factors were statistically significant with respect to door-to-needle time.

The analysis revealed the time associated with acquiring the initial EKG was the only factor that affected door-to-needle time in a statistically significant manner. The quicker this occurred, the faster a thrombolytic was administered. None of the clinical characteristics—day of week or shift—statistically affected door-to-needle time.

Improve

Based on the results of the analyze phase, the team streamlined the process of acquiring the initial EKG, eliminated redundant and non-value-added process steps identified on the process map, and fixed problems ranked high on the failure modes and effects analysis. After the ED staff were trained on the new process and the process improvements were implemented, data were collected to ascertain if an improvement was realized. The results verified that the process changes were effective:

- Average (minutes): 24.8
- Standard deviation (minutes): 2.8
- Defect rate (proportion of patients with door-to-needle time = 30 minutes): 5.0 percent

Control

A control plan was formulated and implemented to ensure that the process was continually monitored and that unacceptable performance was addressed immediately.

If implemented correctly, the Six Sigma methodology has repeatedly demonstrated its effectiveness in fixing myriad process problems in a variety of industries, including healthcare. However, Six Sigma is not a panacea for all of an organization's process-related problems. Instead, Six Sigma should be considered as one component of a comprehensive, integrated process management system. That is, Six Sigma should be incorporated with other process-management methods such as Malcolm Baldrige guidelines, root cause analysis, lean manufacturing, and Kaizen Events. Just as a physician selects the best treatment for a patient's circumstances, an organization should choose the most appropriate process improvement method to achieve effective reorganization of its structure, processes, and services.

REENGINEERING

As the contributing author, Robert Sutter, noted in the section above, healthcare organizations attempt to demonstrate the results of their performance improvement efforts by pursuing such awards as the Malcolm Baldrige National Quality Award or the American Hospital Association's Quest for Quality Award or by seeking certification by demonstrating compliance with the ISO 9000 series of quality management system standards.

Those who have implemented a reengineering process within their institution recognize the need to continuously improve. Reengineering requires you to focus on the customer's needs. By doing so, you are always looking to the customer (patient) for indicators of process modification. Once you begin reengineering, you really cannot stop. You continuously improve and inevitably reach a point when your patient requirements change. Then guess what? You will want to reengineer again, especially in healthcare, with its changing parameters and its constant reaching for better outcomes and measures (Deloitte & Touche 1996b).

Deloitte & Touche's (1996b) *Health Care Review* identified potential reengineering questions for healthcare organizations:

- What is the best way to care for patients?
- What is the best way to organize the work involved in acquiring members?

- What is the best way to manage care across the continuum?
- What is the best way to acquire and distribute materials in the hospital?

Reengineering has the potential to recreate organizations to improve quality and customer responsiveness, reduce costs, and streamline operations. It, too, relies heavily on employee teams coordinated by management to accomplish the change.

Technological, competitive, industry, and funding changes force department managers to rethink their organizational structure and work flow. Given the changes in the workplace, the administration, managers, and supervisors will be called on to initiate programs that redefine the organizational structure, reporting relationships, chain of command, and processes throughout the organization.

Reorganization may take place to overcome existing deficiencies. For example, in the past, many nurses found themselves burdened with too much secretarial and clerical work that kept them away from actual patient care and bedside nursing. This was an undesirable situation because the thrust of their education and purpose was the care of patients. Eventually, it became apparent that many of these functions could just as effectively be performed by someone else without a nursing education. This led to a job redesign and enlargement of jobs held by unit assistants. The care of non-patient-related things was assigned to these unit assistants, whereas the care of people reverted back to the nurses.

The success of this reorganization was evaluated by the industry. As nursing shortages continued to threaten healthcare facility viability, job design and work redesign occurred and patient care technicians evolved. These multiskilled individuals performed some of the patient care duties previously performed by nurses. Some tasks were eliminated, such as nightly backrubs. By employing patient care technicians, the number of nurses needed decreased, the cost of patient care staff plateaued or declined, and the talents of nurses were used for those patient care activities requiring nursing education.

Once this or any other type of reorganization approach has been decided on, it can be implemented in various ways. A gradual, long-term plan provides for a period of adjustment as the organization changes. This approach is less disturbing than sudden, extensive changes, sometimes referred to as the "earthquake" or "shake-up" technique to organizational change.

Learning the techniques, putting them to use, and continuously seeking input from employees all take time. Moreover, encouraging employees to be open to and share constructive criticisms about processes established by their supervisors and encouraging supervisors to not react negatively to the criticisms have been major hurdles that only a few enterprises have successfully overcome. For healthcare organizations to flourish, this type of equal exchange between employees and their supervisors must occur.

It is anticipated that employees in the future will expect to participate more in the decisions that affect their daily work routines, thus requiring managers to consider redesign activities that result in job enrichment.

DOWNSIZING AND RIGHTSIZING

Reengineering is often confused with downsizing and reorganizing. Reengineering is initiated to cause dramatic improvements in services, while *downsizing* or reduction in force, and rightsizing are meant as a means for moderate to high cost reduction. Each is a top-down approach, in contrast to total quality management or performance improvement that seeks changes from the bottom up. Reengineering's focus is strategic—that is, long term with a vision of sustained improvements. However, the focus for reorganizing through downsizing is to cut costs. These approaches can be painful to the staff involved. Not only are coworkers laid off, but layers of management can be collapsed, resulting in new management structures. Additional disadvantages include loss of a recallable pool of talent because the layoffs affect white- and blue-collar workers, hidden costs associated with poor morale, loss of knowledgeable and experienced employees and historians, and potential loss of customers who have established rapport with certain employees.

In reengineering, the employees become members of teams to determine how to do a job better. Because the team approach is employed, reengineering may take two to four years to implement, while downsizing and rightsizing are quickly initiated, usually with the assistance of external consultants and with little input, if any, from the employees.

Alternatives to Downsizing

Through employee input, a variety of alternatives have surfaced to address the fiscal crisis that often leads to downsizing. Some of these include timesizing, cross training (job rotation), lowering wages, attrition, reassignment, leaves, and buyouts. Timesizing is popular in some organizations because it can be applied across the board to all levels of the organization. This technique requires all staff to take a designated number of hours off, with or without pay. No one loses their job, but everyone contributes to the fiscal situation by either using up accrued paid time off or taking time off at no cost to the company. Attrition is another favored approach, whereby a position is not filled when an individual leaves. This approach requires the supervisor and his or her team to reassess the work of the department and reorganize to accomplish the efforts required with the remaining staff. Doing so may involve reassignments, job enlargement, job enrichment, and job rotation.

In any reengineering endeavor, circumstances often drive the approach that an organization must take.

Changes are always disturbing to those who are affected by them, regardless of how well intended the changes are. A manager who frequently changes the department's organizational structure runs the risk of damaging the morale of the subordinates. To the supervisor suggesting the reorganization, it might seem trivial, but to the subordinates it probably appears frightening because it implies changes in their working environment, status, and security. The wise supervisor knows how to strike a balance in the desirable amount with respect to organizational change. In most instances, the supervisor probably finds that most subordinates quickly adjust to change if it is properly explained, if the employees have input or even recommend it, and if the need for change is demonstrated. A more detailed discussion of the introduction of change appears in Chapter 22.

RECENTRALIZATION OF AUTHORITY

As you know, from time to time it is necessary to review the degree of authority that has been delegated. The supervisor may believe that he or she has lost control over certain activities and that it has become necessary to tighten up or to recentralize. Another reason to tighten or recentralize is the significant reorganization of an entity, such as might result from a merger. In a merger many site-specific services are no longer needed at each location. For example, human resources, materials management, accounting, patient financial services, and even telecommunication departments are frequently centralized at one location. This centralization effort streamlines the services, reduces staff, and requires the realignment of authority held by the remaining incumbents. Often reengineering tools are used to redesign critical systems and processes to accommodate the "new" organization. Clearly, involvement of some of your staff is necessary when such drastic organizational changes occur.

SUMMARY

In this chapter, we considered the organizing process from the supervisor's point of view. Drastic reorganization is called reengineering. This reorganizing approach focuses on the customer (the patient in the healthcare setting). Reengineering endorses the involvement of employees in the restructuring efforts. It differs from reorganizing that uses downsizing, which primarily focuses on the cutting of costs and elimination of jobs.

A vast number of tools are available to assist management in assessing reorganization options for the structure of the entity, the department, a service, and even a procedure. Employee involvement is necessary to ensure that a broad range of ideas and opinions is collected about the change and to gain buy-in.

After a change in the organizational structure has been accomplished or at least planned, the supervisor can proceed to delegate or redelegate authority in accordance with the departmental structure or modified process.

NOTES

1. Smart toilets: http://www.aahsa.org/pubs_resources/presidents_messages/2003/cow_chips_smarttoilets.asp.

2. Nielsen, Merry, Schyve, and Bisognano, pg. 9.

3. Ibid, pg. 5.

4. This section is contributed by Michael T. Troncone.

5. As viewed 2/12/06 at http://www.wordwebonline.com/en/TEAM.

6. V. Clayton Sherman has not been discussed in this book. However, Mr. Sherman authored *Creating the New American Hospital*. This book and his teachings have been embraced by many hospitals nationwide. He provides guidance for healthcare managers to balance the regulatory environment and monetary restrictions with the principal purpose of the organization—providing patient care. He encourages building an organization that is driven by customer satisfaction.

7. This section is contributed by Robert Sutter.

REFERENCES

Barry, R., A. C. Murcko, and C. E. Brubaker. 2002. *The Six Sigma Book for Healthcare: Improving Outcomes by Reducing Errors*, 7. Chicago: Health Administration Press.

Chandler, A. D., Jr. 1962. *Strategy and Structure: Chapters in the History of the American Industrial Enterprise*. Cambridge, MA: The MIT Press.

Deloitte & Touche. 1996a. "Interview with Michael Hammer." In *Health Care Review*. Washington, DC: Deloitte & Touche, LLP.

———. 1996b. "Facts and Fallacies About Reengineering: A Change Agent at a Critical Time in Health Care History." In *Health Care Review*, 2. Washington, DC: Deloitte & Touche, LLP.

Deming, W. E. 1986. *Out of the Crisis*. Cambridge, MA: Massachusetts Institute of Technology, Center for Advanced Engineering Study.

Dlugaz, Y. D. 2004. "Six Sigma Adds New Dimension to Quality Management." *Journal of Healthcare Quality* 26 (5): 2, 46.

Frankel, H. L., W. B. Crede, J. E. Topal, S. A. Roumanis, M. W. Devlin, and A. B. Foley. 2005. "Use of Corporate Six Sigma Performance-Improvement Strategies to Reduce Incidence of Catheter-Related Bloodstream Infections in a Surgical ICU." *Journal of the American College of Surgeons* 201 (3): 349–58.

Journal of Accountancy. 2000. "Golden Business Ideas." *Journal of Accountancy* (July): 124.

Lenaz, M. P. 2004. "Added Value in Health Care with Six Sigma." *Managed Care Interface* 17 (6): 50–51, 54.

Nielsen, D. M., M. D. Merry, D. Martin, P. M. Schyve, and M. Bisognano. 2004. "Can the Quality Gurus' Concepts Cure Healthcare?" *Quality & Healthcare*, supplement to *Hospitals & Health Networks* (September): 1–12.

Rice, B. 1984. "Square Holes for Quality Circles." *Psychology Today* (February): 17.

Spath, P. L. 2001. "Applying the Pareto Diagram to HIM." *For the Record*, February 5, 23–24.

Thomas, E. C. 2002. "The Challenges of Cutback Management." *Public Policy & Practice* 1 (2). [Online article; retrieved 10/4/05.] http://ipspr.sc.edu/ejournal/cutbackmanage.asp.

Torres, E. J., and K. L. Guo. 2004. "Quality Improvement Techniques to Improve Patient Satisfaction." *International Journal of Health Care Quality Assurance* 17 (6): 334–38.

Witt, J. D. 1996. "How to Implement Changes from Your QI Team." *Occupational Health Management* 6 (7): 77–78.

Woodard, T. D. 2005. "Addressing Variation in Hospital Quality: Is Six Sigma the Answer?" *Journal of Healthcare Management* 50 (4): 226.

Yound, D. 2004. "Six Sigma Black-Belt Pharmacist Improves Patient Safety." *American Journal of Health System Pharmacist* 61 (19): 1988, 1992, 1996.

CHAPTER SEVENTEEN

Committees as an Organizational Tool

CHAPTER OBJECTIVES

After you have studied this chapter, you should be able to do the following:

1. Explain the need for committees in today's organizational setting.
2. Describe the purpose and authority of committees.
3. Discuss the various types of committees and their functions.
4. Describe the benefits and limitations of committees.
5. Discuss the major considerations to bring about effective committee operation.
6. Discuss the importance of the chair's role.

A COMMITTEE IS a formal group with defined purposes and relationships within an organization. For example, the healthcare center's board of directors has a permanent position and a defined structure and purpose at the top of the management hierarchy. Although individual members may change, the nature of the group is stable.

We find committees, boards, task forces, commissions, and teams everywhere—in business, government, schools, churches, and certainly in healthcare organizations. An institution's growth in size and specialization makes its administration and coordination by the CEO and associates increasingly difficult and, at the same time, more necessary. One method to cope with this difficulty is to establish committees to whom to turn over specific problems to address.

Committees are an organizational tool that, if used properly, can be of great help in the smooth functioning of an enterprise. A committee is a group of people who function collectively by working together, whether their purpose is to make a decision, submit a recommendation, solve a problem, conduct an investigation, or manage a government agency. It differs from other units of management insofar as committee members normally have regular full-time duties in the organization and devote only part of their time to committee activities.

The amount of time management spends in committee activities is increasing. According to the Successful Manager's Handbook, managers spend between 25 percent and 75 percent of their working hours in group meetings (Davis et al. 2000). There are several reasons for the growing emphasis on committee meetings. First, because most enterprise activities have become more complex and specialized, a need has arisen to tap the specialized expertise of staff throughout the organization. Complexity has created an urgent need for coordination and cooperation. Conferences and meetings have proved to be a good means of answering these needs. Second, administrators now understand the fact that people are more enthusiastic about carrying out directives and plans they have helped to devise rather than those handed down from above. Thus, committees are an additional means for effectively combining the formal and the acceptance theories of authority, giving employees more freedom, greater delegation of authority, and more motivation.

Although we often hear people complain that there are too many meetings and that they take up too much time, committees are still a widely used device in all organizations, especially in healthcare organizations. They seem to have no substitutes. Without committee meetings, it would be almost impossible for an organization of any size to operate efficiently and effectively. Of the many ways of obtaining ideas and opinions on how to handle certain problems, there is really no better way than by holding a meeting. The real criticism of meetings is probably not that there are too many but that the results produced often do not warrant the time and effort invested.

No doubt you have sometimes been annoyed at being tied up in a meeting in which the chair (or one of the committee members) rambled along in all directions without any purpose whatsoever. In the meantime, more important work accumulated on your desk. It is very likely that the chair had not properly prepared for the meeting and that the performance did not increase your respect for his or her managerial ability. After an experience of this type, you can quickly see how important it is for supervisors to acquaint themselves with committee meetings and with committee or conference leadership techniques. In other words, supervisors should learn how to run committees well and how to obtain effective participation. Meetings then become increasingly interesting and stimulating because the participants have the satisfaction of knowing that the meeting is accomplishing something.

There may be occasions when the supervisor finds it necessary to establish an intradepartmental or interdepartmental committee or to chair a committee. At other times, the supervisor may only be an ordinary member of the committee.

THE NATURE OF COMMITTEES

A committee is a formal group of people with defined purposes and reporting relationships within the organization to whom certain matters have been committed. The committee meets for the purpose of discussing matters that have been assigned to the group. Committees have the following characteristics:

- Committees function collectively, and their members normally have other duties, making their committee work merely a part-time assignment. Because committees function only as a group, they differ considerably from other managerial devices.
- Committees can be found at all organizational levels, and at some time a committee likely exists or existed for every organizational activity.
- Committees can have line or staff capacity. The committee works on the problem to which it is assigned. In a line capacity, the committee makes a decision when a solution is reached. In a staff capacity, the committee makes a recommendation after analyzing and debating the problem at hand.
- Committees can be classified as standing or temporary. A standing committee has a formal, permanent place in the organization. Typically, it deals with the same set of recurring issues on an ongoing basis. In a hospital, for instance, the performance improvement, surgical review, infection control, pharmacy and therapeutics, and safety and new products committees are considered standing committees. The nature and purpose of a permanent committee remain the same although the individual members may change. A temporary committee, on the other hand, is one that is appointed for a particular short-term purpose and is dissolved as soon as it has accomplished its task. This type is also known as an *ad hoc* committee, and at times, it is called a task force or a team. The employee awards committee may be an ad hoc committee.

FUNCTIONS OF COMMITTEES

Most committee meetings may be described as either informational or discussional. In an *informational meeting*, the leader or chair does most of the talking to present certain information and facts. Assume, for example, that a supervisor wants to make an announcement about the new snow day policy. A meeting is called as a substitute for posting a notice or speaking to each employee separately. It may be expensive to take the entire workforce away from the job, but having an informational meeting guarantees that everyone in the department is notified of the subject at the same time. Such a meeting also gives subordinates a chance to ask questions and discuss the implications of the announcement. Care should be taken, however, that questions from participants are largely confined to further clarifications of the supervisor's remarks so that the meeting does not stray from its purpose.

In a *discussional meeting*, the chair encourages more participation of the members to secure their ideas and opinions. The supervisor could ask the individuals singly for suggestions, but it is probably better to call a meeting to allow them to make recommendations. Although it is up to the supervisor to make the final decision and to determine whether to incorporate some of the employees' suggestions, employees in such meetings nevertheless derive great satisfaction from knowing that their ideas have been considered and may even be used. The employees are likely to offer good suggestions and may most likely implement changes more enthusiastically if they participate in finalizing the decisions. In this case the committee acts in a staff capacity.

Many questions in a healthcare organization are of such magnitude and affect so many departments that it is far better to have the decision made by committee members representing several functions and specialties than by one individual alone. The same situation can exist within a department. For example, employees are frequently dissatisfied with the vacation schedule and weekend work, regardless of the supervisor's efforts to be fair. Naturally the supervisor can make a decision for the employees on these matters, but it would be better if staff could find a solution themselves. In such a case, management is not really concerned with what decision is made so long as it falls within the limits set—for example, that not all individuals who perform a single function are allowed to take vacation at the same time. By letting the group make this type of decision, it will come up with an acceptable solution. Even if such a solution is merely adequate and not necessarily the best, it is still better if it is implemented by the group with great enthusiasm than a "perfect" decision that is met with resistance.

BENEFITS OF COMMITTEES

A group of individuals exchanging opinions and experiences often comes up with a better answer than any one person thinking through the same problem. This is perhaps the major benefit of group discussion. Various people bring to a meeting a wide range of experience, backgrounds, information, perspectives, and ability far beyond what an individual can offer; as new members join the group, they bring new ideas and perceptions. All of this would not be available if the problem is delegated to an individual decision maker. Indeed, many problems are so complicated that a single person could not possibly have all the necessary knowledge to come up with a wise solution. The forum for evaluating alternatives and ideas among several people stimulates and clarifies thinking.

Group deliberation can also be very helpful in promoting coordination and cooperation. Members of the committee often become more knowledgeable of and considerate of the problems of other employees, supervisors, and administration. They become more aware of the advantages of and the need for working together to seek solutions. By being involved in the analysis, logic, rationale, and solution of a problem, individual members are more likely to accept and implement what has been decided. In reality, it matters little how much a person actually contributed to the plan, as long as this individual was a member of the committee and sat in on the meeting. Probably the most significant benefit of committees in healthcare organizations is promoting coordination and cooperation among the various units of the institution.

Committees have a number of additional benefits. They produce continuity in the organization; few committees replace all their members at the same time. Furthermore, they are a good environment for junior managers and executives to learn how decisions are made, to absorb the philosophy and thinking of the hospital, and to see how the organization functions. It provides a forum for potential leaders to be identified. Also it gives representatives from the various departments a chance to be heard and get involved in the affairs of the organization.

DISADVANTAGES OF COMMITTEES

Despite all these beneficial features, the committee has often been abused. Sometimes committees are created to delay action, and many people have come to think of the committee as a debating society. Jokes about committees are numerous, such as a group "that keeps minutes but wastes hours" and "where the unwilling appoint the unfit to do the unnecessary." Remarks are often made that meetings go all day long and leave no time for anyone to get real work done.

Indeed, one of the most often voiced complaints about committees is that they are exceedingly time consuming. Each member is entitled to have his or her say, and often certain individuals carry on too long about how valid their points are. According to Nelson and Economy (1996), meetings represent 25 percent of the average businessperson's working hours, 40 percent of the middle manager's, and 80 percent of the executive's. In addition to their cost in terms of time, committees also cost money. Time spent in committee meetings obviously is not spent otherwise on other productive activities. Thus, every hour taken up by a meeting costs the institution. Furthermore, expenses might be incurred for travel and preparation for meetings.

Another shortcoming of committees is that there are limitations to the sense of responsibility that they evoke. When a problem is submitted to a committee, it is submitted to a group and not to individuals. Responsibility does not weigh as heavily on the group's shoulders as it would on an individual's shoulders. The committee's problems become everybody's responsibility, which in reality means they are nobody's responsibility. It is difficult to criticize the committee as a whole, or any single member, if the solution proves to be wrong because each person may be quick to say that the committee made the decision. Members are willing to settle for less than the best solutions and blame the committee if the solution does not work. This dilution of responsibility is natural, and there is no way to avoid it.

The dangers of a weak compromise decision and tyranny of the minority are other shortcomings of committees. It has become a tradition in many organizations to reach decisions of unanimity based on politeness, cooperative spirit, mutual respect, and other considerations; committees, in this instance, use the lowest common denominator instead of the optimum solution. This often leads to committee action that is a weak, watered-down, undesirable compromise. Also, in their efforts for unanimous or nearly unanimous conclusions, committees may be tyrannized by a minority or a dominant individual who holds out as long as possible for the solution he or she advocates. Finally, the majority might allow itself to be dominated by such a minority or a dominant personality because of lack of time, interest, or sense of responsibility. This may even lead to a strain in working relationships outside of the committee.

Another danger is that committee members may become victims of the groupthink phenomenon. *Groupthink* is a way of thinking in which one's deliberations are dominated by a desire to concur with the group at any expense, even if the facts point to another conclusion. Pressure for unanimity may overwhelm some members, causing the group to overlook or negatively appraise alternative solutions. Under this influence, the group is likely to make decisions that are not in the best interest of the organization just to avoid conflict and dissent.

THE EFFECTIVE OPERATION OF A COMMITTEE

Most healthcare facility administrations have established a number of committees because, ultimately, they contribute to the smooth functioning of today's sophisticated organizational climate. A number of these committees exist to fulfill the requirements of JCAHO, Healthcare Facilities Accreditation Program, or the National Committee for Quality Assurance.

Therefore, supervisors must familiarize themselves with the means for ensuring effective committee operation and conference leadership. It is not easy to make committee meetings and conferences a success because the goals are numerous and difficult to achieve. As we have already indicated, the goals of committee meetings are (1) to develop the best suggestions or solutions for the problem under consideration; (2) to arrive at suggestions or solutions with a majority or, ideally, unanimity or consensus; and (3) to accomplish objectives in the shortest time. It is a challenge for any committee to fulfill these goals, but the following discussion offers a guide for effective committee operation and conference leadership.

Scope, Functions, and Authority

The first thing a committee must have is a mandate; it must know its scope and functions to operate effectively. The executive establishing the committee must define the subjects to be covered and the functions to be fulfilled; there must be a description of the committee's job. How the committee relates to other units within the organization must also be stated; this prevents the committee from floundering and enables the manager to check on whether it is meeting the expectations.

In addition to its functions and scope, the degree of authority conferred on the committee must be specified (see Figure 17.1). As briefly mentioned earlier, it must be made clear whether the committee is to serve in an advisory (staff) capacity or decision-making (line) capacity. For example, in many hospitals the human research committee (sometimes referred to as the investigational review

Figure 17.1: Example of Formalized Scope of Authority for a Medical Policy and Peer Review Committee of a Managed Care Organization

Criteria for Physician Committee Members and Committee Composition

Each physician appointed to this committee must have an initial organization medical efficiency estimate of at least 80%. Committee members and the physician committee chair are appointed by the chair of the board of directors. This physician committee is composed of nine Partners in Quality physicians representing a cross-section of physician specialties and central region geographic areas. At least six committee physicians must be present for the committee to make recommendations.

Medical Policy

The medical policy and peer review committee will recommend to the executive committee of the board of directors medical policy intended to promote high-quality, efficient medical care.

Organization's medical policy is used both in determining medical benefits payable to members and as criteria in retrospectively estimating an individual physician's medical efficiency displayed in medical practice patterns observed through data-based physician profile reports, focused medical chart audits, and all other relevant information from other sources.

In formulating medical policy, there will often be preliminary review and full development of medical policy issues by ad hoc specialty physician committees composed of the organization's specialty physicians. These ad hoc committees will recommend medical policy to the medical policy and peer review committee.

Medical Efficiency Estimates and QIS Score Based Physician Reimbursement

This committee will become familiar with all aspects of retrospective medical efficiency estimates and recommend various improvements likely to improve the accuracy of medical efficiency estimates.

The chair of the medical policy and peer review committee will recommend to the executive committee "best estimates" of medical efficiency ratings (QIS scores) for all organization physicians.

These QIS scores, when approved by the executive committee, will become the basis for physician reimbursement. The committee is also asked to address other issues touching on the terms of an individual physician's participation in the various organization physician networks serving various organization product lines and membership groups.

Any changes in an individual organization physician's QIS score will also be recommended to the executive committee by the medical policy and peer review committee.

Committee Meetings: Time, Place, and Minutes

The medical policy and peer review committee will meet as often as needed to accomplish the work of the committee but no less frequently than monthly. Committee members will be reimbursed for each meeting plus any travel expense. The place of meetings will be the organization's board room unless otherwise determined by the committee. The minutes of the committee meetings will be prepared by organization staff and approved and signed by the committee chair. The chair of the medical policy and peer review committee will typically present the recommendations of the committee to the executive committee (or full board of directors).

board) has line authority to make decisions on whether a proposed research project should be approved. In reaching the decision, this committee clearly has line authority. On the other hand, in most hospitals the medical executive committee acts in an advisory (staff) capacity when it deals with a physician's or surgeon's application for hospital privileges. This committee makes a recommendation to the board of directors, and the board in turn decides. In such an instance, the medical executive committee clearly acts as a staff committee. Committees may have been delegated hybrid authority—that is, having line authority for some actions and staff authority for others. The medical staff's executive committee may have line authority to remove an impaired surgeon from the operating room and have staff authority to recommend to the board what additional action should be taken relative to this surgeon.

For a formal, standing committee, all such information should be set down in writing in the organizational manual. Documents stating all this information for the various committees are also usually required by JCAHO. For a temporary committee, scope, functions, and authority must also be explicitly stated but perhaps not so formally. It is extremely important that an ad hoc committee only be established for a subject worthy of group consideration. If a topic can be handled by one person or over the phone, there is no need to establish a committee.

Composition

Because the quality of committee work is only as good as its members, care should be exercised in choosing people to serve on committees. Members should be capable of expressing and defending their views, but they should also be willing to see the other party's point of view and be able to integrate their thinking with that of the other members. Depending on the purpose of the committee, members with certain expertise or knowledge may need to be selected. For example, it would be wise to select a minister or priest to sit on a bioethics committee. If possible, members should be from approximately the same organizational rank so that they can contribute freely without the complications of a direct superior-subordinate relationship. If committee members are chosen from different departments, the problems of rank are more easily overcome. Sometimes the composition of a committee is dictated by outside regulations.

The committee device provides a good opportunity for bringing together the representatives of several different interest groups. Specialists of different departments and activities can be brought together in such a way that all concerned parties are properly represented. This results in balanced group integration and deliberation. The various representatives are then assured that their interests have been heard and considered. Administration should ensure that this concern with proper representation is not carried too far. It is more essential to appoint capable members to a committee than merely representative members. The ideal solution is to appoint to the committee a capable member from each

Figure 17.2

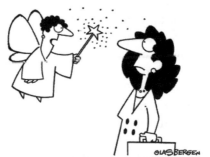

"I'm your Corporate Fairy Godmother with three wishes!
I wish you'd get to meetings on time, I wish you'd stop
interrupting other people, and I wish you'd
contribute something besides cynicism!"

pertinent activity. Finally, asking others to participate on a committee carries with it an obligation; you want them to know that the time they invest will be put to good use.

Size

No definite figure can be given as to the ideal size of a committee for effective operation. The best that can be said is that the committee should be large enough to provide for thorough group deliberation and broad resources of information. It should not be so large, however, that it becomes unwieldy and unusually time consuming. Usually, smaller committees with about four to ten members seem to work best. If the nature of the subject under consideration requires a very large committee, it might be wise to form subcommittees that can consider the various aspects of the problem. Then the entire committee can meet to hear subcommittee reports and decide on a final answer.

Effective Conference Leadership

Because the success of any meeting depends largely on the chair's ability to handle it, he or she must be familiar with effective conference or committee leadership techniques to guide the meeting to a satisfactory conclusion. The individual members of a committee undoubtedly bring to the meeting their individual patterns of behavior and points of view. The chair must know how to fuse the individual viewpoints and attitudes so that teamwork can develop for the benefit of the group. It takes considerable skill, time, and patience on the chair's part to create a closely knit group out of a diverse membership, but having such a group is generally the best way to achieve integrated group solutions.

The Role of the Chair

The chair is the most important member of the committee. This person is expected to play and succeed in two roles: (1) bring about the fulfillment of the task and (2) build and maintain successful group interaction. Because the committee is made up of individuals, great skill is required to help these individuals interact productively. The chair facilitates this interaction.

The first step, once the committee has convened, is to ask for volunteers to serve as the recorder and timekeeper. Next, the chair needs to help the members agree on the nature of the problem under discussion so that everybody understands the issues. Too often, people think first of how a new proposition affects them and their own working environment, which can lead to unnecessary friction in a committee setting. Also, people tend to see the same facts differently. Words can mean different things to different people. Thus, the chair has to find out what the participants think the issues are to be able to learn whether the participants understand the issues as they actually are. Committee members are reminded not to compete with other members and to give others' ideas precedence over theirs.

Finding out everyone's interpretation of the issues is easier said than done. A frequent comment about committees is that the issues on the conference table are really not as difficult to deal with as the people around the table. Individuals at a meeting often react toward each other rather than toward their ideas. For instance, just because Person A talks too much, everything he or she suggests may be rejected; Person B may automatically reject whatever someone else suggests; and Person C may be that member of the committee who never speaks. If you are running the meeting, listen to everyone. Paraphrase what participants have said when appropriate, but do not judge the merits of their comments. Avoid putting anyone on the defensive. As the meeting leader you must assume that everyone's ideas have value.

It is the chair's job to minimize these personality differences by using the legitimate tools of parliamentary procedure. Attempt to control the dominant people without alienating them. The speaking time of each participant can be limited so that one person does not monopolize the entire meeting. Also, one should be especially careful to call on people who seldom speak. Eventually, with the help of such leadership techniques, the committee will start reacting toward the meeting content and not the individuals around the table. For a meeting to be successful, the various members need to forget about their personalities and outside allegiances and work together as a team toward a meaningful solution of the problem at hand. In all this, the chair plays a critical mediating role.

The quality of the solution also depends to some extent on the amount of time spent in reaching it. Too much haste probably does not produce the most desirable solution. On the other hand, most meetings have a time limit. Ideally, time periods are assigned to each topic on the committee's agenda. By doing so, you are giving the timekeeper the limits for discussion. If there are no limits, you may risk members becoming bored and frustrated.

As the chair, your levels of interest and alertness are contagious. It is the chair's job to give every member a chance to participate and voice his or her suggestions and opinions. This is especially important when the committee members are also expected to execute the decisions they make. Then the chair may need to persuade the minority to go along with the decision of the majority. On other occasions, the majority might have to be persuaded to make concessions to the minority. All this takes time and may result in a compromise that does not necessarily represent the best possible solution. If the solution has been arrived at democratically, however, the chair's leadership abilities have been demonstrated and the major purpose of the meeting—finding a solution—has been accomplished.

It is important to keep all participants informed about the committee's actions. The recorder keeps notes during the meeting on a flip chart or board that everyone can see. This helps members to keep track of what they have discussed and what has been decided. At the end of each meeting, the recorder distributes, in advance of the next meeting, copies of the minutes and decisions made at the meeting with a reminder of the next meeting, date, time and location, and any assignments made during the meeting. In some organizations, the format of the minutes may be predefined by the organization for all committees.

The Chair's Opinions

It has often been stated that the function of a good chair is to help the members of the group reach their own decisions, to work as a catalyst to bring out the ideas present among the committee members. If the chair expresses his or her own views, the members of the committee may hesitate to argue further to express their opinions, especially if they disagree. This is even more likely to occur if the chair also happens to be their boss or holds a position higher up in the hierarchy. On the other hand, in many situations it would be unwise and completely unrealistic for the chair not to express his or her views. This individual may have some factual knowledge or a sound opinion, and the value of the deliberations is lessened if these facts were left unknown to the members of the committee.

On the whole, it is best for the chair to express his or her opinions last and, at the same time, to let participants know that his or her opinions are subject to constructive criticism and suggestions. After all, silence on the leader's part may be interpreted to mean that he or she cannot make a decision or does not want to do so for fear of assuming responsibility. On certain occasions, however, the chair must use sensitive judgment on whether or to what extent his or her opinions should be expressed.

The Meeting Set Up

At least initially, one should attempt to set a time when all the members are available. Once the committee has met several times at a consistent time and its schedule is established, members should take it on themselves to book the time in their schedules to attend future meetings. Always allow sufficient time between meetings to prepare for the next meeting and gather any information required.

Select a location that is convenient to all attendees. The room should be comfortable and stocked with supplies required to conduct the meeting effectively, such as a white board, flip chart, and markers. Set up the room to maximize participation, either around a table or in a semicircle so that all participants can see each other and hear the comments shared.

Today, many meetings are held via the telephone, thus eliminating the need for a conference room. These audioconferences (with sound only) or videoconferences (with sound and view of other participants) often serve committee members who are geographically dispersed. These approaches expedite the work of the committee and contain the costs of travel to a common location. However, this format presents its own challenges as the chair may not be able to judge member understanding of the issues or concerns because the visual advantage is not available. Members may be distracted by other work on their desk or e-mails that pop up on their PCs; as a result, they may be less participative in the discussion at hand.

Agenda and Task Control

Successful committee work requires good preparation. First, the chair must carefully outline the strategy and establish an agenda before the meeting. He or she should list the discussion topics in the proper sequence and decide how long the meeting will last. The chair may even want to establish, for his or her own guidance, an approximate time limit for each discussion item to ensure better control of the situation. If possible, the agenda should be distributed to the members before the meeting so they can better prepare themselves for the coming discussion.

Working with a well-prepared agenda is the best way to keep members on task. Although the agenda sets the overall strategy and sequence, it must not be so rigid that there is no means for adjusting it. The chair should apply the agenda with a degree of flexibility so that if a particular subject requires more attention than originally anticipated, the time allotted to some other topic can be reduced. In other words, staying close to the agenda should not force the chair to be too quick to rule people out of order. What seems irrelevant to him or her may be important to other committee members. Some irrelevancies at times actually help create a relaxed atmosphere and relieve tension that has built up. Because it is the chair's job to keep the meeting moving along toward its goal, it is a good idea to pause at various points during the meeting to consult the agenda and remind the group of what has been accomplished and what still remains to be discussed. A good chair knows the opportune time for summarizing one point and for moving on to the next item on the agenda.

The agenda should state the purpose of the meeting and any specific goals that need to be achieved. It should also state the starting and ending times with consideration given to employees' work hours. Occasionally, a meeting may not progress as planned. If the meeting does not appear that it will end as scheduled, ask the group if they wish to extend this meeting or to table discussion of the remaining topics. If the latter is chosen, you as the chair must make sure these topics appear on the next agenda. To assist the members and the chair to remain on schedule, some chairs establish time limits for the topics. Using the agenda as a guide and referring to it often keep the group aware of the time and their progress.

Advance Preparation

Furthermore, additional background information should be gathered either by the chair, the committee's own staff, or by designated committee members. This information should be distributed to the members before the meeting for their perusal and study. Meetings should be planned far enough in advance to give the members adequate notice and time to review any materials that will be discussed. This preparation allows the committee members to minimize conflicting responsibilities as they often serve on several committees.

Last, but not least, is making specific arrangements for the room, setup, equipment, and food. Confirm the arrangements at least once before the meeting and again, in person, on the day before the meeting. Nothing is more frustrating than to arrive at a meeting room only to find it is not set up properly or, worse yet, is occupied by another committee.

THE COMMITTEE MEETING

Now that you are familiar with some of the guidelines for effective committee operation, the discussion turns to examining how these guidelines can be applied in a typical committee meeting. In short, we discuss how a diverse group of people can, with the help of an effective conference leader, hold a meaningful discussion and arrive at satisfactory answers to the problems under consideration.

Always start the meeting on time. After a few introductory remarks and social pleasantries, the chair should make an initial statement of the problem to be discussed. This opens up an opportunity for all members of the meeting to participate freely. Any member should be able to bring out those aspects of the problem that seem important to him or her, regardless of whether they seem important to everyone else. The chair should facilitate the discussion to eventually get to the relevant points.

There are always some members at the meeting who talk too much and others who do not talk enough. One of the chair's most difficult jobs is to encourage the latter to speak up and to keep the former from holding the floor for too long. There are various ways to do this. For example, after a long-winded speaker has had enough opportunity to express his or her opinions, it may be wise not to recognize that member again, giving someone else the chance to speak. It might also help to ask him or her to please keep the remarks brief or to arrange the seating at the conference table so that it is easy not to recognize his or her request to have the floor. Most of the time, however, the other members of the committee find subtle ways of indicating that those members who monopolize the discussion are hindering others.

This does not mean that all members of the meeting must participate equally. Some people know more about a given subject than others, and some have stronger feelings about an issue than others. The chair must take such factors into consideration but should still stimulate overall participation. The chair should accept everyone's contribution without judgment and create the impression that everyone should participate. Controversial questions may have to be asked merely to get the discussion going. Once participation has started, the chair should continue to throw out provocative, open-ended questions that ask why, who, what, where, and when. Questions that can be answered with a simple yes or no should be avoided.

Another technique that the chair can use is to start at one side of the conference table and ask each member in turn to express thoughts on the problem. The major disadvantage of this technique is that instead of participating in the discussion spontaneously, members sit back and wait until called on. The skilled chair watches the facial expressions of the people in the group, as this may provide a clue about whether someone has an idea but is afraid to speak up. Then, the chair makes a special effort to call on that person.

If a meeting involves many participants, it may be advisable for the chair to break it up into small discussion groups, typically known as buzz sessions. Each of the subgroups holds its own discussion and reports back to the meeting after a specified period. In this way, people who hesitate to say anything in a larger group are more likely to participate in the smaller groups. Buzz sessions are usually advisable whenever there are more than 20 participants.

In using all these techniques to encourage general participation in the discussion, the chair should try to stick to the agenda and see that the discussion is basically relevant. Sometimes a chair who is inexperienced at holding meetings is so anxious to have someone say something that much discussion occurs merely for discussion's sake. This usually is not desirable because it confuses the issues and delays the even more important decision-making phase of the meeting.

Group Decision Making

Once a problem has been considerably narrowed down and understood in generally the same sense by all members of the group, try to determine the facts as objectively as possible. Only by looking at all the relevant facts is the group able to suggest alternative solutions. The chair knows that the best solution can only be as good as the best alternative considered. Therefore, the members at the meeting should be urged to contribute as many alternatives as they can possibly think of so that no solution is overlooked.

A popular and highly interactive group-discussion and decision-making technique is brainstorming. Brainstorming encourages the participants to be spontaneous and creative and have complete freedom of expression, regardless of how far out the suggestion is. Brainstorming is used to help a group create as many ideas as possible in as short a time as possible.

Brainstorming comes in two formats:

1. *Structured.* In this method, every person in a group must give an idea as their turn arises in the rotation or pass until the next round. It often forces even shy people to participate but can also create a certain amount of pressure to contribute.
2. *Unstructured.* In this method, group members simply give ideas as they come to mind. It tends to create a more relaxed atmosphere but is also open to domination by the most vocal members.

In both methods, the general rules are the same:

- Never criticize ideas.
- Write every idea on a flip chart or whiteboard. Having the words visible to everyone at the same time prevents misunderstandings and reminds others of new ideas.
- Everyone agrees on the question or issue being brainstormed. Write it down too.
- Record the exact words of the speaker on the flipchart; do not interpret.
- Do it quickly; 5 to 15 minutes works well.

The next step in this approach is to determine which idea to work on. GOAL/QPC (1988, 70–71) describes a commonly used technique known as the *nominal group technique* (see Figure 17.3).

The next step is to evaluate the alternative solutions and discuss the advantages and disadvantages of each. In so doing, the field can eventually be narrowed down to two or three alternatives on which general agreement can be reached. The committee members, by unanimous consent, can probably eliminate the other alternatives. The remaining options must be discussed thoroughly to bring about a solution. The chair should try to play the role of a mediator by working out a solution that is acceptable to all members of the group.

Often the best procedure is to find a solution that is a synthesis of all the important points raised by the members. Throughout this process the chair has the difficult job of helping the minority to save face. It is easier to placate the minority if the final decision of the group incorporates something of each person's idea so that everyone has a partial victory. This can be a long and tedious process, and, as we have said, such a compromise may not always be the strongest solution.

FIGURE 17.3: NOMINAL GROUP TECHNIQUE

When selecting which problems to work on and in what order, it often happens that the problem selected is that of the person who speaks the loudest or who has the most authority. This often creates a feeling in the team that "their" problem will never be worked on. This feeling, in turn, can lead to a lack of commitment to work on the problem selected and the selection of the "wrong" problem in the first place. Nominal Group Technique tries to provide a way to give everyone in the group an equal voice in problem selection. The steps in the process are as follows:

1. Have everyone on the team write (or say) the problem that he or she feels is most important. If members of the team do not write the problems out, have someone write on a flip chart or blackboard (or somewhere visible) the concerns as they are being communicated. If people do produce written problems, collect them when they are finished. Everyone may not feel comfortable writing, but it may make them feel safer by talking about sensitive problems at the beginning.

2. Write the problem statements where the team can see them.

3. Check with the team to make sure that the same problem is not written twice (slightly different words may be used for the same problem). If a problem is repeated, combine the two listings into one item.

4. Ask the team members to write on a piece of paper the letters corresponding to the number of problem statements the team produced. For example, if you ended up with five problem statements, everyone would write the letters A through E on the paper.

5. Make sure that each problem statement has a letter in front of it. Then ask the team members to vote on which problem is most important by putting a "5" next to that problem's letter. For example:

The problem list would look like this:

A. Space
B. Safety
C. Housekeeping
D. Quality Going Down
E. No Preventive Maintenance

So, if someone thought "quality is going down" was the #1 problem, it would look like this:

A. _____
B. _____
C. _____
D. ____5____
E. _____

Each member's paper would look like this:

A. _____
B. _____
C. _____
D. _____
E. _____

Everyone then has to complete the list by voting the second most important, third most important, etc.

A. 2, 5, 2, 4, 1
B. 1, 4, 5, 5, 5
C. 4, 1, 3, 3, 4
D. 5, 2, 1, 1, 2
E. 3, 3, 4, 2, 3

(continued on following page)

Figure 17.3: *(continued)*

An alternate ranking approach involves the "one-half plus one" rule. Especially when dealing with a large number of items, it may be necessary to limit the items to be considered. This rule suggests ranking only one-half of the items plus one. For example, if 20 items were generated, team members only rate 11 ideas.

6. Add up each line of numbers across. The item with the highest number is the most important one to the total team. In this case, B (Safety) is the most important item with a total of 20. Add up the numbers for each item, and put them in order.
7. You then work on Item B first, and then move through the list.

Source: Reprinted from The Memory Jogger.™© 1988, GOAL/QPC, Salem, NH. www.goalqpc.com. Used with permission.

Sometimes the group may not be able to reach a compromise or to come to any decision on which the majority agrees. This happens more often when the group is hostile. In such a situation the chair has to find out what is bothering the group and discuss it. Committee participants may think first of what is objectionable about a new idea rather than think of its desirable features. Discussing such objections may dispel unwarranted fears and may allow participants to see the positive aspects of a certain alternative. Also, the objections may be strong enough to void the proposition. In any case, the group must have a chance to voice negative feelings before a positive consensus can be reached.

Taking a Vote

The chair is often confronted with the problem of whether a vote should be taken or whether the committee should keep on working until the group reaches a final, unanimous agreement, regardless of how long it takes. Offhand, many people would say that voting is a democratic way to make decisions. Voting does accentuate the differences among the members, however, and once a person has made a public commitment to a position by voting, it is often difficult to change his or her mind and still save face. Also, if this individual is a member of the losing minority, he or she cannot be expected to carry out the majority decision with great enthusiasm. Therefore, whenever possible, it is better not to take a formal vote but to work toward a roughly unanimous agreement, even though it may take more time.

However, the price of unanimity is often a solution that is reduced to a lower common denominator and may not be as ingenious and bold as it would have been otherwise. The situation and the magnitude of the problem involved determine whether unanimity is worth this price.

The skilled chair can usually sense what the members are feeling, and all he or she needs to say is that a particular solution seems to be the consensus of the group. At this point, especially in a small meeting, the group can probably dispense with parliamentary procedure and a formal vote. In a large meeting, of course, unanimity may be an impossible goal, and decisions should be based on majority rule.

FOLLOW-UP OF COMMITTEE ACTIONS

Regardless of whether a committee is acting merely to come up with a recommendation or whether it has final decision-making authority, its results need a follow-up. After the chair has reported the committee's findings to the superior who originally channeled the problem to the committee, it is the superior's duty to keep the chair or the committee posted about what action has been taken. It is common courtesy to give the committee some explanation; inadequate statements or no statements at all cause the committee to lose interest in its work. When the committee has had authority to make a final decision, the chair generally keeps the committee members abreast of actions being taken in response to the committee's decision. Depending on the extent of the line authority granted, the committee may be responsible for carrying out the decision, or the particular executive who normally deals with the matter at hand may execute the decision. In any event, the committee members must be kept informed of any developments.

SUMMARY

Every supervisor has probably been involved in committees either as a member or as an organizer. Committees have become an extremely important device for augmenting the organizational structure and the functioning of an enterprise. They allow the enterprise to adapt to increasing complexity without a complete reorganization. They permit a group of people to function collectively in areas a single individual could not handle. The advantages of committees are offset to a certain extent by their limitations and shortcomings. Despite the disadvantages and other criticisms leveled against committees, they can be of great value if properly organized and led.

Committee meetings are called either to disseminate information or to discuss a topic. If discussion is involved, a distinction should be made between whether the committee is to arrive at a final decision on the question under discussion and take action based on this decision, or whether it is to make recommendations to the line manager who appointed the committee. A committee can be in a line or staff capacity.

Regardless of the committee's purpose, it is likely that group deliberation produces more satisfactory and acceptable conclusions than one formally handed down from above. Decisions are carried out with more enthusiasm if members of the organization have had a role in making them or in making recommendations. For group decisions and recommendations to be of high quality, however, it is necessary that the committee members be carefully selected. In composing a committee, one must ensure representation of as many interested parties as possible. The people chosen as representatives should be capable of presenting their views and integrating their opinions with those of others. As to the size of a committee, there should be enough members to permit thorough deliberations, but not so many as to make the meetings cumbersome.

In addition to these factors, the success of committee deliberations depends largely on effective committee or conference leadership. This means that the chair's familiarity with effective group work makes the difference between productive and wasteful committee meetings. The chair's job is to produce the best possible solution in the shortest amount of time and, it is hoped, with unanimity. In trying to achieve these goals, the chair is constantly confronted with the problem of running the meeting either too tightly or too loosely.

The chair has to depend on his or her perception of the mood and climate of the meeting to know exactly how to lead it and bring it to a successful conclusion. Thus, the chair has to sense when there has been enough general participation in the discussion, when alternative solutions have been properly evaluated, and when and if a vote is necessary to arrive at a group decision. In all these matters, the conference leadership abilities of the chair are of utmost importance.

REFERENCES

Davis, B. L., L. W. Hellervik, C. J. Skube, S. H. Gebelein, L. A. Stevens, and D. G. Lee. 2000. *Successful Manager's Handbook*, 266. Minneapolis, MN: Personnel Decisions International.

GOAL/QPC. 1988. *The Memory Jogger: A Pocket Guide of Tools for Continuous Improvement*. Methuen, MA: GOAL/QPC.

Nelson, B., and P. Economy. 1996. *Managing for Dummies*. Foster City, CA: IDG Books Worldwide.

CHAPTER EIGHTEEN

The Informal Organization

CHAPTER OBJECTIVES

After you have studied this chapter, you should be able to do the following:

1. Discuss the origins of the informal organization.

2. Describe how informal small groups evolve.

3. Describe the structure, benefits, and costs of the informal organization for its members and the power it can exert on the functioning of the formal organization.

4. Suggest ways the supervisor can react to informal groups and their leaders to improve relationships, thereby achieving increased organizational effectiveness.

IN ALMOST ALL enterprises, informal structures arise evolving from personal interactions, social activities, sentiments, friendship, common interests, and needs. This invisible, shadow organization produces intricate patterns of influence beyond and communication between the lines of the formal organization. These informal structures are not written down, nor do they have manuals, charts, or titles. But they are very influential on the functioning of the formal organization and can be supportive of or disruptive to managerial authority.

Whenever people work together, informal relationships exist and become a powerful source of influence on the formal organization. The formal task structure, goals, and functioning of the organization are affected by a social subsystem known as the *informal organization.* Early scholars maintained that an inherent conflict exists between the goals of the formal organization and informal relationships. Today we know that both formal and informal relationships are essential subsystems of a complex system and that the informal relationships help the functioning of the formal organization by providing individual satisfaction and group morale, which otherwise would be lacking.

THE GENESIS OF THE INFORMAL GROUP

The informal organization found in almost all enterprises is closely related to the workings of groups, committees, and group participation, but its origin is quite different. The informal organization is a powerful source of influence that interacts with and modifies the formal organization. Although many managers conveniently overlook its existence, they readily admit that to understand the nature of organizational life fully, it is necessary to "learn the ropes" of the informal organization. In almost every institution, such an informal structure develops. It reflects the spontaneous efforts of individuals and groups to influence their working conditions. For example, two or three people who do not work in the same area may meet daily for lunch because they enjoy each other's company, or people may join together because they have similar ideas about how a task could be improved and they want to approach their supervisor to discuss changing it. Whenever people associate with each other, social relationships and groupings result. The informal organization can make a positive contribution to the smooth functioning of the enterprise or can be disruptive. It also serves as a source of information for the grapevine discussed in Chapter 5. Therefore, the manager must understand, respect, and even nurture the workings of the informal organization.

To be more specific, informal structures arise from the social interactions of people as they associate with each other. Such interactions may be accidental or incidental to organized activities, or they may arise from personal desire or gregariousness. At the heart of informal organization are people and their relationships, whereas at the heart of formal organization are the organizational structure and the delegation of authority. Management can create or rescind a formal organizational structure that it has designed, but it cannot rescind the informal organization because management did not establish it.

At the base of all informal organization is the small group, consisting of a few people (five, for example) who share physical proximity and contact; this brings about an interplay of sentiments and interaction—sharing ideas, feelings, and opinions. The group interacts regularly to accomplish a common goal or purpose (Homans 1950). The first question that comes to mind is why people join such groups. We may wonder what advantages they gain from groups, as they are already members of a department in which their duties are specifically assigned, channels of communication exist, a line of authority has been established, and they are a significant part of a formal organizational structure. The answer to this question is that employees have certain needs they would like to satisfy but that the formal organization apparently leaves unsatisfied. One of the needs is for achievement, and the other is for emotional satisfaction. People have a basic need to associate with others in groups small enough to permit intimate, direct, and personal contact among individuals. The satisfaction derived from these types of relationships generally cannot be obtained from working within a large organization. Thus, the small group provides the individual with fulfillments that are uniquely different from those that can be obtained from any other source.

BENEFITS DERIVED FROM GROUPS

People join groups for various reasons, including interpersonal attraction, group goals, group activities, and social needs. First, group participation provides a sense of satisfaction. An individual in a group is usually surrounded by others who share similar values. This reinforces his or her own value system and interests and gives him or her confidence because it is always more comfortable to be among people who think along the same lines. The group also fulfills the need for friendship and companionship. The employee needs and enjoys the social contact with fellow workers, with whom he or she shares experiences and jokes and in whom he or she finds a sympathetic listener. The group thus fulfills the need for belonging and the need to associate with others who have similar attitudes, personalities, economic standing, and purposes and goals.

Another need satisfied by belonging to a small group in many instances is the need for balance and protection. Social interaction may balance routine and tedious work, but a small group offers protection from what the members may think of as an imposition or an encroachment by management, such as protection against increased output standards, changes in working conditions, or reduced benefits. We are all familiar with the old saying, "there is strength in numbers." In this respect the small group is a source of security, support, and collective power. Often people who enter an organization for the first time are anxious; the surroundings are unfamiliar and much uncertainty exists. When several people are in the same circumstance, they may form a small group on this basis alone, providing temporary support to each other in an unfamiliar environment. New employee orientation programs encourage the creation of these groups. Whenever people sense the need for protection, they form small groups.

An additional need that a small group fulfills is achieved status or acceptance, because the group enables an employee to belong to a distinct, small organization that is more or less exclusive. It also gives the individual an opportunity for self-expression and an audience of sympathetic listeners. Another reason why people join groups is to have access to the informal communications network and to secure information to reduce their uncertainties. This informal communications network is known as the grapevine. The grapevine works very effectively in small groups, providing speedy, although at times inaccurate, information. The network or pattern of communication often has no resemblance to the formal chain of command. Groups tend to form around an individual who seems to be the focal point in a communications network. An individual who has information is able to satisfy the communication needs of others, even though the information transmitted may be false or distorted.

In addition to these emotional needs, there exists the need for achievement, for getting things done. Groups are a means of getting a task accomplished by interacting, communicating, and collaborating. Informal groups help employees accomplish tasks that may be impossible to accomplish alone. They also serve to bring the goals of these tasks more into the realm of the employee. The objectives and goals of the formal organization may appear remote and meaningless to the average employee. It is much simpler to identify with the objectives and goals of one's immediate work group. Often employees readily forego some of their own goals and replace them with the goals of the group.

One of the reasons people form small groups is the need for information to reduce their uncertainties. These groups provide their own unofficial channel of communication—the grapevine—and access to it. This manifestation of the informal organization has already been fully discussed in Chapter 5. Briefly, however, the grapevine is the major connecting link of the informal organization, just as communication through regular channels serves to link the formal organizational structure. The informal organization influences the behavior of employees, regardless of the status they occupy within the informal group. This is important for a supervisor to remember because one cannot hope to understand individual behavior without understanding the behavior of the organizational forces that shape it.

By recognizing all these needs, the supervisor will understand the many reasons why employees tend to join informal groups and attempt to use these groups constructively.

THE INFORMAL ORGANIZATION

Small informal groups, as mentioned, are the basis of informal organization, and all small informal groups have the potential to become informal organizations existing in and interacting with the formal structure of the institution. In every organization, unless it consists of only a few individuals, an informal or invisible organization exists. The informal organization probably differs from the lines of the formal organization, but it is a functioning entity (see Figure 18.1).

The informal organization develops when small groups acquire a more or less distinct structure and a set of norms and standards, as well as ways to exert pressure for conformity and procedure and to invoke sanctions to ensure conformity to those norms. The informal organizational structure is determined largely by the different status positions that people within the small group hold. This is known as the "pecking order."

Status Positions

Generally, there are four *status positions*: the informal leader, members of the primary group, members who have only fringe status, and members who have out status. The informal leader of the small group is the person around whom the primary members of the group cluster; their association is close, and their interaction is intense. This is normally considered the small nucleus group of which newcomers would like to become members.

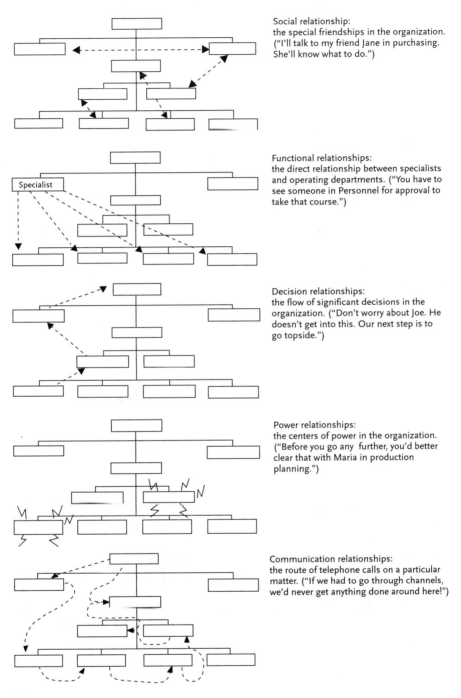

Social relationship:
the special friendships in the organization.
("I'll talk to my friend Jane in purchasing.
She'll know what to do.")

Functional relationships:
the direct relationship between specialists
and operating departments. ("You have to
see someone in Personnel for approval to
take that course.")

Decision relationships:
the flow of significant decisions in the
organization. ("Don't worry about Joe. He
doesn't get into this. Our next step is to
go topside.")

Power relationships:
the centers of power in the organization.
("Before you go any further, you'd better
clear that with Maria in production
planning.")

Communication relationships:
the route of telephone calls on a particular
matter. ("If we had to go through channels,
we'd never get anything done around here!")

Source: *Administrative Organization* by Pfiffner and Sherwood, © 1960. Reprinted with permission of Pearson Education, Inc., Upper Saddle River, NJ.

These newcomers are usually new employees of the department. They remain on the fringe of the group while they are being evaluated by the small nucleus for acceptance or rejection. Eventually these individuals either move into the nucleus, are gradually integrated, and become bona fide members of the small group or move into the outer shell because they have been rejected.

People in the outer shell are still a part of the department, although they have not been accepted as members of the core group. Such rejection, however, can have serious behavioral effects, especially if a person strongly wishes to belong to the nucleus group. This is true because, in essence, the group is a system of interactions that causes members to modify their own behavior and to significantly affect the behavior of persons in the fringe shell or the outer shell. If the rejection is mutual, the person in the outer shell can survive very well on his or her own.

The person who plays the role of the informal leader is usually the dynamic force of the group. As with the committee chairperson, this individual engages in leadership activities, crystallizes opinions, and sets objectives. This group leader is generally democratically chosen by the group. The leadership role is created by consensus. This person usually possesses communication skills, sensitivity, and intelligence and helps the members achieve their tasks and emotional needs. The informal leader gains status, although without rank, and satisfies the group members' need for a leader to whom they can turn for support. Occasionally one might find small groups in which the leadership is shared and in which different leaders perform different functions, sometimes only for a brief time. For example, one leader may deal with administration, whereas another may deal with the union, and another may try to maintain internal cohesiveness and morale. Most of the time, however, there is only one informal leader with whom the supervisor will have to deal.

Norms and Standards

Besides status positions, norms and standards are in place that regulate group behavior. Norms are expectations about how members of the group ought to behave. They define the boundaries between acceptable and unacceptable behavior (Feldman 1984). In addition to these standards for behavior between group members, norms relate to quality and quantity of work and to many other areas such as honesty and loyalty. Norms promoting high performance, creativity, and an honest day's work are clearly desirable, whereas cheating, leaving work early, and limiting output are not beneficial. One should not assume that the norms of one group cannot be generalized to another group.

To be admitted to the group, the employee must be willing and eager to comply with such standards, instead of or in addition to his or her own. Because groups are capable of granting or withholding the advantages of membership, individuals must modify their behavior so that it corresponds to that of the group. This is why the informal organization has such a significant influence over the behavior and work of employees who are primary group members. In addition, the interactions between primary group members also influence the behavior of those who are in the fringe shell and even possibly someone in the outer shell because all of them are members of the total system.

Sanctions

Along with norms, there must be an effective procedure for invoking sanctions if a group member does not conform to the standards set. If individuals violate group norms, group members exert pressure on them to conform to the norms. These sanctions can range from being elusive and evasive to being overt. At first, sanctions can be very mild; the group may try to bring the nonconformist back in line by friendly communication. If this does not produce the desired results, friendly comments may stop, and threats, ridicule, or possibly physical abuse may follow. The most powerful sanction is rejection. Employees who consistently do not comply with the group's norms are soon pushed to the outside shell. Their life can then be made miserable, their work can be sabotaged, and eventually they may want to leave the institution completely. All these sanctions of the informal organization, whether subtle or strong, serve to ensure that group members adhere to the group's ideas of correct on-the-job behavior.

Resistance to Change

Another characteristic of the informal organization is inflexibility, especially resistance to change. It resists especially those changes that could be interpreted as a threat to the informal group. Over time, the small group has developed very satisfying social relationships, and any change that may challenge its equilibrium and stability is greeted with resistance. This resistance can take the form of complaints, work slowdown, excessive absenteeism, and reduction in the quality of the job performed. It is essential for a supervisor to understand the dynamics of these types of group behavior to introduce change successfully. This is discussed further in Chapter 22.

Interaction Between Informal and Formal Organizations

It might appear that the informal organization makes the job of the supervisor more difficult. Because of the interdependence between informal and formal organizations, the attitudes, goals, norms, and customs of one affect the other. Informal organizations do frequently give life and vitality to the formal organization, but this is not always the case. Informal organizations can have either a constructive or hindering influence on the formal organization and on the realization of departmental objectives. The way the supervisor manages the informal structure has much to do with whether that influence is positive or negative.

The supervisor must respect the informal organization for the power it has; it cannot be ignored, and attempts to suppress it should not be made. It is important for the supervisor to be aware that these informal groups are very strong, and they may often govern the behavior of employees to an extent that interferes with formal supervision. Sometimes it can even go so far that the pressure of the informal group frustrates the supervisor in carrying out objectives that the superior manager expects the supervisor to achieve. The wise supervisor, therefore, should make all possible efforts to gain the cooperation and goodwill of the informal organization and the informal leader and to use them wherever possible to further the departmental objectives.

Both formal and informal relationships are part of the system, and they interact, each modifying the other. They may be mutually reinforcing or conflicting. The supervisor should remember that informal groups provide the satisfaction of some needs that the formal organization leaves unsatisfied. Informal relationships make a contribution to the organizational climate; they keep the organization flexible and can promote strong alliances.

THE SUPERVISOR AND THE INFORMAL ORGANIZATION

One way the supervisor can put the informal organization to the best possible use is to let the employees know that its existence is accepted and understood. Such an understanding enables the supervisor to group employees so that those most likely to comprise a good team can work with each other on the same assignments. The supervisor's understanding of how the informal organization works also helps him or her avoid activities that would unnecessarily threaten or disrupt the informal group. The manager should do his or her utmost to integrate the interests of the informal organization with those of the formal organization.

The supervisor should exhibit this positive approach because he or she knows that there are positive attributes in a cohesive informal group. Morale is likely to be high, turnover and excessive absences tend to be low, and the members work smoothly as a team. This can make supervision much easier because the supervisor avoids hearing a lot of bickering; it can also ease the burden of communication because the group provides its own effective, although informal, channels.

Supervisors who encourage informal group leaders and informal relationships are likely to make their own job easier by gaining allies. However, supervisors who suppress informal relationships risk creating enemies and retaliation. By integrating formal and informal organizations, effectiveness is increased.

Group Decision Making

A supervisor can do even more to bring out the positive aspects of informal groups by sharing decision-making authority with them—that is, by practicing group decision making (Maier 1983). When problem solving demands a diversity of viewpoints and skills and when broad-based acceptance is needed, group decisions usually are superior. They enable the group to exercise control over their own activities and to make certain that all their interests are taken into account, with the result that no one comes out a loser. The advantages and disadvantages of group decision making are similar to those of committees discussed in Chapter 17.

The supervisor should establish certain ground rules for a group decision-making process; otherwise, it could bring about results that are opposite from those intended. First, the supervisor must sincerely believe in group decision making and want to use it. Second, the topic must be clearly set. For instance, if the group is to arrange its own vacation schedule, it should be stated how many employees with a special skill must always be present, what the time limits are, and so forth. Third, it must be clear whether the group is merely asked for suggestions or whether the authority to find a solution and make a decision has been delegated. Finally, the supervisor should choose a problem in which the enthusiastic acceptance and execution are at least as important as, if not more important than, the specific elements of the decision itself. Under these conditions, group decision making can be an additional means of bringing out the positive aspects of the informal organization. These techniques can be equally beneficial in a task force or ad hoc committee in which group input and broad-based acceptance of a new process, policy, or the like, are necessary.

The Supervisor and the Informal Group Leader

Informal leaders are powerful because of their status and power of authority; they can be a great help when they work in the best interest of the institution. When informal leaders work against the goals of the organization, however, they can cause great difficulties. Therefore, supervisors should maintain a positive attitude toward the informal group leader. Instead of viewing this person as a "ringleader," supervisors should consider this individual as someone "in the know" and respect and work with him or her. In an effort to build good relations with the informal leader, supervisors can pass information on to that person before giving it to anyone else. They can ask for advice on certain problems and, particularly if a rearrangement of duties is under consideration, may want to discuss the problems with the informal leader first to get some feedback. Supervisors may also ask the informal leader to "break in" a new employee in the department, knowing that the leader would have done so anyway.

In taking this approach, the supervisor must be careful not to cause the informal leader to lose status within the group because working with the supervisor means working with management. In other words, the supervisor should not extend too many favors to the informal leader, as this would ruin the latter's leadership position within the group at once. This discussion assumes that an informal group leader is easily visible in the department. Often it is difficult, however, for a supervisor, especially a new supervisor, to identify the informal leader of a group. Observation is probably the best means to find out.

The supervisor should look for the person to whom the other employees turn when they need help, who sets the pace, and who seems to have influence over the other employees. The supervisor must continually and closely observe this because the informal group occasionally shifts from one leader to another, depending on the purposes to be pursued. Regardless of who the leader is, the supervisor should do all that he or she possibly can to work with the informal leader instead of against that person.

SUMMARY

In addition to the formal organization, there exists in every enterprise an informal organization based on informal groups. These groups satisfy certain needs and desires of their members, which apparently are left unsatisfied by the formal organization. For example, an informal group can satisfy the members' social needs. It gives them recognition, status, and a sense of belonging. Informal information transmitted through the grapevine provides a channel of communication and fulfills the members' need and desire to know what is going on. The informal organization also influences the behavior of individuals within the group and requests them to conform to certain norms the group has set up. Informal organization can be found on all levels of the enterprise, from the top to the bottom. It exists in every department, regardless of the quality of supervision.

Informal organization can have either a constructive or hindering influence on the formal organization. To make the best possible use of informal organization, the supervisor must understand its workings and be able to identify its informal leaders. Then the supervisor can work with them in a way that helps accomplish the objectives of the department. Instead of dwelling on the informal organization as a source of conflict, the supervisor should remember that both the formal and the informal organizations are part of a complex system and interact with each other. Instead of viewing it as something antagonistic, the supervisor should approach it positively and emphasize its potential for the good of the enterprise. One way to emphasize the positive is to practice group decision making by the informal groups. The supervisor must not suppress the informal relationships. Formal and informal relationships should be integrated to increase organizational effectiveness.

REFERENCES

Feldman, D. C. 1984. "The Development and Enforcement of Group Norms." *Academy of Management Review* 9 (1): 47–53.

Homans, G. C. 1950. *The Human Group.* New York: Harcourt Brace Jovanovich, Inc.

Maier, N. P. R. 1983. "Assets and Liabilities in Group Problem Solving: The

Need for an Integrative Function." In *Perspectives on Business in Organizations, Second Edition*, edited by J. R. Hackman, E. E. Lawler, III, and L. W. Porter, 385–92. New York: McGraw-Hill Book Co.

Pfiffner, J. M., and F. P. Sherwood. 1960. *Administrative Organization.* Upper Saddle River, NJ: Prentice-Hall.

PART V

Staffing: Human Resources Management

CHAPTER NINETEEN

The Staffing Process

CHAPTER OBJECTIVES

After you have studied this chapter, you should be able to do the following:

1. Define the staffing function as the sum of activities required to attract, develop, and retain people who have the knowledge and skills needed to achieve departmental objectives.

2. Describe how equal opportunity laws and fair employment regulations affect the staffing function.

3. Describe the relationship between the human resources department and line management.

4. Discuss the growing influence of the human resources staff in managerial decision making.

5. Explain the steps in human resources planning.

6. Describe the importance of job description and job qualifications based on job analysis.

7. Identify recruitment and staffing alternatives.

EOPLE ARE THE most important and valuable asset of an organization, not sophisticated equipment, facilities, or buildings. *Staffing* is the managerial function concerned with the procurement and maintenance of human resources to fulfill the institution's goals. It is the sum of activities needed to attract, develop, and retain people who have the necessary skills and knowledge to achieve departmental objectives. Once goals are determined, departments are set up, and duties and task relationships are established, people must be placed to give life to what would otherwise be an empty structure. It is the manager's responsibility to vitalize the department by staffing it properly.

Human resources management begins with planning for the present and future human resources needs. Staffing begins with recruitment and selection. *Recruitment* is the process of locating qualified candidates, and *selection* is the process of choosing from the pool of applicants. Staffing also involves making sure the department's subordinates are properly oriented, placed, trained, developed, compensated, and given benefits. Some of these activities are handled by the human resources manager, while others are handled directly by the employee's supervisor or manager. The manager's staffing duties also include judging employees' work and evaluating their performance, promoting them according to effort and ability, rewarding them, transferring them, and, if necessary, disciplining or even discharging them. Only if a manager performs all these duties can one say that the managerial staffing function has been truly fulfilled.

Staffing is a difficult task, and the importance of human resources management has expanded greatly in recent years. Good resource planning and maintenance have a major impact on the performance of the organization. Poor resource planning can result in severe shortages, and improper recruiting practices can lead to embarrassing situations. Much of these shortages or improper practices are caused by today's complex legal environment affecting human resources management. Thus, the supervisor depends heavily on the expertise of the human resources (or personnel) department. Most organizations with more than just a few employees usually have a department of human resources to assist the line managers in their task.

Many supervisors may believe that some of the previously mentioned duties are the responsibility of the human resources department. In many healthcare facilities some of these activities are performed by that department. In such institutions, the human resources or personnel department has very broad jurisdiction. Nevertheless, good management still considers human resources management the responsibility of all operating managers. Although the supervisor may be assisted by the human resources staff in performing these functions, they are still the supervisor's responsibility. For example, the human resources department does the recruiting and the initial screening, but the final hiring should be made by the supervisor of the department. The evaluation of the employees' performance should be made by the line supervisor, although the system, procedures, forms, and so forth are designed by the human resources staff.

THE STAFFING FUNCTION AND THE HUMAN RESOURCES DEPARTMENT

Throughout this chapter, the terms human resources department and personnel department are used interchangeably. This department is a staff department as defined in our discussion of line and staff capacity. Its usefulness and effectiveness depend largely on its ability to develop a good working and sharing relationship with line supervisors. This relationship is governed in part by how clearly and specifically the CEO has outlined the activities and authority of the human resources department. In determining the human resources department's scope and relationship to the staffing function of line supervisors, it is necessary for line managers to understand the historical place of the personnel department in organizations. Only then will supervisors be able to establish a structure that is meaningful in terms of current needs and environment.

Historical Patterns

The personnel department started primarily as a record-keeping department. It kept all employment records for the employees and managers, all correspondence pertaining to hiring, application blanks, background information, various positions held within the enterprise, dates of promotions, salary changes, leaves of absence granted, disciplinary penalties imposed, and other information on the employee's relationship to the enterprise.

Proper maintenance of these clerical records is still of great importance today, especially with the growing emphasis on equal opportunity employment, pensions and benefits, insurance programs, unemployment claims, seniority provisions, and promotional and developmental programs. By assigning such clerical service activities to the personnel staff, the administrator knows that the tasks will be handled competently and efficiently because of the department members' specialization. If such a service were not provided by the personnel department, each supervisor would have to keep these records for his or her own department, which is a time-consuming task for which consistency throughout the organization could not be assured.

In the 1920s, many managers in industry believed unionization might be thwarted if the industries gave to or supported for employees such benefits as cafeterias, better recreational facilities, bowling teams, and company stores. Management thought that these additions would make the employees happier and less resentful. Because none of these activities fit into the regular line departments of the enterprise, the personnel department took responsibility for many of them.

During the 1930s, another shift in the emphasis of the personnel department took place. With the increase of union activities, the personnel department was expected to take direct charge of all employee and union relations. It often assumed full responsibility for hiring, firing, handling union grievances, and dealing with general labor problems. In other words, management believed that by having a personnel department, all personnel questions could be handled by the department, leaving the line supervisors with practically no staffing function.

This led to serious difficulties, however, because while the duties and power of the personnel department increased significantly, the standing of the supervisor as a manager decreased. The more power the personnel director acquired, the weaker the supervisor's relationship became with his or her own employees. The demoralized supervisor justifiably complained that it was impossible to manage the department effectively without having the power to select, hire, discipline, and reward the employees. The employees no longer regarded the supervisor as their boss. Because someone in the personnel department hired the employees; established their wages; and promoted, disciplined, and fired them, employees looked to someone in the personnel department as their leader. The evolution of the unity of command concept forced management to clearly differentiate between the functions of the personnel department in a staff capacity and the supervisor's role as the department's operating manager.

Current Patterns

During recent decades, most organizations have recognized the need for constant interaction and proper balance of influence and authority between the line managers and the human resources staff. Good management dictates that supervisors and human resources staff must work together and share the burden because their work is intertwined; however, their areas of authority and their roles must be clearly stated. Sound management principles advocate that the primary job of the human resources department is to provide the line supervisors with advice, suggestions, and counsel and support concerning fair and equitable employee practices and personnel problems. Going beyond this could lead to a fragmentation of the supervisor's job and make it difficult for the supervisor to be an effective manager. Of course, the supervisor must manage within the framework of the organization's personnel policies, procedures, and regulations. Line supervisors should take full advantage of the expertise and assistance that is available within the human resources department, but they must retain the basic responsibility for managing their department.

Figure 19.1 is an excerpt from *The Management of Human Resources* (Cherrington 1991). The passage emphasizes the distinction between management and human resources.

Because it is the supervisor's job to ensure the work is accomplished within the department, he or she must make managerial decisions that concern the department's employees. Generally, this means that the supervisor defines the specific qualifications expected from an employee who is to fill a specific position. It is the human resources department's function to develop sources of qualified applicants within the local labor market. This department must let the community know what jobs are available and, in general, create an image of the organization as an employer. These activities are known as recruiting. *Recruiting* is the process of attracting and seeking a pool of applicants from which to choose a qualified candidate. This can be accomplished by fostering good community relations and recruiting from high schools, training schools, colleges, and other sources of employees. To promote the organization, the human resources department may tout the comprehensiveness of the benefits package in its open-position advertisements, mentioning benefits such as flex-time or job sharing, telecommuting options, insurance coverage, and paid days off.

When individuals apply, the human resources department should conduct screening interviews with the applicants to determine whether their qualifications match the minimum requirements of the job (e.g., education, certification, basic skills) as defined by the supervisor. The department also conducts testing

WE DON'T HAVE AN HR DEPARTMENT

An article in the Personnel Administrator described Nucor Corporation as the most productive steel mill in the world. When students in a human resource management class heard that a Nucor mill was located nearby, they thought it would provide an excellent field trip. One of the student leaders, Rebecca, called to arrange the visit. When she phoned she asked to speak with their human resource manager.

"I'm sorry, we don't have a human resource manager."

"Then could I speak with your personnel director?"

"We don't have a personnel director either."

"Then what do you call that position?"

"I'm sorry ma'am, but we simply don't have that position."

Assuming they had a special title for the position, Rebecca asked, "Who handles your compensation and benefits?"

"Our benefits are managed by our controller but our compensation is directed by a payroll clerk. Would you like to talk with her?"

"Is she also the one who manages the recruiting, hiring, and performance evaluation?"

"No, those activities are performed by our supervisors. Is there something I could help you with?"

Finally, Rebecca realized that they did not have a human resource manager or a personnel department. Eventually her call was directed to the general manager, who explained how the personnel functions were performed at that steel mill. Although Nucor Steel did not have a human resource manager at each mill, they had a manager of personnel services at the corporate headquarters who was responsible for creating personnel policies and programs for the mills.

The general manager explained that 335 employees worked at that location and all but 55 of them were directly involved in producing steel. These 55 included the supervisors, the clerical support staff, and six vice presidents. Although none of these people had the title human resource manager, they all performed various human resource functions. Wages, salaries, and benefits were distributed by the payroll clerk; health and accident insurance was supervised by an insurance clerk. The supervisors were responsible for most of the remaining personnel functions, including interviewing, hiring, discipline, safety, and training. Recruiting was not assigned to anyone since they had a long waiting list of job applicants and turnover was negligible.

The supervisors received a salary for 52 weeks per year, plus an annual bonus, while production workers received hourly pay plus generous productivity bonuses that were calculated daily and weekly. Everyone also participated in an annual profit-sharing plan. The productivity bonuses generally accounted for over two-thirds of the production workers' pay. Employees who came to work late forfeited their daily production bonus, and if

(continued on following page)

they were absent they lost their weekly production bonus. Consequently, tardiness and absenteeism were not problems at this mill.

Rebecca asked if it would be possible to bring the student group on a field trip to visit the plant.

"I'm sorry, but we cannot accommodate you. It's not that we dislike visitors or want to be secretive, we simply don't have anyone to show you around. We are in the business of producing steel, not guided tours."

Nucor Steel is good at making steel. The top five steel mills in the United States average 347 tons of steel per employee per year, while the top five integrated steel mills in Japan average 480 tons of steel per employee per year. Nucor produces approximately 950 tons of steel per employee per year.

Source: Management of Human Resources, Third Edition, by Cherrington, © Reprinted by permission of Pearson Education, Inc., Upper Saddle River, NJ.
Note: For current information about Nucor's continued success, visit www.Nucor.com/AboutUs.htm.

(e.g., keyboarding speed and accuracy, spelling, math) if the position requires it or if the organization mandates certain types of skill or administers personality assessments such as Management Skills Profile or Meyers-Briggs. This department should make necessary reference checks about previous employment dates and positions held, verify certifications and past records, and should not further consider those applicants who do not meet the minimum job requirements. Candidates who meet the stated requirements should be referred to the supervisor.

It is up to the supervisor to interview, select, and hire from among the qualified available candidates. The manager normally makes the final decision, often in collaboration with the direct line superior or team leader for whom the individual will work. The supervisor assigns the new employee to a specific job and has the responsibility of judging how this new employee's skills can best be used and developed. It is the human resources department's job to inform the new employee about the healthcare organization's benefits, general rules, shifts, and hours. This is typically done during an employee orientation program. The supervisor, however, should introduce the employee to the specific details about the department or section in which he or she will work and about the job (i.e., wages, departmental rules, hours, and rest periods). This department-specific orientation covers introductions to coworkers; a department tour; specifics about the assignment; and issues such as safety, security, computer passwords, and confidentiality. The supervisor either arranges to have another person, such as a department trainer, instruct and train the new employee on the job or does the training himself or herself. The supervisor assesses the new employee's performance to determine whether he or she should be retained or possibly retrained. The supervisor also monitors compensation within the pattern of remuneration and later decides whether this person should eventually receive a pay adjustment or be promoted into a better job. If the need to take disciplinary measures should arise, it is clearly the supervisor's duty to do so. During the time an employee is with the organization, the complete employment record is maintained by the human resources department.

Throughout the entire staffing process, the supervisor is greatly aided by the human resources department. The latter maintains all the records. As previously mentioned, this is particularly essential because of the importance of complying with nondiscriminatory employment, insurance, pension, promotion, and other practices as well as the added standards of accreditation and other regulatory agencies. The human resources department also provides expertise, advice, counsel, and guidance whenever personnel problems arise. In making decisions, the supervisor can follow, ignore, reject, or alter the personnel department's advice and counsel. In today's societal and legal environment regarding the staffing function, however, the input of the human resources employees has become vital and has a strong impact on the practice of management.

Sometimes supervisors welcome the human resources department's willingness to help them out of a difficult situation. Frequently supervisors ask the personnel department to make a decision for them so that they do not become burdened with so-called personnel problems. Supervisors gladly accept the department's decision, believing that if the decision is wrong, they can always excuse it by saying the decision was made by the personnel department. As a supervisor, "passing the buck" is not an option. All supervisors must remember that it is their responsibility to execute the staffing functions.

Although it is understandable that the supervisor may be reluctant to question and disregard the advice of the human resources staff expert, he or she must bear in mind that the staff person sees only a small part of the entire picture and is not responsible for how the department performs. Many other factors that affect the department are usually involved in the overall picture; factors with which the human resources staff are not as familiar as the line supervisor. The supervisor cannot always separate his or her functions between personnel problems and performance problems. Every situation has certain personnel implications, and it is impossible to separate the various components of each problem within the department. Only the supervisor is likely to see the broad picture.

Staffing and Legal Implications

During recent years, the staffing function has become more complex as a result of numerous federal, state, and local laws; executive orders and guidelines; and court decisions. Employment practices and policies must comply with these regulations, which in general prohibit discrimination against applicants and employees on the basis of race, sex, color, religion, or national origin. Also, employers cannot use age as a criterion of selection among applicants between 40 and 70 years old. Other laws might request that an organization hire handicapped persons and veterans. Affirmative-action programs might dictate that the institution give hiring preferences to minority members who are qualified or have the potential to fill available jobs.

A detailed discussion of labor laws is beyond the confines of this book; however, supervisors must be aware that information on these regulations is readily available from your human resources department or on the U.S. Department of Labor's web site. Figure 19.2 is a partial listing of the major labor laws and their respective enforcement agencies. Other legislative and regulatory issues have been discussed in Chapter 6.

It would be impossible for a line supervisor to keep abreast of all employment-related laws. This is where the expertise of the human resources department comes into play. The human resources department must make sure the organization complies with the multitude of laws and regulations. Of course, it is always desirable for the human resources director to disseminate current information regarding fair employment practices to all first-line supervisors. For example, the department of human resources should familiarize the supervisors with recent issues and government provisions. Also, the various possibilities of conscious and unconscious discriminatory practices and sexual harassment should be brought to the attention of the supervisors, and supervisors should understand the meaning of affirmative action. Ideally this information is disseminated and discussed at a new supervisors orientation program, either annually as a refresher or update course or regularly at management meetings.

FUNCTIONAL AUTHORITY AND THE HUMAN RESOURCES DEPARTMENT

The beginning of this chapter stated that the human resources department is attached to the organization in a staff position, which means that staff's job is to advise and assist line managers. During the last few years, however, many CEOs of healthcare institutions, industry, and businesses have decided to limit the supervisor's authority to terminate an employee. Thus, all dismissals have to be approved by the human resources director or designated liaison. Such a change is necessary to protect the organization from expensive wrongful discharge suits. The top-level administrator has the authority to make such a provision, and in this instance functional staff authority, as discussed in Chapter 15, has been conferred on the human resources department. In other words, top-level administration wants human resources to make the final decision on whether an employee who has been working in the institution longer than the customary probationary period should be dismissed. Many administrators have removed this portion from supervisors' authority and conferred it on the human resources department.

There must be solid reasoning behind such a decision because it clearly runs counter to the principle of unity of command and weakens the authority

FIGURE 19.2: LEGISLATION CHART

Legislation	Concern or Content	Administrative or Enforcement Agency
Fair Labor Standards Act of 1938	Minimum wage, overtime pay, and record keeping	U.S. Department of Labor
Equal Pay Act of 1963	Compensation relative to the sex of a worker	Equal Employment Opportunity Commission
Title VII of the Civil Rights Act of 1964[†]	Sex, color, race, religion, and national origin	Equal Employment Opportunity Commission
Age Discrimination in Employment Act of 1967 (amended 1978)	Age (protection for those 40 to 70 years old)	Equal Employment Opportunity Commission
Occupational Safety and Health Act of 1970	Workplace safety	Occupational Safety and Health Administration
Rehabilitation Act of 1973	Handicapped persons	U.S. Department of Labor
Employee Retirement Income Security Act of 1974	Pension plan rules	U.S. Department of Labor
Immigration Reform and Control Act of 1986	Employment eligibility verification	U.S. Department of Labor
Employee Polygraph Protection Act of 1988	Prohibits use of polygraphs by most private employers	Secretary of Labor
The Americans with Disabilities Act of 1990	Handicapped persons	Equal Employment Opportunity Commission
Family and Medical Leave Act of 1993	Permits unpaid leave for certain reasons	Employment Standards Administration
Health Insurance Portability and Accountability Act of 1996	Health insurance coverage	U.S. Department of Labor
Nursing Relief for Disadvantaged Areas Act of 1999	Permits temporary employment of alien/foreign RNs	U.S. Department of Labor

Note: This is a partial list of laws, regulations, and administrative agencies that govern employment policies and decisions. The list is effective at the time of preparation of this book.
[†] As amended by the Equal Employment Opportunity Act of 1972 and the Pregnancy Discrimination Act of 1978.

of the line manager's position. While the CEO may have other reasons for delegating final authority to the director of human resources, he or she may make such a decision based on the need and desire to comply with all possible fair and nondiscriminatory employment practices and regulations. Furthermore, administration should explain the importance of documentation, and line supervisors should be urged to keep meaningful personnel and recruitment records that they and the institution can refer to if necessary. If supervisors are kept up-to-date on these issues, it is unlikely that, for example, they will contemplate discharging an employee unless all possible ramifications have already been considered. Under these circumstances the director of human resources probably will go along with a proposed dismissal because the supervisor has a well-documented and substantiated case that can become a valid defense. It is desirable, therefore, that the personnel director, who has been given the final authority on discharge and other issues, uses his or her discharge authority with discretion.

Finally, the human resources department often has sole responsibility for many other activities such as maintaining personnel records, complying and keeping current with equal employment opportunity/affirmative action regulations, overseeing insurance benefits administration, conducting exit interviews, negotiating and complying with union contracts, setting wage ranges, handling outplacement service, initiating and maintaining employee assistance programs, developing safety programs, and conducting attitude surveys.

THE SUPERVISOR'S STAFFING FUNCTION

The staffing function is an ongoing activity for the supervisor, not something that is required only when the department is first established. More typically, the supervisor has to staff a department that already has an existing number of employees. In this case, although there is a nucleus of employees to start with, staffing is still needed as the composition of the department rarely stays the same for long. Because every supervisor depends on employees for the department's results, it is his or her responsibility to make certain that there is a supply of well-trained employees to fill the various positions.

Determining the Need for Employees

To make certain that the department can perform the jobs required, the supervisor must determine both the number and type of employees who will be needed for the department. By type, consider what competencies staff must possess that are most significant to the department's success. Some behavior competencies may be achievement orientation, customer service orientation, flexibility, teamwork, conceptual thinking, self-confidence, assertiveness, persuasive ability, professional aspirations, and developing others. Skill competencies may include proficiency with PCs, highly specialized monitoring equipment, printing machines, radiology equipment, air conditioning systems, or dishwashing units. Once the competencies are known, the supervisor can design a competency-based interview approach and query applicants in these areas.

If the supervisor has set up the structure of the department, he or she has designed an organizational structure in which the functions, competencies, and jobs are shown in their proper relationships. If the supervisor takes over an existing department, it is necessary to become familiar with the organizational structure by drawing a chart of the existing jobs and functions and assessing the competencies of the current incumbents. For example, the supervisor of the maintenance department may find that there are groups of painters, electricians, carpenters, and other tradesmen within the department. After taking this inventory of personnel, the supervisor should create a "staffing table" to determine how many skilled positions there are and should be within this department, what shifts need to be covered, and if the current incumbents are able to support the department's needs, considering budgetary constraints. The working relationships between these positions should also be examined and defined by the supervisor.

After determining the needs of the department, the supervisor may have to adjust his or her ideal department design temporarily to existing limitations. Several positions may have to be combined into one if there is not enough work for one employee. Then the competencies of the employee must be assessed to determine if he or she needs additional training to be able to perform successfully in the restructured position. Only by studying the organizational setup of the department can the supervisor determine what and how many employees are needed to perform the various jobs.

To fill the various positions with appropriate employees, the supervisor needs to match the available jobs in the department with the qualifications of prospective employees. The supervisor makes such a match with the help of *job descriptions* and *job specifications* (see Figure 19.3). Often these documents are included in the departmental manual. The job description tells exactly what duties and responsibilities are contained within a particular job. It describes what the employees do, how they do it, and what the working conditions are. A job specification, also at times referred to as job qualification, identifies and describes the minimum acceptable qualifications required of a person holding a job; it typically contains general qualification requirements such as experience and training, education, and knowledge and skills. Often, human resources departments create a single document that includes both the job description and job specification components.

Job descriptions and job specifications are based on *job analysis*—a study of the jobs within the organization. This consists of analyzing the activities the employee performs; the equipment, tools, and work aids the employee uses; and the working conditions. The supervisor who is taking over an already established department often finds a set of job descriptions available. If none is available, the human resources director will help establish a set. However, no one is better equipped to describe the content of a job than the supervisor. He or she is responsible for the accomplishment of the department's tasks and knows (or should know) the content of each position. Although the final form of the job description may be prepared in the personnel office, the supervisor should determine its specific content. Even when job descriptions are available, it is the supervisor's duty to become familiar with them to make sure they are realistic, accurate, and up-to-date.

Only by closely analyzing the job requirements is it possible to ascertain the skills necessary to perform the job satisfactorily. Even if the position is already in operation, it is still advisable to determine the major duties and responsibilities. Several questions you may ask yourself as you are analyzing a position appear in Figure 19.4. If the older job description no longer fits the current content

---

FIGURE 19.3: EXAMPLE OF A JOB DESCRIPTION/PERFORMANCE APPRAISAL FORM

Employee Name _____

Employee Number _____

Department/Unit _____

Job Title: Cook   **Job Number:** 24   **Salary Grade:** 7

Reports To: Immediate supervisor   **FLSA Status:** Non-exempt

Date Prepared/Revised: December 6, 2000   **Licensure/Certification:**

Job Summary: Reviews menus for upcoming meals, pulls meats for thawing and prepares and cooks meats; prepares and cooks baked goods and desserts, vegetables, and soups; and cleans up cook's area.

Education and/or Experience: At least one year experience as a cook and the ability to speak, read, and write English is required; high school diploma or G.E.D. is preferred.

Environmental Conditions: Work occurs inside; work involves frequent exposure to extreme cold conditions and hot and elevated surfaces; work involves occasional exposure to extreme hot and wet conditions, high dust and noise levels, low light levels, confined space, hazardous materials and sharps.

Physical Requirements: Work requires frequent standing, walking, stooping/bending, lifting up to 25 pounds floor to waist (25 to 50 pounds with assistance), up to 20 pounds waist to shoulder, and pushing/pulling up to 400 pounds (with wheels); work requires the ability to taste and perceive colors.

Drivers License Required? No   **CPR Required?** No

(continued)

Ratings for first four sections:

5	4	3
Much more than acceptable—significantly exceeds criteria for successful job performance	More than acceptable—exceeds criteria for successful job performance	Acceptable—meets criteria for successful job performance

2	1
Less than acceptable—generally does not meet criteria for successful job performance	Much less than acceptable—significantly below criteria required for successful job performance

Core Dimensions	Key Actions	Rating	Comments
Adaptability	• Tries to understand changes in work tasks, situations, and environment • Approaches change or newness positively • Adjusts behavior		
Building customer loyalty	• Uses Key Principles • Acknowledges the person • Clarifies the current situation • Meets or exceeds needs • Confirms satisfaction • Takes the "heat"		
Teamwork/ Collaboration	• Builds relationships (using Key Principles) • Exchanges information freely • Volunteers ideas freely • Builds on others' ideas • Supports group decisions • Puts group goals ahead of individual/own goals		
	Average Rating		

Role Dimensions (Skilled Role)	Key Actions	Rating	Comments
Managing Work (includes time management)	• Prioritizes • Makes preparations • Schedules effectively • Leverages resources • Stays focused		

(continued on following page)

Job-Specific Tasks		Standards	Rating	Comments
Tasks:	*% of time*			
Reviews menus for upcoming meal(s).		• Completely • In appropriate amount of time for meat to thaw		
Pulls meats for thawing.		• Accurately • In a timely manner • According to policies and procedures		
Prepares and cooks meats.		• Safely • According to written or verbal instructions based on type of meat • Consistently • By time required		
Prepares and cooks baked goods and desserts.		• Correctly, according to package directions or recipe • By time required		
Prepares and cooks vegetables.		• Correctly • Appropriately • By time required		
Prepares and cooks soups.		• Correctly • Completely • Thoroughly		
Cleans up cook's area.		• Thoroughly • Completely • Practicing "clean as you go"		
		Average Rating		

Other Job Objectives (Optional)	Accomplishment	Rating	Comments
	Average Rating		

(continued)

	Average Rating	Multiplied by:	Weighted Average	
Dimensions (50%)				
1. "Core Dimensions"		$\times$ 0.25	=	
2. "Role Dimensions"		$\times$ 0.25	=	
Performance (50%)				
3. "Job-Specific Tasks"		$\times$	=	If **no** Optional Job Objectives, multiply Average Rating by 50% (0.50).
4. (Optional) "Job Objectives"		$\times$	=	If **has** Optional Job Objectives, assign a percentage value, at your discretion, to "multiply by" in rows 3 & 4 to equal 50% (0.50).
Average Rating of All Previous Sections		(This column needs to total to 1.00)	(Add these averages to get the final rating)	

Ratings for this section only:

Expert—*can use the knowledge or skill independently and is also able to assess others and/or teach the knowledge or skill*

Competent—*can use the knowledge or skill independently*

Novice—*little or no experience with the knowledge or skill; needs training and/or assistance*

Knowledge and Skills (Job-Specific Technical/ Professional Dimension)	Results	Rating **E**-Expert **C**-Competent **N**-Novice	Comments
Knowledge of department policies and procedures.	Policies and procedures are followed.		

(continued on following page)

FIGURE 19.3: *(continued)*

Expert—*can use the knowledge or skill independently and is also able to assess others and/or teach the knowledge or skill*

Competent—*can use the knowledge or skill independently*

Novice—*little or no experience with the knowledge or skill; needs training and/or assistance*

Knowledge and Skills (Job-Specific Technical/ Professional Dimension)	Results	Rating E-Expert C-Competent N-Novice	Comments
Knowledge of safe food handling practices.	Safe food handling practices are followed.		
Ability to use basic mathematics.	Calculations are correctly made.		
Ability to operate cooking equipment.	Equipment is operated correctly and safely.		

Total number of Expert ratings _____

Total number of Competent ratings _____

Total number of Novice ratings _____

List any Corrective Actions received during the past twelve months and discuss progress to date with employee:

Key development (knowledge or skill) needs, including for a future responsiblity: (Ask the employee to complete an "Individual Development Plan" for a future discussion)

Key strengths:

Has employee completed annual requirements (m3 and PPD test) within the last twelve months? _____

Employee Signature _____

Reviewer's Signature _____

Date _____

Source: Courtesy of Deaconess Hospital, Oklahoma City, OK (adapted for use).

FIGURE 19.4: JOB DESCRIPTION WORKSHEET

Main Job Tasks:

1. What is the main purpose?
2. What are the essential duties?
3. What are the main priorities?
4. With whom will this candidate interact?
5. What deadlines does this job have?
6. What equipment does this job use?

Must-Have Requirements:

1. What basic skill requirements must the candidate have?
2. What special skills should the candidate have?
3. What kind of experience should the candidate have?
4. How much experience is needed? (One month? One year?)
5. What level of education is needed?

Preferred/Personal Skills:

1. How much stamina is required?
2. What work characteristics are important? (Ability to work unsupervised? Manual dexterity? Detail orientation?)
3. What level of communication skills is needed? (Written, public speaking, etc.)
4. How long would you like a person to remain in this positon?
5. What additional requirements are preferred, but not mandatory?

Source: McGill, A. *Hiring the Best.* 1993. Reprinted with permission of the McGraw-Hill Companies.

---

of the job, the supervisor should update it. Even if the job in question is a new position, the supervisor should proceed along similar lines. The supervisor should determine the job's duties and responsibilities and, with the help of the personnel department, draw up a new job description. Once the content of the job has been listed, the supervisor should specify the knowledge, education, degrees, experience, and skills required of the prospective employee. Asking current staff to provide input (see Figure 19.5) may surface not only content overlooked by the supervisor but also retraining and job redesign needs.

Equal employment opportunity laws and rulings require that job descriptions must not discriminate against certain classes (e.g., age greater than 40 [ADEA], disability [ADA], national origin [Civil Rights]) and must be job related. The supervisor should consult the human resources department for guidance on these laws. To comply with these laws and regulations, many personnel departments have assumed responsibility for the final review of the draft of the job descriptions. If they are kept current, position descriptions prove invaluable to many people throughout the organization. They inform the incumbent (and whoever needs or wants to know) what he or she is supposed to do, which

1. What is the primary purpose of your job? How does it contribute to the facility?
2. What are the essential functions of your job, and how much time do you spend on those tasks?
3. What are the peripheral functions of your job or tasks that someone else could do?
4. What amount of education and experience do you believe is needed for your job?
5. What skills are needed to perform your job?
6. How much reasoning is needed in your job?
7. What are the physical demands of your job?
8. What are the visual requirements of the job?
9. Please describe the noise level you experience in your job.

Source: Adapted from "Need Job Descriptions? Let Staff Start Them Off via a Questionnaire." May 2002. p. 3–4. Reprinted with permission from *Law Office Administrator*, P.O. Box 11670, Atlanta, GA 30355. (404) 367-1991.

includes some statement of authority and informational relationships; serve as a basis to recruit applicants for open positions; and evaluate incumbents in the position.

In every job, an employee must know certain facts before he or she can perform the job effectively. For example, a certain position may require the ability to read simple blueprints or perform basic or higher-level mathematics. If a knowledge of mathematics is needed for a certain job, the specific type of mathematics required should be clearly defined. The word mathematics could imply knowledge far beyond a working knowledge of simple arithmetic, or a knowledge of simple arithmetic might be all that is required in the job. The more precisely you define the required job knowledge, the easier it is for you to select from among available applicants.

When stipulating the skills needed for a particular job, the supervisor should not ask for a higher degree of skill than is absolutely necessary. One way to avoid this is to check the requirements drawn up with the qualifications of employees who are doing the same or similar work. Such an investigation may quickly reveal the minimum level of education necessary for a certain job. There is no need, for instance, to specify a certain number of years of formal education and experience if all that is required is simply job know-how. The job specifications should not ask for less than what is needed but should specify the requirements realistically. If the requirements are set too high, you may end up employing an overqualified person who may prove to be unhappy and bored with the position. It is just as disastrous to ask for less than the necessary requirements.

The human resources department can guide you in developing or drawing up these job descriptions. Once these job descriptions have been drafted, the supervisor should consult with some of the people who are holding these jobs to compare the job descriptions with the actual positions in question. After you have completed the draft, if this is the first time you have created a job description, it is wise to have it reviewed by the human resources department. Once all discrepancies have been resolved, these job descriptions are reviewed one final time by human resources and possibly by your boss.

The final, approved description is maintained in the human resources department and also in the supervisor's file. This is necessary because the job description is constantly referred to when the human resources department recruits candidates, when the supervisor hires new employees, when the employees' performance is appraised, and when establishing equitable wage patterns within the department or comparing wage scales with other organizations that have similar jobs. As a new employee is hired into the position, he or she should receive a copy of the job description.

If staffing decisions are to be valid, they must be based on comprehensive job descriptions that are systematically revised to reflect the current job situation as accurately as possible. Furthermore, they must reflect the current requirements of equal employment opportunity and nondiscrimination laws.

Position Titles

No standard agreement exists on the use and meaning of titles, especially in the upper echelons of healthcare organizations. This is because of the recent trend toward the use of corporate titles for the top-level person. The role of the most senior executive has evolved from superintendent to hospital administrator to executive director to CEO to president. (Throughout this book the terms president, chief executive officer, and administrator have been used interchangeably.) The job of the CEO in larger hospitals is no longer concerned only with the internal operations of the hospital but also with the external relations in the larger field of community responsibilities. This title communicates to patients, relatives, visitors, physicians, and the public that the president is the CEO in the organization.

Following corporate usage of titles, where the president is the CEO, implies that an executive vice president is on the second level, several senior vice presidents (e.g., for patient care and for fiscal affairs) are on the third, and vice presidents are on the fourth level (e.g., vice president of nursing, of professional services, of human resources, of environmental affairs).

Supervisors should not assume that every healthcare organization uses the same titles. A nursing home may use administrator, while a home health agency may use executive director for its top employed position. Physician groups often use executive director or practice administrator for their top employed position. Although the titles of the upper echelons vary from one healthcare institution to another, there must be internal consistency. Similarly, titles must be consistent across a healthcare system that may include a hospital, several ambulatory clinics, a home health agency, a durable medical equipment company, and a freestanding ambulatory surgery center. One way to do this is to use a basic title, such as director, and add adjectives to indicate the rank and area of activity (executive, associate or assistant director, nursing, medical and surgical; or chief technologist, radiology, ambulatory services).

How Many to Hire

Normally, the supervisor is not confronted with the situation in which many employees have to be hired at the same time. However, such a situation could exist when a new department is created and the supervisor has to staff it completely, if a strike is anticipated, or if part-time armed services personnel are called from their peacetime jobs to serve in a military action. More typically, the question of hiring a single employee will occur.

A supervisor usually needs to hire a new worker when one of the employees leaves the department voluntarily, is dismissed, or leaves for some other reason. Each vacancy should be considered an opportunity for the supervisor to revisit the department's or section's organization and reanalyze the job and related jobs for possible process improvements that may negate the need to replace the person or transition the department's structure closer to the ideal organization. Occasionally changes in the technical nature of the work take place, and manual labor may be replaced by machinery or sophisticated instruments. In this case a replacement may not be needed, or a new employee with the necessary technical skills will be hired unless an existing member can be trained. Opportunities may surface from the supervisor's study of the processes and organization to use volunteers or to consider outsourcing the effort to a contract service, either of which may be more cost effective than hiring a new employee.

Other situations arise for which additional employees have to be added. For example, when departmental activities have been enlarged or when new duties are to be undertaken and no one within the department possesses the required job knowledge and skill, the supervisor has to go to the open market and recruit employees. Sometimes a supervisor is inclined to ask for additional help if the workload is increased or if the supervisor feels added pressure. Before requesting additional employees under those conditions, the supervisor should make certain that the persons currently within the department are working up to capacity and that additional people are absolutely necessary. As a result of these shifting situations, the manager is involved in the staffing function much of the time.

In sum, the actual hiring decision is not to be made in the human resources office but rather by the supervisor of the department in which the employee is to work. Whether the job is non-skilled, semiskilled, or skilled, it is up to the supervisor to hire the employee or identify an alternative approach to getting the work done. Because all applicants are screened by the human resources department, the supervisor knows that all those sent to him or her possess the minimum qualifications prescribed for the job. It is the supervisor's job to pick out the one who can best fill the job. This is not an easy task, but the supervisor gains more and more experience in selecting the "right" applicant over time. The selection process is discussed below and in Chapter 20.

FINDING THE RIGHT PERSON

The pressure continues to mount on human resources departments to find qualified healthcare workers in the present tight labor market. Many of today's employees are members of the *sandwich generation*—that is, baby boomers whose professional livelihoods are "sandwiched" between personal responsibility to their children and their elderly parents. Baby boomer employees tend to have the most experience, but their personal stressors focus their attention on direct compensation, benefits, and flexible work schedules that support a work-life balance (Belliveau 2003). Nurses are not lining up for night shift positions and unskilled labor is not knocking at employers' doors for $12-an-hour jobs anymore. The unskilled pool can find jobs that pay them more and give them free food at the vast number of fast-food restaurants in every community.

Finding individuals that have the basic skill competencies adds another dimension to the recruiting problem. According to a 1998 Snelling Report, 60 percent of the human resources executives surveyed reported that current workers lack basic math skills, 55 percent cite serious deficiencies in workers' basic writing and comprehension skills, and 63 percent feel employees lack positive work habits (i.e., arriving on time and staying at work all day) (Snelling 1998).

The tight job market and the need for workers with both basic and advanced skill competencies have created a demand for older workers and volunteers. More older Americans have remained in the labor force, and this is for several reasons, including staying healthier longer, financial pressures, desire for more income for leisure activities, and the work is less physically demanding. If the tight job market continues, with unemployment rates averaging approximately 5.5 percent, human resources specialists and managers will need to rethink the recruitment process. One suggestion offered by Jeffords, Scheidt, and Thibadoux (2000) for filling those positions requiring college degrees is to develop a work relationship with a student as soon as possible. This may mean that supervisors need to tap local colleges and universities and offer to serve as training, internship, or cooperative work arrangement sites for their undergraduates while the student progresses through the curriculum. By participating in an ongoing program, the hospital has first choice of employees who are knowledgeable about the job and compatible with the department's culture.

The first step in establishing an internship program is to approach nearby technical schools, colleges, and universities to determine if they have an interest in doing so. Approaching the faculty in those curricula that produce the graduates you need most should be your target; examples may be nursing programs, physical therapy programs, heating and cooling technician programs, and radiology technician programs. Together with human resources, you may need to establish a part-time employment arrangement to compensate the student for the services he or she performs. The school may need to permit flexibility in class scheduling to allow the student to be at work, or you may need to modify the standard work schedule to allow the student to attend school. This arrangement will test your skills as a mentor as you will need to work one-on-one with your intern, share the "tricks of the trade," and continually encourage him or her to continue his or her education. At the end of the internship, you may even be required to complete a performance evaluation, including an assessment of his or her skill level, knowledge, and maturity.

Another arrangement similar to an internship or cooperative work arrangement is an externship. The externship is typically a short-term arrangement whereby the student spends from a few days up to a few weeks observing the work of others, working closely with one worker, or both. This option allows the student to determine if this is really the career he or she wishes to pursue.

Internal initiatives can assist with finding the right staff for your jobs. Some organizations have created their own internal "schools" to develop and educate needed staff. An example of this "growing-your-own" approach might be providing medical terminology, anatomy and physiology, and coding courses to groom coding technicians for filling health information, registration, clinic, and patient accounts positions. Cox Medical Center in Springfield, Missouri, established a state-certified school to train medical transcriptionists because the hospital had such difficulty hiring these specialized professionals.

Another alternative is to develop an in-house temporary agency that maintains a roster of individuals interested in part-time or temporary work on an as-needed basis. When a need arises, the agency coordinator starts down the list, calling those on the roster until one or more are able to fill the vacancy for the designated period of time or until a permanent replacement is found. Often these workers do not wish to have a permanent or full-time position but have the skills and are willing to fill in. Occasionally, these in-house agencies include staff who, because of health reasons, are on limited-duty restrictions or employees whose jobs were recently eliminated. Both of these groups of employees have knowledge of the organization, have contributed to the organization's goals, and wish to provide continued service to the facility.

Reevaluating the older-employee option is yet another alternative. Studies have found that older workers have better attendance records, are much less likely to file workers' compensation claims, use less healthcare benefits, and display a sincere willingness to learn new skills (Prenda and Stahl 2001). While some organizations thought it unwise to invest in retraining older workers, AARP revealed that employees in the 50 to 60 age bracket stay on the job an average of 15 years (Prenda and Stahl 2001).

Last, but not least, is a relatively popular approach for human resources recruiting efforts—offering perquisites such as sign-on bonuses, flexible work hours, and options for telecommuting. The candidates you most wish to hire are probably considering offers from competing healthcare organizations. Coupled with low unemployment is the bleak reality that only 35 million people were born between the years of 1964 and 1978 (Generation Xers), considerably fewer than the baby boom generation, who competed for work with 85 million contemporaries early in their career (Jennings 2000). While you have jobs for talented staff, there are not sufficient bodies to go around to fill those jobs. The few

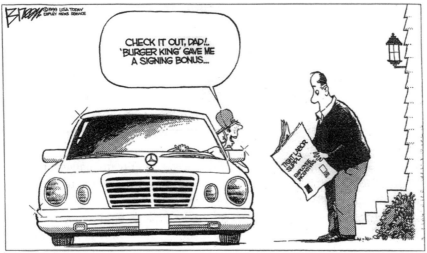

By Steve Breen, Asbury Park (N.J.) Press, for USA TODAY, Nov. 16, 1999.

Source: Courtesy of Steve Breen.

applicants that are available "want to wear khakis to the office, or don sweats and telecommute from home. They want immediate authority, independence and a voice in major decisions. They are technologically savvy and can probably teach you a thing or two about the software programs you use every day" (Jennings 2000). Luring recruits to your organization may require offering sign-on and continued employment bonuses, incentive plans, significant shift differentials for evening, night, and weekend shifts, and, if you are a for-profit healthcare organization, profit sharing or stock options. The clever comic shown in Figure 19.6 depicts how desperate employers may be. You must discuss your staffing needs and difficulties with human resources and together create an innovative recruitment plan to meet the departmental objectives.

Transfers

Transfers are another internal source of recruitment. A *transfer* is a reassignment of an employee to another job of similar pay, status, and responsibility. It is not a promotion because it is a horizontal move, whereas a promotion is a vertical move in rank and responsibility. Transfers take place either because the organization makes it necessary or because the employee requests it. Employees may want a transfer for various reasons—for example, to gain broader experience or to avoid some friction in a department. If an employee has problems that are causing friction, a transfer is not always the right solution unless it clearly resolves the problems. Sometimes technological changes in one department free a number of employees for transfer into a unit where needs for employees are expanding.

Transferring an employee from one position to another within the healthcare institution often results in greater job satisfaction. For example, a nurse's aide may consider a job as an aide in the operating room to be more prestigious than being an aide on the medical-surgical floor. The pay is the same and one cannot call it a promotion, but to the aide such a transfer means greater job satisfaction and constitutes an achievement. Transfers also provide employees with the opportunity to gain broader knowledge of the institution's activities. It is necessary, therefore, that a healthcare institution have sound transfer policies and procedures, always considering equal employment opportunity provisions, so that those who desire a lateral transfer are given the opportunity to do so. The director of human resources together with the various line managers should design these policies and procedures and ensure that employees are prepared to make successful transfers.

It is probably best for the human resources department to act as a clearance center for interdepartmental transfers. If the responsibility is given to supervisors, the supervisee may be reluctant to request interdepartmental transfers. Some supervisors may be understanding in these matters, whereas others may be resentful and not give their consent. Whatever procedure is instituted must have provisions that the employee inform the immediate supervisor of the desire to transfer. It is only fair that the present supervisor should be aware of the employee's intent. In the event that the immediate supervisor does not recommend the transfer, the employee should be able to appeal this decision to a higher line officer or possibly to the personnel director.

Provisions must also be in place dictating whether transfers are to be made only within departments, only between departments, or both. The procedure must state whether the employee carries previous seniority credits with him or her, and it must make provisions for the situation when two or more persons want to transfer to the same job. For example, should length of service be the sole determinant, or should capacity to handle the job also be taken into consideration? Good transfer policies and procedures must cover many additional aspects such as equal employment opportunities. In any event, the opportunity must exist for employees to be transferred, as this provides more job satisfaction and motivates employees in much the same way as a promotion.

Outsourcing

When traditional recruitment efforts are not successful in supplying your labor needs, you may need to consider *outsourcing*, or contracting out a part or an entire function area to a third party who supplies the appropriate staff. The growth in outsourcing in the healthcare industry has increased tremendously. U.S. outsourcing expenditures increased from $100 billion in 1996 to $345 billion in 2000. Future outsourcing expenditures are projected to grow exponentially (Kotabe 2005). You may be a supervisor for such a contracted third party. If so, your duties are not any different; in fact, you now have one additional burden—keeping your client, the hospital, or healthcare facility satisfied with your work.

Why has outsourcing grown? The reason is succinctly stated in *Controller Magazine* (1997): "The successful organization of the past was heavily departmentalized and layered, driven largely by tasks and transactions that move, for the most part, up and down the complex strata of management and supervision. But the organization of the present and future is much different: It has been streamlined by downsizing, decentralized to meet . . ." regional or "global needs, networked for fast and efficient communications, and reengineered from a departmental task orientation to an enterprise-wide process orientation that's designed to address" rapidly changing "corporate goals and objectives."

Hospitals have recognized that they cannot provide every service to every patient. Thus, they are reengineering their structures and focusing on their core competencies. Those activities that are not in the patient care realm become ideal candidates for outsourcing. For example, food service, housekeeping, patient billing, laundry and linen, security, clinical equipment management, information systems, and other activities are now outsourced by many hospitals. In fact, some hospitals are outsourcing clinical areas as well. A Healthcare Financial Management Association (HFMA 2000) newsletter indicates that healthcare executives expect to increase clinic outsource spending from 16 percent to 44 percent, and areas such as pharmacy, rehabilitation, perfusion, emergency, laboratory, and radiology are being targeted. If the outsourcing firm specializes in the service area needed, the hospital benefits from their expertise.

Often-cited reasons for outsourcing given by Controller Magazine (1997) and AHA News (Boothby 1998) include the following:

1. the function is difficult to manage or is currently out of control,
2. resources (labor and expertise) are not available internally or externally,
3. there is a need to reduce and control operating costs,
4. the organization desires to improve its focus,
5. the organization desires to improve patient satisfaction,
6. the function will result in budget flexibility,
7. the organization wants access to world-class capabilities or expertise,
8. the organization will become more competitive, and
9. the organization wants to free resources for other purposes.

Supervisors may find that evaluating outsourcing firms may be just one approach to filling jobs in the workplace. Supervisors who choose to investigate outsourcing possibilities and eventually recommend them must take into consideration the duties and roles the outsourcing firm may have in their departments and the parameters in which they are required to function. Some of these duties may include quality improvement, productivity and other reporting requirements, accreditation preparation, patient or customer satisfaction expectations, achieving expected savings, employee training, waste management, increasing staff morale, and smoothing interdepartmental relationships.

Outsourcing has its disadvantages as well. When a healthcare organization outsources a function, its existing employees may or may not be retained. Other employees will watch how you implement an outsource arrangement and possibly fear for their future employment. This fear could lead to increased turnover for the organization in other departments. The outsource firm may not be as cost effective as initially thought, and costs may rise more quickly than anticipated. Given the terms of the contract, you may or may not be able to terminate the services of the firm. If you do terminate, your recruitment woes return. Careful consideration must be given before proceeding with this alternative, and a supervisor is wise to include his or her boss and human resources in these deliberations before approaching any outsourcing firms.

SUMMARY

Staffing is the managerial function of procuring and maintaining the department's human resources, a function every supervisor has to perform. Staffing means to attract, select, place, train, retain, evaluate, promote, discipline, and appropriately compensate the employees of the department. All this is the supervisor's line function. The human resources department aids the supervisor in fulfilling this duty. In most enterprises, this department is attached to the organization in a staff capacity, and its purpose is to counsel, inform, and service all other departments of the enterprise. Sometimes, to be of service to the line manager, the human resources department may be inclined to take over line functions such as hiring and disciplining. Supervisors must caution themselves not to turn over any of their line functions to the personnel department, although at times it might seem expedient to let them handle the problems.

Before the manager can undertake the staffing function, the number and types of employees and competencies needed in the department must be clarified. The organizational chart combined with job descriptions will help the supervisor decide what workers are needed to fill the various jobs. In addition, the supervisor must consider the amount of work to be performed and the positions allocated in the budget. In all these supervisory duties, the human resources department is available for assistance and service.

During the most recent decades, numerous federal, state, and local laws and regulations as well as executive orders have been enacted regarding equal employment opportunities, fair employment practices, and nondiscriminatory practices. All staffing practices and policies must comply with these requirements. Making sure the organization is complying with these regulations is best handled by specialists in the human resources department. Because of the vast impact this has made on the activities of all managers and because of the importance of compliance, the influence of the human resources department within an organization has increased substantially. The CEO recognizes and deals with the need for a proper balance of influence and authority between the line managers and the human resources staff.

In a number of organizations, functional authority has been conferred on the human resources department, especially when the problem involves dismissals and fair employment practices. The average line supervisor could not possibly remain aware of new laws, court decisions, and so forth. Therefore, it makes good sense that the authority of the human resources department has been greatly increased, even if this means narrowing the supervisor's line authority.

Because of the tightened labor market, recruitment efforts have been stifled. To recruit qualified staff, various incentives may be offered, but these provide no guarantee of employee commitment. Managers have had to consider other options for getting the work done. One option growing in acceptance in healthcare has been outsourcing a function or part of a function to a third-party contract firm that has expertise in the function's duties and access to talented staff. Before proceeding with this option, however, management must consider the positive and negative aspects for the organization as a whole.

REFERENCES

Belliveau, P. 2003. "The Not-So-Young and the Restless." *HR Solutions* 28 (5): 36–38.

Boothby, S. 1998. "The Three Cs Make Outsourcing an 'In' Thing for Many Hospitals." *AHA News* (September 7): 5.

Cherrington, D. J. 1991. *The Management of Human Resources, Third Edition*, 2–3. Boston: Allyn & Bacon, a division of Simon & Schuster, Inc.

Controller Magazine. 1997. "Outsourcing and the Bottom Line." Special Report. *Controller Magazine* (November): 4.

Healthcare Financial Management Association (HFMA). 2000. *HFMA Wants You To Know*. Westchester, IL: HFMA.

Jeffords, R., M. Scheidt, and G. M. Thibadoux. 2000. "Securing the Future." *Journal of Accountancy* 189 (2): 49.

Jennings, A. T. 2000. "Hiring Generation X." *Journal of Accountancy* 189 (2): 55.

Kotabe, M. 2005. "Outsourcing and Financial Performance: A Negative Curvilinear Effect." The Fox School of Business and Administration. Temple University. [Online article; retrieved 9/27/05.] www.London.edu/assets/documents/MichaelMolpaper.pdf.

McGill, A. M. 1994. *Hiring the Best—Business Skills Express Series*, chapter 2, pp. 16–17. New York: McGraw-Hill.

Prenda, K. M., and S. M. Stahl. 2001. "The Truth About Older Workers." *Business and Health* 19 (5): 30–37.

Snelling Report. 1998. *The Skilled Workforce Shortage: A Growing Challenge to the Future Competitiveness of American Manufacturing.* Dallas, TX: Snelling.

CHAPTER TWENTY

The Selection Process

CHAPTER OBJECTIVES

After you have studied this chapter, you should be able to do the following:

1. Discuss the selection process.

2. Describe the purpose of the interview.

3. Discuss the difference between and purposes of the directive (structured) and nondirective (unstructured, counseling) interviews.

4. Discuss the importance of concluding the employment interview and making a decision.

S O FAR WE have discussed staffing as the sum of activities required to attract, develop, and retain people who have the knowledge and skills needed to achieve departmental objectives. We have learned how to successfully integrate the efforts of the human resources staff with our supervisory efforts to identify viable candidates for our positions. In this chapter, we discuss the selection process. The purpose of the selection process is to hire the best employees available for the organization. As Quicken (2000) says, "Hiring an employee is truly [about] making an investment in your organization. When you hire someone to work for you, you will invest time, money, training, and trust. If you do it right, your organization can move forward much faster than ever before; if you do it wrong, not only can you lose your investment, but you could be subject to lawsuits that might cause you to lose much more."

The selection process involves choosing the candidate who best meets the job demands, is likely to perform well, and also will stay with the organization. Candidates for a position may come from within or outside the organization. Because selecting the right employee contributes significantly to the effectiveness of the department, the final decision should rest with the candidate's prospective superior. In so doing, the selector can be completely responsible for how the selected candidate performs. Opinions of others, such as the selector's superior, those who have a working relationship with the candidates, and specialists from the human resources department can help the supervisor make his or her decision. The final decision on selection, however, rests with the department supervisor.

After all the preliminary work has been performed by the human resources department, such as recruitment, preliminary screening interviews, obtaining reference data, and relevant testing, the pool of applicants is reduced to three to five possible candidates. Line managers then interview these applicants, see them, talk to them, and select the one who will best fill the vacant job. The personal interview between the supervisor and applicant is an essential and crucial part of the selection process. It is a decisive step for the candidate and the supervisor and is the moment when the supervisor must match the applicant's personality and capability with the culture of the department and the demands of the job, the authority and responsibility inherent in the position, the working conditions, and the rewards and satisfactions it offers.

Equally important is the applicant's decision to apply. For the candidates, the process may be a considerable risk. The internal candidate may have had to obtain his or her current supervisor's permission to interview, and past performance evaluations are made available to the interviewer. The external candidate probably needs to take time off from his or her current job to interview.

Although some people question the interview as a reliable means of selection and as a predictor of performance, it is an almost universally used selection device. It involves two-way communication, enabling the interviewer to learn more about the applicant's background, interests, and values and enabling the applicant to ask questions about the institution and the job. The interview is not a precise technique, and it is difficult to interview skillfully. Because no fixed criteria exist for success or failure, prejudiced interviewers too easily evaluate an applicant's performance according to their own stereotypes. Job applicants may react differently to different interviewers. As a primary means for deciding, however, interviews are probably more valid for predicting employee behavior than decisions made on tests alone.

INTERVIEWS

It is not easy to appropriately appraise someone's potential during a brief interview. Interviewing is much more than technique; it is an art that can and must be developed by every supervisor. The supervisor will come to learn that there are several types of interviews, including preemployment (or selection) interviews between the supervisor and prospective employees, discussions when employees are fired, and counseling sessions during which the abilities and deficiencies of an employee are discussed. Other interviews occur when an employee voluntarily leaves the job as well as when an employee wants to discuss complaints, grievances, and any other problems. In general, all these can be grouped into two kinds of interviews: directive (structured) and nondirective (unstructured or counseling). Some interviews have aspects of both categories. For example, the appraisal interview (see Chapter 21) is primarily a directive interview, but the discussion may take on some aspects of a nondirective counseling interview.

Directive Interviews

A *directive interview,* also known as a structured interview, is a discussion in which the interviewer knows beforehand the goals, objectives, and areas of discussion. In a structured interview, a predesigned format is followed. The interviewer tries to obtain the necessary information by first encouraging the interviewee to volunteer as much as possible and then by asking the interviewee additional direct questions. The interviewer frequently follows a standardized list of questions, resulting in consistent, job-related, nondiscriminatory questioning. The benefit of structured interviews is that all pertinent aspects are covered and that the contents of all interviews can be compared.

Nondirective Interviews

In a *nondirective,* or counseling, interview, no checklist is used, and the format develops as the interview unfolds. In this interview, the interviewer encourages the interviewee to express his or her thoughts freely.

This type of interview is usually used in problematic situations in which the supervisor is eager to learn what the interviewee thinks and feels. The supervisor may conduct a nondirective interview when an employee has a grievance or an off-the-job problem. The supervisor may use this approach in an exit interview when the employee voluntarily leaves the job. Another reason a nondirective interview may be held is to obtain opinions about the overall operation of the department or employee satisfaction with recent changes. The interview is usually held with the supervisor of the subordinates; occasionally, however, a level of supervision is skipped and the department manager may meet one-on-one with subordinates of a supervisor. Affording your subordinates the opportunity of counseling interviews is a vital aspect of good supervision.

Counseling interviews can often be very time consuming. Although the supervisor is under many pressures and may not have much time for listening, time for such interviews must be made. By listening, a supervisor's relationship with subordinates is improved, and fewer personnel problems are likely to arise.

Skillful listening is an art that can be learned with training and experience. It can be learned better by practice, which the supervisor gains almost every day on the job, than by reading books on the subject. Eventually the supervisor can develop a system of listening that is comfortable, fits his or her personality, and at the same time puts the employee at ease. A common purpose of both directive and nondirective interviews is to promote mutual understanding and confidence. Neither is a cure for all human relations problems.

The Employment Interview

The *employment interview,* also known as the preemployment or selection interview, is an example of the directive, or structured, interview. The interviewer knows ahead of time what facts will be discussed, what the objectives will be, and what areas will be covered. The structured interview is conducted using a set of standardized questions asked of all applicants; this produces data that can be compared and provides a basis for evaluating the applicants. The interviewer should prepare the questions in advance. This does not mean that the structured interview must be rigid. Although the questions preferably should be asked in a logical sequence, the applicant should have ample opportunity to explain the answers. At times, the interviewer has to probe until a full understanding has been reached. The supervisor wants to learn as much as possible, first by letting the interviewee volunteer information and then by asking direct questions.

Preparing for the Employment Interview

Because the purpose of the directive employment interview is to collect facts and reach a decision, the supervisor should prepare for it as thoroughly as possible. First, it is essential that the supervisor become acquainted with the available background information. By studying all the information assembled by the human resources staff, the supervisor can sketch a general impression of the interviewee in advance.

Before conducting any interviews, the supervisor should re-review the position description and identify the competencies the ideal candidate must have. For example, if the supervisor is interviewing for a lead laboratory technologist for the chemistry section, some competencies may include the ability to develop and train others, technical expertise with several chemistry analyzers or other equipment used, good customer relations, a positive perspective, a history of high quality and productivity, and the desire to do things right the first time. Given these competencies, the supervisor should structure his or her questions to encourage the applicants to discuss issues and experiences related to these competencies. This also is the time to clarify any questions that may concern results of skill and aptitude tests given by human resources before the interview.

The Application Form

The *application* is a form that seeks information about the applicant's background and present status (see Figure 20.1). The completed application supplies a number of facts such as the applicant's schooling and degrees; training; previous work experience, including nature of duties, length of stay, and salary; and other relevant data. The candidate completes the application on his or her first visit to the human resources department, and the data are evaluated to decide whether the applicant merits further consideration.

The information contained in a completed application is somewhat limited because of laws, regulations, and court decisions regarding equal employment opportunities and discrimination. Generally, except under certain bona fide, job-related circumstances, federal regulations and guidelines prevent employers from requiring applicants to state religion, sex, ancestry, marital status,

EMPLOYMENT APPLICATION - Anywhere Ambulatory Surgery

General Information

NAME (LAST, FIRST, M.I.)			DATE	
PRESENT ADDRESS	CITY		STATE	ZIP CODE
PERMANENT ADDRESS	CITY		STATE	ZIP CODE
TELEPHONE NUMBER		SOCIAL SECURITY NUMBER		

Are you younger than 18 years of age?   If yes, birth date | Available start date: | Salary requirements:
☐ Yes   ☐ No

Employment status desired: | Shift preference: | Can you work weekends/holidays?
☐ Full-time ☐ Part-time ☐ Temp ☐ Per-diem | ☐ Day ☐ Evening ☐ Night ☐ Rotation | ☐ Yes ☐ No

POSITION DESIRED
1) _____   2) _____

Have you ever applied or worked for this facility before?   ☐ Yes ☐ No

If yes, facility _____   Date(s) _____ Position(s) _____
Supervisor(s) _____   Under what name(s) _____

Education

SCHOOL	NAME AND LOCATION	YEAR ATTENDED	DID YOU GRADUATE?	SUBJECTS STUDIED
High School				
Vocational/Technical				
College/Univeristy				
Graduate/Other				

Special courses, training, military service, or experience acquired.

Skills

OFFICE SKILLS	SOFTWARE PROGRAMS	EQUIPMENT
☐ Typing wpm ☐ Dictaphone ☐ Shorthand wpm ☐ PBX ☐ Ten key by touch ☐ Word processor ☐ Medical terminology ☐ Personal computer		

Licenses

LICENSES, CERTIFICATIONS, OR OTHER	STATE	ID NUMBER	EXPIRE DATE

We are an equal opportunity employer and do not discriminate on the basis of race, color, religion, sex, national original, age, disability, or veteran status as provided by law.

(continued on following page)

EMPLOYMENT INFORMATION
(List below your employment history beginning with the most recent employer.)

Employment History

Employer	Address: City: State: Zip:			Telephone number
Your position title	Dates employed From: To:	Starting salary	Ending salary	Supervisor's name and title
Describe your duties:				Reason for leaving

Employer	Address: City: State: Zip:			Telephone number
Your position title	Dates employed From: To:	Starting salary	Ending salary	Supervisor's name and title
Describe your duties:				Reason for leaving

Employer	Address: City: State: Zip:			Telephone number
Your position title	Dates employed From: To:	Starting salary	Ending salary	Supervisor's name and title
Describe your duties:				Reason for leaving

References

Please give two references (not relatives or persons previously listed) who are acquainted with your training or activities during the past five years. If recent college graduate, professors and faculty advisors in your field of concentration are particularly helpful.

Name	Address	Telephone number	Occupation	Years known

Other

Have you ever been convicted of a misdemeanor or felony (other than a parking violation)?   ☐ Yes   ☐ No

If yes, explain _____

The type and seriousness of the crime, along with your entire work history, education history, and the position for which you are applying will be considered. A "Yes" response to the above question will not automatically disqualify you from consideration for employment.

Comments

Make any comments that you feel are important in regards to your application.

I certify that the responses given above are true and correct to my knowledge. I have not withheld any fact which might adversely affect my application, and understand that any omissions of fact or any false or misleading statements will be considered just cause for immediate dismissal, no matter when discovered. I further understand that I may be required to pass a physical examination prior to final acceptance of employment.

_____   _____
Applicant's signature   Date

age, birthplace of the applicant or parents, and other personal data. Matters concerning what questions an interviewer is allowed to ask the interviewee are discussed later in this chapter.

An application may provide the supervisor with a sample of the candidate's abilities to write, organize thinking, and present facts clearly. The application indicates whether the applicant's education has been logically patterned and whether there has been a route of progression to better jobs. Also, it gives the interviewer points of discussion for the interview and references to contact.

While studying the completed application before the interview, the supervisor should keep in mind the job for which the applicant is being interviewed. If some questions arise while studying the application, the supervisor should write them down and ask them during the interview. For example, all previous jobs are stated in chronological sequence; however, these data might reveal a gap of six months during which the applicant did not work. Careful questions about this may reveal that the candidate spent the time unemployed, recovering from an illness or assisting a family member with an illness, traveling abroad, or attending a specialized course of study.

Scheduling Interviews

Not all interviews must be conducted in person. You may find, after careful review of a batch of applications and the accompanying human resources research, that six or seven candidates meet your requirements. You may choose to do a brief telephone interview with them. Be careful not to call them at work. If you call them at home and connect to an answering machine, you may wish to be somewhat vague about your call—for example, "Hello, this is Mr. Smith calling from Littletown Ambulatory Surgery Center. This message is for Suzanne McKnight. We received the information you sent us and would like to speak with you further about the materials. You may reach me at 555/444–1212. I look forward to speaking with you." The applicant may not have shared the fact that she was looking for a new job with her family or roommate.

To avoid interrupting candidates at work, try to arrange telephone interviews when they are at home or a private location. Furthermore, schedule the interviews with them ahead of time. It is only fair that they have time to prepare as you have. From the telephone interview, you may select two or three people to interview in person. You may wish to send these candidates a copy of the job description in advance. If they do not like what they see, they may not come in and you will not waste an hour or more of your time and the time of others who participate in interviews.

Because the purpose of the employment interview is to gather information to make a hiring decision, the supervisor should prepare a schedule or plan for the interview. The interviewer should jot down all those areas that need further clarification. Having thought out the various questions in advance, the supervisor can devote much of the attention to listening and observing the applicant, and writing the questions down helps ensure all the key points are covered in the interview. A well-prepared plan for the employment interview is worth the time spent on it.

Finally, the supervisor should be concerned with the proper setting for conducting the interview. Privacy and some degree of comfort are normal requirements for a good conversation. If a private room is not available, the supervisor should create an aura of semiprivacy by speaking to the applicant in a corner or in a place where other employees are not within hearing distance. Privacy is a necessity. If it can be arranged, precautions should be taken to avoid any interruptions during the interview by phone calls or other matters that could distract your attention from the applicant. Placing your telephone line on "do not disturb" or "busy" and posting a sign on the door "interview in progress" give the interviewee additional assurance of the importance the supervisor places on this interview.

Conducting the Interview

In conducting the employment interview, the supervisor should make certain that a leisurely atmosphere is created and that the applicant is put at ease. The good supervisor thinks back to when he or she applied for a job and recalls the stress and tension connected with it. After all, the applicant is meeting strangers who ask probing questions and is likely to be under considerable strain. It is the supervisor's duty to relieve this tension. The applicant might be put at ease by opening the interview with brief general conversation, possibly about the weather, traffic, or some other topic of broad interest. To put the applicant at ease and to build rapport, the interviewer may offer a bottled water or cup of coffee or may employ any other social gesture such as walking the applicant through the work area. A good starting question is, "How did you learn about this job opening?"

This informal warming-up approach should be brief, and the interviewer should move the discussion quickly to job-related matters. Excessive non-job-related informal conversation should be avoided. Studies have shown that sometimes the interviewer makes a selection decision in the first minutes of the interview, and it would be inappropriate to do this without having discussed job-related matters.

In addition to obtaining information from the applicant, the interviewer should ensure that the job seeker learns enough about the job to help in the decision whether he or she is the right person for the position. The supervisor, therefore, should discuss the details of the job, such as working conditions, wages, hours, vacations, information about the immediate supervisor (if he or she is not present and participating in the interview), and the job's relationship with other jobs in the department. The supervisor must describe the situation completely and honestly. In his or her eagerness to make the job look as attractive as possible, especially to professionals who are in short supply, the supervisor conceivably may state everything in terms better than they actually are. The supervisor must be careful not to oversell the job by telling the applicant the

Appropriate

1. What did you like best about your present (most recent) job? Why? What did you like least?
2. What special assignments have you taken on in the past (or your current job) that will make you successful here?
3. Have you ever been convicted of any crime or misdemeanor other than parking violations?
4. Is there anything that would preclude you from traveling out of town overnight or working overtime?

Inappropriate

1. Were you born in Cuba or the United States?
2. Will your husband (wife) have any problems with your working hours?
3. Have you ever been arrested for any crime?
4. Do you have babysitters arranged for your children?
5. Do you dislike your current job because you are reporting to a woman?

benefits or advantages that are available only to exceptional employees. If the applicant turns out to be an average worker, this may lead to disappointment.

After outlining the job's details, the supervisor should ask the applicant what else he or she would like to know about the job. If the interviewee has no further questions, the supervisor should proceed with questioning to find out how well-qualified the applicant is. The supervisor will have some knowledge about the applicant's background from the application, so there is no need to ask him or her to restate information already given. However, the interviewer will need to know exactly how qualified the interviewee is for the job. By this time, the applicant has probably gotten over much of the tension and nervousness and is ready to answer questions freely. Most of this information is obtained by the supervisor's direct questions. The interviewer should be careful to phrase these questions clearly for the applicant. In other words, only terms that conform with the applicant's language, background, and experience should be used. Questions should be asked in a slow and deliberate form, one at a time, so as not to confuse the applicant.

Be careful not to ask questions that could be considered discriminatory or illegal. Your human resources department can assist you in designing your questions to avoid certain pitfalls. Examples of appropriate and inappropriate questions appear in Figure 20.2.

Some employers publish guidance for their managers in policy manuals or on web sites. The University of Maryland Eastern Shore (2001) advises its managers, "A structured interview may include four different types of questions

Figure 20.3: Sample Interview Questions

The best predictor of future behavior is past behavior. Typically, a wide variety of questions can be used to help gain information that targets a specific job's skill requirements. Remember to probe until the question has been answered to your satisfaction.

1. Considering your previous positions, describe the work you enjoyed doing the most.
2. Considering your previous bosses and without giving me any names, which one did you like the least and why?
3. If a physician starts to yell at you because you failed to chart something for him or her, what would you do? How would you respond?
4. Have you had to change the way you did your work in the past because a new procedure or policy was implemented? What would you do if you didn't agree with the change?
5. Describe a situation where you did not agree with the supervisor's directive.
6. What would you do if you found two of your employees fighting?
7. Give me an example of a new process or system change you proposed and tell me how you convinced your supervisor that it was the right thing to do.
8. What experience from your prior positions will help you perform this job?
9. Why did you choose to apply to this healthcare facility?
10. If you found a copy of a patient's bill on the floor in the hallway, what would you do with it?

---

concerning job knowledge, job samples/situations, work requirements, and handling various situations." Your organization may provide you with sample interview questions similar to those shown in Figure 20.3. Many sample questions are available on the Internet for you to incorporate in your screening process.

The interviewer should take care not to ask leading questions that suggest a specific answer. The interview is a setting for dialog and for determining whether you and the candidate are a good match. The supervisor should refrain from questions such as, "Do you have difficulty adjusting to authority?" or "Do you daydream frequently?" This form of questioning may lead to antagonism and does not encourage dialog between the interviewer and the candidate. Better questions are those that leave an open ending—for example, "Could you describe how you handled the flooding disaster last fall?" "How do you view the nurse's right to not participate in a surgical abortion?" "Which responsibilities of this position are of most concern to you?" "What were the reasons you left your prior position?"

Frequently, supervisors take notes during or, preferably, immediately after the interview. This can be helpful, especially if several candidates are being interviewed. It is difficult to remember in such a situation what each of the applicants said and not to get their statements confused. There is no need to take notes on everything; only the key factors should be jotted down.

All questions the supervisor asks should be pertinent and job related. This brings up the area of questioning that, although not directly related to the job itself, can become relevant to the work situation. Problems of a personal nature, although only indirectly connected with the job, may be relevant. A supervisor has to use good judgment and tact in this respect, as the applicant may be sensitive about some of the points to be discussed. By no means should the supervisor pry into personal affairs that are irrelevant and removed from the work situation merely to satisfy his or her own curiosity.

Additional information about candidates can also be gained from a reference check. These are obtained from previous employers and are best handled by the human resources department; special care is advisable because of privacy regulations and potential exposure to damage claims. The points to be checked should be job related. All reference checks should be done with the knowledge and permission of the applicant. Figure 20.4 is a typical mail-out reference check form often used by human resources departments. However, a supervisor may wish to contact the applicant's former supervisor(s) for more specific, job-related information. Figure 20.5 presents some tips to consider when doing a telephone reference check as well as sample questions to ask.

Some applicants are skilled at designing, or should we say inflating, their resumes. You should warn candidates that you intend to check references very carefully. Even if a colleague recommends a candidate, the supervisor is wise to check other references given by the candidate. Further, if human resources has not checked education credentials, you should.

Equal Employment Opportunity Laws

Before the 1960s, the interviewer could ask almost any question that was job related in some way. Today, interviewing has become far more complicated and sophisticated because of the many laws, executive orders, and court decisions that affect equal employment opportunities, discrimination, and affirmative action. A number of questions are still perfectly lawful; for example, the interviewer can ask for the applicant's first and last names, current address, previous employment, and educational background. Questions that are for the most part unlawful include those about race or color, sex, religion, birthplace, and arrest record. Some questions are potentially unlawful to ask. For instance, it is certainly lawful to ask the applicant what other languages he or she speaks, as it is desirable, even sometimes necessary, in many healthcare positions to be bilingual. However, this question should not lead to asking the applicant's native language and the one used at home.

It would be presumptuous to provide a comprehensive list of what to ask and not ask in this book because each situation could involve legal restraints and has to be judged in the local context, relativity to the job, and the particular circumstances of the work environment. It is far better for supervisors to consult with the human resources department periodically to learn what can be asked, in which way, and what should not be asked. The laws and regulations are

FIGURE 20.4: SAMPLE AUTHORIZATION FOR REFERENCE CHECK

Deaconess Hospital

Authorized Release of Personal Data: Deaconess Hospital may request information regarding an applicant's education and work history from previous employers and educational facilities. Therefore, I, the undersigned, hereby authorize and request any present or former employer, educational institution, law enforcement agency, financial institution or other persons having personal knowledge about me to furnish Deaconess Hospital and/or its agents, with any and all information in their possession regarding me, in connection with any application for or retention of employment. Further, I hereby release from liability and hold harmless all persons and corporations supplying this information to Deaconess Hospital and/or its agents. A photocopy of this authorization is as effective as the original.

Signature: _____ Date: _____

Release Authorization: I authorize the company and/or its agents, including consumer reporting bureaus, to verify any of this information including, but not limited to, criminal history and motor vehicle driving records. I hereby release without reservation all persons, schools, companies and law enforcement authorities from any liability for any damage whatsoever for issuing this information.

Today's Date: _____ Signature: _____

The following must be filled out completely for your application to be considered. PLEASE PRINT.

Last Name: _____ First: _____ MI: _____

Home Address: _____

City: _____ State: _____ Zip: _____

Social Security No.: _____ Date of Birth: _____

Driver's License No.: _____ Driver's License State: _____

If you have ever attended school or been employed under any name other than the one listed above, please indicate the name(s) used: _____

Source: Adapted and excerpted from the Deaconess Hospital Application for Employment and related materials. Courtesy of Deaconess Hospital, Oklahoma City, OK.

FIGURE 20.5: TELEPHONE REFERENCE CHECK CHECKLIST

1. Identify yourself immediately, explain your position with the organization, and tell the reference party why you are calling about the applicant.
2. Ask if this is a good time to discuss the candidate. If not, arrange a time to discuss the applicant.
3. Assure the reference that any discussion you have will be held in confidence.
4. Offer to have the reference call you back collect or toll-free if you sense that the person doubts the legitimacy of your call.
5. Try to establish rapport with the reference you are calling to encourage freer exchange of information.
6. Tell the reference about the position for which the applicant is being considered. Ask the reference party, "How do you think the candidate would fit into our vacancy?"
7. Ask questions about the candidate's relationship with the reference:
   - How is it that you know the applicant?
   - What are his or her strengths? Weaknesses?
8. How did he or she get along with peers? Supervisors? Physicians?
9. Did the applicant meet commitments? Deadlines?
10. Did you observe the applicant in any stressful situations? How did she/he handle her/himself?
11. What type of support will we need to provide him/her to ensure he/she will be successful in this position?
12. Why do you think the applicant is interested in this position?
13. Does the applicant work best alone or with a team?
14. How was the applicant's attendance?
15. Did you find him or her to be honest and trustworthy?
16. Compared to others, how would you assess this person's professional/clinical knowledge and skill?
17. How would you describe the individual's communication skills?
18. Did you observe this individual working with subordinates? If so, could you describe that interaction?
19. Would you rehire the applicant?
20. Is there anything else you think I should know about the applicant?

---

numerous and ever changing and, in some cases, may be state specific. New decisions are made by the courts and administrative agencies almost daily, so it is a full-time job to stay abreast of them. The staff in the human resources recruiting division is usually familiar with the most recent developments and proper current practices. The interviewer should consult with them to learn which questions are appropriate, lawful if properly worded, and unlawful. The interviewer may also receive some suggestions as to how to obtain information that is necessary but cannot be asked directly. For example, rather than asking,

"How would your spouse feel about you traveling a lot or working long hours?", the supervisor may try to get the same information from questions such as, "Can you be away from home overnight if the job requires it?" or "Will your home responsibilities permit you to work around the clock?"

Closing the Interview

Candidates, no doubt, have questions they wish to have answered so that they, too, may make an informed decision. Some may ask questions throughout the interview, while others may wait until you have finished asking yours. Regardless, it is important for you to ask the applicant if he or she has any questions. This provides you and the applicant an opportunity to clarify anything that had been discussed beforehand. It also provides you with a snapshot of how interested this candidate may be in the position. Did he prepare questions? Are these questions that popped into his head during the interview? Are the questions well structured? Do the questions seek specific information?

This closing period of the interview also permits you to tell the applicant your next steps. These options are discussed in the next section; suffice it to mention here that you should give the applicant an idea of when he or she may expect a decision about his or her candidacy for the position.

EVALUATING THE APPLICANT

The chief problem in employment interviews is how to interpret the candidate's employment and personal history and other pertinent information. It is impossible for supervisors to eliminate completely all their personal preferences and prejudices. Interviewers should face up to personal biases and make efforts to control them. A supervisor cannot claim that he or she has no biases and should be able to clearly write down the reasons one applicant has been selected over another. It is essential that the interviewers take great care to avoid some of the more common pitfalls while sizing up a job applicant (Bynham 1984). Also, a supervisor may overlook something on an application or a resume that may be caught by another set of eyes. For all these reasons, it may be beneficial to ask another peer supervisor to participate in the interview or to interview the candidate separately. Some organizations encourage the team peers to conduct an interview with the final one or two candidates that the supervisor prefers. The purpose for having multiple interviewers is to help the supervisor avoid the following pitfalls.

The first of these pitfalls is making snap judgments. It is difficult not to form an early impression and look for evidence during the rest of the interview to substantiate this first impression. The interviewer should collect all the information on the applicant before making a judgment. This also helps the interviewer not to become a victim of the halo effect, which occurs when an interviewer lets one prominent characteristic overshadow other evidence. It means basing an applicant's entire potential for job performance on one or two characteristics and using this impression as a guide in rating all the other factors. This may work either favorably or unfavorably for the job seeker. In any event, it is wrong for the supervisor to form an overall opinion of the applicant based on a single factor, such as the ability to express himself or herself fluently. If an applicant is articulate, there is no reason to automatically assume the rest of his or her qualifications are top notch. A glance at the employees in the department will remind the supervisor that there are some very successful employees whose verbal communications are rather poor.

Another common pitfall is that of overgeneralization. The interviewer must not assume that because an applicant behaves in a certain manner in one situation he or she will automatically behave the same way in all other situations. There may be a special reason why the applicant may answer a question in a rather evasive manner. It is wrong to conclude from this evasiveness in answering one question that the applicant is underhanded and probably not trustworthy. The halo effect is a factor if the interviewer lets, for example, an applicant's alma mater overshadow other aspects of his or her profile. Remember that people are prone to generalize quickly.

Judging the applicant by comparisons with current employees in the department is another common mistake. The interviewer may wonder how this applicant will get along with the other employees and with the manager of the department or other supervisors, and how the candidate will fit into the corporate culture. The interviewer may believe that any applicant who is considerably different from current employees is undesirable. This thinking may do great harm to the organization because it only leads to uniformity, conformity, and thus mediocrity. This should not be interpreted to mean that the interviewer should make it a point to look for "oddballs" who obviously do not fit in the department. Simply because a job applicant does not exactly resemble the other employees is no reason to conclude that the person will not make a suitable employee.

If a team interview is conducted, the team members may see attributes in this candidate that you as the supervisor would have never discovered. Team members can delve into the specific expectations of doing a job and find weaknesses or strengths in a candidate that the supervisor may not. The benefit of team interviews, however, is after the hiring. If the team was in favor of selecting the candidate, the team will support the candidate when he or she starts work. The contrary may be true as well: if the team is not favorably inclined toward this candidate, it may provide less enthusiastic support when he or she starts to work. The latter scenario is a disadvantage of team interviews.

As the principal interviewer, you must beware of a candidate who has all the right answers. The interviewer should realize that the applicant may often give responses that are socially acceptable but not very revealing. The job seeker knows that the answer should be what the interviewer wants to hear. For example, if the interviewer asks a nurse what his or her aspirations are, the reply probably will be to be a head nurse one day. He or she settles for aspiring to be a head nurse rather than the director of nursing to avoid appearing conceited or presumptuous because the applicant knows that a certain amount of ambition is socially acceptable. Asking a candidate how his former boss would describe him may yield a reply that describes him as hard working, motivated, willing to do what it takes, and a good team player. Each of these attributes is what every supervisor desires in an employee. They are also the answers that are written in every guide on how to interview.

To avoid receiving "canned" or rote answers, the questions posed should require the applicant to explain how he or she handled a difficult situation such as an unexpected patient death, the observed theft of patient cash, the loss of electricity to the operating rooms, preparation for JCAHO accreditation, or the registration of a blind or deaf patient. According to *Medical Office Manager* (2001), some supervisors offer scenarios to see how an individual may respond to the circumstance—for example, "Suppose you ask a staffer in your group to do some task differently. The staffer—who is a top performer—says no and gives a reason. What would you do?" Even these answers lend themselves to some embellishments, but they are less likely to be "memorized" answers. The supervisor also may consider giving the candidate a copy of the job description and asking, "Which of these points can you do?" and "Is there anything here that you cannot do?" (*Medical Office Manager* 2001).

Another hazard for the interviewer to avoid is giving undue merit to excessive qualifications. Eager to get the best person for the job, the supervisor may look for qualifications that exceed the requirements of the job. Although the applicant should be qualified, there is no need to look for qualifications in excess of those actually required. An overqualified applicant may make a poor and frustrated employee, who may quickly become bored with the job.

Testing the Applicant

You may wish to have human resources test applicants for certain skills prior to considering their applications. Such skill testing may be for spelling, alphabetizing, working with numbers, aptitude for math, or typing. Several products are available for this type of basic testing. Beyond that, what if you want to test someone on a specific job, say, on performing a screening mammogram or writing a specialized diet? The American Health Information Management Association (AHIMA) published information about this type of preemployment testing to screen applicants (see Figure 20.6).

Prescreening tests can provide you with additional information about a candidate's ability to perform the job, but caution must be used to avoid discrimination charges. Putting the effort in at the beginning of the process to develop a sound and justified test may save you turnover and recruitment expenses in the long term.

Making the Decision

The final step in the selection process is choosing an individual for the job. It can be difficult to make a judgment based on the information gathered. However,

FIGURE 20.6: PRE-EMPLOYMENT TESTING

The Equal Employment Opportunity Commission (EEOC) enforces the myriad of federal Equal Employment Opportunity laws. The EEOC does not provide guidelines for validating pre-employment tests. In fact, the EEOC does not take action unless a discrimination charge is filed. Once a discrimination charge is filed, the test in question is analyzed by an EEOC investigator and an industrial psychologist who measure it against accepted industry standards.

There is no formal organization or service that provides validation for pre-employment tests. Any organization looking for assistance in developing pre-employment tests should seek the advice of a human resources consultant or an industrial psychologist. There are also a number of published resources available.

There are five basic steps to a valid test:

1. Job analysis: The test writer must develop a "core competency model" for the open position, in which the knowledge, skills, and abilities needed to perform the actual job are identified. For example, someone interviewing for a coder position should never be tested on codes for conditions that are not treated at the facility.

2. Test blueprint: The test writer should develop a test plan (or outline) that accurately reflects the competencies identified as essential to performing the open position. The test plan should be grouped by categories of performance. Each performance category should be weighted based on its importance to performing the job.

3. Item writing: The test writer should eliminate any question that carries an ethnic, gender, socioeconomic, or geographic bias. Questions should only be written that reflect the actual tasks that are performed as part of the job.

4. Field testing: The completed pre-employment test should be field tested before it is given to any potential job applicants. Your current employees may be a good test group. The field testing process is an excellent opportunity to "fine tune" the test questions so that they accurately test for the job being offered.

5. Item Analysis: Once the test is administered to job applicants, it is vital to refine and validate it as test data is collected and evaluated. Issues that the test writer should consider during evaluation include: Are any questions too difficult? Do any of the test questions show a pattern of discrimination? Does the test correlate to the overall knowledge, skills, and abilities needed to perform the job?"

Source: Courtesy of the Journal of AHIMA, Vol. 70, No. 4 (April 1999). © AHIMA.

if the above suggestions have been followed, the chances of making a successful decision are improved. The discussion is based on the assumption that it is within the supervisor's sole authority to decide and that the organization's policies and procedures do not require authorization from the line superior or someone in the human resources department. However, in many organizations, the immediate supervisor may not actually extend the offer of employment or establish the starting wage. Today, more and more human resources departments have this functional responsibility. This transfer of responsibility has occurred to ensure consistency in hiring practices and equity in pay to avoid favoritism and discrimination claims.

At the conclusion of the employment interview, the supervisor will likely choose among three possible actions: recommend hiring the applicant, defer the decision, or reject the applicant. The applicant is eager to know which of these actions the supervisor is going to take and is entitled to an answer within a reasonable period of time.

No particular problem exists if the supervisor decides to recommend hiring a particular applicant. However, the supervisor must recognize that the human resources department may require additional tests such as a preemployment physical that may include a drug screen. Additionally, human resources staff may conduct criminal checks once the supervisor's recommendation has been submitted. It is not until after the candidate has successfully passed these additional screens that the human resources department establishes, with your cooperation, the start date and initial orientation for the candidate.

The supervisor also may decide to defer a decision until several other applicants for the same job have been interviewed. In this case, it is necessary and appropriate for the supervisor to inform this person that he or she will be notified later. Preferably, the supervisor will set a time limit within which the decision will be made. Such a situation occurs frequently, but it is not fair to use this tactic to avoid the unpleasant task of telling the applicant that he or she is not acceptable. Under such circumstances, telling the applicant that the interviewing supervisor is deferring action raises false hopes. While waiting for an answer, the applicant may not look for another job and consequently may let some other opportunities slip by. It is unpleasant to tell an applicant that he or she is not suitable, but if the supervisor has decided that an applicant will not be hired, he or she should be told in a clear but tactful way. Although it is much simpler to let the rejected applicant wait for a letter that never arrives, the applicant is entitled to an honest answer. If the job seeker does not fulfill the requirements of the job, it is preferable to say so.

It is better not to state the specific reasons for rejection beyond a general phrase. Supervisors may have experienced that stating reasons for not hiring someone encourages arguments and comparisons and can lead to many other problems, especially because the chances for being misquoted and misunderstood are great. It is best to turn the applicant down by stating, in a general way, that the match between the applicant's qualifications and the needs of the job is not sufficient. It is also not fair to tell the applicant that he or she will be called if something suitable opens up if the interviewer knows that no hope exists.

Supervisors should avoid rejecting candidates too quickly. One should wait until the chosen candidate has accepted the job, and in some cases you may wish to wait until after the candidate has started the job, before sending a rejection letter to your second-best candidate. However, you should promptly notify those applicants you would never consider hiring, those whose salary expectations are above the rate range permitted at your organization, or those who definitely do not have the skill set you are seeking.

The supervisor should always bear in mind that the employment interview is an excellent opportunity to build a good reputation for the institution. The applicant knows that he or she is one of several candidates and that only one person can be selected. A large percentage of applicants are not hired. The way they are turned down, however, can have an effect on their impression of the institution. Often, the only contact the applicant has with the organization is through the supervisor during the employment interview. Therefore, the supervisor should remember that the interview will make either a good or a bad impression of the institution on the applicant. It is necessary, therefore, that an applicant leaves the interview, regardless of its outcome, at least with the feeling that he or she has been courteously and fairly treated. Every supervisor should bear in mind that it is a managerial duty to build as much goodwill for the organization as possible and that the employment interview presents one opportunity to do so.

Documentation

In recent years, the need for documentation has become increasingly evident, as supervisors' hiring decisions are increasingly challenged. The interviewer must write down the reasons for not hiring a certain applicant and why one was hired in preference to the others. This documentation is essential because the supervisor could not possibly remember all the various reasons, and he or she may be asked to justify the decision months later.

Generally speaking, the department of human resources informs the line managers how to document the selection process. In some cases, supervisors might be pressured by the human resources department, peer supervisors, or higher management to give preferential hiring considerations to minorities or women. Supervisors should realize that the organization might have to meet certain affirmative action goals. Again, only by careful documentation are supervisors able to justify their decisions. Notes on a separate piece of paper and attached to the application serve this purpose.

Temporary Placement

Sometimes, although the applicant is not the right person for a particular job, he or she may be suitable for another position for which no current opening exists. The supervisor might be tempted to hold this desirable employee by offering temporary placement in any job that is available. The applicant should be informed about this prospect by the supervisor. At times, however, temporary placement in an unsuitable job causes misunderstanding and disturbance within the department. It is usually strenuous for an employee to mark time on a job that he or she does not care to perform while hoping for the proper job to open up. Normally such strain causes dissatisfaction after some time, which is usually communicated to other employees within the work group. Also, the expected suitable job may not open up. Therefore, generally speaking, interim placements should be approached with great care.

SUMMARY

Available job openings may be filled in two ways: hire someone from the outside or promote someone from within the organization. In hiring from outside, the supervisor is aided by the human resources department because it performs the services of recruiting and preselecting the most likely applicants. For internal candidates, the human resources department provides screening for minimum job requirements but usually encourages employment from within and may, in effect, be less stringent on the referral of internal candidates. It is the supervisor's function and duty, however, to interview the various candidates appropriately and to hire those who promise to be the best ones for the jobs available. To accomplish this, the supervisor must acquire the skills needed to conduct an effective interview. The employment interview is primarily a directive (or structured) interview, in contrast to the nondirective interview often encountered in the supervisor's daily work.

During the employment interview, the supervisor tries to determine whether the applicant's capability matches the demands of the job. To carry out a successful interview, the supervisor should become familiar with background information, list points to be covered and questions to be asked, be prepared in advance, and have the proper setting. In addition to securing information from the applicant, the interviewer should discuss with the interviewee as many aspects of the job as possible. There will be a number of additional questions and answers before the interviewer is ready to conclude the employment interview, evaluate the situation, and make a decision. All this must be accomplished while giving proper attention to the many aspects of equal and fair employment practices and other legal considerations.

In addition to conducting directive interviews, the supervisor is often called on to carry out nondirective interviews. This form of interview usually covers problematic situations and gives the employees the opportunity to freely express their feelings and sentiments. Many sources of frustration exist within and outside the working environment that can easily lead to a variety of undesirable responses. Giving subordinates the opportunity for a counseling interview is another vital duty of the supervisory position.

REFERENCES

American Health Information Management Association (AHIMA). 1999. "Pre-Employment Testing." *Journal of AHIMA* 70 (4): 54.

Bynham, W. C. 1984. "The Ten Most Common Interviewing Mistakes." *Personnel Journal* (June): 10–12.

Medical Officer Manager. 2001. "Finding the Right Job Candidate." *Medical Officer Manager* XIV (5): 6–8.

Norfolk and Norwich University. 2003. Hospital Recruitment Guidelines. [Online information; retrieved 9/26/05.] http://195.224.49.93/docs%5Ctrustdocs%5C74.pdf.

Quicken Company. 2000. "CCH Business Owner's Toolkit." *Small Business Newsletter,* June 29. [Online newsletter.] www.quicken.com/small_business/cch/text/?article=P05_0001.

University of Maryland Eastern Shore. 2001. Human Resources Policies. [Online information; retrieved 2/17/01.] http://www.admin.umes.edu/manual/admin500.html; http://www.admin.umes.edu/manual/admin511.html.

CHAPTER TWENTY-ONE

Performance Appraisals, Promotions, and Transfers

CHAPTER OBJECTIVES

After you have studied this chapter, you should be able to do the following:

1. Describe the purpose of periodic performance appraisals.
2. Discuss the role of the supervisor in performing the appraisal.
3. Outline problems in performance ratings.
4. Review the relationship between wage and salary structure and employee retention and recruitment.
5. Describe the purpose and methods of promotion.

THE PERFORMANCE APPRAISAL system is the ongoing process of gathering, analyzing, evaluating, and disseminating information about the performance of employees. These appraisals not only guide management in selecting certain individuals for promotion and salary increases but also are useful for coaching employees to improve their performance. Appraisals are an important part of long-range personnel planning and the supervisor's staffing function. In addition, well-identified and -described appraisal methods and procedures contribute to a healthy organizational environment of mutual trust and understanding. This type of atmosphere is necessary if the health-care organization wants to bring about increased productivity and better patient care. A performance appraisal system helps identify work requirements, performance standards, analysis and appraisal of job-related behaviors, and recognition of those behaviors.

Performance appraisals are central to organizational and management development. Their purpose is to provide a measure of the employee's job performance that leads to counseling (motivation) and his or her further development (training). Because a *performance appraisal* is a formal system of measuring, evaluating, and influencing an employee's job-related activities, it identifies the types of training experiences that may enhance the employee's performance. In addition, as we discussed in Chapter 19, the tight labor market has created recruitment difficulty for many organizations. Difficulty finding individuals with specific skills has caused many organizations to train individuals on the job.

Performance appraisal is a control system that serves as an audit of the effectiveness of on-the-job training programs, of supervisory coaching, and of each employee. Decisions regarding an employee's continued employment, promotion, demotion, transfer, salary increase, or possible termination are made on the basis of the performance appraisal. Performance appraisals are important to maximize employee motivation and productivity (Figure 21.1) and to minimize the chances of litigation. In the typical organization, every employee is subject to a periodic performance appraisal; every organization needs valid information that enhances management's effectiveness in directing human resources.

THE PERFORMANCE APPRAISAL SYSTEM

The appraisal of an employee's performance is central to the supervisor's staffing function. It points to the need for further development, shows how effectively various subordinates contribute to departmental goals, and helps management identify those employees who have the potential to be promoted into better positions. It is important for a supervisor to be in a position to assess objectively the quality of the employees' performance in the department. Therefore, most organizations request that their supervisors carry out the provisions of the institution's formal appraisal system and periodically appraise and rate their employees (see Figure 21.2). This formal appraisal system is also known as employee evaluation, employee rating, annual review, or merit rating. For the purposes of this book, assume that the system has been designed so that it is legally defensible and not discriminatory in any way.

According to Michael Holzschu (2001), preparing the performance review can be both stressful and nonproductive: "sometimes the fault lies with the format of the appraisal instrument. A review should give an accurate appraisal of how well a staff member has done then show the person where and how to improve." This chapter provides guidance in this important management responsibility.

Performance Appraisal Methods[1]

Performance appraisals take many forms. The written essay, the simplest appraisal method, is a written narrative assessing an employee's strengths, weaknesses, past performance, and potential and provides recommendations for improvement. Other types of performance appraisal methods include comparative standards (e.g., simple ranking, paired comparison, forced distribution; see below) and absolute standards (e.g., critical incidents, BARS, 360-degree feedback).

FIGURE 21.1: HOW AM I DOING?

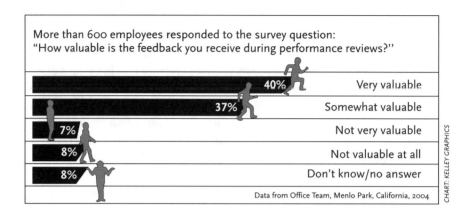

More than 600 employees responded to the survey question:
"How valuable is the feedback you receive during performance reviews?"

40%	Very valuable
37%	Somewhat valuable
7%	Not very valuable
8%	Not valuable at all
8%	Don't know/no answer

Data from Office Team, Menlo Park, California, 2004

CHART: KELLEY GRAPHICS

Source: Courtesy of Office Team, Menlo Park, CA.

Comparative standards, or multi-person comparison, is a relative assessment method that compares one employee's performance with that of one or more others. In group rank ordering the supervisor places employees into a particular classification such as top one-fifth and second one-fifth. If a supervisor has ten employees, only two could be in the top fifth, and two must be assigned to the bottom fifth. In individual ranking the supervisor lists employees from highest to lowest. The difference between the top two employees is assumed to be equivalent to the difference between the bottom two employees. In paired comparison, the supervisor compares each employee with every other employee and rates each as either the superior or weaker of the pair. After all comparisons are made, each employee is assigned a summary or ranking based on the number of superior scores received.

Other performance appraisal methods include critical incidents, graphic rating scale, and behaviorally anchored rating scales (BARS). For critical incidents assessment, the supervisor's attention is focused on specific or critical behaviors that separate effective from ineffective performance. The *graphic rating scale* lists a set of performance factors such as job knowledge, work quality, and cooperation that the supervisor uses to rate employee performance on an incremental scale. *BARS* combine elements from critical incident and graphic rating scale approaches. The supervisor rates employees according to items on a numerical scale.

The last method discussed here is the *360-degree feedback method.* This multi-source feedback method provides a comprehensive perspective of employee performance by using feedback from the full circle of people with whom the employee interacts, including supervisors, subordinates, and coworkers. It is effective for career coaching and identifying strengths and weaknesses.

Many other methods can be used for performance appraisals. As a supervisor, you probably use pieces of some described here and others you may discover throughout your career. Regardless of the method(s) you choose, your goal is to ensure a comprehensive and factual evaluation.

Performance Appraisal Purposes

The performance appraisal system serves many purposes. It can provide a guide for possible promotion, further development, and a basis for merit increases. It can also translate the performance, experience, and qualities of an employee into objective terms and allow comparison with the requirements of the job. The formal appraisal system is designed to consider such criteria as job knowledge, ability to follow through on assignments, judgment, attitude, cooperation, dependability, output, housekeeping, and safety. Such a system of evaluations helps the supervisor take many factors into account when considering merit increases or a promotion. It also provides a rational basis for decision making, as it reduces the chances for personal bias.

Such a formal appraisal system forces the supervisor to observe and scrutinize a subordinate's work not only from the standpoint of how well the employee is performing the job but also from the standpoint of what can be done to improve the employee's performance. Such judgments are difficult to make in most healthcare settings because one is not dealing with concrete performance measures, such as units produced, but with concepts of leadership, teamwork, and cooperation. Because an employee's poor performance and failure to improve may result from inadequate supervision, a formal appraisal system is also likely to determine the extent of supervisory qualities and lead to improvement.

A formal evaluation system also serves another purpose. Employees have always expected security from their work. In addition to that, they seek satisfying and interesting work that enables them to grow. Often employees are provided copies of their job descriptions but may not know exactly what is expected of them. A well-designed appraisal system reduces ambiguity concerning job requirements and uncertainty by providing employees with information about what is expected from them (see Figure 19.3) and feedback on how they have performed.

Every employee has the right to know how well he or she is doing and what can be done to improve his or her work performance. One can assume that most employees are eager to know what their supervisors think of their work. In some instances, the employee's desire to know how he or she stands with the boss can be interpreted as asking for reassurance about his or her future in the organization. In other instances this expressed desire may be interpreted differently. For example, a supervisee may realize that he or she is doing a relatively poor job but hopes to find that the boss is not aware of it. On the other hand, another subordinate who knows that he or she is doing an outstanding job may wish to make certain that the boss is aware of it. This employee will want to receive more recognition.

Regular appraisals are important incentives to the employees of an organization. In a large, complex organization, employees can easily feel that they and their contributions are forgotten and considered insignificant. Regular appraisals assure employees that the potential exists for improving oneself in the position and that one is not lost within the enterprise; they assure employees that supervisors and the entire organization care about them.

Some organizations are experimenting with an approach known as empowerment. *Empowerment* permits individuals within a work team to make certain decisions about their work assignments, schedules, and other related items. When teams were discussed earlier in the book, this decision-making freedom was explored in the context of delegation and authority. If you and your subordinates are working in an environment that supports empowerment and team structures, it may be appropriate to allow team members to prepare or contribute to the performance appraisal of a member of the team. Team members often know the strengths and weaknesses of a fellow team member better than the supervisor. Caution must be exercised against overly criticizing or praising an individual without adequate substantiation of the facts.

The performance appraisal is a critical tool at the disposal of the supervisor, as it influences all personnel functions. It is a determinant in the planning, developing, and recognition of the organization's human resources. Performance appraisals motivate employees, which benefits the organization. Because the appraisal interview is a directive or structured interview, you need to prepare in advance the guidance you intend to give the employee to consider. The guidance should help him or her improve his or her performance, meet your expectations, and improve his or her position in the department or the organization. This process is a component of your mentoring duties. Furthermore, this constructive dialog, held privately between you and the employee, helps build trust.

In addition to creating a healthy organizational climate of trust, performance appraisals help management with the following:

- make decisions about compensation and employees' developmental and training needs,
- provide an inventory of employees suitable for promotions,
- aid the supervisor by showing whether an employee is in the right job,
- identify for the boss those employees who are moving ahead and those who are not progressing satisfactorily, and
- show whether the supervisor is succeeding in the job as a coach and teacher.

A skills inventory may also result from the development section of performance appraisals. In the development section, both the employee and supervisor discuss the individual's skill strengths and weaknesses; skills used both on the job and off the job should be noted. In this way the strengths of all staff are captured in the inventory. Strengths may include "Internet skills," "bilingual," "public speaking experience at the Chamber of Commerce," "pilot in training," and "databases experience." The benefit of a skills inventory for the organization is obvious: it allows the organization to search within the organization for individuals with new or unusual skills before filling a position with an external applicant.

As mentioned, an appraisal program also has many advantages for employees. It reflects the quality of their work and gives them a sense of being treated fairly and not being overlooked. The employee knows what he or she can do to be promoted to a better job. Appraisals give the subordinate an opportunity to express concerns, personal goals, and ambitions. In this respect, appraisals are motivational because they create a learning experience for subordinates that inspires them to improve.

Timing of Appraisals

Appraisals must be conducted regularly to be significant to the employee and the organization. A one-time performance measure is of little use, so the supervisor should formally appraise all the employees within the department at regular intervals at least once a year, which is generally considered to be sufficient. If an employee has just started in a new or more responsible position, it is advisable to schedule an initial appraisal within three to six months.

Ideally, employees should be evaluated several times throughout the year to ensure that they receive timely feedback on their performance and to separate the performance review from the timing of a wage adjustment; this separation helps the supervisor focus on performance improvement and not the economic situation of the employee. However, often supervisors do not have the luxury of the time it takes to conduct this amount of structured counseling. Therefore, they must take advantage of opportunities to give immediate feedback when they observe appropriate and inappropriate actions. An advantage of doing these on-the-spot counseling sessions throughout the year with team members is that at evaluation time, there should be no surprises.

Periodic appraisals assure the employee that whatever improvement was made will be noticed and that he or she will be recognized for this progress. As time goes on, periodic ratings and reviews become an important determinant of an employee's morale. It reaffirms the supervisor's interest in the employees and in their continued development and improvement.

Annual formal appraisals and the review of these appraisals do not replace the feedback on performance that is part of the day-to-day coaching responsibilities of the supervisor. Employees should receive feedback daily; it is well known that performance feedback is most effective when it occurs immediately after the event to which it relates. This applies equally to feedback on below-par performance and to recognition of above-par performance. Without this ongoing daily feedback, formal, once-a-year appraisals do not suffice.

Who Is the Appraiser?

A major difficulty in effective performance appraisal is that we as human beings can only make subjective appraisals. This creates intellectual and perceptual problems, leading to the rater's own interpretation of reality and not necessarily absolute reality. To minimize these shortcomings, some organizations devise an appraisal system in which the employee is evaluated by various appraisers. This may include self-appraisals and peer appraisals; in some systems, the appraisals are subject to reviews by those higher up in the administrative hierarchy. A few organizations have assessment centers for evaluating employees for their future potential as managers. (This concept is discussed more fully toward the end of this chapter.)

With the exception of team-cultured organizations, almost all organizations, however, have come to the conclusion that the appraisal is best conducted by the individual's immediate supervisor. Formal authority inherent in the managerial hierarchy means, among many other aspects, the supervisor's right to make decisions in reference to the subordinate's performance. Among all other appraisers, the immediate supervisor is the person who should know the duties of the jobs within the department best. The immediate supervisor has the best opportunity to observe the appraisee on the job and provide feedback. Furthermore, most subordinates want to receive performance-related feedback from their immediate superior and feel more comfortable in discussing the appraisal with him or her.

Sometimes it may be necessary for the first-line boss to call on the next higher supervisor for assistance in making appraisals. In some institutions the appraisal is made by a committee composed of the first-line supervisor, his or her boss, and possibly one or two other supervisors who have adequate knowledge of the performance of the person being rated. This approach has the advantage of reducing some of the immediate supervisor's personal prejudices or biases. Alternative sources to supervisory appraisals are particularly necessary in situations in which the superior has little opportunity to observe the employee on the job; this is a problem concerning all enterprises that have employees who work around the clock, in a matrix organization, in project management roles, or in remote facilities or telecommuting.

Self-appraisal, or self-rating, is an alternative source of appraisal input. There are several advantages to self-ratings: they (1) often contain less "halo" error (employee self-ratings tend to be more critical than those done by supervisors), (2) show the supervisor how the employee perceives the responsibilities and problems of the position, (3) help identify differences of opinion, and (4) are particularly useful when employees work in isolation. However, self-appraisal can often lead to a situation fraught with conflict if the supervisor's appraisal differs significantly from an inflated self-rating by the employee. When this occurs, the supervisor should prepare for an in-depth discussion with the employee. By asking the employee to explain his or her rationale for the self-ratings, the supervisor may learn about achievements of which he or she was previously unaware.

Once the employee shares his or her opinions and justifications, the supervisor must show the employee the data collected since the time of the last evaluation and how these actual occurrences vary from the expectations set forth. That is why the appraisal system often combines self-appraisals and supervisory appraisals into one comprehensive performance appraisal.

At times, peers are used as appraisers. They can provide valuable information about their colleagues because of their daily interactions if they have close contact with one another. They can observe how an employee interacts with them, the subordinates, and the boss. Peer appraisals offer independent judgment and have often proved to be good predictors of performance when used as a basis for promotion.

However, some powerful influences in organizational life may distort or cloud a peer's perception. Most employees have a strong need for security and work for present and future rewards from the employer. If someone else receives additional rewards, the chances for additional rewards become smaller for everyone else because the resources are limited. This competition for current or future employer rewards, whether readily apparent or not, could distort a peer's perception of a colleague's performance and potential. In addition, friendships and stereotyping may bias the rating. Friendship relates not only to individuals but also to groups. For instance, the appraiser may evaluate some peer in a group of which he or she was once a member. The appraiser may be tempted to rate members of that particular group higher than individuals in another group. Also, at times peers are not willing to evaluate each other, considering it to be an inducement to snitching on one another. Some union contracts forbid peer participation in the evaluation process.

For all practical purposes, appraisal done by the immediate supervisor should suffice, and in most organizations the immediate supervisor is the primary, if not the only, appraiser of employee performance. However, the use of multiple sources of appraisals is likely to obtain a more comprehensive evaluation.

PERFORMANCE RATING

To minimize and overcome the difficulties in appraising an employee, most enterprises find it advisable to use some type of appraisal form (see Figure 21.2). These appraisal forms are prepared by the personnel department, often in conjunction with outside consultants and with the supervisors' suggestions. As mentioned, great care must be exercised to make certain that the system used is legally defensible.

Although many types of appraisal forms are available, most of them specify job-related and other important criteria for measuring job performance, intelligence, and personality traits. In addition to determining criteria, standards must be clarified to determine how well employees are performing. The instruments most used in the appraisal process are based on both behavior and traits. Some are objective, whereas others are subjective.

The following are qualities and characteristics that are most frequently rated. For non-supervisory personnel, typical qualities include the following:

- quantity and quality of work produced,
- job knowledge,
- dependability,
- cooperative attitude,
- amount of supervision required,
- maintenance of work area and equipment,
- unauthorized absenteeism and tardiness,
- safety, and
- personal appearance.

For managerial and professional employees, typical factors include the following:

- analytical ability,
- judgment,
- initiative,
- leadership,
- quality and quantity of work produced,
- knowledge of work,
- attitude,
- dependability,
- teamwork, and
- emotional stability.

For each of these factors the supervisor is charged with selecting the degree of achievement attained by the employee. In some instances, a point system is provided to arrive at a numerical scoring (see Figure 19.3)

Despite the outward simplicity of some rating forms, the supervisor will probably run into a number of difficulties. First, not all supervisors agree on what is meant by a simple adjective rating scale such as unsatisfactory, marginal, satisfactory, above average, and superior. It is advisable, therefore, that the form contain a descriptive sentence in addition to each of these adjectives, such as the following:

- For unsatisfactory, "performance clearly fails to meet minimum requirements"
- For marginal, "performance occasionally fails to meet minimum requirements"
- For satisfactory, "performance meets or exceeds minimum requirements"
- For above average, "performance consistently exceeds minimum requirements"
- For superior, "performance clearly exceeds all job requirements"

FIGURE 21.2: SAMPLE PERFORMANCE APPRAISAL

Performance Appraisal   Date: _____

Employee Name: _____ Title: _____

Department: _____ CC: _____ Emp. No. _____ DOH: ___/ ___/ ___

Appraisal Period: _____ to: _____

Instructions: Carefully evaluate employee's work performance in relation to current job requirements. Check rating box to indicate the employee's performance. Indicate N/A if not applicable.

Definition of Appraisal Ratings:

Outstanding (O): Performance is exceptional in all areas and is recognizable as being far superior to others.

Very Good (VG): Results clearly exceed most position requirements. Performance is of high quality and is achieved on a consistent basis.

Good (G): Competent and dependable level of performance. Meets performance expectations of the job.

Improvement Needed (IN): Performance is deficient in several areas. Improvement is necessary.

Unsatisfactory (U): Results are generally unacceptable and require immediate improvement.

N/A: Not applicable to this person's job.

Appraisal Factor	Rating
Applies past experiences to new problems?	
Retains information? Does not repeatedly ask the same questions or make the same mistakes?	
Follows instructions and takes notes when necessary?	
Has gained the skills necessary to navigate the computer system for the functions for which he/she is responsible?	
Takes care of equipment?	
Uses supplies wisely?	
Follows department procedures?	
Completes assigned work when expected?	
Completes assigned work accurately?	
Completes volume required?	

(continued on following page)

Appraisal Factor	Rating
Makes efficient use of time?	
Meets accuracy requirements?	
Completes assigned work with little or no dependence upon others?	
Handwriting legible?	
Does not transpose numbers?	
Willing to work overtime?	
Requires minimum supervision?	
Improved in all areas that were marked "improvement needed" or "unsatisfactory" in last appraisal?	
Achieved goals outlined in last evaluation?	
Maintained strengths in same areas as last evaluation?	
Days of absence?	
Tardies?	

Area(s) for Improvement:

Strengths:

Goals:

1.

Target Date: _____ Employee's Initials: _____

2.

Target Date: _____ Employee's Initials: _____

Employee Comments:

Employee's Initials: _____

Employee's Signature: _____ Date: _____

Supervisor's Signature: _____ Date: _____

Manager's Signature: _____ Date: _____

Instead of the adjective, the supervisor might choose from descriptive sentences the one that most adequately describes the employee.

For example, in rating a nurse's degree of emotional stability, the appraiser may select among the following choices the phrase that is most descriptive:

1. "Unreliable in crises; goes to pieces easily; cannot take criticism"
2. "Unrealistic; emotions and moodiness periodically handicap his or her dealings; he or she personalizes issues"
3. "Usually on an even keel; has mature approach to most situations"
4. "Is realistic; generally maintains good behavioral balance in handling situations"
5. "Self-possessed to a high degree; has outstanding ability to adjust to circumstances, no matter how difficult"

Problems in Performance Rating

Performance rating of an employee is frequently subject to a number of errors and weaknesses because it is a subjective process. Some of these errors are more common than others. The supervisor should be aware of these pitfalls to minimize the errors in processing, storing, and recalling observed behavior.

Some supervisors have a tendency to be overly lenient in their ratings, rating appraisees higher than normal. They are afraid they might antagonize those being evaluated if they rate them low, thus making them less cooperative.

Other supervisors are overly harsh in rating their employees and appraise them lower than the average appraiser. To give consistently low ratings is equally as damaging as being too lenient. A low evaluation rating for an individual may also reflect the supervisor's own inability to motivate his or her subordinates.

For example, if the nursing personnel on one station are consistently appraised higher than those on the next station, it is difficult to determine whether this is because of one head nurse's strictness or the other's leniency or whether this reflects real differences in the employees' abilities and performance.

Another common error is central tendency, in which the appraiser rates the employees consistently as average or around the midpoint in the range, although an employee's performance warrants a higher or lower rating. Such a supervisor is often reluctant to rate employees high or low, a tendency that shows that the supervisor may be unprepared for the formal appraisal and avoids being decisive. Another subjective error of the appraiser is to be influenced by the halo effect (discussed in Chapter 20), which is the tendency to let the rating they assign to one characteristic influence their rating on all subsequent characteristics. This works in two directions. Rating the appraisee as excellent on one factor influences the rater to give the employee another high or higher rating on other qualities than he or she actually deserves. On the other hand, rating the employee as unsatisfactory on one factor influences the appraiser to give the appraisee another low or lower-than-deserved rating on other factors. One way to minimize the halo effect is to rate all employees on a single factor or trait before going on to the next factor. In other words, the supervisor only rates one factor of each employee at a time and then goes on to the next employee for the same factor, and so on. This enables the supervisor to standardize the ratings. Additionally, it is not necessary that the distribution of ratings resemble a normal, or bell-shaped, curve.

Some raters are tempted to judge more favorably those employees whose attitudes resemble their own; this is the similar-to-me appraisal tendency. A further distortion can be caused by interpersonal relations and bias. The ratings may be influenced by the supervisor's likes and dislikes about each individual working in the department. This is especially apparent when objective standards of performance are difficult to determine or not available.

Organizational influences, or the way administration uses the ratings, may give rise to another source of difficulty. Often raters are lenient when they know that pay raises and promotions depend on the appraisals. If the organizational emphasis is on further employee development, appraisers are inclined to be harsh and emphasize weaknesses.

The supervisor's judgment must be based on the total performance of the employee. It is unfair to appraise a subordinate based on only one assignment on which he or she had done particularly well or poorly. The evaluation should be based on the employee's performance during the entire appraisal period, not just on the appraisee's most recent behavior. If periodic appraisals are performed at intervals throughout the evaluation period, a supervisor is less likely to judge an individual on the most recent experience. Employees know when their appraisal is due and will act accordingly. As a supervisor you may notice the halo effect just prior to an evaluation period.

Compiling the information you need for an appraisal is no simple task. If your facility requires you to prepare evaluations of all your team members at the same time, you have much work ahead of you. Because memory tends not to go beyond about two months, it is to your advantage to keep dated notes throughout the year of observations, good and bad, and conversations you have had with staff members. These notes can simply be dropped in a folder for each employee. Another source for recall may be e-mail messages you have sent to employees acknowledging their accomplishments throughout the year. By printing and dropping these in your folder or saving them in an e-mail folder, they, too, will serve as memory joggers. This approach provides you with a year-long basis from which to develop the appraisal and impress your staff that you took such care in preparing their evaluations. Also, supervisors may find it beneficial to use a performance analysis checklist (see Figure 21.3) or performance problem-solution checklist (see Figure 21.4).

Supervisors must caution themselves not to let random or first impressions of an employee influence their judgment, which should be based on the employee's total record of performance, reliability, initiative, skills, resourcefulness, and capability. Obtaining input from peers and customers served by the employee and combining these observations with the supervisor's impressions result in fairer assessment of the individual's performance.

Figure 21.3: Performance Analysis Checklist

1. Whose performance is at issue?

2. What is the performance discrepancy? What is actually happening? What should be happening?

3. Is the problem worth solving? What would happen if you ignored it?

4. Can we apply fast fixes? Are expectations clear? Are resources available and adequate? Is quality of performance easily observed?

5. Are the consequences appropriate? Is desired performance punishing to the performer? Is poor performance rewarding to the performer? Are consequences arranged effectively?

6. Do they already know how? Could they do it if their lives depended on it? Could they do it in the past? Are the tasks performed often?

7. Are there more clues? Can the task(s) be simplified? Can obstacles to performing be removed? Can the performer(s) learn to perform?

8. Describe solutions.

9. Calculate the cost of each solution.

10. Select the most practical of the cost-effective solutions.

11. Implement the solution(s).

Source: © 1997, The Center for Effective Performance, Inc., 1100 Johnson Ferry Road, Suite 150, Atlanta, GA 30342. www.cepworldwide.com 1-800-558-4237. Reprinted with permission. All rights reserved. No portion of these materials may be reproduced in any manner without express written consent from The Center for Effective Performance, Inc.

Supervisors also should not allow past performance appraisal ratings to influence current ratings unjustly either way. An aid to minimize these errors and biases is to document employee behavior as soon as possible after each occurrence. When the formal appraisal takes place, supervisors can refer back to the documentation and minimize such biases and other pitfalls in rating.

Observing all these problems in rating helps supervisors overcome subjectivity in processing, storing, and recalling observed behavior when evaluations are made. Although the results are not perfect, many human errors can be significantly reduced and counteracted by top-level administration's emphasis on training for those who do appraisals. Such training is necessary because appraisals that are biased, inaccurate, or distorted do not increase an employee's motivation. These errors may lead to poor promotion and retention decisions, and even possibly to charges of discrimination. Training supervisors in how to observe behavior is an ongoing process. The success of the performance appraisal largely depends on the supervisor's ability to obtain accurate information and then to discuss it with the appraisee in a nonthreatening and constructive manner. The evaluation interview that follows the appraisal fulfills this function.

FIGURE 21.4: PERFORMANCE PROBLEM-SOLUTION CHECKLIST

Problem	Solutions
They can't do it, and . . .	
the skill is used often:	Provide feedback
	Simplify the task
the skill is used rarely:	Provide job aids to promote desired performance
	Simplify the job
	Provide periodic practice

Training will be required if the above remedies are inadequate

Problem	Solutions
They can do it, but . . .	
doing it right leads to punishment:	Remove the sources of punishment.
doing it wrong is more satisfying:	Remove the rewards for incorrect performance
nobody notices when they do it right:	Apply rewards to the performer for doing it right
there are obstacles to performing as desired:	Remove the obstacles (or help people work around them)

THE APPRAISAL INTERVIEW

The second step in the appraisal procedure, the appraisal interview, takes place when the immediate superior who has prepared the formal evaluation sits down with the individual being evaluated to discuss the appraisee's performance. Some supervisors prefer not to have to tell their subordinates how they stand in the department and what they should do to improve. They are reluctant because, unless it is done with great sensitivity, this type of interview can lead to hostility and even greater misunderstanding. However, every employee is entitled to an honest, accurate, comprehensive, and fact-based performance evaluation. Many employees distrust anything that relates to their review, starting with the validity of the measuring instrument used and the appraiser's ability to observe.

Staffing: Human Resources Management

Employees may be reluctant to discuss their workplace behavior. However, this discussion is absolutely essential to ensure effective appraisals.

The institution should provide supervisors with learning opportunities to conduct appraisals in such a way that they are effective. Many facilities provide training in such forms as practice sessions, behavior modeling training programs, role-playing experiences, in-basket exercises, and assessment centers. All this is done to increase the supervisors' effectiveness in dealing with those being evaluated, to improve their observer accuracy, and to aid them in carrying out appraisal interviews effectively. The four major formats for this interview are (1) the tell-and-sell approach, (2) the tell-and-listen/listen-and-tell format, (3) the problem-solving approach, and (4) a mixed interview combining all these formats.

Doing the Appraisal

Although experienced supervisors probably do not need to follow a formalized system, administration often suggests that all supervisors follow a standardized outline.

At the outset of the appraisal, the supervisor should state the purpose of the evaluation procedure and the interview; state that the interview is to be a constructive and positive experience for both the person being appraised and the appraiser; and indicate that it is being conducted for the benefit of the employee, the supervisor, and the institution. As part of this warm-up, the supervisor may wish to comment on the progress the worker has made since the preceding counseling interview and compliment the supervisee on achievements. The discussion then covers areas that need improvement. Be aware that the formula of starting with praise, following it up with criticism, and ending the interview with another compliment is not necessarily the best method. Good and bad may cancel each other out, and the worker may forget the criticism. A mature employee is able to take deserved criticism when it is appropriate. By the same token, when praise is merited, it should be expressed. It is not always possible to mix praise and criticism effectively.

Because the idea of being rated imposes some extra tension and strain, feelings of friendliness and privacy in the interview are probably more important than at any other time. As personal feelings and opinions most likely will be brought out in the discussion, the appraisee must be assured of privacy and confidentiality. The supervisor should not discuss specifics of the interview with the appraisee's coworkers even though some issues may have arisen in the session that will require further action or investigation. The employee should be assured that the content of this counseling session will be held in confidence.

The supervisor should next proceed to a discussion of the evaluation itself. The subordinate's strong points and then the weak points are stated, followed by a general discussion that allows the employee an opportunity to state his or her opinions and feelings. This is the tell-and-listen format. The supervisor should stress that everyone in the same job in the department is rated according to the same standards and that the employee has not been singled out for special scrutiny. He or she should be in a position to support the rating by citing specific, documented instances of good and poor performance. The supervisor should be careful to relate the measured factors to the actual demands of the job. The rating must be geared to the present qualities of the employee's performance.

This last point is particularly important if some employees are already doing good work and the supervisor is tempted to leave well enough alone; these are probably the very employees who are likely to make further progress, and to tell them simply to keep up the good work is not sufficient. These employees may not have major problems, nevertheless they deserve thoughtful counseling. Such employees are likely to continue to develop, and the supervisor should specify future development plans. The appraiser must be familiar, therefore, with the opportunities available to the employee, requirements of the job, and the employee's qualifications. Whenever he or she is discussing a subordinate's future, the supervisor should not make promises for promotion that may not be possible to keep.

Another possible procedure is to let subordinates appraise themselves first. This gives the appraisees the opportunity to state their side of the story first. It is easier for many subordinates to criticize themselves than to take criticism from the supervisor. After reviewing the employee's self-rating, the supervisor offers his or her comments on the subordinate's strengths and weaknesses. The interview should end with a discussion of what the subordinate can and wants to do about any deficiencies and what the supervisor will do for the employee in this regard. This is the listen-and-tell format.

The tell-and-sell format requires the supervisor to do much of the communicating. Often, it is used when a subordinate believes he or she did nothing wrong and the supervisor is placed in a position of "selling" his or her evaluation and performance improvement plan to the employee. This approach does not have to have a negative result, however. The format may be acceptable to subordinates when a supervisor is trusted and is known for his or her expertise and his or her insight is valued by the subordinates.

The problem-solving approach is most often used when a single issue concerns the supervisor, such as the subordinate's excessive tardiness. Both the supervisor and subordinate will discuss how this problem will be solved.

When using any of these approaches, supervisors should remember to avoid using the word "I" in the interview. This is a time to discuss your employee's performance—what he or she has done, not how you feel about it or how you performed that job in the past. As supervisors gain experience, they will devise their own plans, and each supervisee probably will be approached in an individual manner.

Preparing for the Interview

Everything regarding general techniques of interviewing (see Chapter 20) is applicable to the appraisal interview. Additional skills are necessary as well because the direction of evaluation interviews cannot be predicted. At times it may be very difficult for the supervisor to carry on this interview, especially if the subordinate shows hostility when the supervisor discusses some negative evaluations. Of course, employees need to know if and where their performance is inadequate. Positive judgment can be communicated effectively, but it is difficult to communicate criticism without generating resentment and defensiveness. It takes much practice and insight to acquire skills for handling the evaluation interview.

Some supervisors do not believe they need to conduct an evaluation interview because they are in daily contact with their employees. These supervisors claim that their door is open at all times, but this approach is not enough. Many employees want a formal appraisal in which they receive a substantiated report on their performance and one that is in writing for others to see should the employee apply for an advanced position. Also, employees may have some things on their mind that they do not want to discuss in the everyday contacts with the supervisor in the open office.

The supervisor must be well prepared for this review session. The appraiser must know what should be covered and achieved in this meeting and gather all the information relevant to the discussion. The various events that occurred during the evaluation period must be clear in the interviewer's mind. It may be advisable to prepare an agenda for this meeting. Thorough preparation enables the appraiser to be ready for any direction the discussion will take.

Predicting what will happen in this review session is difficult. It may be an uneventful meeting, and the appraisee's responses may be minimal—an occasional yes or no, or a nod of the head. Another meeting, however, may end up as a major bitter confrontation. Because of the importance and sensitivity of the performance review, the appraiser must also be skilled in interviewing and counseling. The reviewer must ask the right question at the right time and be a constructive listener. In the review session, information must be shared. The appraisee must feel that his or her concerns are important. Success of this review session can be improved if the appraiser has empathy, listens constructively, asks the right questions at the proper time, and observes keenly. Lastly, the appraiser must allow enough time to conduct the interview and ensure that no distractions or interruptions are allowed to occur during the session.

Management by objectives (MBO) has been discussed on several occasions in this book. The underlying concept of MBO is that identified, measurable, and workable objectives are agreed on by the supervisor and the employee, which leads to improved performance and a motivating environment. MBO creates a participative climate because the subordinates help decide what their goals are. Although MBO is primarily a planning tool and a process that goes beyond performance appraisals, it can be logically and conveniently linked with performance evaluation and appraisal interviews. The review lends itself well to measuring the quality of an employee's on-the-job performance, achievements, and participation in setting new objectives. These new goals are to be achieved during the next period and will be appraised and reviewed at the end of the period. Thus, the subordinate is judged by standards he or she helped determine.

The Appraisal Agenda

The appraisal interview should be held shortly after the appraisal has been prepared, and, as stated before, supervisors should refresh their memories regarding the reasons for the opinions expressed in the appraisal. Appraisees should be given enough notice so that they can prepare for the interview as well. The agenda for the appraisal interview or conference should aim to do the following (Allen 2000):

1. communicate the evaluation,
2. resolve any misunderstandings,
3. seek acceptance of the rating,
4. identify areas for improvement, and
5. secure commitment to future goals.

Closing the Evaluation Interview

The interview should also give the employee an opportunity to ask questions so that the supervisor can answer them fully. Any misunderstanding cleared up at this time may avoid future difficulty. The appraiser should also clarify that further performance ratings and interviews are regular procedures with the enterprise. The supervisor should always remember that the purpose of the appraisal interview is to help employees to see their shortcomings and aid them in finding solutions. The real success of the interview lies in the employees' ability to see the need for their own improvement, stimulating in them a desire to change.

Because the appraisal interview is the most important part of the evaluation procedure, the supervisor should make certain that at its termination, the employees are clear on their performance expectations and the ways in which they can improve. They also should come away with a desire to improve. It is hoped that employees will establish goals that are mutually satisfying to both themselves and the supervisor. An employee's commitment provides some measurable goals against which future performance can be judged. Furthermore, the supervisor must agree to set aside time to retrain the individual on processes that are not being performed well or coach the individual on ways to enhance the appraisee's performance. Figure 21.5 is a tool used to capture the goals of the training or coaching session. At the end of the next appraisal period, both supervisor and subordinate will meet to evaluate how well the goals have been achieved and what the next objectives will be. This gives the subordinate a custom-made standard for evaluation. It provides him or her with a specified goal within a specified period. The employee will be that much more motivated because the goal was a commitment on his or her part.

FIGURE 21.5: POST-TRAINING FOLLOW-UP

Date of Training: _____ Date of Return to Work: _____

Skills/knowledge learned: _____

_____

Remember the following:

1. Be a Coach: Be clear how the worker's performance should have improved from the training and encourage the worker to use these new skills and knowledge.

EXAMPLES OF WHERE AND HOW THE SKILLS/KNOWLEDGE SHOULD SHOW UP:

_____

_____

2. Allow PRACTICE, PRACTICE, PRACTICE: How will you schedule the worker's next month to fully use these skills?

3. Know what "IMPROVEMENT" looks like: You know what mediocre is—now do you know what "best" looks like? Be specific with your worker on what highest quality looks like in the area they received training—then look for it.

EXAMPLES OF EXEMPLARY PERFORMANCE IN THE AREA TRAINED ARE:

_____

4. Reinforce Performance: Do not forget to reinforce the worker when performance is at the level expected.

Custom requires that the person being appraised sign the evaluation form on completion of the review. Usually a statement appears above the signature line saying that the employee's signature merely confirms that the interview occurred and that the appraisee in no way approves or disapproves of the statements contained in the evaluation.

With this understanding, the subordinate will probably sign. If, however, the appraisee would like to state personal views, no harm is done in letting him or her do so. Many employees will not verbalize their disagreement with the rating, and signing the forms with such feelings can create resentment against the organization. The real purpose of the signature is to document for the supervisor's boss that the evaluation interview took place. As stated, many supervisors have mixed reactions about the appraisal interview. Because it provides essential feedback on the entire evaluation procedure, administration must make certain that it occurs, and the signature is the simplest way to confirm this. At this time, you may wish to review the performance evaluation checklist that has been included in Exhibit 21.1.

PROPER WAGES, SALARIES, AND BENEFITS

Some experts strongly advocate that the annual performance appraisal review be separate from salary review. They suggest that discussing one's past performance, future potential, and further education and development as well as the coaching and counseling taking place should not be tainted by discussing pay and compensation. Whether a salary adjustment will be made does not depend only on the performance but also on the financial condition of the enterprise, wages paid elsewhere, the economic conditions, and many other factors. Most likely if both reviews are done together, the appraisee will interpret everything that is said in relation to future reward opportunities and possible promotions. A proposed solution is to have two separate review sessions. The first may be concerned with the review and employee development, and the second session (four to eight weeks later) may cover the compensation issue.

Although people want more from their jobs than just a wage or salary, the latter are basic necessities. Pay provides more than the means of satisfying physical needs; it provides a sense of accomplishment and recognition. Most people at work consider relative pay as very important, and real or imagined wage and salary inequities are frequent causes of dissatisfaction, friction, and low morale. It is top-level management's duty to pursue a sound policy of wage and salary administration throughout the entire organization; the goal is to have a nondiscriminatory compensation structure. By setting wages high enough, the healthcare organization is able to recruit satisfactory employees and motivate their present employees to work toward pay increases and promotions. Reducing inequities among employees' earnings raises morale and reduces friction.

In most healthcare institutions and other organizations, wage rates and schedules are set by top-level administration, and the supervisor's authority in this respect is quite limited. Nevertheless, it is a part of the supervisor's staffing function to make certain that the employees of the department are properly and equitably compensated. It is every manager's job to offer the amount of compensation that will retain competent employees in the department and, if necessary, attract good workers from the outside. Monetary rewards are an exceedingly important factor for all employees. However, many employees are much more concerned about how their salaries compare to the earnings of others than they are about their absolute earnings. No doubt many wage rates and schedules follow historical patterns, whereas others are often accidental or due to exceptions. For example, certain wage rates can be distorted when positions are difficult to fill, when individuals are retained because of certain knowledge or skill, or when the administration prefers different wage scale philosophies. In the long run such situations cannot be tolerated.

It is the supervisor's duty to see that the wages paid within the department are properly aligned internally and externally. Internal alignment means that the jobs within the department and institution are paid according to what they are worth. Internal consistency based on equity provides a system of compensation that is acceptable to the employees involved, resulting in satisfaction and a desire to be promoted and to remain with the present employer. External alignment means that the wages offered for the work to be performed in the department compare favorably with the going rate in the community and area. External competitiveness refers to the pay relationships among organizations and the competitive positions reflected in these relationships. If wages do not compare favorably, the supervisor knows that some of the most experienced workers will leave and that attracting new ones from the outside will be difficult. All of this applies also to an appropriate benefits program, often called fringe benefits.

Internal Alignment

To pay the various jobs within the department according to what they are worth, the supervisor should call on the help of the human resources department to conduct a job evaluation. Job evaluation is a method of determining the relationships between pay rates and the relative monetary value of jobs within a department. In such a procedure, a committee guided by the human resources staff evaluates the jobs according to various factors, such as competence, problem solving, and accountability, then devises an appropriate wage rate based on the worth of each job and institutes an appropriate wage schedule. Of course, some questions will arise about what to do with exceptional cases—that is, those employees who are receiving either excessively high or exceedingly low salaries in relation to others. Once a plan has been designed, it is necessary to maintain it properly so that no new inequities arise.

The supervisor might request a job evaluation from the human resources department for his or her department if one has not been performed recently. Sometimes the help of an outside consultant is used. There are several methods of job evaluation. Although they are systematic, they are not totally precise because they involve questions of human judgment. In addition to the most widely used point system, other methods, such as ranking, factor comparison, and job classification, are typically used.

External Alignment

If the wage and salary policy of the institution is to be externally competitive, pay rates must be approximately the same as those prevailing in the community. Thus, accurate wage and salary data must be collected through surveys. Job evaluations establish differentials between jobs based on different job content; wage surveys provide management with information on whether the organization's wage level is competitive externally and aligned. A wage survey involves collecting data on wages paid in the community for similar key jobs in similar or related enterprises. The jobs that are similar in every healthcare organization are called *benchmark jobs*. Examples of benchmark jobs are dietitian, housekeeper or custodian, registered nurse, health information director, and patient billing clerk. The benchmark positions in your organization are adjusted based on data from these surveys. Then the job evaluations of the other positions that have equal weight or points can be adjusted accordingly, causing what some term the "ripple effect." These routine adjustments are important. Without proper external alignment, the supervisor cannot recruit competent employees or prevent present employees from leaving for better-paying jobs.

To conduct such a survey is a rather costly and sophisticated procedure; performing one's own survey probably produces the most meaningful results. Many sources publish reliable surveys, including government agencies such as the Bureau of Labor Statistics, professional healthcare associations (see Figure 21.6), and metropolitan hospital associations. The area usually considered in the survey is the geographic region within which workers seek employment and employers recruit workers without necessitating a change of residence.

Most enterprises also provide benefits for employees, such as pensions, insurance, education reimbursement, healthcare, dental plans, maternity leave, daycare, vacation time, and pay for time not worked. These are often called fringe benefits, although at this time these benefits often account for 25 to 35 percent of the cash payroll. Most of these additional benefits are established by top-level administration as institutionwide measures. The supervisor has little to do with such benefits other than to make sure that the individual who has been evaluated understands how benefits operate and that each receives his or her fair share. It is advisable to include this information in any wage survey.

To determine whether the rates offered by the department are competitive, the supervisor should request that the human resources department undertake a wage and salary survey unless recent reliable information is available. By comparing this information with outside wage patterns, the supervisor can determine if the wages are properly aligned externally. A sound wage and salary pattern should always be of great concern to the CEO. Although the supervisor has very little direct authority in this area, pointing out such inadequacies and inconsistencies may cause the administrator to launch an evaluation of other positions.

In most instances, supervisors do not have enough authority to make wage and salary adjustments except within the framework of the departmental wage scale. However, they should definitely plead their case to upper management when multiple vacancies occur because of employees leaving to assume similar positions at other hospitals, or in other departments within the facility, or when the type of person required to fill a position is in short supply. To make an intelligent presentation, the supervisor must know the value of the various jobs within the department and also the going rate within the community. As every supervisor knows, proper compensation of employees is a significant aspect of the employee's continuing satisfaction and motivation. Without a sound wage and salary pattern, it is almost impossible for a supervisor to recruit competent employees or keep the subordinates motivated.

FIGURE 21.6: EXAMPLE OF A SALARY SURVEY

	All surveyed hospitals		Year-to-year change, same hospitals	
	Average annual base salary	Average annual total cash	Salary increase, 1997-98	Total cash increase, 1997-98
Admitting	$46.40	$46.90	4.0%	4.2%
Ambulatory services	72.50	73.60	6.1	6.2
Biomedical engineering	57.50	58.10	3.2	3.4
Case management	63.80	64.80	N/A	N/A
Compensation and benefits	57.70	58.30	5.0	5.2
Computer operations	65.70	66.30	6.9	7.1
Contracting	74.70	75.70	N/A	N/A
Controller	77.00	78.60	4.7	4.8
Critical care	63.30	64.10	N/A	N/A
Dialysis unit	58.20	58.80	2.8	2.6
Dietary and food service	58.20	59.10	3.3	3.6
Emergency services	64.70	65.40	4.0	3.8
Facilities / plant operations	68.20	69.30	5.0	5.4
Home health	64.60	65.40	5.8	6.0
Housekeeping / environmental services	48.50	49.10	4.5	4.8
Imaging / radiology (nonmedical)	63.90	64.70	3.6	3.5
Labor relations	67.70	68.20	1.6	1.7
Laboratory	63.80	64.60	3.8	4.0
Management services organization	94.70	97.70	N/A	N/A
Marketing	68.90	70.90	7.5	8.5
Maternal / child / nursery	63.90	64.80	N/A	N/A
Medical group management	75.70	77.40	N/A	N/A
Medical / surgical	64.10	65.10	N/A	N/A
Medical records	58.10	58.80	4.4	4.5
Nursing services	79.20	81.00	5.2	5.1
Occupational health	59.60	60.10	5.1	5.0
Occupational therapy	59.80	60.20	3.6	3.7
Operating room service	67.10	67.90	5.1	5.2
Pastoral care	52.60	53.50	3.9	4.1
Patient accounting / business office	59.70	60.40	6.1	6.1
Personnel services	61.50	62.50	6.2	5.4
Pharmacy	78.10	79.20	4.0	4.1
Physical therapy	65.80	66.20	3.2	3.4
Physician-hospital organization	86.90	88.00	N/A	N/A
Physician network development	90.80	92.50	4.8	3.4
Physician services	61.10	62.50	2.3	2.5
Planning and development	91.80	96.00	13.4	15.9
Public relations / communications	58.60	59.30	7.2	7.3
Purchasing / materials management	62.00	62.80	3.5	3.6
Quality management	63.00	64.10	4.6	4.9
Radiation therapy	63.20	63.90	4.2	4.2
Rehabilitation services	71.70	72.80	3.1	3.3
Reimbursement	65.50	65.90	3.2	3.3
Respiratory therapy	56.10	56.80	2.8	3.0
Risk management	61.60	62.40	6.6	6.6
Skilled nursing facility	56.10	57.00	N/A	N/A
Social services	56.00	56.50	4.8	4.7
Utilization review	54.40	54.80	3.7	3.7

*All figures in thousands of dollars.   Source: *1998 Hay Hospital Compensation Survey*

Source: Reprinted from *Hospitals & Health Networks*, Vol. 72, No. 17, by permission, Sept. 5, 1998. © 1998 by Health Forum, Inc.

PROMOTION

Promotions provide an internal source of potential applicants. A promotion is the reassignment of an individual to a position higher in rank. This higher-level job entails more demands on the individual but results in higher pay, more authority and responsibility, more privileges, higher status, increased benefits, and greater potential for advancement. A promotion may also carry symbols of higher status, such as a more important job title, a larger cubicle or office, a bigger desk, or a secretary. Although some people do not want to advance, promotions are sought by most people who have a high level of aspiration. It is part of our culture to start at the bottom of the ladder and rise in status and income as one grows older. Because most people in our society look on promotions in this way, it is essential that organizations develop and pursue sound promotion policies.

Promotion from Within

Organizations depend heavily on promoting their own employees into better and more promising positions. The policy of promoting from within the organization is one of the most widely practiced personnel policies today. It helps achieve the organizational objective of being a good employer and a good place to work. The latter is undoubtedly one of the many goals of all healthcare centers.

Establishing and maintaining a policy of promotion from within versus external recruitment is important to the enterprise and the individual employee. For the enterprise, it ensures a constant source of trained people for the better positions; for the employees, it provides a powerful incentive to perform better. After an employee has worked for an enterprise, much more is known about that person than even the best potential candidate from outside the organization.

Internal promotion often is less expensive to the institution in time and money than luring applicants from the outside. Additional job satisfaction results when employees know that with proper efforts they can work up to more interesting and more challenging work, higher pay, and more desirable working conditions. Most employees like to know that they can get ahead in the enterprise in which they are working and feel more secure in a setting that provides future job opportunities. All this provides strong motivation. On the other hand, little motivation exists for employees to do a better job if they know that the better and higher-paying jobs are always reserved for outsiders.

The internal promotion policy should be applied whenever possible and feasible. Most organizations are aware that under special circumstances outside people must be hired; sometimes strict adherence to internal promotion does harm to the organization. For example, if no qualified candidates are available or appropriate for the job, the internal promotion policy cannot be followed. Also, an organization may be forced to look outside because employees with inadequate potential for promotion have been hired in the past.

At times the injection of "new blood" into an organization may be necessary because it keeps the members of the enterprise from becoming too complacent. Bringing in new people is important primarily in high-level managerial jobs and for highly trained professionals but is less important in hourly paid jobs.

Another reason the enterprise may have to recruit employees from the outside is that the organization cannot afford the expense of training and educating current employees. A particular position may require a long period of expensive and sophisticated schooling, and the institution simply may not be able to afford this type of upgrading program. Only large organizations can usually afford such expenses.

Another problem with promotion from within is that the organization must continue to live amicably with those who were bypassed. Such a problem, however, does not exist with an applicant from the outside who was rejected. In all this, as mentioned throughout this discussion, considerations of equal employment opportunity and possibly affirmative action must be included.

On the other hand, the supervisor should remember that not every employee wants advancement; many people know their limitations. Some employees are quite content with what they are doing and where they are within the enterprise. They prefer to remain with employees whom they know and responsibilities with which they are familiar. These employees should not be pressured by the supervisor into taking or seeking better positions. The supervisor should also bear in mind that what he or she may consider a promotion may not seem like a promotion to the employee. An ultrasound technician may believe that a promotion to administrative work is a hardship and not an advancement. He or she may find the administrative activities less interesting than direct patient care duties and may be concerned about his or her loss of skills over time. The supervisor has to provide promotional opportunities that do not entail compromising professional aspirations.

Sometimes a supervisor sees an employee as indispensable and does not want to release him or her to take a better job in another department. Often the opportunity for an employee's advancement is a reflection of the supervisor being extremely good at developing subordinates; for example, as a patient accounts manager develops outstanding billers and collectors, they are generally promoted out of that department to become assistant physician practice managers. The patient accounts manager may believe that the department suffers because of the loss of these outstanding professionals. In such a situation, administration should give credit to this manager for consistently developing promotable employees and should assure him or her that good employees will continue to enter the department from other hospital areas.

At times, the supervisor may be inclined to bypass someone for promotion within his or her department because the supervisor faces extra work for replacing the promoted employee and training a new one. The supervisor may fear that the productivity of the department will suffer. This is shortsighted, as promotion from within is a prime motivator for employees to excel. Supervisors who are tempted to think this way should ask themselves where they would be today if their former superiors had had this attitude.

Basis of Promotion

Despite the objections just stated, usually more employees apply for promotions than openings exist within the organization. Because of this, it is important for the organization and supervisors to formulate a sound basis on which employees are chosen for promotion. Because promotions are considered an incentive for employees to do a better job, it follows that the employee who has the best record of quality, productivity, and skill should be promoted. In many situations, however, it is difficult to objectively measure some employees' productivity, even though the supervisor has attempted to do so through merit ratings and performance appraisals. The most important criteria for choice are merit (current performance), ability (potential future performance), and seniority (experience).

Merit and Ability

Because promotion is an incentive for good performance, the best-performing employees should be promoted. Our discussion of performance appraisals emphasized the difficulty in measuring performance. The differences in merit among different employees in a healthcare job are also often difficult to measure precisely.

Ability

Ability and potential to assume the responsibilities of a higher-level position are additional criteria to consider. Perhaps an employee has extensive public speaking experience outside of your organization in his or her volunteer role as chairperson of the local Chamber of Commerce. This may be a skill that was captured during the skills inventory or development section of the performance appraisal. Now consider whether this person or another without public speaking skills is better for a promotion into a public relations position. Perhaps an individual has a baccalaureate degree in science and a master's degree in gerontology. The person's education adds depth to his or her set of core competencies. If the organization decides to open or manage a continuing care community, this individual may have the competency to fill a top position in this endeavor, even though his or her current position does not utilize these competencies.

The performance appraisal process is a major source of information; it is central to all organizational and management development. Generally, performance appraisals are used as a means of measuring performance in the past, but just as important is the appraisal of an employee's potential. Appraising a person's potential is based on the process and personal resources the employee uses to achieve results—that is, intellect, maturity, and the ability to lead. In appraising potential and future performance, the supervisor should evaluate the employee's oral and written communication skills, flexibility, and his or her decision-making, leadership, and planning abilities.

Some of the shortcomings of traditional methods used for selecting candidates for a position have been discussed above. In response to these shortcomings, thousands of industries and some healthcare organizations have adopted an assessment center approach for evaluating and selecting managers (Sullivan, Decker, and Hailstone 1985). An assessment center uses a process in which current employees seeking promotions to managerial jobs are administered individual and group exercises. The exercises and activities include job-related simulations such as interviews, in-basket exercises, tests, questionnaires, videotape exercises, and group problems. These exercises are designed to bring forth skills the organization considers critical to success. As the candidates go through these exercises, they are being observed by a group of specially trained observers (assessors, evaluators) who are members of the institution's management group. After the session, the candidates are evaluated by this panel of assessors to make selection recommendations or placement decisions or to determine a candidate's future promotability. Generally, the composite performance evaluation is communicated to the candidate.

Seniority

The exclusive use of merit and ability, which are to a great degree subjective criteria, often gives employees the feeling that promotions are not made fairly. Also, because many factors beyond an employee's control may affect productivity and performance, basing a promotion solely on these factors would be unfair. Frequent charges of favoritism, bias, and possible discrimination have caused managers to search for more objective decision criteria that would not create morale problems. However, as it is difficult to find objective criteria that completely eliminate favoritism and possible discrimination, the only objective criterion is length of service. Supervisors generally believe that their relations with their employees will be easier if they promote on the basis of seniority. Therefore, all organizations give some weight to seniority, whether they have a union or not (unions stress that employees should be promoted on the basis of seniority). This approach is now regularly accepted even by those enterprises that do not deal with unions and is applied to those jobs not covered by union agreements.

Basing promotion on the length of service assumes that the employee's ability increases with service. Although this may be questionable, with continued service the ability to perform and the knowledge about the organization probably do increase. If management is committed to promotion based on length of service, it is likely that the initial selection procedure of a new employee will be made carefully and that the employee will get as much training as possible in various positions. Most managers believe that an employee's loyalty is expressed by the length of service and that, consequently, this loyalty deserves the reward of promotion. On the other hand, some good employees may become discouraged and leave the organization, realizing that their chances for promotion are slim because many long-service employees may be ahead of them in line for such promotion.

Balancing the Criteria

Good supervisory practice attempts to strike a "happy medium" between the criteria of merit and ability on the one hand and length of service on the other. When the supervisor selects from among almost equally capable subordinates, the one with the longest service will no doubt be chosen. If an employee with less seniority stands head and shoulders above one with longer service, the employee with more core competencies will probably be promoted. As much as this selection process seems to make sense, these decisions are difficult, and it is easy to see why some supervisors have finally resolved to make length of service the sole determinant of selection for promotion. However, the ideal solution is to combine both factors. Rarely does a supervisor choose a person with the greatest merit and ability from all eligible candidates without giving any weight to length of service.

Selection for promotion also depends on the type of work involved, demands of the position to be filled, degree requirements prescribed by accrediting and professional associations, and many other factors. Most likely more and more emphasis is placed on merit and ability when the position to be filled is a demanding and sophisticated job on a higher level, whereas more weight can be given to seniority for promotion into a lower-level position. Every organization must decide on the relative weight of these factors in each case when deciding who is to be promoted.

SUMMARY

Performance appraisals are central to organizational and management development. They are formal evaluations of employees' job-related activities. Such a system not only guides management in gathering and analyzing information, it also provides guidance for merit increases, promotions, and coaching of employees. The purpose of the appraisal system is to provide a measure of the employee's job performance that leads to counseling and further development. An evaluation system consists of rating the employee and the appraisal interview, which usually occurs later. Although the appraisal interview between the supervisor and the employee may be awkward or difficult, the entire performance appraisal system is of no use if this aspect is ignored and not carried out appropriately.

An important source of candidates for job openings is the reservoir of employees who are currently with the institution. Whenever possible, promotion from within is one of the most rewarding personnel policies any enterprise can practice. It is of great benefit to the enterprise and to the morale of the employees. Although it is difficult to specify clearly the various criteria for promotion, it is normally acknowledged that merit and ability factors should be balanced with length of service. To be able to assess the ability, merit, and future potential of the employee, supervisors must remain aware of the employee's performance. Therefore, the supervisor must regularly appraise the performance of the employees in the department. A further internal source of recruitment is available from transfers.

In addition to all these duties, the staffing function includes making certain that the employees of the department are properly compensated and have a benefits program. Although much of this is out of the supervisor's domain, it is a supervisory duty to make certain that good internal wage alignment exists, meaning that each job is paid in accordance with its worth and difficulties. The wages paid must be high enough to attract people from outside the organization, if necessary, and to prevent present employees from leaving for higher wages. To do this, the supervisor must be familiar with the rates being paid in similar occupations in the community. Such information can be obtained by wage and salary surveys conducted by the human resources department.

NOTE

1. The Performance Appraisal Methods section is adapted from Allen (2000).

REFERENCES

Allen, G. 2000. "Evaluating-Performance Appraisal Methods," *Supervision, Second Edition*. Denton, TX: RonJon Publishers.

Holzschu, M. 2001. "Here's What Makes Job Reviews Successful—and Also Why They Fail." *Law Office Administrator* (January): 5.

Sullivan, E. J., P. J. Decker, and S. Hailstone. 1985. "Assessment Center Technology: Selecting Head Nurses." *The Journal of Nursing Administration* (May): 13–18.

Exhibit 21.1: Performance Evaluations

The objective of every performance evaluation is to identify staff strengths and weaknesses and create a plan for career development. Because performance evaluations can be uncomfortable, particularly when the employees being evaluated have performance problems, the process sometimes fails to receive the attention it deserves. This can result in errors in job assignment and training decisions.

Following are some essentials for conducting an effective performance evaluation.

BEFORE THE EVALUATION:

- Training sessions for all evaluators that include review preparation, evaluation methods, techniques for identifying obstacles to success and recommendations for ways to remove them, methods for creating goals, and identification of relevant legal issues
- Evaluation forms that have space for comments and descriptions
- A clearly written, up-to-date position description and an employee manual that have been distributed to staff
- Documentation of all relevant employee behavior throughout the review period so that the evaluation is not influenced solely by recent performance and provides no surprises to the employee
- Thorough review of the employee's personnel file, including previous evaluations and any other information that may apply, such as information from clients and other employees
- A carefully planned evaluation meeting
- Notice to staff that the meeting is a two-way discussion (Provide the employee with a copy of the completed evaluation form.)
- Communication of how performance is measured and how it is compared with policies and procedures

THE EVALUATION MEETING

- A meeting that begins with a discussion of the employee's strengths, gradually moves to development needs, and concludes with a positive comment (Use as many examples as possible when discussing strengths and weaknesses.)
- A meeting that is free of interruptions (Allow at least one hour to perform the evaluation.)
- An atmosphere that is relaxed and as informal as possible (An employee should be encouraged to voice his or her opinions on performance-related matters and know that those opinions will be heard.)
- A focus on the employee's performance, not on his or her personality (Avoid comparisons with other employees. If a personality conflict exists, discuss how it has negatively affected performance without attributing anything to the employee's personality.)
- Minimal criticism of performance, with a focus on the future, emphasizing counseling and development (A performance appraisal is not the time to raise specific instances of past employee shortcomings. Provide constructive criticism to an employee when the situation arises.)
- Measurement criteria that apply to traits as well as skills, such as the ability to work with others and leadership
- Comments/conclusions pertaining to professional responsibilities and achievement of goals that are specific, unambiguous, and delivered in such a way that they motivate the employee to work harder in the future

- Clearly written professional responsibilities and quantitative goals (with a deadline for completion) that are effectively communicated to staff; established goals that are realistic yet challenging
- Observations that neither overemphasize shortcomings nor provide undeserved praise
- Recommendations, such as training, that can overcome obstacles to achieving goals
- Separation from salary reviews (Although performance evaluations and salary reviews are linked, avoid discussing them at the same time. If the employee begins to discuss salary, respond that the amount of any raise depends on how well goals have been met.)

AFTER THE EVALUATION

- Documentation of the important issues raised during the evaluation
- Confirmation that both the evaluator and employee understand the employee's development needs, future goals, and plan for career guidance
- Staff feedback on how well the evaluation was performed; solicit recommendations from other employees on how the evaluation process could be improved
- Review of an employee's ongoing performance before his or her next evaluation

Source: Adapted from *Management of an Accounting Practice Handbook,* published by the American Institute of CPA. © 1997 from the *Journal of Accountancy* by the American Institute of Certified Public Accountants, Inc. Opinions of the authors are their own and do not necessarily reflect policies of the AICPA. Reprinted with permission.

PART VI

Influencing

CHAPTER TWENTY-TWO

Giving Directives and Managing Change

CHAPTER OBJECTIVES

After you have studied this chapter, you should be able to do the following:

1. Define the managerial function of influencing.

2. Describe the essential characteristics of good directives.

3. Compare and contrast the major techniques and theories of directing.

4. Describe the role of teams as a motivational instrument to achieve the work of the organization.

5. Review tools for group decision making

6. Relate the function of influencing to changing environments.

I NFLUENCING IS THE managerial function by which the supervisor evokes action from others to accomplish organizational objectives. It is the process that management uses to achieve goal-directed action from subordinates and colleagues in the organization and is vital to implementing change. The influencing function when used in the context of human resources is particularly concerned with behavioral responses. William Drayton states, "Change starts when someone sees the next step,"[1] while Nathaniel Branden says, "The first step toward change is awareness. The second step is acceptance."[2] The role of the supervisor is to draw the next step for the employees to see and motivate them to accept it.

The influencing function is also known as leading, motivating, directing, and actuating. Regardless of the terminology, it is the managerial function that the supervisor exercises to get the best and most out of the subordinates. At the same time, the supervisor strives to create a climate in which the subordinates find as much satisfaction of their needs as possible. In the past, managers depended largely on negative persuasion, disciplinary action, and a few incentive programs to influence their employees. The notion of organizational hierarchy dominated managerial thinking until the behavioral sciences brought about new understanding of human motivation and taught us better methods of influencing. Today every manager must understand some of the psychology involved in interpersonal relations.

It is the role of every supervisor to influence to get the work done through and with the help of employees. Influencing is the managerial function that initiates action. In most work settings, very little may be accomplished without influencing by the manager. Influencing includes issuing directives, instructions, assignments, and orders as well as guiding and overseeing employees. It also addresses the problems of how to motivate one's employees.

Moreover, the manager should consider the influencing function as a means not only for getting the work done and motivating the employees but also for developing them. The most effective way to develop employees is diligent coaching and teaching by their immediate superior. Thus, influencing is more than just giving orders or supervising the employees to make certain that they follow directives. Influencing means building an effective workforce and inspiring its members to perform their best, in effect getting the employees to work in a large enterprise as effectively as possible and with the same enthusiasm that they would display if they were working for themselves, either in their own enterprise or at a hobby.

Influencing is the job of every manager, from the CEO of a healthcare facility to the supervisor of one of its many departments. The amount of time and effort a manager spends in this function varies, however, depending on the level, number of employees supervised, and other duties. The supervisor of a department spends most of the time influencing and supervising, more so than the administrator of the institution does.

Influencing is a continuous function of the supervisor that covers the day-to-day activities within the department. It is interconnected with the other managerial functions. Planning, organizing, and staffing can be considered preparatory managerial functions; the purpose of controlling is to determine whether the goals are being achieved. The connecting and actuating link between these functions then is the managerial function of influencing.

Influencing is largely affected by the type of employee the supervisor has selected while performing the staffing function. The plans that the supervisor has made and the organization has drawn up also have a bearing on the influencing function. The controlling function is likewise affected by influencing, inasmuch as control often involves identifying the causes of variances to plans, some of which may be human problems.

To get the job done, every supervisor spends much time and effort in giving directives to subordinates. Recall the principle of unity of command, which means that in each department only one person has the authority to make decisions appropriate to his or her station and can give directives to the employees. Each employee has a single immediate supervisor, who is in turn responsible to his or her immediate superior, and so on up and down the chain of command. This also means that a subordinate is responsible to only one supervisor.

As discussed in Chapter 12, in healthcare organizations the unity-of-command principle may be violated by the presence of two sets of instructions: one from an immediate administrative supervisor and another from a patient's attending physician. Most times these instructions do not conflict, but if they do, the subordinate should refer the conflict to the supervisor. The supervisor or manager should confer with the physician and the administrator if necessary to resolve the issue. If time does not permit such deliberations, which is often the case in healthcare, the action that delivers the most appropriate clinical care to the patient should occur—that is, the instructions that benefit the patient should be followed.

CHARACTERISTICS OF GOOD DIRECTIVES

Because issuing directives is such a basic and integral part of the supervisor's daily routine, it has often been taken for granted that every supervisor knows how to give orders. This is, in fact, a skill that must and can be learned; some ways to issue directives are more effective than others. The experienced supervisor knows that faulty or bad order giving can easily upset even the best-laid plans and can create a general state of chaos, instead of coordination of efforts.

To the uninitiated outsider, it may seem that some supervisors can get excellent results even though they appear to break every rule in the book. Other supervisors may use all the best techniques of order giving and phrase their requests in the most courteous ways and still get only grudging compliance. The question of the most appropriate method of order giving depends on the employees concerned, the work situation, the supervisors and how they view their job, their attitude toward people, and many other factors.

Specific techniques for giving orders exist, and because the supervisor's own success depends largely on how the subordinates carry out the orders, the manager must possess the knowledge and skill for good directing. In other words, because directing is the fundamental tool employed by supervisors to start, stop, or modify activities, it is necessary for every supervisor to become familiar with the basic characteristics that distinguish good and accomplishable directives from those that are not. These characteristics are fulfilled when directives are reasonable, intelligible, worded appropriately, compatible with the objectives, and posed within reasonable time limits.

Reasonable Directives

The first essential characteristic of a good directive is that it must be reasonable—that is, you can reasonably expect compliance. Unreasonable orders not only undermine morale but also make controlling impossible. The requirement of reasonableness immediately excludes orders pertaining to activities that physically cannot be done or are dangerous. In judging whether a directive can be reasonably accomplished, supervisors should not only appraise it from their own point of view but should also try to place themselves in the position of the employee. The supervisor should not issue a directive if the capacity or experience of the employee is not sufficient to comply with the order. This becomes particularly important in the case of recent graduates who may have had an excellent education in many areas but lack working experience and even some of the basic knowledge required. Supervisors should not forget the value of their own on-the-job training.

A supervisor may indeed issue unreasonable instructions. For instance, to please the superior, a supervisor promises the completion of a job at a particularly early time and then issues such an order without considering whether the employee who is to carry it out can actually do so. In this situation, the supervisor should make it clear that he or she will try to get the job done in time, but unreasonable pressure should not be put on the subordinate. The supervisor should place himself or herself in the position of the subordinate and ask if compliance reasonably can be expected under these limits. The decision will depend on many factors prevailing at the time. In some cases the directive may actually be intended to stretch the subordinate's capabilities a little beyond what had previously been requested. Then the question of reasonableness becomes a question of degree. Generally, however, a primary requirement of a good directive is that it can be accomplished by the employee to whom it is assigned without undue difficulty.

Intelligibility

Another requirement is that a good directive should be intelligible to the employee—that is, the employee should be able to understand it. The subordinate cannot be expected to carry out an order that he or she does not understand. For example, a directive in a language not intelligible to the subordinate cannot be considered an order. The same also applies if both speak English but the supervisor uses words that the employee does not comprehend. This, then, becomes a matter of communication (see Chapter 5). The supervisor must make certain that the employee understands, and it is his or her duty to communicate in words that the employee actually understands and not merely should understand.

Appropriate Wording

Every good supervisor knows that the tone and words used in issuing directives significantly affect the subordinates' acceptance and performance of them. A considerate tone is likely to stimulate willing and enthusiastic acceptance, which is preferable to routine or grudging acceptance or outright rejection. In the patient care field, the word "order" in connection with the attending physician's directives is normally used without unpleasant connotations. However, most supervisors should refrain from using the term order as much as possible and instead use such terms as directives, assignments, instructions, suggestions, and requests. A directive followed by a sincere thank you is always appropriate.

Requests

Phrasing orders as requests does not reduce their character as a directive, but there is a major difference in the reaction a request inspires as compared to a command. With most subordinates, a request is all that is usually needed and used. It is a pleasant and easy way of asking an employee to get the job done. For example, "Mary, as time permits this morning, could you help Tina with her backlog of physician orders so that she is caught up by 10:00 a.m.? Thanks for your assistance." This style of directing works well, particularly with those employees who have been working for the supervisor for some time and who are familiar with the personality of the supervisor, and vice versa. A request works best with this type of employee, and it usually does not rub anyone the wrong way.

Suggestions

In other instances it might be advisable to place the directive in the form of a suggestion, which is an even milder form than a request. For example, the supervisor might say, "Mary, we are supposed to get all of this work done before noon and we seem to be a bit behind. Do you think we can make up for it?" Suggestions of this type accomplish a great deal for the supervisor because they are understood and accepted by responsible and ambitious employees. Such employees like the feeling of not being ordered around and of being on their own to get the job accomplished. This suggestive type of order, however, is not advisable when dealing with new employees. They simply do not have the background of the department and have not been around long enough to have received sufficient training and familiarity with its activities. Suggestion is also not the proper way of giving orders to those employees who are less competent and less dependable.

Commands

Some subordinates must be told what to do simply because a request or suggestion might invite an argument as to why they should not do it, or they will never get around to doing what was requested. For example, "Mary, I need the status on those two patient bills I gave you last Friday by 10:00 a.m. Before you go on break today, stop by my office with your report. Thanks." The command or directive style leaves no room for questioning expectations.

Sometimes the command type of order is the only way to get things done. Everyone remembers commands from parents and school teachers as part of growing up. Most people, however, think that once they are adults, commands are no longer necessary. Thus, the best rule for a supervisor is to avoid commands whenever possible but to use them when necessary.

Compatibility with Objectives

A good directive must be compatible with the purposes and objectives of the organization. If the instructions are not in accordance with these objectives, the subordinate may not execute them adequately or may not execute them at all Thus, when issuing directives that appear to conflict with the organizational objectives, the supervisor must explain to the employee why such action is necessary, or the supervisor should explain that the directive merely appears to be but actually is not contrary to the institution's objectives. Instructions must also be consistent; they must not be in opposition to orders or directives previously given unless there is a good explanation for the discrepancy.

Ethics

Similar to compatibility issues is the resistance to directives that, in the mind of the employee, are not ethical. Ethical theories offer a means to explain and justify actions and serve as guides for making moral decisions (Munson 1992) and, thus, influence behavior.

Some organizations have written codes of ethics (see Exhibit 22.1 and Figure 6.1) to provide a roadmap for staff of ethical practices and expectations. Supervisors encounter enticements from equipment manufacturers and others to purchase their products. Sometimes the enticement is so subtle it goes unrecognized as something that could bias the supervisor's decision, such as tickets to a baseball game, or perhaps an overly zealous public relations manager slightly overstates the capabilities of the hospital. Regardless of the reason, inaccurately stating the organization's licensure, capability, and resources is fraudulent.

Furthermore, with the federal government's push for compliance, many organizations have increased staff education in this topic. So when a supervisor issues a directive that appears contrary to the organization's published practices, staff should resist. In these situations, the supervisor must clearly explain his or her rationale to staff and possibly include his superior or the organization's compliance officer to ensure that staff recognizes that the requirement being placed on them is not unethical.

Ethics has roots not only in published guidelines but also in cultures, religions, and families. Therefore, a supervisor in a culturally diverse environment may encounter resistance because of perceptions of those team members who grew up in a different culture or during a different period in time. Consider the younger generation of today. The morals under which they practice differ substantially from those that predominated 40 years ago. Many factors affect healthcare today, including genetic testing, cloning, abortion, and privacy, that you must effectively address and gain support from your staff to deal with; many of these issues may cause ethical discomfort for some of your staff.

Time Limit

An additional characteristic of a good directive is that it specify the time within which the instructions should be carried out. The supervisor should allow a reasonable amount of time and, if this is not feasible, must realize that the quality of performance is only as good as can be produced under the time limit. In many directives, the time factor is not stated, although it is probably implied that the assignment should be carried out within a reasonable time.

Because the performance of the employee depends to a great extent on the format and content of directives given, the supervisor should make certain that the directive is in accordance with these most essential characteristics.

MAJOR TECHNIQUES OF DIRECTING

In previous chapters, various theories were discussed describing the supervisor's underlying managerial attitudes, such as Theories X and Y, autocratic and democratic leadership, participation in decision making, and broad or narrow delegation of authority. The following is a more detailed discussion of how these managerial attitudes manifest themselves in the daily working environment in which the supervisor depends on the subordinates to get the job done.

Generally the supervisor may choose from two basic techniques of direction: autocratic, or close supervision and consultative, or participative general supervision. This discussion clearly distinguishes between these two extremes, but in practice the supervisor usually combines and blends the techniques. For example, the manager might use the autocratic technique for one situation and the democratic technique for another. The supervisor might consider it more advisable to use one method for only some employees. No one form of supervision is equally good in all situations. Whether it is better to apply a more autocratic or a more democratic type of supervision depends on many factors, including the type of work; current situation; attitude of the employee toward the supervisor; personality and ability of the employee; and personality, experience, and ability of the supervisor. A good supervisor is sensitive to all these factors and to the needs of each situation, so the style of supervision should be adjusted accordingly.

Autocratic (Close) Supervision

When the autocratic or close technique of directing is employed, the supervisor gives direct, clear, and precise orders to the subordinates with detailed instructions as to exactly how and in what sequence things are to be done. This allows little room for the initiative of the subordinate. The supervisor who normally uses the autocratic technique delegates as little authority as possible and believes that he or she probably can do the job better than any of the subordinates. The supervisor relies on command and detailed instructions, followed by close supervision. An autocratic supervisor believes that subordinates are "not paid to think"; they are expected to follow instructions. The boss alone is to do the planning and decision making. This type of supervisor does not necessarily distrust the subordinate but believes that without detailed instruction the subordinate could not properly carry out the directive. This person believes that only he or she can specify the best method and that there is only one way, the supervisor's way, to get the job done. In other words, Theory X management is practiced.

With most people, the consequences of autocratic supervision can be disastrous. Employees lose interest and initiative; they stop thinking for themselves because no need or occasion arises for independent thought. They are obedient but silent and lack initiative and ingenuity. It becomes difficult for the subordinates to remain loyal to the organization and to the supervisor, and they secretly rejoice when the boss makes a mistake. This form of supervision tends to make the employees somewhat like robots. Freedom is curtailed, and it is difficult for them to learn even by making mistakes. They justly conclude that they are not expected to do any thinking about their job, and, although they perfunctorily perform their duties, they find little involvement in the work. They are certainly not motivated.

Shortcomings of the autocratic technique of supervision are obvious. Generally, men and women who have been brought up in a democratic society resent autocratic order giving. It is contrary to our traditional democratic way of life in the United States. No ambitious employee will remain in a position where the supervisor is not willing to delegate some degree of freedom and authority. Any subordinate who is eager to learn and progress will resent being constantly given detailed instructions that leave no room for his or her own thinking and initiative. Frequently, this type of management is referred to as micromanaging because the supervisor directs every detail of the subordinate's action. The employee is stifled and eventually will leave the enterprise if possible. This method of supervision does not produce good employees and only chases away those who have potential.

On the other hand, one must not forget that under certain circumstances and with certain people a degree of close supervision may be necessary. This is the exception, however, not the rule. Suppose, for example, that the subordinate is the type of person who does not want to think for himself or herself and prefers to receive clear orders. Firm guidance gives reassurance, whereas loose and general supervision may be frustrating. Some employees lack ambition and imagination and do not want to become involved in their daily job. Other employees have been brought up in an authoritarian manner and their previous work experience leads them to believe that general supervision is no supervision at all. Moreover, a work setting sometimes is so chaotic that only autocratic techniques can bring order. Also, the autocratic supervisor usually makes the basic Theory X assumption that the average employee does not want to do the job and that close supervision and threats of loss of the job are needed to get people to work. Such a supervisor believes that if he or she were not on the job and "breathing down their necks," all the subordinates would stop working. Under these conditions, they probably would. Autocratic, or close, supervision is not conducive to motivating employees to perform their best; general supervision, however, is conducive to achieving maximum work potential. Aside from these rather unusual situations, however, it can generally be assumed that autocratic, or close, supervision is the least desirable and effective method.

Consultative (Participative) Supervision

The opposite of autocratic supervision is consultative supervision. Consultative supervision is also known as participative, democratic, or permissive supervision. It is similar to the concept of general supervision referred to earlier. Its basic assumption is that employees are eager to do a good job, have the motivation to perform their best, and are capable of doing so. The supervisor behaves toward them with this basic assumption in mind, and the employees in turn tend to react in a manner that justifies the expectation of their supervisors.

This democratic approach to the directing function manifests itself in the practice of general supervision when it comes to routine assignments within the department. When new jobs have to be performed and new assignments made, the democratic method of supervising appears in the consultative, or participative, technique of directing. Both have the underlying assumption that employees are more motivated if they are left to themselves as much as possible.

The essential characteristic of consultative supervision is that the supervisor consults with employees concerning the extent, nature, and alternative solution to a problem before the supervisor makes a decision and issues a directive. The supervisor who uses the consultative approach before issuing directives is earnestly seeking help and ideas from the employees and approaches the subject with an open mind. More important than the procedure is the attitude of the supervisor. A subordinate can easily sense superficiality and is quick to perceive whether the boss genuinely intends to consult him or her on the problem or only intends to give the impression of doing so.

Some supervisors are inclined to use such pseudo-consultation merely to give employees the feeling that they have been included in the decision-making process. Supervisors often ask for participation only after they have already decided on the directive. Here the supervisor is using the consultative technique as a trick, a device for manipulating people to do what he or she wants them to do. The subordinate will quickly realize that he or she is not being taken seriously and that this participation is not real. The results achieved will be much worse than if the superior had used the most autocratic method. To practice actual consultative management when issuing new directives and assignments, the supervisor must be ready to take it seriously and be willing to be swayed by the employees' opinions and suggestions. If the manager is not sincere, it is better not to apply this technique at all.

If the subject matter concerns only the supervisor and one employee, the consultative or participative method can be carried out informally. Numerous occasions arise during the day to hold such private consultations; however, if this approach is used all the time, the subordinates may begin to doubt whether the supervisor has any opinions of his or her own and is able to make any decisions. Although some supervisors are incapable of making decisions, many go too far in using this philosophy of direction and, while implementing the technique of participation, cannot retain the atmosphere of managing.

To reinstate the atmosphere of managing, one should recall that consultative direction does not lessen or weaken formal authority, as the right of decision making still remains with the supervisor. Moreover, the supervisor using this approach is just as concerned with getting the job done economically and expeditiously as the manager who uses another approach. Although the supervisor must not dominate the situation to the exclusion of any employee participation, this does not mean the supervisor cannot express an opinion. It must be expressed in a manner that indicates to the employee that even the supervisor's opinions are subject to critical appraisal. Similarly, participative consultation does not mean that the suggestions of the employee cannot also be criticized or even rejected. True consultation implies a sharing of information between the supervisor and employee and a thorough and impartial discussion of alternate solutions, regardless of who originated them. Only then can it be said that the manager really consulted the subordinate.

For such consultative practices to be successful, it is not only necessary that the supervisor be in favor of them, but the employee must also want them. If the employee believes that "the boss knows best" and that making decisions and giving directives is none of his or her concern, the opportunity to participate is not likely to induce better motivation or morale. The supervisor must also keep in mind that the problems involved must be consistent with the subordinate's ability. Asking for his or her participation about topics that are outside the employee's scope of experience makes the employee feel inadequate and frustrated instead of being motivated.

In using consultation, the danger exists that at the end of an extended discussion the employee may not have a clear idea of the solution. It is therefore desirable and even necessary for the supervisor or subordinate to summarize the conclusions to avoid such a pitfall. This is even more essential if several employees participated in the consultation.

The consultative approach is comparable to the 4 Es approach developed at Humana, Inc. and described by LeTourneau (2004). While the approach was developed to help clinicians communicate better with patients, the concepts apply to communication between supervisors and staff, whom they wish to encourage to accept changes and take action in a defined way. The first E is *engage*: "The goal of the engage stage is to introduce and generate interest in the change"; this step introduces the subject and encourages dialog and awareness. The second E is *empathize*; during this step, the supervisor's role is to listen and empathize with employee concerns and gather their questions and comments about the proposed change. The third E is *educate*, during which the supervisor explains how the change will be implemented, taking into consideration the comments and concerns that were raised and, ideally, responds to the various questions raised. During this process, education takes place and the approach can be collaboratively "tweaked." LeTourneau states that "As change progresses, the teaching process should continue to include the skills and information needed for success." Finally, the fourth E is *enlist*: "Early involvement with engagement and empathy help to entice" employees to "become involved with the change. The process of explaining, listening, answering questions, and listing and addressing concerns is the start of enlisting them in the change process. When [employees] become drawn into planning and developing a change, it is much more likely to meet their needs" and influence their actions (LaTourneau 2004).

One of the obvious advantages of the consultative or 4 Es approach is that the emerging directive does not appear to the employee as an order but rather as a solution in which he or she participated. This ensures the subordinate's cooperation and enthusiasm in carrying out the directive. It imparts a feeling of importance because the ideas evidently were desired and valued. Active participation also provides an outlet for reasoning power and imagination and an opportunity for the employee to make a worthwhile contribution to the organization. As there is considerable talent among employees, their ideas often prove to be valuable in improving the quality of directives. The approach may even bring the employee closer to the supervisor, which will make for better communication and understanding between them. Looking at these impressive advantages, it becomes apparent that consultation is by far the best method to use whenever the supervisor has to issue new assignments, directives, and instructions.

This democratic, participative approach to directing subordinates leads to what we have already referred to as general or loose supervision when making routine assignments and carrying out the daily tasks involved in each employee's job. General supervision means allowing the subordinate to work out the details of the job and make decisions on how best to do it. Through this process, workers gain great satisfaction from being on their own and from having a chance to express themselves and make decisions. Instead of having a specified, detailed list of orders to comply with, the supervisor generally indicates what the end result needs to be and makes a few suggestions as to how to go about it. In so doing, the supervisor assumes that given the proper opportunity, the average employee wants to do a good job. The supervisor is primarily interested in the results. Once the subordinate is told what is to be accomplished and goals are established and limits defined, the employee is left on his or her own. This form of thinking and supervision usually leads to higher motivation and morale and ultimately better job performance. It gives employees the opportunity to satisfy their needs for self-expression and being their own boss. In this atmosphere, team management thrives.

Explaining Directives

The supervisor who practices general supervision creates an atmosphere of understanding and mutual confidence in which the employee feels free to call on the boss whenever the need arises without fearing that his or her call for help may indicate incompetence. Such a supervisor takes the necessary time to explain to the workers the reasons for general directives. Knowing the purpose behind the directives, the employee is able to understand the environment of the activities. This makes the employee better informed, and the better informed the subordinate is, the better he or she can perform the job.

In many enterprises, a common complaint is that subordinates are kept in the dark most of the time and that supervisors hoard knowledge and information that they ought to pass on. In most instances, it is exceedingly difficult to issue directives so completely as to cover all factors and issues involved. If the person who receives the directive knows the purpose behind it, however, he or she is in a better position to carry it out than one who does not. This enables the worker to put the environment in total perspective and make sense out of it so that he or she can take firm and secure action. Without such knowledge, employees may feel anxious. Also, subordinates may run into unforeseen circumstances; if they know why the directive was given, they probably can use their own good judgment and carry out the directive in a manner that brings about proper results. They could not possibly do this if they were not well informed.

Sometimes a supervisor can overdo a good thing, however, and instead of clarifying the situation, provide so much information that the subordinate is utterly confused. Explanations should include only enough information to get the job done. If the directive involves a very minor activity and not much time is available, the explanation should be brief. Supervisors must use their own judgment in deciding how detailed their explanations are. They should take into consideration such factors as the capacity of the subordinates to understand, the training they have had, the content of the directive, the underlying managerial attitude, and the time available. After evaluating these factors, the supervisor is in a better position to decide what constitutes an adequate explanation.

GENERAL SUPERVISION COMPARED WITH NO SUPERVISION

As mentioned, general supervision is not the same as no supervision at all. General supervision requires that the employee be given a definite assignment, but one that is definite only to the extent that the employee understands the results expected. It is not definite regarding the specific instructions that state precisely how the results are to be achieved. General supervision does not mean that subordinates can set their own standards. Rather, the supervisor sets the standards and makes them realistic—high enough to be a challenge, but not higher than possibly can be achieved.

Although general supervision excludes direct pressure, employees know that their efforts are being measured against these standards, and this knowledge alone should lead them to work harder. By setting the standards reasonably high, the supervisor does apply a degree of pressure, but it is quite different from that exerted by "breathing down someone's neck."

General supervision requires the supervisor to keep developing the potential of the employees. Everyone knows that active learning is more effective than passive learning. Employees learn more easily when they work out a solution for themselves than if they are given the solution. It is also known that employees learn best from their own mistakes. In general supervision, ongoing training of employees is an absolute necessity; the supervisor spends considerable time teaching employees how to solve problems and make decisions as problems arise at work. The better trained the employees become in basic problem-solving methods, the less need there will be for supervision. One way to judge the effectiveness of a supervisor is to see how the employees in the department function when the boss is away from the job.

General supervision, however, is a way of life that must be practiced over time, and the supervisor cannot expect instantaneous results if general supervision is introduced into a situation in which the employees have been accustomed to close supervision. It takes time before the results can be seen. The supervisor who uses a generalist approach is just as interested in results as any other supervisor, but he or she is also interested in the employees' individual development, which differentiates him or her from the autocratic supervisor.

Although the supervisor may be a firm believer in general supervision and practices it whenever possible, under certain conditions firmness, fortitude, and decisiveness must be shown. Certain employees simply may not thrive under loose supervision. This, again, is the exception and not the rule. Although general supervision is not a cure-all for every problem, most research studies indicate that it is more effective than close supervision in terms of productivity, morale, and achievements. General supervision permits the employee to acquire pride in the work and in the results achieved. It helps develop the employee's talent and capabilities and permits the supervisor to spend less time with the employees and more time on overall management of the department. General supervision provides the motivation for the employees to work on their jobs with enthusiasm and energy, thus deriving full satisfaction from their work.

TEAM MANAGEMENT

Teams are mentioned throughout this book. They can play a major role in influencing the action of others in the department. Teams may be established to temporarily address an issue or as a formal structure within a department or organization. Temporary teams such as quality improvement teams are cross-functional and gather workers from various parts of an organization to focus on a process or problem. Departments or organizations that have established self-directed teams as part of the formal structure have long-term purposes that are related to producing a product or delivering a service.

One advantage to establishing teams is that it places authority in the hands of those closest to the product or service to make decisions that will affect that product or service. Employees often appreciate being given this level of authority. It shows that management acknowledges their wisdom and trusts them to do the assignment. Another advantage is that it allows the supervisor's span of control to be enlarged because some of the decision-making efforts have been pushed down the ladder of the organization. By expanding the span of control, supervisors can oversee more employees, or, conversely, fewer supervisors are required. Improvement in both the quality and cost of processes is yet another advantage. Kodak and Texas Instruments both use teams and successfully implemented change with their employees. For example, at Kodak, the changes implemented by teams slashed cycle time—the amount of time it takes for a product to move from invention to store shelves. What once took ten years to develop now takes five. Similarly, Texas Instruments improved annual revenue per employee from $142,000 to $227,000 in two years (Neuborne 1997).

Teams fail as well. The most commonly cited reasons for failure are having unclear goals, changing objectives, lack of accountability, lack of management support, lack of role clarity, ineffective leadership, low priority of team, and no team-based pay (Neuborne 1997). One can see that several of these reasons for failure are directly related to communication. All employees need some degree of clear direction.

Even teams that do not fail are not without disadvantages. Conflict between team members is a disadvantage that could affect morale of an entire department when coworkers take sides with one team member or another. Conflict within the team can also affect the product or service, especially if the team cannot come to agreement on the method to produce the product or deliver the service.

Staff sometimes need a decision maker. As the supervisor, you must take these advantages and disadvantages into consideration when you establish short- and long-term teams and recognize symptoms of team breakdown that may lead to poor results.

CHANGE AND INFLUENCING

All organized activities are under continuous pressure for change. There are various reasons for change, but the most common are scientific and technological developments, people, competition, and communication.

Supervisors' effectiveness in the influencing function is extremely important whenever they are faced with change. Because every enterprise operates in a larger context and a dynamic environment than itself, change is inevitable and is a part of everyday life. In fact, the growth of most undertakings depends largely on the concept of change and the ability to accommodate it. Communicating the reasons for change may reduce to some degree rejection and hostility. Changes are often the result of outside events that force the enterprise to alter its practices. Sometimes changes must occur for the enterprise to stay alive.

Although all organized activities are subject to change, the degree and complexity of change vary considerably from one activity to another. This is particularly true in the healthcare field. The healthcare organization as a social system produces an ever-shifting equilibrium of forces because of the amazing and beneficial changes in medical sciences and technologies and in the social and economic environment. The supervisor's own department is a small social subsystem, interdependent on the larger system of the healthcare center. Any change imposed from outside is likely to shift the equilibrium of forces within each individual department as well as within the organization as a whole.

The departmental supervisor is at the forefront of change because he or she is the one in the daily work environment who has to make it a reality. The supervisor must sell the idea of change to the subordinates. Most often the supervisor has had little to do with the decision to make the change or with its timing; it originated higher up in the administration or outside the organization. However, the supervisor should understand and accept the change because now his or her duty is to introduce it, explain it to the subordinates, and implement the alterations in processes. The supervisor encounters reactions from the employees that range from ready acceptance to outright rejection and hostility; these should be reported when they occur.

Resistance to Change

When it comes to jobs and interpersonal relations, many people tend to resist change. This is important to realize because if an enterprise, especially in healthcare, is to survive, it must be able to react to the prevailing forces. The main reasons for resistance to change are uncertainty, perception, loss, self-interest, and insecurity. The short rhyme, "I hate learning new stuff all the time. And I hate change. It makes me feel so insecure. Why can't things just stay the same?" (Grattan 1999) likely sums up the feelings of many of your staff. That is why it is important to recognize that one of the important factors of internal inflexibilities is psychological. Supervisors and employees may develop patterns of thought and behavior that are resistant to change. Supervisors are often frustrated in instituting a change by the unwillingness or inability of people to accept it. To overcome these inflexibilities, the supervisor must realize that it requires patiently selling the idea, educating the staff, carefully disseminating information, providing good leadership, and developing a tradition of change among the department's members. The supervisor must not fail to realize that even a small and seemingly insignificant change may cause strong reactions within some of the employees.

This difficulty is further complicated because of different perceptions. For example, employees may believe that a new organizational arrangement will result in their loss of control or influence. This belief will cause resistance to change. The fact that the new structure will in no way reduce staff's influence does not diminish staff resistance as long as they feel threatened or attacked.

To a large degree these sources of resistance to change center around a major consideration—uncertainty about the effects of change. An impending change is likely to cause anxiety and nervousness. The employees may worry about their being able to fulfill the new job demands. Also, the change may be fraught with weaknesses that have been overlooked or brushed aside by those who planned its implementation.

Another reason for resisting change is that it disturbs the equilibrium of the current state of affairs. The assumption is that before the change, the employee exists within an environment that is highly stable; the change may threaten, prevent, or decrease satisfaction with the environment. Therefore, it is natural for some employees to do whatever possible to thwart the introduction of a change. A further reason for resisting change is that any change is seen as a potential threat to the employee's security and self-interest. The subordinate must give up the known familiar routine for something new and unpredictable. For example, a new apparatus in the cardiopulmonary lab could make some of the technologists' previous skills unnecessary. The change may require the technologists to upgrade their skills, and they may not be sure they can master the new responsibilities.

Change may also threaten the employee's status within the organization and the existing social networks. The employee may fear that his or her status will be lowered and someone else's will be raised; such feelings of loss are common when mergers occur. A merger announcement can appear to be threatening and expected to produce changes in the reporting relationships and status of numerous employees.

Often threats of an economic nature provide another reason for resistance to change. The subordinate may fear that the change will affect his or her job economically. Many years ago Dutch hand-weavers in the Low Countries of Europe (Belgium, The Netherlands, and Luxembourg) tried to destroy mechanical looms by throwing their wooden clogs (sabots) into the machinery (hence the word sabotage) because they feared that the machines would destroy their jobs and income. The same fears of loss prevail today.

In general, a change that causes great disturbance to one person may create little disequilibrium for another. The severity of the reaction that occurs in a particular situation depends on the nature of the change and the person concerned. The important factor for the supervisor to recognize is that changes do disturb the equilibrium of the employee and that, when individuals become threatened, they develop behaviors that serve as barriers to the threat (see Figure 22.1). Therefore, it is the supervisor's duty to facilitate the inevitable process of adjustment when changes are necessary.

Overcoming Resistance to Change

In his book, *Resistance*, Pritchett (1996) offers the following analogy that serves as our starting point for ways to overcome this condition:

> Resistance is the most common side effect of change. If you don't encounter it, you have to wonder if you've really changed things much. Here's how it works. Change triggers the organization's immune system. People start to resist, trying to fight off the change. It's sort of like antibodies attacking some organism that invades a person's body. This just seems to be the natural order of things. Upset the status quo, and here comes the opposition. Look at it this way, and

FIGURE 22.1: RESISTANCE TO CHANGE

Nature of Resistance	Common Staff Reactions	Reactions Caused By	Approaches to Reduce Resistance
Psychological	Anxiety Nervousness	Uncertainty	• Communicate • Educate staff
Perception	Anxiety Disinterest in organization activities Inattention to work	Loss of status Loss of control Loss of job satisfaction	• Sell idea(s) • Provide information • Lead by example • Facilitate change • Upgrade skills
Economic	Sabotage Strike Leave job	Uncertainty Insecurity Instability	• Involve staff • Initiate change often

you see how resistance can be a valuable protective device. For example, strong resistance to change might cause a company to ditch some dangerous new plan or project, just like your body's white blood cells fight off an infection. Resistance can defend the health of organizations as well as individuals.

The supervisor should always remember that employees seldom resist change just to be stubborn. There usually are valid reasons for resistance. Subordinates resist because the change affects their equilibrium socially, psychologically, and possibly economically. One of the factors that is particularly important in gaining acceptance of change is the relationship that exists between the supervisor who is trying to introduce the change and the employee who is subject to the change. If a relationship of mutual confidence and trust exists between the two, the employee is much more likely to go along with the change.

The supervisor should assume that a considerable amount of time is necessary to implement a change; a rigid timetable for change is unrealistic. The change must be planned far in advance, and its impact on each position and job should be anticipated. Even if the change is well thought out and carefully planned, some ramifications will probably be overlooked. With the proper attitude and the right techniques, the supervisor can facilitate the introduction of change. Involving subordinates in change discussions and decisions helps to overcome the various types of resistance.

Explanation and Communication

As noted earlier, the most important aspect in facilitating the introduction of change is the supervisor's duty to explain the change to the employees in advance. This should begin long before the change is to be initiated. It must be clear to the employees what the organization is trying to achieve with its change initiative and how it connects with the organization's goals. There should be ample time before the changeover to familiarize the employees with the idea, allow them to think through the implications, and ask questions for more clarification. They must understand the reason for the change. In other words, there must be sufficient time for feedback and additional communication.

In explaining the change, the supervisor should put himself or herself into the subordinate's position and discuss its pros and cons from the subordinate's point of view. Referring to our earlier discussion on consultation or the 4Es, this discussion should explain what will happen and why. It should clarify the way in which the change will affect the employee, what it means to that person, and, if applicable, how it will even improve the present situation.

In this process of communication, the manager might want to interject what is often referred to as the *force-field analysis*, an approach to overcome resistance to change. In every change process forces act for and against the change. The supervisor should comment on the pluses and minuses connected with the change from the employee's point of view, then try to tip the balance toward acceptance so that the forces for the change outweigh the forces against the change. All this information should be communicated to the entire department, both to employees who are directly involved and to those who are indirectly involved. It is essential to be absolutely truthful. Pritchett (1996), in fact, says one should promise problems. Even the best planned change will encounter some unpredictable problems. Insinuating that there will be no problems is risky. The supervisor cannot afford a credibility gap.

The supervisor must also try to communicate, and if necessary, over communicate, explaining to the employees what they consciously and subconsciously want and need to know to resolve prevailing fears. Only then can employees assess and understand what the proposed change means in terms of their positions and activities. The supervisor must help the subordinate understand the need for the change. If the goals are easy to see and identify an endpoint that is better for the team, department, or organization, staff will perceive that the struggle to make the change is worthwhile. The subordinate who has been informed of the reasons for change, recognizes that the change is purposeful, and knows what to expect and why will be committed to the change. Instead of blind resistance, intelligent adaptation to the instructions will occur; instead of insecurity, a feeling of security will emerge. It is not the change itself that leads to so much misunderstanding but it is the manner in which the supervisor introduces the change. In other words, resistance to change that comes from fear of the unknown can be minimized by supplying an appropriate explanation.

Participation

Another effective way of reducing resistance to change is to permit participation in planning and implementing it. Playing a part in planning the change reduces uncertainty and removes some of the fears and threats to social relationships and self-interests. Furthermore, those who are affected by the change may have something to contribute, as they are close to the situation and may see some weaknesses in the change proposal that management might have overlooked. Last, if the plan for change is their plan, acceptance by the employees is greater.

This participation may be in the form of consultation, whereby criticism and suggestions are sincerely solicited from the employees in relation to the contemplated change. In face-to-face conversations, the supervisor discusses problems, asks questions, and tries to get the employees' ideas and reactions. Management can then incorporate as much of this into the change as possible, and the employees can consider themselves partners in the change. A change imposed from above without participation is likely to generate resentment.

A more advanced stage of participation occurs when the supervisor lets the employees make the decision about how to resolve the problem. The supervisor defines the problem and sets the limits but allows the subordinates to develop the alternatives and choose between them. Group decision making could also produce a better decision because pooled expertise is likely to identify and evaluate more alternatives than an individual could; those who are involved in this process are probably more deeply committed to the alternative selected. Therefore, group decision making is an effective means for overcoming resistance to change. Such an approach recognizes that if the employees who are threatened by a change have the opportunity to work through the new ideas and methods from the beginning and can be assured that their needs will be satisfied in the future, they will accept the new ideas and methods as something of their own making and will support the changes. Group decision making also makes it easier for each member to carry out the decision once it is agreed on, and the group will put strong pressure on those who have reservations or who do not want to go along.

Both types of participation should be encouraged because they help facilitate the introduction of change. Of course, in trying to implement change in the department, the supervisor makes use of all means available, including persuasion, discussion, participation, and group decision making. Participation is not always possible, however; in extreme situations, it may be necessary to make unpleasant changes unilaterally, impose them, and then help the subordinates understand and accept them.

Survival During Change

Even though you, the supervisor, buy into the reasons for change, and even if you are successful in influencing your staff to accept the change, adjusting to new circumstances can drain you. The desire to successfully pull off a major change in your department can result in exhaustion, irritability, dissatisfaction, and insomnia. These are all symptoms of stress. They are the hormonal and mental reactions to internal and external pressures. Practicing stress management techniques and maintaining a sense of humor will help you get through this challenging time.

SUMMARY

The influencing function of the manager forms the connecting link between planning, organizing, and staffing on one side and controlling on the other. Issuing directives is perhaps the most important part of the influencing function because without them, very little would be achieved. Certain prerequisites ensure that a directive is properly carried out. A good directive must indicate who, what, where, when, how, and why. It should be accomplishable, intelligible, properly phrased, and compatible with the objectives of the enterprise. In addition, a reasonable amount of time should be permitted for its completion.

In issuing directives, the supervisor may employ two major techniques: (1) the autocratic technique, which brings about close supervision, and (2) the consultative technique, which is characterized by general supervision. For certain occasions, employees, and conditions the autocratic technique is probably more effective, but for most situations it is far better for a supervisor to apply consultative techniques to produce the highest motivation and morale among employees. This means that in the case of new assignments, the supervisor consults with the employees about how the job should best be done.

In directives primarily concerned with routine assignments and the daily performance of the job, the supervisor employs a form of general supervision instead of close supervision. In so doing, the supervisor gives the employees the freedom to make their own decisions on how the job is to be done, after he or she has set the goals and standards to be achieved. This also gives employees the freedom to use their own ingenuity and judgment; experiences of this type offer continuous room for further training and improvement. In addition, general supervision motivates employees to the extent that they find satisfaction in their jobs. All indications are that general supervision produces better results than close supervision.

The general supervision environment provides an appropriate setting for teams to function. Team members influence themselves to achieve the organization's objectives. Teams can be long term or short term in nature. Long-term teams (such as self-directed work teams) are part of the formal organizational structure. Short-term teams often work on quality or process issues and as such require a cross-functional representation. These teams may be called quality improvement teams, do-it groups, quality circles, or any title that encourages a teamwork attitude. Teams have advantages such as reducing cost for additional layers of management, improving processes that result in cost-effective and efficient ways of delivering services or products, and improving morale. They also have disadvantages in that team discontent can result in production delays, damaged morale, and conflicts with management. Clear communication of the team's purpose and its authority is necessary to guard against these disadvantages.

Because the healthcare field is dynamic, necessitating constant and often substantial changes, the supervisor is confronted with the problem of how to introduce change. To cope successfully with average employees' normal resistance to change, the supervisor must realize that there are valid social, psychological, and possibly economic reasons for this resistance. By involving employees in change discussions and decisions, much of the resistance can be overcome. The supervisor is in the front line, and it is his or her responsibility to accommodate change and make it reality.

NOTES

1. Think Exist.com. Viewed 2/21/06 at
   http://en.thinkexist.com/quotes/william_drayton/.

2. Bradley, Darlene. "Nursing Leadership In Practice." 6/14/2005 California Emergency Nurses Association. Viewed on the internet at http://www.enw.org/CAL-ENA-LeadershipInPracticeCommittee.htm on 2/21/06.

REFERENCES

Grattan, M. 1999. "Becoming Comfortable with. . . . Uncomfortable," *Office Hours* (May): 1.

LeTourneau, B. 2004 "Communicate for Change." *Journal of Healthcare Management* 49 (6): 354–57.

Munson, R. 1992. *Intervention and Reflection: Basic Issues in Medical Ethics, Fourth Edition,* 2. Belmont, CA: Wadsworth Publishing Company.

Neuborne, E. 1997. "Companies Save, But Workers Pay." *USA Today,* February 25, p. 2B.

Pritchett, P. 1996. *Resistance,* 1. Dallas, TX: Pritchett & Associates, Inc.

Exhibit 22.1: Code of Ethics

Guide to Ethical Behavior for the Staff of Anytown Hospital

This guide for acceptable conduct was developed to give all employees, physicians, suppliers, lenders, customers and prospective customers, and the members of Anytown's general public an understanding of how Anytown Hospital's staff is expected to conduct the operations of this hospital and its affiliated services. For purposes of these guidelines, the use of Anytown Hospital means the hospital, its clinics, home health center, rehabilitation center, ambulatory surgery center, and physician practices.

All members of the Anytown Hospital staff (employee, board, auxiliary, medical, and volunteer staffs) are expected to carry out their activities responsibly; comply with all state, federal, and local rules and accrediting agency regulations; avoid any behavior that could reasonably appear to be improper or that could injure their own or Anytown Hospital's reputation for honesty and integrity in all its activities; and follow the policies listed below.

Failure by staff members to comply with these ethics guidelines; other codes provided upon employment, appointment or reappointment, or election; and acceptable standards of business conduct set forth by the hospital places it in a position of risk. When appropriate, the violator could be subject to disciplinary procedures, up to and including termination of the relationship the individual has with Anytown Hospital.

Alleged violation of or related dilemmas arising from these guidelines shall be referred to one or more of the following bodies for further action:

- Ethical issues related to patients or patient care shall be referred to the Bio-Ethics Committee;
- Ethical issues related to physicians or medical staff services are referred to the Executive Committee; and
- Ethical issues related to employees, suppliers, or any other not otherwise specified group or entity shall be referred to the Human Resources Director, unless Human Resources is at issue, then the referral shall be to the Administrator.

Employee Conflict of Interest

Employees should refer to the Compliance Manual and the Code of Conduct received upon employment. One should have no personal, business, or financial interest that could compromise the objectivity, responsibility, and loyalty owed to Anytown Hospital. It is not possible to identify every activity that might cause a conflict of interest or an appearance of such conflict. Following are some examples of practices and circumstances in which conflicts might occur:

Dealing with Suppliers and Customers: Our goal must always be to obtain goods and services and promote Anytown Hospital services on terms most favorable to the hospital when buying and selling. Neither you nor any of your immediate family members should (1) have or acquire by gift, inheritance, or other means, any interest in a supplier, customer, or its business (other than owning a small—five percent or less—percentage of the stock of a publicly held corporation); or (2) perform services for such a firm, unless properly disclosed. You should disclose any such holding or relationship to your immediate supervisor, department director, clinical service chief, or administrator, as such a relationship could appear to have the potential for biasing your judgment or activities.

Dealing with Competitors: You must disclose to your immediate supervisor, department director, clinical service chief, or administrator if you or any of your immediate family members: (1) receive by gift, inheritance, or otherwise, an interest in a competitor or its business; or (2) are performing services for a competitor of Anytown Hospital other than serving as a member of the medical staff of a competitor hospital.

Compensation, etc., from Others: You or any of your immediate family members should not accept compensation or entertainment having more than nominal value, commissions, property or anything else of personal financial advantage from any outside parties in connection with any transactions involving the hospital. This does not apply to personal loans from a recognized financial institution made in the ordinary course of business on usual and customary terms. At no time shall staff accept cash or gifts of more than nominal value from patients or their families.

Giving or Receiving Gifts: No gift (regardless of value) or other thing of value shall be given to or received from a supplier, lender, or customer representative with the intent to corrupt or bias that person's or the employee's conduct.

Political Payments: No funds or assets of Anytown Hospital shall be used for, or in aid of, any candidate or nominee for local, state, or federal political office in the United States or for, or in aid of, any political parties or committees in connection therewith unless allowed by law and authorized by the Administrator of Anytown Hospital. These prohibitions cover direct contributions and indirect assistance such as the furnishing of goods, services, or equipment to candidates, political parties, or committees.

Accounting Systems: Books and Records

Anytown Hospital policy requires that its books and records shall accurately reflect transactions and disposition of assets. Books and records will be kept in accordance with Generally Accepted Accounting Principles (GAAP) in the United States. No false, artificial, or misleading statements or entries shall be made in Anytown Hospital's books or records including, but not limited to, time reports, accounts, and financial statements. No unrecorded "slush" funds or secret assets of any kind shall be maintained for any purpose whatsoever. Staff is expected to follow the hospital financial and information management policies regarding retaining documentation in their area of responsibility.

Patient Billings and Records: All initial patient billings shall be itemized. Patients are entitled to receive an itemized bill upon request. Patients are also permitted to receive a copy of their record in accordance with the Health Information Management Department policies and procedures.

At least annually, Patient Financial Services and Health Information Management will have an external agent audit a sample of accounts to ensure proper billing and coding practices have been followed and that adequate documentation exists to justify the billings.

From time to time, Administration will evaluate its charges against the prevailing charges in the region to ensure its charges are consistent with others providing similar services.

CHAPTER TWENTY-THREE

Leadership

CHAPTER OBJECTIVES

After you have studied this chapter, you should be able to do the following:

1. Define the concept of leadership.
2. Discuss the major leadership theories.
3. Compare and contrast different leadership styles.

BECAUSE LEADERS CAN have a substantial impact on performance, leadership is one of the most popular and important topics in the field of management. It is a key process in any organization, and an organization's success or failure is largely attributed to it. *Leadership* is an essential component of the organizational climate; the term leadership has been mentioned repeatedly throughout this book, but merely in passing to this point. Ultimately, management leadership is responsible for establishing the type of climate that facilitates motivation and the successful performance of the institution.

The concept of leadership is of great importance because every organization is concerned with attracting and developing people who will be effective leaders. Leadership plays an important role in organizational life. It serves many areas not covered by organizational design or manuals by providing greater organizational flexibility, facilitating coordination and personal needs satisfaction, and ultimately making the difference between an effective and an ineffective organization.

Leadership can be defined as a process by which people are imaginatively directed, guided, and influenced in choosing and attaining goals. It is helpful to look at leadership in an organizational setting as a behavior, as something one person does to influence others (Steers 1988). Kouzes and Posner (1987) define leadership as a shared responsibility and state the difference as "managers . . . get other people to do, but leaders get other people to *want* to do." For the purposes of this book, *leadership* is the process by which one person influences others to do something voluntarily rather than out of fear or as a result of coercion. This voluntary aspect is different from other processes such as influence by authority or power.

In any organized activity a leader mediates between organizational and individual goals so that the degree of satisfaction of both is maximized. A manager also plays this mediating role, but not necessarily in the same manner as a leader. Although the terms manager and leader are often used interchangeably, they are not synonymous. A person who has formal positional authority may use formal legitimate authority and power to get things done; this individual certainly is a manager but may not be the leader. On the other hand, the individual who has no position of formal authority, such as the informal leader, may use the leadership influence but is not the manager. Therefore, a manager can do a reasonably good job of managing without being a leader. From the view of organizational effectiveness, however, it is desirable for the manager to also be the leader. Thus, it is essential to learn what other qualities and prerequisites must be evident to be a leader as well as a manager. Many theories have been formulated as to what constitutes a good leader and what enables some people to be a leader and not others.

The Early Genetic Theory

For hundreds of years observers recognized leadership as the ability to influence people in such a manner that they willingly strove toward an objective. It was believed that this ability was something apart from official position. This view held that certain people were born to be leaders, having inherited a set of unique traits, characteristics, or attributes that could not be acquired in any other way. This position, also known as the "great man" theory of leadership, concluded that leadership qualities were inherited simply because the leadership phenomenon emerged frequently within the same prominent families. In reality, however, strong class barriers made it impossible for anyone outside these families to acquire the skills and knowledge required to become a leader. In the beginning of the twentieth century, this belief in inherited leadership characteristics lost ground, although the belief in the significance of leadership attributes remained a factor.

The Trait, or Attribute, Theory

In the 1920s and 1930s, as social and economic class barriers were broken down and leaders began to emerge from the so-called lower classes of society, the early genetic theory was modified. This modification primarily occurred because in the first half of the twentieth century behavioral scientists began to contribute to the literature on leadership. Rather than considering leadership only as a function of inherited characteristics, they held that it could also be acquired through experience, education, and training. Efforts were made to identify all the traits, whether inherited or acquired, that were found in individuals regarded as leaders. These traits frequently included physical and nervous energy, above-average height, a sense of purpose and direction, willingness to accept the consequences of their actions, enthusiasm, friendliness and affection, integrity, technical mastery, decisiveness, verbal fluency, assertiveness, initiative, originality, intelligence, teaching skill, faith, ambition, and persistence.

The inadequacy of this approach soon became obvious. No satisfactory answer could be reached about which traits were most essential for leadership or whether a person could be a leader if certain traits were lacking. Also, how to isolate and identify all the specific traits common to leaders was not clear. A further weakness of the trait approach was that it did not distinguish between those characteristics needed for acquiring leadership and those necessary for maintaining it.

Although the trait approach is partially discredited today, a considerable body of research shows that leaders have in common certain general characteristics. Some of these are intelligence, communication ability, and sensitivity to group needs. Such traits are interwoven in the personality of the leader. These studies led researchers to question the validity of the trait approach as the predictor of leadership. Subsequent research determined that leadership style varies based on the managerial situation being confronted, the types of employees or skill levels they may have, or both.

The Contingency Approach

In their search for other variables, behavioral scientists discovered the importance of situational factors that make it easier for certain persons to acquire positions of leadership. This theory assumes that leadership behavior varies in accordance with the situation (Fiedler 1967; Vroom and Yetton 1973). This approach, also known as the contingency model of leadership effectiveness, points out the interdependence between leadership style and the demands of the situation. Consider the role that Lee Iacocca played when he took over the dying Chrysler Corporation in the late 1970s. Chrysler turned to him in its time of need, and he brought a "broad, popular, and galvanizing vision" to the table that changed Chrysler's future (Peters 2001).

Proponents of the situational approach do not deny that the characteristics of individuals play an important part in leadership, but they point out that leadership is also the product of situational factors. Fred Fiedler (1967) studied these relationships for nearly 40 years. His contingency theory states that there is no best way for managers to lead. Leadership in one group differs from leadership in another group; in one situation a certain person might evolve as the leader, whereas under different environmental conditions someone else would emerge as the leader. For example, in a political meeting someone with good public speaking ability may rise to the top. In other words, the leadership characteristics and behavior needed are a function of the specific situation.

In their desire to deemphasize the traits approach, however, some behavioral scientists may have ruled out the possibility that at least some characteristics predispose people to attain leadership positions or at least increase their chances of becoming leaders. Both characteristics and the situation are involved in the concept of leadership.

The Follower Factor

A still better understanding of leadership incorporates the input contributed by groups and followers. This theory maintains that the followers and the makeup of the group must also be studied because essentially it is the follower who perceives the leader and the situation and accepts or rejects leadership. Proponents of this approach further maintain that followers' persistent motives, points of view, and frames of reference determine what they perceive and how they react to it. The follower approach emphasizes the importance of the group at a particular point, but it also acknowledges that certain characteristics help one person emerge as the leader over another person. Satisfaction of the followers' needs then is an important aspect.

More specifically, the follower factor stresses the idea that the leadership function must be analyzed and understood in terms of a dynamic relationship, a social-exchange process between the leader and the followers. They bring to the situation their personalities, needs, motivations, and expectations. The leader appears to the followers as the best means available for the satisfaction of their needs, whether those needs are emotive or task oriented. A leader is essential for influencing a group to act as a unit to move toward task accomplishment. The members look at this individual as their leader not only because he or she possesses certain characteristics, such as intelligence, skill, drive, and ambition, but also because of his or her functional relationship to the members of the group.

LEADERSHIP ROLES

Most of us have had occasion to observe individuals and the different roles they play in groups. One person may organize the group to achieve goals, whereas another plays the "devil's advocate," raising a stream of objections, and yet someone else is a "synthesizer," who puts together the ideas of all group members. These roles and many others are essential for group life. They fulfill the needs of the individual members of the group and are vital to the group's accomplishments. The group's leader is not necessarily expected to assume all these roles, but he or she is expected to fulfill some of them. Generally, leadership roles fall into two broad classifications, task-oriented roles and emotive leadership roles, geared toward satisfying each of these types of needs.

Task-oriented roles are those used by the leader to organize and influence the group to achieve specified objectives. Usually in an organized activity these objectives are imposed on the group from above. In groups that arise spontaneously, however, tasks and objectives are generated from within the group itself. In both instances, the leader must facilitate the accomplishment of the group's goals; that is, the leader plays the role of getting the group to fulfill its tasks.

Emotive leadership roles are just as important as task roles. In this approach, the leader takes on some of the traits exhibited by the character of George Bailey in "It's a Wonderful Life," in which he lives by a motto of treating customers and employees with generosity and consideration with the result that good deeds always came back to you. Emotive leadership roles are employee centered and provide satisfaction for the individual needs of the group's members. The emotional needs of people are of a social and psychological nature. A leader in the emotive role helps members of the group to gain satisfaction of these needs and at the same time prepares the way for task performance.

Frequently the ideal leader is one who plays both roles effectively. In some instances, however, leadership of a group can be shared without diminishing the group's performance or morale. In such a case one person plays the task role and another takes the emotive role. This is not an unusual situation in a large healthcare institution. The formal organization of such an institution often forces a supervisor to be primarily concerned with getting the job done. He or she must concentrate largely on task leadership. Under these conditions, the groups probably select another individual, the informal leader, who can function in the emotive role. The supervisor should not object to the informal leader's role. Rather, the supervisor should realize that it is a necessary part of the leadership process, one that fulfills important human needs and is an essential component of high employee morale.

Schein (1996) describes paradoxes of leadership when stating that leaders of the future will be persons "who can lead and follow, be central and marginal, be hierarchically above and below, be individualistic and a team player, and, above all, be a perpetual learner." Deming (1994) says the primary responsibility of leaders is to manage the transformation of the organization. Another leadership role is to ensure that the organization works effectively with respect to the interactions between individuals, groups, and business units both within and outside the organization and that behaviors meet accepted standards for business ethics. Finally, Warren Bennis (1994) defines the difference between managers and leaders as doing the right thing (leadership = effectiveness) versus doing things right (management = efficiency).

LEADERSHIP STYLE

Leadership style is of great importance because it influences acceptance of managers by subordinates. According to Peters (2001), "The best leader is rarely the best pitcher or catcher. The best leader is just what's advertised: the best leader. Leaders get their kicks from orchestrating the work of others—not from doing it themselves." As introduced in Chapter 22, leadership styles can generally be classified into broad categories such as autocratic and democratic.

Autocratic Leadership (Theory X)

Autocratic leadership usually reflects tight supervision with a high degree of centralization and a narrow span of management. The autocratic style is repressive, and this type of supervisor normally withholds communication except that which is absolutely necessary for doing the job. Autocratic management leaders make decisions unilaterally and do not consult with the members of the department. Therefore, the autocratic style of leadership minimizes the degree of involvement by subordinates.

In more specific terms, autocratic leadership is described by Douglas McGregor (1985) as *Theory X*. According to McGregor, a Theory X manager leans toward an organizational climate of close control, centralized authority, authoritarian practices, and minimum participation of the subordinates in the decision-making process. One may consider this the "big stick" approach. A Theory X manager makes certain assumptions about human behavior, including the following:

1. The average person dislikes work and will avoid it to the extent he or she can.
2. Most people have to be forced or threatened by punishment to make the effort necessary to accomplish organizational goals.
3. The average individual is basically passive and therefore prefers to be directed rather than take any risk or responsibility. Above all else, he or she prefers security.

Democratic Leadership (Theory Y)

The democratic style emphasizes a looser type of supervision and greater individual participation in the decision-making process. Authority is delegated as far down as possible, and a wide span of management is advocated. A free flow of communication is encouraged among all members of the department so that a climate of trust and confidence can be established.

In McGregor's terms, the democratic style is represented by *Theory Y*. The Theory Y manager operates with a completely different set of assumptions regarding human motivation. He or she maintains that an effective organizational climate uses more general supervision, greater decentralization of authority, democratic techniques, consultation with subordinates on departmental decisions, and little reliance on coercion and control. The assumptions on which this type of organizational climate is based include the following:

1. Work is as natural to people as play or rest, and therefore it is not avoided.
2. Self-motivation and inherent satisfaction in work will be forthcoming when the individual is committed to organizational goals; thus, coercion is not the only form of influence that can be used to motivate.

3. Commitment is a crucial factor in motivation, and it is a function of the rewards coming from it.
4. The average individual learns to accept and even seek responsibility given the proper environment.
5. The ability to be creative and innovative in the solution of organizational problems is widely, not narrowly, distributed in the population.
6. In modern businesses and organizations, the intellectual potential of employees is only partially utilized.

McGregor underscores the notion that theories X and Y are beliefs held by management about the nature of human beings. As such, they constitute the foundation on which the organizational climate is built. The supervisor who follows Theory X has a basically limited view of people and their capabilities. He or she believes that individuals must be controlled; closely supervised; and motivated by money, discipline, and authority. Thus, the autocratic manager believes that the key to motivation is in the proper implementation of approaches designed to satisfy the lower-level needs of people.

The Theory Y supervisor, however, has a much different opinion of the capabilities and potential of people. He or she believes that if the proper approach and conditions can be presented, people exercise self-direction and self-control toward the accomplishment of objectives. The Theory Y manager recognizes that the supervisor's activities must fit into the scheme of each employee's own set of needs. He or she also believes that the higher-level needs of people are more important in terms of personality and self-development. Bill Bradley (2005), retired U.S. senator from New Jersey and former professional basketball player, once said, "The business of leaders, of heroes, is tricky. Leadership is not something that is done to people, like fixing your teeth. Leadership is unlocking people's potential to become better." Thus, the supervisory skills are used to enable employees to achieve at least partial satisfaction of their needs for esteem and self-actualization on the job.

Theory Z Approach

A different managerial approach that is gaining in popularity is William Ouchi's *Theory Z* approach, influenced by practices in Japanese industry, the success of which has been attributed to a managerial philosophy about people and organizations that is different from that generally accepted in the United States (Ouchi and Jaeger 1978; Ouchi 1981). The Japanese organizational climate is based on lifetime employment, slow evaluation and promotion paths, nonspecialized careers, consensual decision making, collective responsibility, informal controls, and a holistic concern toward the firm. From this basis, Ouchi's Theory Z makes certain assumptions about workers, including the notion that workers tend to want to build cooperative and intimate working relationships with those that they work for and with as well as the people who work for them (Flinn 2001). In brief, this approach fosters a trust relationship between workers and supervisors that results in high-quality output because fear of reprisal is absent and emphasis on teamwork dominates the workplace. This is contrary to many current practices in the United States, such as short-run employment expectations, rapid evaluation and promotions, specialized careers, individual decision making and responsibility, severe disciplinary actions for errors, and explicit controls. Although some of the characteristics of this theory are being phased out in Japan, Theory Z is an approach that U.S. managers could use to increase productivity and job satisfaction.

Quality circles and total quality management, discussed in Chapter 16, are an outgrowth of the Japanese approach to management. Ironically, much of the Japanese management approach was taught to them by Americans W. Edwards Deming and Joseph M. Juran after World War II (Walton 1986). Today more healthcare CEOs are pursuing the Theory Z environment in their organizations, and those individuals exhibiting the related leadership traits are being sought.

Free-Rein Leadership

The free-rein style goes beyond Theories Y and Z. It is often called *laissez-faire leadership* because the climate of the organization is such that people are left almost entirely alone to do their jobs. On the assumption that individuals are self-motivated, a minimum amount of supervision is imposed. Although the manager is available as a consultant to help out if necessary, the individuals have enough authority to devise their own solutions. Sometimes this approach is used in self-directed team settings in which an entire department is managed by self-directed teams that receive periodic guidance or direction from an administrator in the healthcare facility whose office is outside the department.

Making a Choice

Tom Peters, contemporary management theorist and author of *In Search of Excellence*, says that we should "think of pre-1990 as the Age of Sucking Up to the Hierarchy," while the "Age of the Promise 'Em Everything Pitch lasted from 1995 to 2000." He states further that the years 2001 through 2006 are the "Age of No-Bull Performance, which means that we're going to see leadership emerge as the most important element of business—the attribute that is highest in demand and shortest in supply." More than ever, leaders are expected to achieve results through people. Obviously, no single leadership style is appropriate for all situations. A leader must be able to call on a whole range of responses. A good manager knows when to use one or another style of leadership to "involve the right people, at the right place and at the right time" (Peters 2001).

Each of these four styles has a place in the practice of management. The free-rein approach is probably the most useful in an organization of professional people who desire and have shown the capacity for independent work. This would apply, for example, to research scientists and professors. The democratic style seems to be appropriate when a relatively unfettered environment is necessary, under which skilled and educated people seem to thrive. This probably includes most activities performed in any healthcare center. It is wrong to state, however, that a democratic leadership style is beneficial for all organizations, regardless of the nature of their activities and skill levels of their employees. In some situations even the autocratic leadership style produces good results, especially among unskilled subordinates who are poorly prepared to participate in decision making and who might be uncomfortable if urged to do so.

In conclusion, leadership style must be adapted to each specific situation. In general a more democratic, open style seems to achieve greater leader acceptance than an autocratic one. Such a style is more humanistic and more optimistic, which also makes it more acceptable to most employees. In addition, much of the research evidence indicates that the Theory Y democratic leadership approach is more likely to achieve better results.

Nevertheless, it is a sign of a good manager and a good leader to be able to use any one of these four techniques or a mixture of one or more whenever the need or occasion arises. Employing the appropriate style largely determines the degree to which the leader can influence others in the performance of a task and with the situation at hand. This is what leading is all about.

SUMMARY

Leadership is a process by which one person tries to influence others in the performance of a common task. Through leadership, subordinates are imaginatively directed, guided, and influenced in choosing and attaining goals. One cannot equate the terms leadership and management; a person does not have to be a leader to be an adequate manager, but it would be far more desirable if the supervisor of the department were also the leader.

Much research has been done on the leadership phenomenon. The early genetic theory maintained that leadership was a function of specific characteristics with which a leader was born. Later the genetic approach was altered to state that leadership was a function of numerous personal traits that could be acquired as well as inherited. More recent studies point out that the situation has significant bearing on who emerges as a leader. Furthermore, the follower factor adds to the concept of leadership the importance of the followers' perception and the group that they constitute. Many variables play a role in the leadership process. The leader is an individual perceived to be in harmony with the needs of the group and responsive to the group situation. However, because leaders must always be recognized as such by group consensus and because managers who are appointed do not necessarily reflect subordinate group choice, they are not generally regarded as leaders at the outset. They may become true leaders of the group, but they do not start out as such. It is desirable from an influencing standpoint that subordinates accept the manager as a leader and not merely as the head of the department. Thus, each manager must adopt a leadership style that facilitates such acceptance.

Four broad categories of leadership style exist: autocratic (Theory X), democratic (Theory Y), quality-trust (Theory Z), and free rein. Managers use these styles in their efforts to emerge as leaders. A manager who is appointed to a position of organizational authority is not generally perceived as a leader at the outset. It is hoped, however, that this person will emerge as a leader of the subordinates, thus becoming a much more effective manager as well.

In the leadership process, it is necessary to fulfill both the task role (influencing the group to achieve its goals) and the emotive role (satisfying the emotional needs of group members). If it is impossible for the leader to fulfill the emotive role, however, one should not object if an informal leader is chosen by the group to substitute for the leader in this role.

Although much about leadership remains to be studied, the research into this concept has given us a better understanding of the types of behavior needed in different settings and the importance of leadership for organizational effectiveness.

REFERENCES

Bennis, Warren. 1989. *On Becoming a Leader*, 40. Reading, MA: Addison-Wesley.

Bradley, B. 2005. Quote. [Online information; 02/21/06] http://www.insightquotes.com/l.html.

Deming, W. E. 1994. *The New Economics*, 116. Cambridge, MA: Massachusetts Institute of Technology.

Fiedler, F. E. 1967. *A Theory of Leadership Effectiveness*. New York: McGraw-Hill Book Co.

Flinn, W. P. 2001. "The Theory XY&Z of Management Theory." [Online article; retrieved 2/9/01.] http://fsosvr.arizona.edu/dickportfolio/dissertation/ToFile/xyz.htm.

Kouzes, J. M., and B. Z. Posner. 1987. *The Leadership Challenge*, 27, 135. San Francisco: Jossey-Bass.

McGregor, D. 1985. *The Human Side of Enterprise*, chapters 3 and 4. New York: McGraw-Hill Book Co.

Ouchi, W. G. 1981. *Theory Z: How American Business Can Meet the Japanese Challenge*. Reading, MA: Addison-Wesley Publishing Co.

Ouchi, W. G., and A. M. Jaeger. 1978. "Type Z Organization: Stability in the Midst of Mobility." *Academy of Management Review* (April): 305–14.

Peters, T. 2001. "Rule #3: Leadership is Confusing as Hell." [Online article; retrieved 3/1/05.] http://www.fastcompany.com/online/44/rules.html.

Schein, E. H. (1996). "Leadership and Organizational Culture." In *The Leader of the Future,* edited by F. Hesselbein, M. Goldsmith, and R. Beckhard, 69. San Francisco, CA: Jossey-Bass.

Steers, R. M. 1988. *Introduction to Organizational Behavior, Third Edition,* 460–86. Glenview, IL: Scott, Foresman & Co.

Vroom, V. H., and P. W. Yetton. 1973. *Leadership and Decision Making.* Pittsburgh, PA: University of Pittsburgh Press.

Walton, M. 1986. *The Deming Management Method.* New York: The Putnam Publishing Group.

CHAPTER TWENTY-FOUR

Motivation

CHAPTER OBJECTIVES

After you have studied this chapter, you should be able to do the following:

1. Outline the major theories of motivation.

2. Describe the motivational processes.

3. Define perceptions, values, attitudes, and the factors that affect each of these.

4. Discuss the supervisor's duty in minimizing frustration and conflict.

MOTIVATING EMPLOYEES IS important to managers because it affects performance. Motivation is closely related to the crucial managerial function of influencing because it deals most intimately with the individual. Thus, we must understand what motivates a person and, more basically, what underlies a person's motivations.

Motivation is the process affecting the inner needs or drives that arouse, move, energize, direct, channel, and sustain human behavior. Generally, the motivational process begins the drive that impels individuals to work toward certain goals they believe will satisfy their inner needs. Once these goals are attained, we judge whether these efforts were worthwhile. If deemed worthwhile, the result is reinforcement, and we continue to pursue these and other needs and drives. Understanding motivation will enable managers to help their employees achieve higher levels of job satisfaction and job performance.

THEORIES OF MOTIVATION

Managers have long been aware of the importance of motivation. It has been a major concern for managers and psychologists, and many theories have attempted to explain how people are motivated. There are several ways to interpret the concept of motivation; two of the major categories of contemporary motivational theories are the content theory and the process theory.

Content theory focuses on the question of what factor or set of factors moves, energizes, and starts the behavior of an individual. This theory discusses the concept of needs or motives that drive people and the incentives that cause people to behave in a particular manner. Some authors call this school of theory *need theory*. A need is anything that is required, desired, or considered useful to obtain an item, feeling, or status. We do not discuss all of the motivational theories in this chapter, but we touch on several in both the content and process arenas. Four of the most publicized content theories of motivation are (1) Maslow's hierarchy of needs; (2) Alderfer's ERG; (3) Herzberg's two-factor approach of satisfiers and dissatisfiers; and (4) McClelland's needs for achievement, affiliation, and power. Each of these four content theories tries to explain individual behavior from a slightly different perspective.

On the other hand, *process theory* examines how and why people choose a particular behavior to accomplish a goal and how they evaluate their satisfaction after reaching the goal. Equity and expectancy are the two major process perspectives on motivation. The first approach stresses the equity of effort in relation to the results; that is, there should be a balance in the amount of effort one must put forth for the resulting rewards—compensation, benefits, and so forth. The other approach emphasizes that one will put forth a certain level of effort if he or she expects to receive some reward, promotion, or recognition. If there is inequity or imbalance, staff will not be motivated. We discuss two process theorists: Victor Vroom (expectancy model) and B. F. Skinner (reinforcement model).

MODEL OF MOTIVATIONAL PROCESSES

Although the complete set of processes is very complex, a generalized model of basic motivational processes is presented in Figure 24.1. This model shows five basic parts of the process: (1) needs or desires; (2) expectations, perceptions, motives, values, and attitudes; (3) tactical behavior action plan; (4) goal; and (5) results or feedback. At any point, individuals are likely to have a mixture of needs, desires, and expectations. For instance, one subordinate may have a strong need to achieve and a desire to earn more money; this person expects that doing the job well will lead to the desired rewards. This expectation is likely to cause behavior that is directed toward specific goals. Achieving the goals serves as feedback on the impact of this behavior and reassures this individual that the behavior is correct to satisfy the needs and expectations. On the other hand, if the action plan fails, it may tell the person that the present course of action is incorrect and should be altered.

This model of motivation is oversimplified because it does not take into account all influences on motivation; however, it shows the basic cyclical nature of the process. People strive to satisfy a variety of needs and expectations, and the success of one effort triggers the pursuit of another need and desire. Once a need has been met, another need or desire emerges and stimulates further action.

FIGURE 24.1: MODEL OF THE MOTIVATIONAL PROCESS

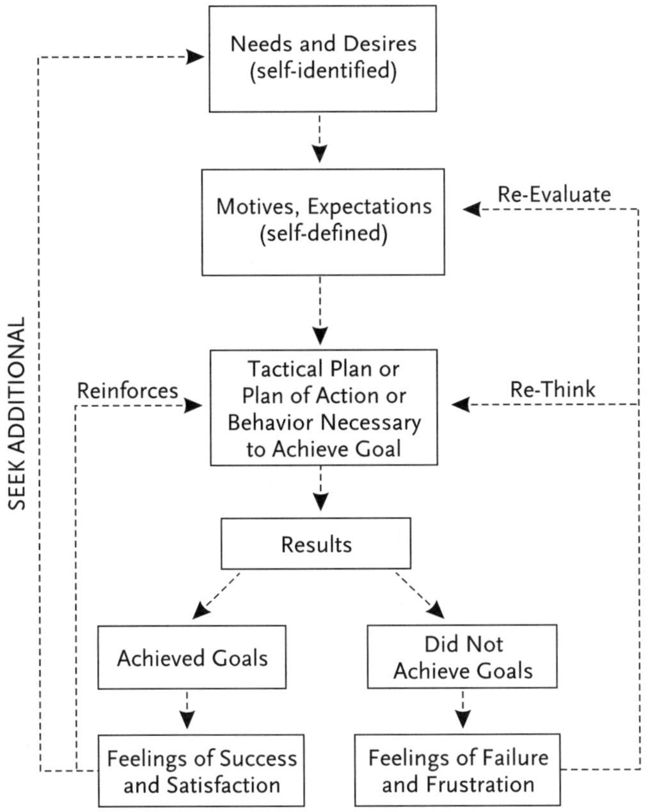

Maslow's Hierarchy of Human Needs (1954)

One approach to employee motivation is based on individual human needs. Every action is motivated by unsatisfied needs. These unsatisfied needs cause human beings to behave in a certain manner and to try to achieve certain goals in hopes of reducing the tensions that arise from unmet needs. A person eats because hunger creates the need for food. Someone else has a strong need to achieve and strives to advance in his or her field of work. In other words, there is a reason for everything that people do.

People are always striving to attain something that has meaning to them in terms of their own particular needs. It is often observed that human beings never seem satisfied; we are continuously fulfilling needs. After the successful fulfillment of one need, we start on another round of pursuits. Indeed, we can say that life is a process in which needs constantly arise and demand satisfaction.

Probably the most widely known and accepted theory of needs and motivation is the model designed by Abraham H. Maslow consisting of deficiency needs and growth needs. Deficiency needs must be satisfied if the individual is to be healthy and secure. They are the physiological needs for food, water, clothing, and shelter; needs for safety; and the feelings of belonging, love, and respect from others. Growth needs refer to development and achievement of one's potential. All needs, however, are not of the same order of importance. Many different kinds of needs exist, and some produce stronger motivation or demand more immediate satisfaction than others. Maslow suggests that these needs are arranged in a hierarchy (Huitt 1998) (see Figure 24.2).

Maslow's model contains five levels of needs that can be visualized as forming a pyramid. The most basic needs are physiological needs. Normally, in organizational settings, adequate wages and the work environment itself enable an individual to obtain the necessities and comforts of life that are vital to fulfilling these physiological needs.

When the physiological needs are reasonably satisfied, needs at the next higher level begin to dominate. These are usually called safety needs, such as safe physical and emotional environments. They are the needs we have for protection against danger and threat. Such needs are natural reactions to insecurity. We all desire more control over and protection from the uncertainties of life. In a work environment, these uncertainties would produce security needs caused by, for example, an unstable economic climate (recession), fear of arbitrary management action (e.g., decision to close a clinic), loss of job, favoritism, discrimination, or unpredictable administration of policy. Most enterprises today offer various programs designed to satisfy and fulfill these safety or security needs. For example, most enterprises have grievance systems, adequate medical and other insurance plans, provisions for retirement benefits, provisions for unemployment compensation, and seniority benefits. Especially during times of economic instability, this need tends to dominate employees' concerns. Therefore, the manager must attempt to respond to security needs when they arise.

Once the physiological and safety needs are satisfied, social and belongingness needs become important motivators. Social needs consist of belonging, association, acceptance by one's peers, and giving and receiving friendship and love. These needs are often identical to the needs people have for a feeling of group identity—that is, being part of a group or team and being accepted and respected by their peers. A supervisor must be aware of the existence of these needs, which can be fulfilled in organizational settings by informal groups. As we know, tightly knit, cohesive work groups generally enable employees to gain greater on-the-job satisfaction and produce a better climate for motivation. This is why the supervisor should look at the positive aspects and strengths of informal groups. Often supervisors go to great trouble to control and interfere with the natural grouping tendency of human beings. This is ill-advised. When a person's social needs are thwarted and frustrated, this individual will behave in ways that are likely to hurt organizational objectives. The manager should

FIGURE 24.2: MASLOW'S HIERARCHY OF NEEDS

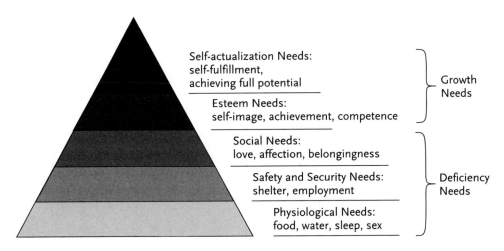

Maslow, Abraham; Frager, Robert (editor), Fadman, James (editor), *Motivation and Personality*, 3rd edition, © 1987. Adapted by permission of Pearson Education, Inc., Upper Saddle River, NJ.

always realize that social needs are fulfilled largely by informal groups and informal organization, as discussed in Chapter 18.

Once the first three needs, also known as deficiency needs, have been satisfied, people generally attempt to satisfy growth needs. These are the needs for esteem and self-actualization. Esteem needs focus on one's desire to have a worthy self-image and receive recognition from others. Self-esteem includes the need for self-confidence, a positive self-image, self-respect, independence, achievement, competence, and knowledge. These needs are often fulfilled by mastery over part of the environment—for example, by knowing that you can accomplish a certain task.

However, a person also needs the esteem and recognition of others for his or her accomplishments. These needs relate to reputation, status, recognition, appreciation, and the deserved respect of colleagues. Many jobs in industrial settings offer little opportunity for satisfaction of such needs. However, many positions in the healthcare field are much more conducive to achieving these needs because of their challenging nature. The manager can satisfy those needs by providing external symbols of esteem such as appropriate titles and offices. Of course, it is desirable that both aspects of the need for esteem are fulfilled. Frequently, however, the esteem of self comes before esteem from others.

The highest level of needs is the need for self-actualization, self-fulfillment, or self-realization. These are the needs for realizing one's own potential, for continued self-development, and for being creative in the broadest sense of the term. It has often been said that this is the need to become what one is capable of becoming. Unlike the other four needs, which probably are satisfied, self-actualization is seldom fully achieved. It is a process of becoming, and as one gradually approaches self-fulfillment, this process is intensified and sustained. Because this need can be met only from within, there is little the manager can do to facilitate the achievement of this need except to provide an organizational climate conducive to self-actualization. The focus of contemporary American lifestyles leaves little time to fulfill this need. Most employees are continuously struggling to satisfy the lower needs and must divert most of their energy to satisfy them. Therefore, the need for self-fulfillment frequently remains unfulfilled.

There seems to be a relationship between the hierarchy of needs and age. Physiological and safety needs are paramount in the life of an infant. As a child grows up, love needs become more important. When the adolescent reaches young adulthood, needs for esteem seem to take precedence. If the person is successful in meeting the lower-level needs in life, the move to self-actualization later in life is likely. Such a step does not necessarily follow because pressing circumstances may arrest the route of progress at the esteem level or at lower levels. Also, as seen in the following discussion, this situation is often the basis of conflict between organizational and individual goals.

Maslow's hierarchy of needs has been and still is popular among managers. Because it is the supervisor's job to create a climate in which employees can satisfy the multitude of needs, this theory makes clear recommendations to management (see Figure 24.3). Some of the specific dynamics of Maslow's theory may still be in question, however, and have been challenged. Nevertheless, Maslow's hierarchy was the first clear theory urging managers to recognize the importance of higher-order needs. It caused a shift from the traditional lower-order motivators to higher motivators. Most healthy and normal employees probably have satisfied the lower-order deficiency needs (they are not hungry, feel reasonably secure, and have sufficient social relationships), but this fact does not negate the possibility of their existence. Consider a dietary worker who is the sole supporter of her extended family, including her husband, three children, one grandchild, and mother. Thefts of food items, such as whole chickens or boxed items, may require management to investigate this employee's lower-order needs.

Supervisors also must emphasize a working climate conducive to satisfying the higher-order growth needs. This means supervisors should stress some variety of duties, delegation of authority, autonomy, and responsibility so that employees can more fully realize their potential and their growth needs. Techniques to empower staff with levels of decision making previously held only by supervisors allow them to satisfy some higher-order needs.

Alderfer's ERG Model (1972)

Content or need theorist Clayton Alderfer did not totally agree with Maslow. He identified three categories of needs—existence, relatedness, and growth (ERG). These needs may surface when frustration occurs. His frustration-regression

FIGURE 24.3: FACTORS AFFECTING JOB SATISFACTION

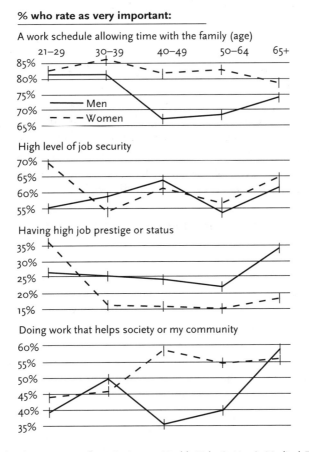

% who rate as very important:

Source: Adapted with permission from *Business & Health*, Vol. 18, No. 8. Medical Economics Co., Montvale, NJ.

hypothesis states that when individuals are frustrated in meeting or achieving higher-need levels, they regress and seek lower-level needs again. Furthermore, more than one level of need can cause motivation simultaneously.

Existence needs are those that are material or psychological desires. These are satisfied by basic support resources such as food, water, shelter, working conditions, and pay. They are items that are divided among people, and one person's gain is another's loss.

Relatedness needs involve relationships. These are satisfied by having friends, family, and coworkers. These friendships allow for sharing feelings and thoughts, being accepted and having one's worth confirmed by others, and understanding.

The last category of need is that of growth. Growth needs encourage a person to be productive or creative. This need is satisfied by one contributing in a problem-solving environment or having opportunities for personal development.

Alderfer's ERG model can be placed on a dimensional plane across Maslow's hierarchical pyramid, revealing a distinction between the degrees of introversion and extroversion. For example, an introvert at the level of relatedness might be more concerned with his or her own perceptions of being included in a group, whereas an extrovert at that same level may pay more attention to how others value that membership (Huitt 1998). More apparent is the correlation between Maslow's and Alderfer's need categories. Maslow's physiological and safety needs tie to Alderfer's existence needs. The social needs described by Maslow compare to Alderfer's relatedness needs. Finally, Maslow's remaining two tiers are consistent with Alderfer's growth needs.

Herzberg's Two-Factor Motivation-Hygiene Theory (1959)

Another approach to the content theory of motivation as a need classification system was developed by Frederick Herzberg. As a psychologist, Herzberg has done much research on job satisfaction and has developed a number of conditions on which satisfaction is based. He distinguishes between those factors at the workplace that are unlikely to motivate employees (hygiene factors) and those that tend to motivate employees (motivators). In essence, he states that the hygiene rewards satisfy what are commonly known as lower-order needs, whereas the motivators satisfy higher-order needs. Herzberg identifies the groups listed in Figure 24.4 as hygiene factors and as motivators.

Herzberg (1966)[1] measures satisfiers and dissatisfiers by how frequently they appear and how long they produce either a significant improvement or reduction in job satisfaction (see Figure 24.5). The five hygiene factors are environmental. When they are at an unacceptable level, they are noticed, and dissatisfaction occurs. When they are at an acceptable level, they are unnoticed, and satisfaction results. The factors most frequently involved in events causing job dissatisfaction (dissatisfiers) are company policy and administration, supervision, interpersonal relations, working conditions, and salary. When these factors are negative or lacking, they are considered to be dissatisfiers. Even when they are positive and appropriate, these factors do not tend to motivate people; they are expected. At this level, they are satisfiers.

This, however, does not mean that the hygiene factors are unimportant. They are essential because whether they exist or not is either satisfying or dissatisfying. Therefore, the manager must make certain that administration and policies are fair and suitable, that pay and benefits are appropriate, that technical supervision is acceptable, that working conditions are safe and healthy, and so forth. By providing these factors at the proper level, the manager does not give the employees the opportunity to feel motivated, but these factors do keep them from being dissatisfied.

FIGURE 24.4: HERZBERG'S TWO-FACTOR MOTIVATION-HYGIENE THEORY

Hygiene Factors	Motivation Factors
The organization's policy and administration	Achievement
Technical supervision	Recognition
Interpersonal relations	The work itself
Working conditions	Responsibility
Salary	Advancement

If managers really want motivated employees, they should use motivators. Herzberg's study indicates that the most frequently mentioned factors in improved job satisfaction are achievement, recognition, the work itself, responsibility, and advancement. These are the factors that, if present, truly motivate people. It is the opportunity for advancement, greater responsibility, and the possibility of promotion, growth, achievement, and interesting work that makes a job challenging, meaningful, and really motivating to subordinates. Watson Wyatt's (2000) survey found that the top three non-monetary rewards for employees under the age of 30 were (1) advancement opportunities (76 percent, up from 60 percent in 1999), (2) flexible work schedules (73 percent, up from 64 percent), and (3) the opportunity to learn new skills (68 percent, up from 62 percent). Interestingly, age and gender define needs that affect job satisfaction (see Figure 24.3). The manager, therefore, should give the employees an opportunity to experience these motivational factors in an environment conducive to growth. Such motivational factors are obviously associated with the higher-order needs of people: they are related to the work content, whereas the hygiene factors relate to the work environment.

Herzberg's findings have important implications for the supervisor. Although management strives for good organizational hygiene through sound wage administration, enlightened supervision, pleasant working conditions, appropriate fringe benefits, and so forth, these factors alone normally do not produce a motivational climate. If properly fulfilled, they merely minimize dissatisfaction. What is actually required to achieve motivation is a two-way effort that is directed first at the hygiene factors and then at the development of motivation. In addition to the need to avoid unpleasantness that comes from largely dissatisfying conditions, the supervisor must produce positive motivation through a more sophisticated set of factors, which is closely related to the concept of self-actualization. Although it is difficult to apply these motivators in some situations, most positions in the healthcare setting provide ample opportunity to stress them. More information on Herzberg's theory appears in Exhibit 24.1.

FIGURE 24.5: FACTORS AFFECTING JOB ATTITUDES

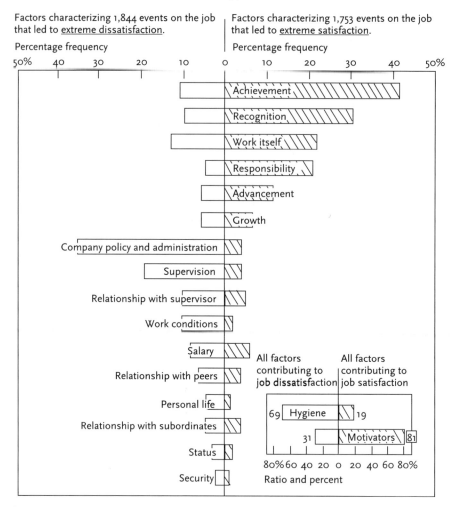

Factors Affecting Job Attitudes*

Factors characterizing 1,844 events on the job that led to <u>extreme dissatisfaction</u>.

Factors characterizing 1,753 events on the job that led to <u>extreme satisfaction</u>.

* As reported in 12 investigations. Figure does not include duration data.
Source: Herzberg (1966). Used with permission.

McClelland's Achievement Theory (1961)

Another approach to the content view of motivation concerns other important needs. David McClelland's (1953) research in organizational behavior led to what he has termed learned needs and is now commonly known as need for achievement (n Ach), need for affiliation (n Aff), and need for power (n Pow).

The need for achievement is a need for personal challenge and accomplishment. It involves the desire to assume personal responsibility and pursue reasonably difficult goals, a preoccupation with the task, and specific and quick feedback as to accomplishment. This *n Ach* is obviously essential for a successful manager; it is critical for development in early childhood and can be used by adults as well. McClelland defines it as behavior toward competition with a standard of excellence.

The need for affiliation is the need for human companionship, support, and reassurance. People with a strong *n Aff* look for approval and reassurance from others, are willing to conform to the norms and wishes of others, and are sincerely interested in the feelings of others. They are likely to do well in situations that include a lot of social interaction. This trait can be distracting and have a negative impact on work performance.

The third need is the need for power, or need for dominance. The *n Pow* is a need to influence others and to lead and control them. Today we call this type of individual a driver. Those with strong *n Pow* are willing to make decisions. One of McClelland's studies concluded all managers tend to have a stronger power motive than the general population and that successful managers tend to have stronger power motives than less successful managers (McClelland and Burnham 1976).

Human behavior is controlled by these three needs. The intensity of desire for each may vary from situation to situation. For example, many of us recognize people who are drivers at work and who suddenly become followers when at home (Figure 24.6).

LEVELS OF ASPIRATION

A person's level of aspiration is closely related to the order of needs. Level of aspiration causes an individual's goals to shift as various needs are satisfied; that is, once the needs on one level are satisfied, the individual tends to aspire to higher levels. For example, suppose an individual is highly motivated by the need to achieve, and attitudes and personality cause this person to look for such satisfaction by working as a laboratory technician in a healthcare center.

This person will not be satisfied for very long by being a phlebotomist. Once the phlebotomist position has been attained, this individual is likely to strive for the next higher position, such as laboratory technician, then laboratory scientist, then laboratory director, and so on. The objectives that present possibilities for the satisfaction of the achievement needs also may shift to something outside the hospital, such as governmental activities, perhaps serving as deputy director of the Centers for Disease Control and Prevention.

This endless search for alternatives to satisfy increasing aspirations is an important aspect of human motivation. If an organization can provide an individual with a wider range of need satisfactions, this person will have a greater commitment to the organization.

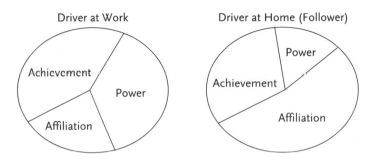

Vroom's Expectancy Model (1964)

Process theorists speculated that motivation was driven by external influences. The theorists Vroom and Skinner assess why and how people choose certain behaviors to meet their needs. Victor Vroom's expectancy model suggests that people tend to act in a particular manner because they anticipate that the behavior will achieve the outcome or goal desired; that is, the amount of effort put forth by a person is directly related to the reward expected and the person's perceived ability to reach the goal. For example, if I pursue this certification program, will I be named the shift supervisor? Expectancy is the belief that if one puts forth effort X, the direct result will be Y. There must be a willingness on the individual's part to exert a high level of effort to reach an objective and satisfy an individual need.

The degree of effort is based on the individual's belief that the probability of achieving the goal will be reached and a reward received. This is the equity consideration each employee gives when doing an assignment. Equity is the perception of fairness in rewards or compensation given. Individuals perceive rewards differently and consequently exert more or less effort to obtain them. If rewards are given out inconsistently, employees may perceive the distribution as inequitable and hold back their contribution of effort. This theory has a significant bearing on facts we must consider when conducting performance evaluations (see Chapter 21) and may identify why some individuals with ability do not demonstrate merit.

Thus, for one to proceed through Vroom's expectancy model, three steps must occur. First, the individual must assess the probability that he or she can complete the assignment or do the job. If that probability is high, he or she will take the second step—evaluate the probability of getting a reward for doing the job. In this step he or she must determine how well the job or assignment must be done to get a reward and try to accurately speculate what the reward will be.

If the desire still exists to pursue the assignment and now the reward, he or she will take step three—do the job and hope that he or she will get what is expected.

B. F. Skinner's Reinforcement Model (1938 and 1953)

Another process theory is that of reinforcement. Reinforcement ties nicely to Vroom's theory because it is the reward that reinforces certain behavior on the part of the employee. However, reinforcement can also be negative. Punishment discourages an employee's behavior, such as counseling for excessive absenteeism or suspension for using inappropriate language.

Skinner, a psychologist, determined that behaviors can be controlled through the use of rewards. He believed that employees who receive rewards for exceptional performance on one assignment are willing to take on other assignments and do well as long as the employee knows he or she will be rewarded. Under Skinner's approach, to get people to behave in a certain way, you must reward them every time. Rewards can be symbolic, monetary, or related to prestige or public recognition. This may explain why programs modeled after the Seattle Fish Market are popular and successful in organizations today: individuals strive to accumulate a large number of certificates or fish charms to demonstrate their exceptional performance. The important point is that a reward is offered that is desired by the employee, it is given as soon as possible after the employee has accomplished the task, and the employee perceives the reward worthy of his efforts. Failure to perform in a way that was expected results in no reward.

Who Is Right?

If we follow Vroom's and Skinner's notions, motivation simply is one of the rewards for good work and deprivation of rewards or punishment for bad work. Clearly, motivation starts with personal recognition and appreciation (*Medical Office Manager* 2000). However, the employee will also apply probability to his decision—that is, his risk in doing or not doing the assignment or the degree of effort he will put forth. The calculating effort is directly related to the realistic level of the work assigned. Just because an employee was able to unbox 40 cases of canned goods in central supply today does not mean that giving him a reward will encourage him to unbox 80 cases tomorrow. Remember that as supervisors you have different needs than your staff. You need higher productivity from your team, but your team desires shorter shifts.

Lastly, supervisors should be motivators, but they can be motivation destroyers too. Remember that rewards do not need to be monetary to be considered rewards by an employee. The simple pat on the back or thank you can motivate an employee to exhibit a certain behavior. Moreover, rewards that show an extra effort by the supervisor, like issuing a certificate or writing a thank you note, can significantly increase motivation levels. Failing to distribute those rewards in a timely and sincere fashion is sure to kill motivation in your workplace.

Delnor-Community Hospital in Geneva, Illinois, used simple rewards as motivators that paid back the hospital handsomely. The organization took the position "that satisfied employees provide better patient care. In a time of national shortage of healthcare workers, the best way to fill vacancies may be by preventing them" (Solovy 2001). The hospital's recognition program was publicized, praise was given publicly in mini-celebrations at the employee's worksite, and coworkers rewarded each other with $5 gift certificates. Departments rated each other, and the ratings were published. When the organization achieved its financial, patient satisfaction, and turnover goals, everyone received a bonus (Solovy 2001).

As you can see, no one motivational technique works all the time. You must recognize that what encourages one employee to do one thing may not be the same technique that would encourage another employee to do the same thing. Much has been written on motivational techniques, and this chapter has not discussed all the theorists. Additional research on your part may yield a theorist who may have the right solution for your situation.

PERCEPTIONS, VALUES, AND ATTITUDES

As we have said, all human behavior is motivated by unsatisfied needs. These needs spring from causes that are deep within the person and, together with other motives, attitudes, and behaviors, form the configuration usually called the personality. From this point of view, the motivation that contributes to personality can be defined as the potential to act to satisfy those needs that are not met. The phrase potential to act implies that some motives are stronger than others and thus more likely to produce action. The strength of motivation is determined by the strength of a particular need, the probability that the act required to satisfy that need will be successful and the rewards forthcoming. An individual is more likely to act if his or her motive is stronger, the probability for success is high, and the reward is significant.

Other factors are also involved in producing human behavior or action. Motives do not stand alone. Closely related to them and significantly affecting their strength are perceptions, values, and attitudes. We are constantly subjected to many stimuli from our environment; all of them compete for our attention. In our daily working environment there are noises, sights, sounds, smells, supervisors' instructions, memos, reports, physicians' directives, coworkers' remarks, people walking by, beepers, phones ringing, posted signs, and so on. All these and many more vie for our attention. The individual therefore has the challenge of interpreting and organizing the more important stimuli and responding to them appropriately.

The individual uses perception to screen, select, organize, and interpret stimuli. This does not necessarily lead to an accurate portrayal of the environment but to a unique picture, influenced by the perceiver's needs, desires, values, disposition, and frame of reference. Through the process of perceptual selectivity, certain stimuli catch one's attention and are selected, whereas one screens out those he or she either does not want to bother with or finds uncomfortable.

The perceptual process plays an important role in all managerial activities, including decision making, appraising employees, communicating orally, and writing. It is important for the manager to understand the perceptual process and to realize that people perceive things differently.

Perceptual organization is how an individual categorizes, groups, and fills in information systematically. Once meaning has been attached to a certain stimulus, the individual can reach an appropriate response. Several barriers to accurate perception, however, can enter into these perceptual processes. Examples of barriers are the frame of reference, stereotyping, the halo effect, biases, and perceptual defense (see chapters 5 and 21). All the perceptual processes affect a person's attitudes and behavior at work.

Attitudes and values also play a role in all behavior. Attitudes are different from values. Values are closely held normative standards; the individual chooses them based on personal preference. "Values carry with them an 'oughtness' component. They are frequently defined as ideas about how everyone should feel or behave" (Mitchell 1982; see also Steers 1988). Values are broader, general, more encompassing concepts than attitudes; for example, most of us value freedom and equality. Our values of equality can be translated into our attitude toward minority groups.

Attitudes can be viewed as "a predisposition to respond in a favorable or unfavorable way to objects, persons, concepts, or whatever" (Mitchell 1982; see also Steers 1988). They are the ways an individual tends to interpret, understand, or define a situation or relationship with others. Attitudes constitute one's feelings about something—likes and dislikes directed toward persons, things, situations, or a combination of all three. They are more than casual opinions, as they are heavily charged with emotional overtones. Attitudes may include feelings as well as intellectual elements. They also include evaluations and value judgments. Attitudes differ in type, strength, and the extent to which they are open or hidden.

Attitudes are revealed in two ways: (1) by the individual's expressed statements or (2) by behavior. An individual may express dislike for his or her manager or he or she may merely demonstrate this attitude by being absent excessively. Although we cannot see perceptions, values, and attitudes, their consequences can be observed in behavior.

Factors Determining Attitudes

Attitudes are learned from prior experiences. An infinite number of factors determine and influence an individual's attitudes. One major influence is a person's biological, or physiological, makeup. Such factors as sex, age, height, race, weight, and physique are important in determining the attitudes that contribute to overall personality structure. In addition, many psychologists believe that the very early years of life are crucial to attitudinal development. Freudian psychologists (those who subscribe to the theories of Sigmund Freud), in particular, believe that early childhood is the most critical period in shaping what a person actually becomes. This theory is often referred to as childhood determinism; it maintains that such factors as feeding patterns, training patterns, and home conditions in early childhood are the primary determinants of personality structure.

Another area that influences a person's attitudes and personality is the immediate environment. Education, employment, income, and many other experiences that confront an individual as he or she goes through life influence who this person is today and what he or she eventually becomes. Furthermore, one should never forget that the broader culture of society also influences a person's attitudes. In the United States, people generally believe in competition, reward for accomplishment, equal opportunities, and other values that are part of the democratic capitalistic society. Individuals learn from their early years to strive for achievement, think for themselves, and work hard; they learn these roads lead to success.

As the United States becomes even more of melting pot, now including people from other cultures, dominant attitudes and beliefs may shift. For example, some people may become willing to compromise the freedom Americans now enjoy to do essentially whatever they want and whenever they want to do it; this is a result of heightened concerns about safety and security that arose in the aftermath of several disastrous incidents in the 1990s (i.e., the Columbine shootings, the damage wrought by the bombs sent through the U.S. Postal Service by the Unabomber, the bombing of the federal building in Oklahoma City, the bomb that detonated in Atlanta, Georgia, at the summer Olympics) and in 2001 (i.e., the simultaneous terrorist airplane hijackings that resulted in deadly attacks against the World Trade Center Twin Towers in New York and the Pentagon in Washington, DC). These events and countless other cultural influences and factors affect a person's attitudes and thus behavior.

Attitudes and Behavior

No matter what factors have caused their development, attitudes become deep-seated attributes of the individual's makeup. They are learned and acquired through a person's life experiences, and they do not have to be rational or logical. We hold firmly to our attitudes and resist forces that attempt to interfere with them. Attitudes can change, but they change very slowly. Attitudes do not exist only within individuals but are also generated within groups. Often individuals accept the attitudes of the group to which they belong as their own.

As shown in Figure 24.1, needs and motives do not stand alone as determinants of behavior. They are also influenced by the underlying attitudes and values of a person. Indeed, we can say that values and attitudes determine the route a person takes for the satisfaction of his or her needs. Although the same basic needs are manifest in every person, attitudes vary greatly and affect individuals' unique responses to their needs. In other words, attitudes help determine what motivates a person to take a certain action to fulfill a certain need. For example, many people may have a strong need for achievement. However, differing attitudes and values motivate one individual to seek fulfillment of that need—one may do this by working in a hospital, another by working in a government agency, yet another by working in a specific industry, and a fourth by teaching in a university or going into politics. Similarly one individual may find fulfillment as a cook in a nursing home's kitchen, while another may find it as a chemist in a research laboratory.

MOTIVATION VERSUS FRUSTRATION

If the individual's chosen route results in goal accomplishment, his or her need is satisfied and the attitudes are reinforced, which serve as feedback. What happens, however, if the chosen course of action does not result in goal accomplishment? What happens when an individual wishes to pursue a certain course of action but is prevented from doing so by an external or internal circumstance?

Generally, actions that do not succeed in obtaining goals result in blocked satisfaction, frustration, and anxiety. As shown in Figure 24.1, feedback notifies the individual that his or her needs are not being fulfilled. Hence, stress, instead of need satisfaction, results, in the forms of frustration and anxiety. People usually resolve the problems of conflict and frustration in five basic ways: (1) problem-solving behavior (the best method), (2) resignation, (3) detour behavior, (4) retreat, or (5) aggression.

Problem-solving behavior is usually the most desirable way of meeting frustration. It is advantageous if a person can look at problems objectively and base his or her decisions on reasoned analysis of the situation. Consider basketball superstar Michael Jordan's experience, for example: "When I got cut from the varsity team as a sophomore in high school, I learned something. I knew I never wanted to feel that bad again. I never wanted to have that taste in my mouth, that hole in my stomach. So I set a goal of becoming a starter on the varsity" (Gilbert 1999). Unfortunately, many people are not capable of assessing a personal obstacle objectively and of problem solving to address frustration; it is the supervisor's duty to help the employees learn problem-solving behavior. This can be started with nondirective interviews, as discussed in Chapter 20.

Using Nondirective Interviews to Overcome Obstacles and Conflict

Supervisors should encourage subordinates to come to them with their problems, both work and aspiration related. Encouraging nondirective interviews for work-related issues shows the employee that the supervisor is willing to hear employees out. Otherwise, minor irritations may turn out to become major problems. The supervisor must realize that inherent in the managerial position is an invisible barrier between the supervisor and the subordinates. Some employees have little difficulty speaking to their supervisors, but many may be more timid. Therefore, the supervisor must make an effort to encourage those who are reluctant to reveal their thoughts. The supervisor should see that time is always available to listen to the subordinates. If time is not available at the moment, the interview may be postponed for a few hours; in this way the supervisor may allow enough time and not rush through the discussion.

The principal function of the nondirective interview is to alert the supervisor as to what the interviewee really thinks and feels and what lies at the root of a particular problem such as excessive turnover, absenteeism, or complaints about work or the department. In addition, it gives the interviewee a feeling of relief and helps the subordinate develop greater insight into his or her own problems, often finding solutions while thinking out loud. Many sources of frustration exist within and outside the working environment, and unless frustration is relieved, it may lead to all forms of undesirable responses such as seeking support from the informal group leader. Another, potentially more detrimental response is for the frustrated employee to begin to exhibit the actions that are irritating him or her, perhaps by being absent from work regularly or openly complaining about his or her employer.

For aspiration-related issues, the principles of the nondirective interview are similar. It is an opportunity for the supervisor to hear where the employee aspires to go within the organization. It is an ideal time for the supervisor to suggest different courses of action for the employee to consider, being careful not to bias or encourage one over the other. Suppose, for instance, that a licensed practical nurse (LPN) is eager to advance to a better position, but all better positions demand the registered nurse (RN) degree as a prerequisite. The LPN is frustrated because he or she keeps running into this obstacle. In this case, an analysis of the situation and a thorough discussion with the supervisor could encourage the LPN to obtain the RN degree through an online program in a way that does not interfere with his or her work schedule. This option will enable him or her to move up within the hierarchy of nursing services. Such a route constitutes intelligent problem-solving behavior.

The interview also may identify work processes or organization policies that are perceived as roadblocks to employees growing within the organization and thus leading them to consider employment opportunities outside. Finally, it provides the supervisor with valuable insight into factors that motivate this and other employees to progress within their department or another unit within the organization if provided a vehicle or opportunity to do so. This is the supervisor's role as a coach and mentor.

The ground rule for conducting a nondirective interview is to let the interviewee say whatever he or she wants to say. Conducting such an interview is more difficult than conducting a directive interview. It demands the concentrated listening and continuous attention of the supervisor. The supervisor must exert self-control and hide his or her own ideas and emotions during the interview. He or she should not interrupt, argue, or change the subject. The supervisor should not express approval or disapproval even though the employee may request it. This may prove exasperating, but it is essential.

In such a counseling interview, the employee must feel like he or she can speak openly. In all likelihood, as soon as all the negative feelings or anxieties have been expressed, the employee may start to find some favorable aspects of the very same issues that he or she had criticized earlier. When the employee is encouraged to verbalize problems and frustrations, he or she may gain greater insight into these troubles or may arrive at an answer or course of action that will help solve the difficulties. The employee must be permitted to work through difficulties alone, without being interrupted and advised by the interviewer regarding the best course of action. If the problem concerns the job, work, and organization, however, the supervisor may have to be directive so that the solution is consistent with the needs of the institution.

If the concerns are personal in nature, the supervisor should exercise great care not to give advice or become burdened with the task of running the subordinate's personal life. Most of the time the interviewee wants a sympathetic or empathic listener and not an advisor. The average supervisor is not equipped to do counseling, and this is not part of the job. If necessary, the subordinate should be referred to trained specialists—for example, one of the institution's social workers or psychologists—or the organization's employee assistance program. This may be necessary when sensitive areas and deep-seated personality problems are involved. The patient-psychiatrist relationship is not applicable to that of subordinate and boss.

When Conflict Goes Unchecked

When employees do not believe they can approach their supervisor or another for guidance, they naturally resort to other alternatives. One such way to solve a conflict is by resignation. Suppose our LPN from the earlier example thinks, "What else can I do? I have to stick it out." The LPN seems resigned to his or her lot. This LPN will keep working for the healthcare institution but may no longer consider himself or herself a part of it. Once an employee has given up in the face of obstacles, it is difficult to rebuild morale to the point at which institutional and departmental goals continue to be really important for this person. Some employees simply stay on the job, listlessly performing their duties until they are able to retire. Such employees who have resigned themselves to their lot are usually passive and resistant to change. They are difficult for the supervisor to deal with because new ideas do not excite or stimulate them. The supervisor may try to restimulate the employee to strive either for past goals or toward some new and desirable goals that address the employee's needs. The supervisor knows that the result of resignation is usually inferior performance on the job, lowering of morale, and a climate that is not conducive to the best performance of the department.

Another alternative way to solve a frustrating situation is to resort to detour behavior. With the direct way of reaching the goal barred, the employee tries to find another way to get there. Such detours, however, are often obscure and sometimes devious. For example, one kind of detour behavior is self-induced illness. Children learn early in life that being sick gives them an acceptable excuse for getting out of doing an unpleasant task. Similarly, employees often avoid conflict by inducing, many times subconsciously, painful and very real physical disorders. Some people can stand conflict and frustration better than others, but sooner or later the strain begins to show and conflict resolution becomes necessary.

Retreat, or leaving the field, is a third way to meet the problems of conflict and frustration. Most people at one time or another have looked at their jobs and have wished that they could quit right then and there. They may believe that they are not getting the satisfaction they thought the position would bring, that no one realizes the difficulties involved in the job, that their supervisor does not appreciate all the things they are doing, and so on. Most people have such feelings sometime in their lives. In many instances an employee finds it necessary to leave the organization and find alternative employment. Whether this reaction to frustration is good or bad, however, depends on the major source of the conflict and frustration. If the major source is the employee's personality and the conflict does not stem from the working situation, leaving the field is not the right answer. In other words, if the frustration is caused by the person's own particular psychological makeup, quitting probably will not bring about the desired result. If, however, the conflict is the result of an unfavorable work situation, leaving may represent a real solution to the problem. Often it is difficult for the individual to determine whether this is the case. Of course, it is not always necessary to quit the job or move to another city to leave the field. "Leaving the field" may be displayed by daydreaming, spending a lot of time in the washroom, surfing the Internet during the workday, developing a high rate of absenteeism, resorting to alcoholism and drug abuse, or using some other form of symbolic escape. All these forms of retreat cause the supervisor additional problems.

Aggression is the fourth way in which people may meet the problem of severe frustration. The individual feels frustrated and cannot find an acceptable, legitimate remedy. Sabotage is one common form of aggressive behavior that serves as a response to frustration. Aggression here does not only refer to overtly hostile behavior aimed at harming other people (such as disgruntled workers returning to the workplace armed with firearms) or to hostile behavior toward inanimate objects, but it also refers to the tendency to commit acts of aggression. This tendency may manifest itself in thoughts or words, or even in feelings that have not yet been put into words. In one situation, the staff of a dietary department used various forms of sabotage to express frustration with management: patients were served raw chicken and in some cases empty, but heated, plates. Their dissatisfaction was clear.

The supervisor should always remember that frustration and aggression are closely linked and that all aggression stems from frustration. As we have said, some individuals can stand more frustration than others and do not respond as quickly with aggressive behavior. The job of the supervisor is to see that frustration is minimized and to provide constructive outlets for it. The supervisor should try to anticipate sources of frustration and eliminate them. If this cannot be done, the supervisor should ensure that the causes of frustration are not aggravated. Often listening patiently helps to ease employee tensions, and it may enable the subordinate to seek the real source of the frustration. A supervisor's talent can be measured by his or her ability to accurately determine when a subordinate needs both patient listening and advice or only patient listening.

Conflicts Between Individual and Organizational Goals

Although many causes of frustration exist, a major cause arises when individual needs and goals conflict rather than coincide with those of the organization or department. Much has been written about the conflict between the individual who seeks action and independence and the climate in a bureaucratic, formalized organization that stifles a person's natural desire for freedom and self-determination. The consequences of such a climate manifest themselves in high turnover, waste, lower productivity, slowdown, lack of innovative and creative behavior, non-acceptance of leadership, and so on. The most serious consequence of a bureaucratic organization, however, is that it blocks the individual from attaining satisfaction of his or her needs.

Managers today are becoming more aware of these consequences and of the necessity for an organization to provide a climate that enables its employees to find personal satisfaction. In fact, the need for an appropriate organizational climate is increasing because of the rising expectations of employees. This is especially true in the healthcare field, in which organizations are confronted with ever-advancing and more sophisticated activity. The highly skilled and educated employees are primarily professionals who expect to fulfill many of their needs right on the job. Because such employees tend to take high wages and appropriate fringe benefits for granted, it should be apparent that the key to long-term motivation for them rests in the satisfaction of the higher-level needs—that is, their esteem and self-fulfillment needs. It is management's duty to develop an organizational climate that produces effective motivation and satisfaction of these needs, thereby helping resolve the conflict between individual and organizational goals. Therefore, the supervisor's knowledge of the basic motivational processes is necessary because it facilitates high levels of job satisfaction and minimizes conflicts.

MODIFYING MOTIVATIONAL TECHNIQUES

Flinn (2001) aptly states, "Achieving a clear understanding of human nature is an important aspect of management in the work place." For managers and staff to work together as an effective and productive unit, staff members must know how they fit into the overall scheme of things. Likewise managers must clearly understand how they can maximize productivity by supporting their employees through the appropriate leadership style. It is also extremely important for managers to realistically evaluate the working environment, as well as the characteristics of the task, to decide how best to deal with employees.

As a supervisor, you likely work with a multigenerational team or workforce. Most working people fall into one of three generations: (1) those born between 1946 and 1964 (baby boomers), (2) those born between 1965 and 1980 (Generation X), and (3) those born between 1981 and 2000 (Generation Y). (Note that generation boundaries are not carved in stone, so you may see in other resources timeframes that vary by a year or two.) Members of each generation are influenced by the cultures, values, and mores of the time in which they are raised. Geography, family dynamics, socioeconomic issues, religion, and other factors play a part as well.

Clearly, the younger members of your team were raised during a time that differed substantially from that of other older team members. Figure 24.7 depicts some of the problems encountered in schools in the 1940s through late 1990s; this listing reflects changes in the U.S. culture over time.

Working with the Generations

A great deal of change has occurred since the 1960s. Technology and telecommunications have shrunk the size of the world and altered international relations. Business has grown from these changes, and so have the perspectives of your staff. As our global economy flourishes, the diversity of our workforce increases accordingly. Team members from different countries and cultures have joined the American workforce and brought with them different values, attitudes, and needs.

Generation X employees grew up in a world in which access to information was relatively immediate and the ability to absorb and analyze this information was imperative. Computing technology advanced as quickly as the Xers were maturing. The year 1969 brought microchips, 1971 brought time-shared computers, 1973 brought microprocessors, and 1977 brought Apple personal computers. The 1980s introduced affordable laptop computers, and since that time computers have become more powerful, smaller, and cheaper. While growing up, members of Generation X were shuttled from one sporting event to another and between home to daycare by dual-career baby boomer parents. These activities taught Gen Xers at least two things: (1) schedule your time wisely so you can fit everything in and (2) learn how to survive in a group, because your family is likely not around.

Furthermore, a trend toward socially conscious employment has become apparent. Recently enacted regulations recognize that workers must be given time to attend to their families and their lives. The Family Medical Leave Act, state initiatives on same-sex marriages, and similar other provisions support the need for organizations to be more sensitive to worker-family requirements. Given these changes, we are seeing more and more organizations abandoning the traditional top-down, rigid, and hierarchical structures. Team involvement in decisions is paramount with the growing level of specialized expertise that is needed in today's healthcare organization. Team leaders and managers must be flexible and ready to deal with changes and have available to them a group of

FIGURE 24.7: TOP PROBLEMS IN PUBLIC SCHOOLS: 1940s VERSUS LATE 1990s

1940	1996–1998
Talking out of turn	Drug/alcohol abuse
Chewing gum	Physical attacks/assault
Making noise	Theft and larceny
Running in the halls	Pregnancy
Cutting in line	Rape
Dress code infractions	Violence/gangs

Sources: Morrison (1997), NCES (2005), Phi Delta Kappa (1998).

advisors, who are often team members, to chart the course through the rapidly changing healthcare environment.

Team members today are probably Generation Xers; in the coming years, they will be from Generation Y. Generation Y members are not motivated by the fear of poverty, economic disasters, or (up until September 11) international terrorism. They grew up during a time in which there were ambitious social programs, higher taxes, and a recovering and flourishing economy that was being infiltrated by foreign firms.

Generation Yers graduated (or will graduate) from high school in the twenty-first century. They know computers, and they are and will be expert at using multimedia, networking, the Internet, and technology not yet developed. Not only do their music preferences differ from previous generations (as expected), but their dress also differs considerably. As far as boomers and the Silent Generation (1925–1945) are concerned, both Gen Xers and Gen Yers do not dress appropriately. To these younger generations, fashion is not used to make a statement, with Generation Yers leaning toward an androgynous look. Unlike boomers and silenters, both Xers and Yers grew up on their own, as both parents worked. Many were reared in divorced and single-parent homes. This has made them independent and desirous of a "better" family atmosphere.

Graeme Codrington (2001a) suggests that the leadership style that is most effective for Generation Xers is consultative; for Gen Yers (or Millennials), it is grand and expansive. In fact, he predicts that Yers are being groomed to be a civic-minded, community-oriented workforce. (Codrington 2001b). (See Figure 24.8 for a listing of generational traits.) Ensman (2000) says these younger employees often seek instant gratification and certainly lack patience and an understanding of workplace fundamentals such as punctuality, terms of formal address, and workplace etiquette. What this means for you as their supervisor is that you need to teach them these skills on the job and during their orientation.

FIGURE 24.8: WHAT MAKES THE GENERATIONS TICK?

Name	Period	U.S. Population	Effects	Values and Characteristics	Management Style
Silenters	1925–1945	75 million	Depression; Pearl Harbor; WWII; radio; manufacturing advances; big band; TV; copier	"Family" values; head of household works; modest income; company loyalty	X
Baby Boomers	1946–1964	76 million	Vietnam; Watergate; Kennedy and King assassinations; rock & roll; space travel	50% Divorce rate; career advancement; entrepreneurs; material items; small families	X/Y
Generation X	1965–1980	17 million	Racial integration; school bussing; rapid tech changes; telecom advances; both parents working/latchkey kids; marijuana	Volunteer work; later-life marriages; better family life; group oriented; career minded; achievement obsessed; may still live at home	Y
Generation Y	1981–2000	60 million	Racial and ethnic diversity; dual-income families; Internet; single parents; cable TV; street drugs; oil spills; terrorism; cloning	Better family life; conservation; ecology; financial responsibility; career driven/fast track; analytical	Y/Z

It is anticipated that younger employees will not remain with you long term. The silenter trait of staying with an employer for 20, 30, or more years only to receive the traditional gold watch at retirement is not apparent with the younger employees. They will move from one job to another for better pay; a better title; or more material benefits such as an office, a car, and an expense account.

According to Ensman (2000), younger employees may voice open-ended complaints or frustrations and may not know how to address problems. He says they might be bothered by things that an older employee would shrug off, and they may appear inarticulate, gruff, whiny, or angry. Their behavior is likely influenced by the impatience of youth and a communication style borne out of e-mail—that is, informal, direct, and often grammatically incorrect. Ensman suggests that when you hear a petty complaint or criticism, explain politely and directly why the situation exists, and if it is significant, investigate it. Furthermore, he suggests dealing with younger employees' problems privately but without offering empathy; rather, address the issues with professionalism. All this being said, your job as a supervisor is to be a role model; both young and mature employees will look to you for the "right" way to approach an issue. You, on the other hand, need to understand their needs and values so that you can motivate them to get the job done.

Temporary Workers

As stated earlier and in Chapter 19, the healthcare organization has had to become more flexible to deal with the economic and technological changes affecting the industry today. To accommodate some of this need, management has employed more part-time and temporary workers. These workers, often categorized as contingent workers, include temporary employees employed by the human resources department or through an agency, independent contractors, leased employees, and part-time employees directly hired by the organization. The American Management Association (2000) "suggests that as staffing issues become more fluid, employers are looking to these workers to provide the flexibility necessary to move their businesses quickly."

These individuals require a different set of motivators. They know they are with your organization for a relatively short period and are considered "fill-in" employees, so they do not feel like they are part of your team. Most individuals want to be part of the family; one thing you can do is to include them in special activities, ad hoc problem-solving groups, and events that are organized for your department. Make sure that notes from department or team meetings are shared with them if they are unable to attend. Give this contingent workforce the training and resources they need. They should be assigned their own equipment and space and not be required to borrow (or beg to use) the equipment of full-time employees.

Training is essential, as you will not want to correct errors made by temporary staff after they leave. Moreover, remember these employees may be a valuable source of future full-time employees. You should build a mentoring relationship with them and learn more about their goals, interests, and skills. Some of these employees may have unique skills that you are seeking. As with all employees, ensure that these part-timers are commended for doing a good job. They need to know that they are appreciated, and for that they will remember your facility as they move on to other organizations. Contingent workers can be your healthcare facility's best promoter in the community.

Lastly, caution should be exercised when sharing company information with contingent workers that is sensitive, confidential, or not for public consumption.

They may not have the loyalty of full-time, permanent employees and therefore may not use the same discretion in sharing information with friends and family.

SUMMARY

Influencing is the managerial function in which the supervisor creates a climate that enables subordinates to find as much satisfaction as possible while getting the job done. The influencing function is particularly concerned with behavioral responses and interpersonal relations. Only by appropriately influencing will the supervisor instill the motivation in the department's employees to go about their jobs with enthusiasm and also to find personal fulfillment of their needs. Therefore, it is necessary for supervisors to understand basic motivational processes.

Motivation is the force that arouses, energizes, directs, and sustains human behavior. All human behavior is caused by unsatisfied needs. These needs eventually stimulate the formation of goals that motivate people to take certain actions. Motivation, however, not only is caused by unmet needs but also is largely influenced by an individual's perceptions, values, attitudes, and entire personality.

An individual's attitudes are formed beginning in early childhood. They affect and are affected by an infinite number of factors in the person's life. Attitudes differ among generations and determine the individual route a person takes for the satisfaction of those needs. Although they vary in strength, most needs are basically the same in all people. Maslow speaks of a hierarchy of needs; in ascending order they are physiological needs, safety, social needs, esteem, and self-fulfillment. A person's level of aspiration is closely related to this hierarchy of needs. People generally move from one level to the next in Maslow's hierarchy.

McClelland focuses on describing other important human needs: achievement, affiliation, and power. Herzberg, in his two-factor approach, stresses the importance of motivators versus hygiene factors. He shows that the more important forces of employee motivation lie in factors related to work content and not work environment, or hygiene factors.

Vroom's expectancy theory espouses the belief that if one puts forth effort X and the risk is appropriately rewarded, the direct result will be Y. The individual must be willing to exert a high level of effort to reach an objective and to satisfy an individual need. Skinner's reinforcement theory ties nicely with Vroom's theory in that he says it is the reward that reinforces certain behavior on the part of the employee.

A person who can understand his or her needs and attitudes fairly well is able to choose courses of action that result in achieving goals. Goal accomplishment serves as feedback to the individual; the need is satisfied and the underlying attitudes are confirmed. If a goal is not attained, however, conflict often sets in because action that does not succeed results in blocked satisfaction, frustration, and anxiety. Most people usually react to conflict and frustration in one of the following five ways: problem-solving behavior, resignation, detour behavior, retreat, or aggression.

It is the supervisor's duty to minimize frustrating situations, especially if they result from a conflict between individual and organizational goals. One way to minimize such conflicts is to realize that in the work environment various factors influence the realization of an employee's expectations. Some of these factors are merely satisfiers and dissatisfiers (Herzberg's hygiene factors), whereas others are motivators and are able to fulfill the higher-level needs and goals of people.

Supervisors will be challenged in the years to come as new generations of workers join the workforce; these younger generations have attitudes and values that differ from their older coworkers. Supervisors will need to change their leadership style and approach with some of these employees to motivate them to adapt to a structured workplace; to accept ideas from their older, possibly less technology-proficient colleagues; and to contribute in a constructive manner to the objectives of the department and organization.

NOTE

1. In 1997, I had the special opportunity to speak with Frederick Herzberg. At that time, an earlier edition of this book cited a magazine article that referenced his work on satisfiers and dissatisfiers. However, based on his guidance and permission to use his work in this book, I now use the original source, *Work and the Nature of Man*, published in 1966. Dr. Herzberg died at the age of 76 in January 2000.

REFERENCES

American Management Association. 2000. "Growing Use of Temporary Workers Driven by Employers' Needs for Flexibility." *Snelling Report* (November): 3.

Codrington, G. 2001a. "Defining Characteristics of Generations." [Online information; retrieved 2/21/06.] http://www.youthpastor.com/lessons/index.cfm/124.pdf?fuseaction=viewdoc&L=124.

———. 2001b. "Definitive Influences on Today's Youth." [Online information; retrieved 1/2/01.] http://home.pix.za/gc/gc12/genx/thesis/ch1.htm.

Ensman, R. G., Jr. 2000. "Working with Young Employees." *Advance for Health Information Professionals* 10 (19): 57.

Flinn, W. P. 2001. "The XY&Z of Management Theory." [Online information; retrieved 2/9/01.] http://fsosvr.arizona.edu/dickportfolio/dissertation/ToFile/xyz.htm.

Gilbert, R. 1999. *Bits & Pieces*. Fairfield, NJ: The Economics Press.

Herzberg, F. 1966. *Work and Nature of Man*. Cleveland, OH: World Publishing.

———. 1987. "One More Time: How Do You Motivate Employees?" *Harvard Business Review* 65 (5): 87–96.

Huitt, W. G. 1998. "Maslow's Hierarchy of Needs." [Online information; retrieved 2/24/01.] http://chiron.valdosta.edu/whuitt/col/regsys/maslow.html.

McClelland, D. C., J. W. Atchison, R. A. Clark, and E. L. Lowell. 1953. *The Achievement Motive*. New York: Appleton-Century-Crofts.

McClelland, D. C., and D. H. Burnham. 1976. "Power Is the Great Motivator." *Harvard Business Review* (March/April): 100–10.

Medical Office Manager. 2000. "Motivating Staff to Do More than the Minimum." *Medical Office Manager* 14 (8): 9.

Mitchell, T. R. 1982. *People in Organizations, Second Edition*, 127–28. New York: McGraw-Hill Book Co.

Morrison, J. L. 1997. "Future Scan 2000 & Beyond." On the Horizon. [Online presentation.] http://www.horizon.unc.edu/projects/presentations/wsf/tsld035.htm.

National Center for Education Statistics (NCES). 1998. "Violence and discipline problems in US Public Schools: 1996–1997." [Online information; retrieved 10/06/05.] http://nces.ed.gov/pubsearch/pubsinfo.asp?pubid =98030.

Phi Delta Kappa. 1998. "The 30th Annual Phi Delta Kappa Gallup Poll of the Public's Attitudes Toward the Public Schools." [Online information; retrieved 10/06/05.] www.pdkintl.org/kappan/kp9809-3.htm.

Solovy, A. 2001. "All the Right Moves." *Hospitals and Health Networks* 75 (3): 30.

Steers, R. M. 1988. *Introduction to Organizational Behavior, Third Edition*, 283–93. Glenview, IL: Scott Foresman & Co.

Wyatt, W. 2000. "HFMA Wants You To Know." E-mail newsletter. Chicago: Healthcare Financial Management Association.

Exhibit 24.1

"ONE MORE TIME: HOW DO YOU MOTIVATE EMPLOYEES?"

by Frederick Herzberg

How many articles, books, speeches, and workshops have pleaded plaintively, "How do I get an employee to do what I want him to do?"

The psychology of motivation is tremendously complex, and what has been unraveled with any degree of assurance is small indeed. But the dismal ratio of knowledge to speculation has not dampened the enthusiasm for new forms of snake oil that are constantly coming on the market, many of them with academic testimonials. Doubtless this article will have no depressing impact on the market for snake oil, but since the ideas expressed in it have been tested in many corporations and other organizations, it will help—I hope—to redress the imbalance in the aforementioned ratio.

"MOTIVATING" with KITA

In lectures to industry on the problem, I have found that the audiences are anxious for quick and practical answers, so I will begin with a straightforward, practical formula for moving people.

What is the simplest, surest, and most direct way of getting someone to do something? Ask him? Tell him? Give him a monetary incentive? Show him? We need a simple way. Every audience contains the "direct action" manager who shouts, "Kick him!" And this type of manager is right. The surest and least circumlocuted way of getting someone to do something is to kick him in the pants—give him what might be called the KITA.

There are various forms of KITA, and here are some of them: Negative physical KITA is a literal application of the term and was frequently used in the past. It has, however, three major drawbacks: (1) it is inelegant; (2) it contradicts the precious image of benevolence that most organizations cherish; and (3) since it is a physical attack, it directly stimulates the autonomic nervous system, and this often results in negative feedback—the employee may just kick you in return. These factors give rise to certain taboos against negative physical KITA.

Negative psychological KITA has several advantages over negative physical KITA. First, the cruelty is not visible; the bleeding is internal and comes much later. Second, since it affects the higher cortical centers of the brain with its inhibitory powers, it reduces the possibility of physical backlash. Third, since the amount of psychological pain that a person can feel is almost infinite, the direction and site possibilities of the KITA are increased many times. Fourth, the person administering the kick can manage to be above it all and let the system accomplish the dirty work. Fifth, those who practice it receive some ego satisfaction (one-upmanship), whereas they would find drawing blood abhorrent.

Finally, if the employee does complain, he can always be accused of being paranoid, since there is no tangible evidence of an actual attack.

Now, what does negative KITA accomplish ? If I kick you in the rear (physically or psychologically), who is motivated? I am motivated; you move! Negative KITA does not lead to motivation, but to movement.

Let us consider motivation. If I say to you, "Do this for me or the company, and in return I will give you a reward, an incentive, more status, a promotion, all the quid pro quos that exist in the industrial organization," am I motivating you? The overwhelming opinion I receive from management people is, "Yes, this is motivation."

I have a year old Schnauzer. When it was a small puppy and I wanted it to move, I kicked it in the rear and it moved. Now that I have finished its obedience training, I hold up a dog biscuit when I want the Schnauzer to move. In this instance, who is motivated—I or the dog? The dog wants the biscuit, but it is I who want it to move. Again, I am the one who is motivated, and the dog is the one who moves. In this instance all I did was apply KITA frontally; I extended a pull instead of a push. When industry wishes to use such positive KITAs, it has available an incredible number and variety of dog biscuits (jelly beans for humans) to wave in front of the employee to get him to jump. But positive KITA is not motivation. If I kick my dog (from the front or the back), he will move. And when I want him to move again, what must I do? I must kick him again. Similarly, I can charge a man's battery, and then recharge it, and recharge it again. But it is only when he has his own generator that he can talk about motivation. He then needs no outside stimulation. He wants to do it.

HYGIENE VS. MOTIVATORS

Let me rephrase the perennial question this way: How do you install a generator in an employee? A brief review of my motivation-hygiene theory of job attitudes is required before theoretical and practical suggestions can be offered. The theory was drawn from investigations using a wide variety of populations (including some in the communist countries). The findings of these studies, along with corroboration from many other investigations using different procedures, suggest that the factors involved in producing job satisfaction (and motivation) are separate and distinct from the factors that lead to job dissatisfaction.

Since separate factors need to be considered, depending on whether job satisfaction or job dissatisfaction is being examined, it follows that these two feelings are not opposites of each other. The opposite of job satisfaction is not job dissatisfaction but, rather, no job satisfaction; and, similarly, the opposite of job dissatisfaction is not job satisfaction, but no job dissatisfaction.

Two different needs of man are involved here. One set of needs can be thought of as stemming from his animal nature—the built-in drive to avoid pain from the environment, plus all the learned drives which become conditioned to the basic biological needs. For example, hunger, a basic biological drive, makes it necessary to earn money, and then money becomes a specific drive. The other set of needs relates to that unique human characteristic, the ability to achieve and, through achievement, to experience psychological growth. The stimuli for the growth needs are tasks that induce growth; in the industrial setting, they are the job content. Contrariwise, the stimuli inducing pain-avoidance behaviors are found in the job environment.

The growth or motivator factors that are intrinsic to the job are: achievement, recognition for achievement, the work itself, responsibility, and growth or advancement. The dissatisfaction-avoidance or hygiene (KITA) factors that are extrinsic to the job include: company policy and administration, supervision, interpersonal relationships, working conditions, salary, status, and security.

A composite of the factors that are involved in causing job satisfaction and job dissatisfaction, drawn from samples of 1,685 employees, is shown in Exhibit 1. (Refer to Figure 24.5.) The results indicate that motivators were the primary cause of satisfaction, and hygiene factors the primary cause of unhappiness on the job. As the lower right-hand part of the exhibit shows, of all the factors contributing to job satisfaction, 81% were motivators. And of all the factors contributing to the employees' dissatisfaction over their work, 69% involved hygiene elements.

Job Loading

In attempting to enrich an employee's job, management often succeeds in reducing the man's personal contribution, rather than giving him an opportunity for growth in his accustomed job. Such an endeavor, which I shall call horizontal job loading (as opposed to vertical loading, or providing motivator factors), has been the problem of earlier job enlargement programs. This activity merely enlarges the meaninglessness of the job. Some examples of this approach, and their effects, are:

- Challenging the employee by increasing the amount of production expected of him. If he tightens 10,000 bolts a day, see if he can tighten 20,000 bolts a day. The arithmetic involved shows that multiplying zero by zero still equals zero.
- Adding another meaningless task to the existing one, usually some routine clerical activity. The arithmetic here is adding zero to zero.
- Rotating the assignments of a number of jobs that need to be enriched. This means washing dishes for a while, then washing silverware. The arithmetic is substituting one zero for another zero.
- Removing the most difficult parts of the assignment in order to free the worker to accomplish more of the less challenging assignments. This traditional industrial engineering approach amounts to subtraction in the hope of accomplishing addition.

These are common forms of horizontal loading that frequently come up in preliminary brain storming session on job enrichment. The principles of vertical loading have not all been worked out as yet, and they remain rather general, but I have furnished several useful starting points for consideration in Exhibit 24.2.

Source: Reprinted with permission of *Harvard Business Review*. From "One More Time: How to Motivate Employees" by F. Herzberg, Sept./Oct. 1987. © 1987 by the Harvard Business School Publishing Corporation, all rights reserved.

Exhibit 24.2: Principles of Vertical Job Loading

Principle Motivators Involved

A. Removing some controls while retaining accountability: Responsibility and personal achievement
B. Increasing the accountability of individuals for own work: Responsibility and recognition
C. Giving a person a complete natural unit of work (module, division, area, and so on): Responsibility, achievement, and recognition
D. Granting additional authority to an employee in his activity; job freedom: Responsibility, achievement, and recognition
E. Making periodic reports directly available to the worker himself rather than to the supervisor: Internal recognition
F. Introducing new and more difficult tasks not previously handled: Growth and learning
G. Assigning individuals specific or specialized tasks, enabling them to become experts: Responsibility, growth, and advancement

Steps to Job Enrichment

Now that the motivator idea has been described in practice, here are the steps that managers should take in instituting the principle with their employees:

1. Select those jobs in which (a) the investment in industrial engineering does not make changes too costly, (b) attitudes are poor, (c) hygiene is becoming very costly, and (d) motivation will make a difference in performance.
2. Approach these jobs with the conviction that they can be changed. Years of tradition have led managers to believe that the content of the jobs is sacrosanct and the only scope of action that they have is in ways of stimulating people.
3. Brainstorm a list of changes that may enrich the jobs, without concern for their practicality.
4. Screen the list to eliminate suggestions that involve hygiene, rather than actual motivation.
5. Screen the list for generalities, such as "give them more responsibility," that are rarely followed in practice. This might seem obvious, but the motivator words have never left industry; the substance has just been rationalized and organized out. Words like "responsibility," "growth," "achievement," and "challenge," for example, have been elevated to the lyrics of the patriotic anthem for all organizations. It is the old problem typified by the pledge of allegiance to the flag being more important than contributions to the country—of following the form, rather than the substance.
6. Screen the list to eliminate any horizontal loading suggestions.

7.   Avoid direct participation by the employees whose jobs are to be enriched. Ideas they have expressed previously certainly constitute a valuable source for recommended changes, but their direct involvement contaminates the process with human relations hygiene and, more specifically, gives them only a sense of making a contribution. The job is to be changed, and it is the content that will produce the motivation, not attitudes about being involved or the challenge inherent in setting up a job. That process will be over shortly, and it is what the employees will be doing from then on that will determine their motivation. A sense of participation will result only in short-term movement.

8.   In the initial attempts at job enrichment set up a controlled experience. At least two equivalent groups should be chosen, one an experimental unit in which the motivators are systematically introduced over a period of time, and the other one a control group in which no changes are made. For both groups, hygiene should be allowed to follow its natural course for the duration of the experiment. Pre- and post- installation tests of performance and job attitudes are necessary to evaluate the effectiveness of the job enrichment program. The attitude test must be limited to motivator items in order to divorce the employee's view of the job he is given from all the surrounding hygiene feelings that he might have.

9.   Be prepared for a drop in performance in the experimental group the first few weeks. The changeover to a new job may lead to a temporary reduction in efficiency.

10. Expect your first time supervisors to experience some anxiety and hostility over the changes you are making. The anxiety comes from their fear that the changes will result in poorer performance for their unit. Hostility will arise when the employees start assuming what the supervisors regard as their own responsibility for performance. The supervisor without checking duties to perform may then be left with little to do. After a successful experiment, however, the supervisor usually discovers the supervisory and managerial functions that he has neglected, or which were never his because all his time was given over to checking the work of his subordinates. For example, in the R&D division of one large chemical company I know of, the supervisors of the laboratory assistants were theoretically responsible for their training and evaluation. These functions, however, had come to be performed in a routine, insubstantial fashion. After the job enrichment program, during which the supervisors were not merely passive observers of the assistants' performance, the supervisors actually were devoting their time to reviewing performance and administering thorough training.

What has been called an employee-centered style of supervision will come about not through education of supervisions, but by changing the jobs that they do.

Concluding Note

Job enrichment will not be a one-time proposition, but a continuous managment function. The initial changes, however, should last for a very long period of time. There are a number of reasons for this:

- The changes should bring the job up to the level of challenge commensurate with the skill that was hired.
- Those who have still more ability eventually will be able to demonstrate it better and win promotion to higher-level jobs.
- The very nature of motivators, as opposed to hygiene factors, is that they have a much longer-term effect on employees' attitudes. Perhaps the job will have to be enriched again, but this will not occur as frequently as the need for hygiene.

Not all jobs can be enriched, nor do all jobs need to be enriched. If only a small percentage of the time and money that is now devoted to hygiene, however, were given to job enrichment efforts, the return in human satisfaction and economic gain would be one of the largest dividends that industry and society have ever reaped through their efforts at better personnel management.

The argument for job enrichment can be summed up quite simply: If you have someone on a job, use him. If you can't use him on the job, get rid of him, either via automation or by selecting someone with lesser ability. If you can't use him and you can't get rid of him, you will have a motivation problem.

Source: Reprinted with permission of *Harvard Business Review*. From "One More Time: How to Motivate Employees" by F. Herzberg, Sept./Oct. 1987. © 1987 by the Harvard Business School Publishing Corporation, all rights reserved.

CHAPTER TWENTY-FIVE

Morale

CHAPTER OBJECTIVES

After you have studied this chapter, you should be able to do the following:

1. Discuss the supervisor's role in motivation and leadership and its bearing on the morale of subordinates.

2. Provide a basis for understanding the factors influencing morale.

3. Discuss the relationships among morale, retention, and productivity.

4. Discuss common techniques to assess and improve morale.

U NDERSTANDING THE supervisor's role in motivation and leadership has much bearing on the *morale* of the subordinates. Some writers do not speak of morale of the individual but refer to job satisfaction, emphasizing the satisfaction of needs. Others stress the social aspects of groups and friendships, and some are particularly concerned with attitudes toward coworkers, the organization, and supervision. Many writers link satisfaction with the needs and attitudes of an individual, whereas morale pertains to the spirit of a group. Although this distinction is precise, it is largely academic because the factors and methods used in measuring group morale are usually the same as those used in measuring an individual's satisfaction.

Although there are many definitions for morale, a particularly useful one is to describe it as a state of mind and emotion affecting the attitudes, feelings, and sentiments of individuals and groups toward their work, environment, administration, and colleagues. Morale is the total satisfaction a person derives from the job, work group, boss, the institution, and the environment. "Morale pertains to the general feeling of well-being, satisfaction, and happiness of people" (Beach 1985). When morale is high, the employees are likely to strive hard to accomplish the objectives of the enterprise; conversely, low morale is likely to prevent or deter them from doing this.

THE NATURE OF MORALE

Supervisors often make the mistake of speaking of morale as something that is either present or absent among their employees. Morale is always present, and by itself has neither a favorable nor unfavorable meaning. Morale can range from excellent and positive, through many intermediate degrees, to poor and completely negative. If the attitude of the subordinates is poor, the morale is also poor. If the subordinates are highly motivated to strive hard for the best possible patient care, their morale is high. Employees with high morale find satisfaction in their position in the enterprise, have confidence in their own and in their associates' abilities, and show enthusiasm and a strong desire to cooperate in achieving the healthcare organization's objectives.

One cannot order employees to have high morale. It can only be created by introducing certain conditions into the work setting that are favorable to its development. High morale is not the result of good supervision and human relations. Rather, it is the result of good motivation, respect and dignity for the individual, realization of individual differences, good leadership, effective communication, participation, counseling, and many other human resources practices. In other words, the state of morale reflects how appropriately and effectively the administration practices good human relations and good supervision.

THE LEVEL OF MORALE

Every manager, from the CEO to the supervisor, should be concerned with the level of morale in the organization. A good supervisor knows it is a supervisory function to promote and maintain the morale of the subordinates at as high a level as possible. The immediate supervisor in day-to-day contact with the employees influences and determines the level of morale more than anyone else. Raising morale to a high level and sustaining it is a long-term project and cannot be achieved solely on the basis of short-term devices such as pep talks or contests. The supervisor will also find that although good morale is slow to develop and difficult to maintain, it can change quickly from good to bad. The level of morale varies considerably from day to day and is far more changeable than the weather.

Bad morale can contribute to staff turnover. Turnover, as we have discussed in prior chapters, can be costly to the organization. The key to keeping employees is to ensure that they have been fully oriented to their new jobs and the department. The orientation is their first introduction to the culture of the department; this is where they become part of the "family." The depth and warmth with which the orientation program is conducted sets the stage for the employee's bond to the department. A good orientation program provides employees with enough information to do their jobs effectively and encourages an open dialog for employees to share ideas about their assignments and work processes. Building confidence and competence in new employees pays for itself in the long run by reducing service errors or patient complaints. The program should acquaint the employees with the history of the organization, a clear view of how their department fits into the organization, and how their jobs contribute to the department's objectives. Your orientation program goal must be to make your employees never want to leave.

No one ever wants to leave a positive and light-hearted environment. You can retain employees by teaching them how to do their jobs well, appreciating their input and ideas, and building high morale by keeping them happy and productive. Keeping humor in the workplace allows everyone to set aside his or her concerns, even if momentarily. Creating an environment that is fun goes a long way toward retaining employees and getting work done. Humor also reduces stress. When staff is less stressed, they are willing to go the extra mile for you. To foster a fun environment, post appropriate jokes and stories throughout the department. Remember, the jokes should not criticize work, management, or the worker. Instead of casual days, spice up the environment with theme days, such as Hawaiian Day or Roaring 20s Day.

Morale is contagious. The higher the degree of individual satisfaction of group members, the higher is the morale of the entire group. This in turn tends to raise the overall level of morale even higher because individuals derive personal satisfaction from being in a high-morale group. Although favorable attitudes spread, unfavorable attitudes among employees spread even more quickly. It seems to be human nature to forget the good quickly and remember the bad (see Exhibit 25.1) (Kelly 1998).

Management is not alone in its desire for a satisfactory level of morale. Each employee of the institution is likewise concerned because bad morale is simply not as satisfying as good morale. A state of bad morale creates an unpleasant environment for the employees of the healthcare organization, and they have as much at stake as the administration. Good morale, on the other hand, makes the employee's day at work a pleasurable and satisfying experience and not a misery. High morale is also important to the patient and the patient's family. They quickly sense whether the employees are operating on a high or low level of morale, and they respond accordingly. What then determines the level of morale?

FACTORS INFLUENCING MORALE

Because morale is a composite of feelings, sentiments, attitudes, satisfaction, well-being, and happiness, almost anything can influence the morale of the employees. Some of these factors are within the control of the supervisor, whereas others are not. Although there are countless morale determinants, we can divide them into two broad groups: (1) those factors that arise primarily from situations external to the institution and (2) those factors that originate mainly within the realm of the supervisor's activities. Many factors were discussed in Chapter 23; examples of both broad groups appear in the Deloitte & Touche survey results shown in Figure 25.1.

Figure 25.1: Decreased Employee Morale

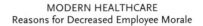

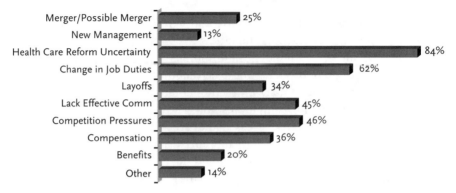

MODERN HEALTHCARE
Reasons for Decreased Employee Morale

Merger/Possible Merger	25%
New Management	13%
Health Care Reform Uncertainty	84%
Change in Job Duties	62%
Layoffs	34%
Lack Effective Comm	45%
Competition Pressures	46%
Compensation	36%
Benefits	20%
Other	14%

Source: Deloitte & Touche LLP—Human Resources Strategies Group, Member of ABC Consulting, Hospital Human Resource Survey—1995.

External Factors

External factors affecting morale—those connected with events and influences outside the work environment and institution—are generally beyond the scope of the supervisor's control. Although they are external in origin, these factors nevertheless concern the supervisor, as everyone takes his or her problems to work and does not check them in the morning at the organization's door or leave them in the car. Examples of external factors are family problems, financial worries, national disasters, car troubles, or a sickness in the family. Consider the impact on morale of those working at the local hospital when the only large employer in town, a mining company employing more than 35 percent of the town, closes or if a large insurer's national billing office outsources its operations to India. What happens away from the job may change the employee's feelings quickly; an argument before leaving home or an accident on the highway causing a long delay may set the emotional tone for the rest of the day. The morning news may be depressing, or it may produce high morale. Clearly, there are many contributors to morale.

In an article in *CIO Magazine,* a CIO offers this insight: "What you need to understand about morale is this: The mood of your employees can be brought down by external factors, such as the state of the economy, but it is your leadership skills—or lack thereof—that will tip the morale scales one way or the other. In tough times such as these, the people you are responsible for are looking for support, leadership and reassurance. If you ignore or underestimate that need, you'll have a morale problem on your hands. Lack of communication and bad management, or lack of confidence in management, are the two biggest causes of low morale" (Kaplan 2005).

The supervisor can indirectly deal with these external factors primarily by communicating honestly and conducting a nondirective counseling interview, as discussed in chapters 21 and 23. The supervisor should try to sense such factors; often they are reflected in the work behavior of the subordinates. If something has happened to lower an employee's morale and if the supervisor is familiar with the cause, he or she should try to get the employee to forget the incident as quickly as possible by supplying an antidote. One of the best ways to help an employee get past a depressing incident is to encourage the employee to talk about it freely. Aside from a nondirective counseling interview and keeping staff abreast of organizational changes that are being implemented to support them through challenging times, however, a supervisor can do little else to counteract outside factors affecting morale. The supervisor must remember that he or she or the institution itself is not the sole cause of shifts in the level of morale.

In recent years, many organizations have developed what is called *employee assistance programs* (EAPs). These are staffed by professional social workers and medical and counseling personnel who are trained in providing confidential, professional assistance to employees and their families. Some programs may also regularly use the services of an outside clinic. The purpose of the employee assistance program is to help employees who have personal problems that may interfere with attendance and job performance; whether this counterproductive behavior is the result of work, home, or outside pressures is irrelevant. Some of the more common problems are caused by alcoholism, drug dependency, financial worries, marriage or family difficulties, stress, and poor health. An employee can seek out this support on his or her own; often supervisors refer an employee to this program, or the referral might come from a medical person or from the union.

Several other techniques that have become popular with organizations to help combat these external pressures, improve morale, and reduce turnover include offering flexible work hours, shared paid-time-off (PTO) banks, and telecommuting opportunities. These programs speak to the employee need to balance external and internal needs—family time and work time. They also help to combat the stress that comes with a fast-paced world that forces us to respond instantaneously to e-mails, faxes, and electronic calendars. Flexible work hours allow individuals to schedule their workweek around other obligations common in dual-career families such as taking children to sporting events or aging parents to their physicians. In 1999, Singer reported that nearly eight in ten major firms offered flextime. However, flextime offerings have dropped to 26 percent according to Baker.[1] This reduction in a perceived "benefit" has been more than offset by the 81 percent of the firms that offer telecommuniting (Baker 2005). Similarly, Singer reported that two out of three offer opportunities to work part time. This option dropped to 23 percent in 2004, but at the same time, 64 percent of the firms reported work-at-home options (Baker 2005). Baker's study did not provide information on job sharing, but Singer reported that four in ten permit job sharing (Singer 1999). PTO banks permit employees to decide when and how the time is used; shared PTO banks allow employees to donate their excess time to a shared bank that can be tapped by coworkers when emergent needs arise. These banks allow the employee to use the time to pay for hours used to attend to personal and family matters, but by doing so, the employee may be left with little or no paid time for vacations. Some of the benefits of telecommuting have already been discussed in prior chapters. Each of these approaches allows the employee to make decisions about his or her work environment, a feature that can certainly contribute to positive morale.

Internal Factors

Many important factors that affect the morale of employees fall within the realm of the supervisor's activities. These include incentives, working conditions, and, above all, the quality of supervision. When considering incentives, the first thing that comes to mind is pay. Making the work environment appealing is the responsibility of all managers. Employees want to feel important and be recognized for what they do for the organization. We have already discussed simple recognition tools such as certificates or a pat on the back for a job well done. This type of incentive program is offered in more than half of the managed care organizations that responded to the 1999 Hay Managed Care Compensation Survey. If the organizational culture supports these techniques, it also may support the establishment of incentive plans. Plans that are productivity based are commonly used in the laundry and health information departments where measurable output, such as pounds of laundry and lines typed, can be objectively measured. Incentive plans reward employees financially, and payments can be based on one's measured performance, such as a laundry worker's pounds of washed laundry, or for an individual's noteworthy accomplishment, such as obtaining certification in respiratory therapy or having a perfect attendance record.

Merit bonuses are a type of incentive program. These bonuses are a flat amount paid in additional to or in lieu of a salary increase. They may vary from one individual to another because they are based on an individual's performance. Some organizations offer organization-wide bonuses for staff. This may be a one-time bonus for achieving an organizational goal such as JCAHO accreditation without any recommendations, or it could be a year-end distribution following favorable financial performance. Finally, incentive-type programs may be based on team performance. This type of program encourages teamwork and may promote peer pressure if a team member is slacking in his or her duties. The Mercer 2001 compensation survey reported that 46 percent of healthcare providers offered short-term incentive plans. Of the hourly clinical and technical staffs, 25 to 27 percent participated in these plans. Of the plans offered, 19 to 24 percent were individual based and 12 to 14 percent were team based.

Incentive programs can be applied in virtually all departments. Developing a plan is not easy and must be well thought out. Management must gather data on employees' performance, track the performance for a reasonable period of time, and set an acceptable goal for the staff to pursue. The published results of an integrated incentive plan, including physicians and hospital surgical staff, demonstrated improved on-time case starts, decreased turnaround time, improved physician satisfaction, and reduced RN and surgical technologist turnover; it also provided staff recognition for aligning their efforts to achieve organization goals (Poole 2004).

However, incentive plans do not need to be complex. In the admitting area the goal might be a reduction in registration errors; in patient financial services it could be a reduction in the days in accounts receivable; and for a patient care area, it could be based on a safety issue such as a reduction in patient falls or needle sticks. Organization-wide, administration could set an incentive goal of increasing patient satisfaction based on the results of patient surveys or cost reduction without sacrificing quality or customer satisfaction. The supervisor's role in developing an incentive plan includes setting targets that are attainable and specific and having appropriate controls in place to avoid any negative patient satisfaction. If employees do not perceive the rewards as meaningful or fair, the plan will fail. Wages are exceedingly important, but aside from wages and fringe benefits, many other aspects are essential to the employee.

Pay-for-performance programs recognize employees for outstanding performance but may discourage others who are unable to achieve targets. Thus, whereas such programs may improve morale of some, they could definitely destroy the morale of others. Other programs demonstrating management's interest in the welfare of its employees are stress-reduction programs, health-risk appraisals, onsite immunization programs, onsite fitness facilities, sponsored athletics, prenatal programs, and well-baby programs. A very nontraditional benefit offered to some employees today is nap time during the workday. According to a poll by the National Sleep Foundation, 27 percent of adults surveyed are sleepy at work two days per week or more, 19 percent made errors at work because of sleepiness, and 2 percent sustained injury as a result of sleepiness (Gemignani 2000). Consider what such a benefit may yield in safety improvements. However, many believe that the most important benefit that an organization can offer its employees, while at the same time boosting morale, is training. It solidifies a sense of commitment between you and your employees at a time when you are most likely asking them to do more with less.

According to Spath (2002), every supervisor is "responsible for ensuring that department personnel are competent. *Competence* is defined as the demonstrated ability to apply knowledge and skills and involves four elements: education, training, skills, and experience. To ensure that people are competent to perform their jobs, it is important they receive proper training that meets the needs of the department and the staff." Known as competency-based training, this approach focuses attention on the employee and his or her job. The employee benefits from better understanding of the job duties and recognizes that the organization is interested in his or her success. The organization benefits because the employee gains the competence needed to achieve the goals of the department.

Considerations such as job security, interesting work, good working conditions, appreciation of a job well done, skill building, chance for advancement, recognition, and prompt and fair treatment of grievances are all necessary components of a high-morale environment (see Chapter 23). Although reasonable monetary incentives may be provided and the quality of supervision is high, morale can still sink quickly if, for example, working conditions are neglected.

One such change that has been highly accepted is casual day. A simple change to working conditions that permits employees to wear jeans every Friday as casual-day attire may both increase the comfort level and reduce an employee's out-of-pocket expenses for dry cleaning. More than 60 percent of human resources professionals say their organizations allow casual dress at least once a week (Perry 2000). As this practice became more prevalent, supervisors found themselves in the position of clothes cop because some employees took advantage of the casual environment. In some cases, the informal atmosphere encouraged a lax attitude toward work and an increase in flirtatious behavior (Perry 2000). Because of these circumstances, some of those same organizations have returned to standard form of business wear and in some organizations, the employees bucked the trend by dressing up rather than down on casual day (Perry 2000). The majority of people who work full time in an office setting have a dress code, according to a BizRate Research study, with just 26 percent allowed to don casual work attire. Most—64 percent—work under a business casual requirement.[2] However, we should not expect a return to the 1950s workplace attire requirement of wearing jackets and ties for men and dresses for women. The important factor is that an honest attempt is made to improve working conditions whenever possible.

Finally, recall the Hawthorne studies. Morale may be affected by the simplest of things. If the employee group is more mature, brighter but diffused lighting and matte surfaces to reduce glare are appreciated. Less noise and warm colors may reduce stress. Thus, simply changing light bulbs and adding a coat of paint may do wonders for improving morale. In many cases, employees work under undesirable conditions and still maintain high morale as long as the supervisor has made a serious effort to correct the conditions.

The Supervisor's Role

Aside from these on-the-job factors that influence morale, the most significant influence is exercised by supervisors in their immediate, day-to-day relationships with employees. The supervisor's overall manner of supervision, directing, leadership, interpersonal skills, and general attitude more than anything else make for good or bad morale. Employees put forth their best efforts when given an opportunity to satisfy their needs through work they enjoy and at the same time to contribute to achieving departmental objectives. Such job satisfaction raises and keeps morale at a high level. It can only be maintained if the supervisor tells the employees how significantly they contribute to the overall goals of the healthcare organization and how their work fits into the overall effort.

Morale can also be maintained if the boss gives them a feeling of accomplishment in their work and allows them to be on their own as much as possible. The supervisor who practices democratic supervision, as discussed in previous chapters, and who "practices what he preaches" is likely to reduce the undesirable features of a job and create an environment in which the employees derive genuine satisfaction from the work they do every day. In addition, the supervisor should not forget the importance of social satisfaction on the job. The employees should have an opportunity to develop friendships and work as a team. In other words, one must not forget the positive contributions that informal groups and informal organization make.

The supervisor should bear in mind that the employees' morale is affected not only by what the supervisor does but also by how it is done. If the supervisor's behavior indicates a feeling of superiority to the employees or the supervisor is suspicious of the employees' motives and actions, only a low level of morale can result. The supervisor should not forget how little it takes to make one's own spirits rise or fall. A word of appreciation from the boss or administrator can change the supervisor's outlook toward the whole work setting. He or she will become more cheerful, and in all likelihood so will the employees.

One may think of this as a mirror effect. If the hospital vice president commends the department director on successfully completing a major project, such as preparing for a JCAHO visit, the director will probably mirror the vice president's actions with those departmental supervisors who participated in accomplishing the project. The supervisors will then most likely mirror the director and share their appreciation with their line staff.

Similarly, attitudes beget similar attitudes. If the supervisor shows worry, the employees tend to follow suit. If he or she becomes angry, others become angry. When the supervisor appears confident in the operation of the department, employees react accordingly and believe that things are going well. This does not mean that the supervisor should only see the good side of departmental operations and refuse to acknowledge difficulties and troubles. The supervisor should show the employees that as a leader he or she has the situation well in hand and that if anything goes wrong, he or she will give them an opportunity to correct the situation and prevent it from happening again.

THE EFFECTS OF MORALE

The question arises as to how high or low morale affects other variables such as turnover, absenteeism, the rate of accidents, teamwork, and productivity. Much research has been done in this area, and some general conclusions can be drawn from it. For example, high morale is moderately related to lower employee turnover. Probably the same holds true for a lowered rate of absenteeism. Furthermore, higher morale most likely also leads to other desirable consequences such as fewer grievances, better mental and physical health, faster learning of new tasks, and possibly a lowered rate of accidents or care errors, although some apparent results have no relation whatsoever to high or low morale. The following considers some other consequences.

Morale and Teamwork

The term teamwork is often associated with morale, but the two terms do not have the same meaning. Morale applies to the attitudes of the employees in the department, whereas teamwork is the smoothly coordinated and synchronized activity achieved by a small, closely knit group of employees. Although good morale is usually helpful in achieving teamwork, it is possible for teamwork to be high, yet morale low. Such a situation could exist in times when jobs are scarce and when the employees put up with close and tight supervision for fear of losing their jobs. Also, teamwork may be absent even though morale is high; in such a case the employee, a solo performer, probably prefers individual effort and finds satisfaction in his or her own job performance.

Morale and Productivity

It is generally assumed that high morale is automatically accompanied by high productivity. Supervisors believe that as long as the morale of employees is high, their output will be correspondingly high. Moreover, some research evidence backs up the contention that there is a small but positive relationship between overall morale or job satisfaction and productivity (Beach 1985). Every supervisor also believes, based on personal experience, that a highly motivated, self-disciplined group of employees consistently does a more satisfactory job than a group whose morale is low. Therefore, supervisors should do everything possible to keep morale high so that the department's performance remains high.

However, many studies show that this general statement does not hold true in all situations. There is proof that the morale-productivity relationship can appear in many forms: low morale and high productivity, high morale and low productivity, high morale and high productivity, and low morale and low productivity. In fact, in the third quarter of 2003, the productivity of American workers grew at a rate of 9.4 percent, the best it had been since mid-1983. However, at the same time employees experienced higher levels of stress and burnout, costing the U.S. economy $344 billion a year; Harris Poll data reflected lower morale reported by 27 percent of the employees surveyed (Ceridian Corporation 2005). Much depends on other factors such as the economic situation, the rewards, the job market, and the mechanical pace of the job. Thus, a supervisor cannot automatically depend on the positive relationship between morale and productivity; however, this is still a controversial issue.

ASSESSING CURRENT MORALE

It is important for management to be familiar with the extent of job satisfaction or dissatisfaction of the employees. Much of the foregoing discussion has assumed that the level of morale is measurable, but one should realize that morale cannot be measured directly. Nevertheless, suitable indirect ways and means exist for determining the prevailing level of morale and its trends. Although some supervisors pride themselves on their ability to detect intuitively low or high morale, the wise supervisor would do better to approach this problem more systematically in either of two ways. One approach is through observation of activities, events, trends, and changes; the other method is to use what is usually referred to as attitude, opinion, or morale surveys. The *Journal of Accountancy* (2001) stated that when conducting a survey of employees, one of the best questions is, "What keeps you from doing your job as well as you would like to?" It not only invites employees to focus on their specific area of knowledge and expertise, it gives them an opportunity to disclose how well they really want to do the job.

Observation

Observation is a tool that involves watching people and their reactions. Although this tool is available to every supervisor, it is often not fully utilized. If the supervisor does observe the employees consciously and systematically, however, their level of morale and major changes in it can be appraised. The manager should watch the subordinates' behavior and listen to what they have to say; he or she should observe their actions and notice any changes in their willingness to cooperate. The supervisor probably finds it fairly easy to recognize through observation the extremes of high and low morale. Finer means of measurement, however, may be required to differentiate among the intermediate degrees. Personal observation can be used for obvious manifestations of morale, such as a facial expression or a shrug of the shoulder; but often these signs are difficult to interpret. It is also difficult to determine how far from normal the behavior must be to indicate a shift in morale. Thus, it takes an extremely sensitive supervisor to conclude correctly from such indicators that a change in morale has occurred or is currently taking place.

Moreover, the supervisor may not be able to make the detailed observations necessary for accurate morale appraisal. Although the closeness of the day-to-day working relationship usually offers much opportunity for supervisors to become aware of morale changes, they are often so burdened with work that they do not have time to look, or if they do look, they do not actually see. At times they may even be afraid to look for fear of what they might find. Although some supervisors may realize that changes are taking place, they are frequently inclined to ignore them. Only later, after a change in the level of morale is openly manifested, will they recall the first indications and admit to noticing them but not giving them much thought at the time.

To avoid such situations, the supervisor must take care not to conveniently brush aside any indicators. The most serious shortcoming of using observation as a yardstick to measure current morale is that when the events causing the low morale are recognized, the change has probably already occurred. The supervisor, therefore, should be extremely keen in his or her observation to do as much as possible to prevent such changes before they take place, or to quickly counteract them if they have already begun. The closer the supervisor's relationship with the employees, the more sensitive he or she is to these changes and the more quickly he or she can act.

Attitude Surveys

The other approach to assessing current morale is the use of attitude surveys, also called opinion or morale surveys. Many institutions use attitude surveys as a way of finding out how employees view their jobs, coworkers, benefits, wages, working conditions, quality of services, supervisors, the institution as a whole, and specific policies. Such a survey is a valuable diagnostic tool for management to assess employee problems. It is like taking the pulse of the organization (York 1985). Surveys provide the most accurate indicators of the organization's human resources, as well as valuable upward communication, because they allow employees to express their feelings about their jobs. As a result, administration is aware of the general level of satisfaction in the institution and which specific areas cause dissatisfaction. The attitude survey shows employees that management is truly concerned and at the same time gives them an opportunity to vent their opinions. This in itself improves morale.

For surveys to be meaningful, however, administration must be committed to this undertaking. This means that management must be willing to invest effort, time, and money. Administration must be willing to follow through with action based on the results of the survey and be ready to communicate the major findings of the survey to the employees. Such a survey requires careful planning and professional development. Unless the institution's human resources department is large and has in-house professionals trained and experienced in attitude surveys, it is advisable to hire an outside consultant. This ensures a well-designed instrument with appropriate validity, reliability, sampling, and statistical methods. The employees may have more confidence in an outside consultant's work than in their own personnel department doing the job. An outside consultant could also help in deciding whether a standardized survey, a customized one, or a combination of the two would be most appropriate.

Administering the Survey

Expressions of employees' opinions are requested in the form of answers to written questionnaires. These questionnaires must be prepared with great care and much thought. A good attitude survey measures the major variables of organizational life, such as leadership, supervision, administration, job satisfaction, job conditions and work environment, coworkers, pay, benefits and rewards, job security, advancement, and stress. The questionnaire should be written at a level appropriate for most of the employees. A cover letter from the CEO should accompany the questionnaire, encouraging the employees' participation and stressing the confidential and anonymous nature of the employees' involvement.

In a healthcare organization, attitude surveys can cover the entire organization. At times, it is appropriate to limit the survey to only one large department, such as nursing services, which usually accounts for half of all the employees. Full-scale attitude surveys should not be given in less than approximately three-year intervals; this allows enough time to indicate significant attitude changes.

Once an institution-wide survey is decided on, the administrator and all other managers must be prepared to endure criticism because dissatisfactions are likely to be expressed. More importantly, however, management must be prepared and willing to act on the complaints once they are revealed. Until the survey is taken, management can always plead ignorance, but after a survey, everyone knows that the administration has heard about the problems causing dissatisfaction. It is hoped that some of the complaints can be adjusted; at least a serious and honest effort must now be made. If the administration is not prepared or willing to act, it is far better not to take surveys: if management asks the employees for their input and ideas and fails to take action, the employees will avoid expressing themselves in the future.

Questionnaires submitted to employees come in a variety of types. Two general forms are used most often. According to the format of the question asked, one can distinguish between objective surveys and descriptive surveys. An objective questionnaire (see Figure 25.2) asks the question and offers a choice of answers; there can be multiple choice or true and false questions. In objective surveys, the employees mark the one answer that comes closest to their feelings. In a descriptive survey, the question is asked, but the employees answer freely in their own words and ways. Because many employees may have difficulty expressing their opinions in writing or may not want to take the time to write out answers, the best results are usually obtained on a form that enables the employees to check the box that seems to provide the most appropriate answer for them.

The survey forms can be filled out on the job or at home. Although there are many advantages to filling out questionnaires at home, a high percentage of them are never returned. It is better to have more meaningful answers, however, even if the number of replies is smaller. Some organizations are concerned that the rate of returned surveys might be low and prefer to distribute and collect the surveys the same day during working hours. The employees complete the survey forms on the premises and on company time. This procedure is likely to maximize the number of completed surveys.

Regardless of whether they are filled out on the job or at home, care must be taken that the questionnaires remain unsigned and that the replies cannot be personally identified. Respondents must be assured that the replies will be kept confidential. Employees are sometimes suspicious of the institution's motives, and they may respond in ways they believe the institution wants. Therefore, it is essential that no individual identification information appears on the survey. However, it may be necessary to ask the employees to identify their work group or to identify their department so management can focus its response to the source of the concern.

Analyzing the Results

Once the forms have been filled out, the results must be analyzed (see Figure 25.3). Even if the survey is well designed, organized, and properly conducted, it can lead to failure if it is improperly or superficially analyzed. The manner in which the data are analyzed is critical for the success of the survey. Only proper analysis will ensure that management gets a clear picture of the results so that the real problems are addressed by action and appropriate solutions. A misdiagnosis of the survey results will lead to ineffective solutions.

A discussion of statistical approaches and concepts such as segmenting the survey, cluster analysis, and so forth is beyond the scope of this book. Briefly, the analysis must be thorough, and instead of simple, straight-run statistics, it should produce more meaningful interpretations. For example, the interaction of organizational and demographic variables must be examined in relation to attitudes. Instead of simply stating that 65 percent of the subordinates have frequent communication with their boss and 35 percent do not, or that 75 percent of the respondents like their jobs and 25 percent do not, it is better to state that of the 75 percent who like their jobs, 85 percent have frequent contact with their boss and 15 percent do not. At the same time, one can learn that among the 25 percent who do not care for their jobs, 55 percent claim that they have infrequent communication with their superiors. Also, for example, the results may determine whether females are more or less satisfied than males, young more than older employees, and so forth.

After a meaningful analysis and interpretation of the survey have been done, the results are presented to the top-level executive team. Then each executive will meet with his or her line managers to analyze and evaluate the survey results. Plans for action to correct the problems that surfaced should be formulated in these meetings. This process then moves downward throughout the hierarchy, first to all supervisors. Then the results of attitude surveys are used as discussion material with the rank-and-file employees in workshop meetings.

Besides this feedback of results to those who filled out the questionnaires, attitude surveys provide top-level administration, department heads, and supervisors with information to guide them in their overall efforts to improve morale. The surveys will reveal certain deficiencies, and specific actions should be taken to rectify them. For example, the questionnaire may show an overwhelming interest in and need for a childcare center where young children are cared for during their parents' working hours. This obviously is an area of dissatisfaction, and administration should take immediate and specific action. Occasionally, however, the results of initial surveys are not so clear. They may raise many

EMPLOYEE OPINION SURVEY
Anytown Health Center
Anytown, USA

Your employer is interested in your opinions and feelings about your work. This survey is one way to obtain your input about various aspects of your work. You should answer the questionnaire items honestly and frankly because it is totally **anonymous and confidential**. No one but you will know how you answered the question items. There are four parts to this survey. After you have completed one part, proceed to the next one until you have completed all four parts. After you have finished all four parts, place this completed form in the locked box at the front of this room and return your materials to the person administering the survey.

The results of this survey will be discussed with you at a later date by your supervisor and/or area manager.

PART B

The following statements concern specific aspects of the organization and your job here. Indicate your level of agreement with each statement by filling in the bubble to the right of the statement. Possible responses are:

1 = Strongly Agree	4 = Slightly Disagree
2 = Moderately Agree	5 = Moderately Disagree
3 = Slightly Agree	6 = Strongly Disagree

For example, if you "moderately agree" with a statement, you would fill in the bubble marked ② under the column marked Moderately Agree.

Again, your answers are anonymous and confidential, so please feel free to answer honestly.

	Strongly Agree	Moderately Agree	Slightly Agree	Slightly Disagree	Moderately Disagree	Strongly Disagree
1 I am proud to work for this organization.	①	②	③	④	⑤	⑥
2 I understand how the success of my department is measured.	①	②	③	④	⑤	⑥
3 My supervisor gives me clear working instructions.	①	②	③	④	⑤	⑥
4 Efficiency is highly valued in my department.	①	②	③	④	⑤	⑥
5 My department head sets clear goals for our department.	①	②	③	④	⑤	⑥
6 Communications among shifts in this organization are good.	①	②	③	④	⑤	⑥
7 I would have to make a bad mistake to be removed from my present position in this organization.	①	②	③	④	⑤	⑥
8 Employee promotions are handled fairly in this organization.	①	②	③	④	⑤	⑥
9 Compared to similar jobs in the community, I feel that I am paid fairly.	①	②	③	④	⑤	⑥
10 The organization's top management will use the information from this survey to make improvements.	①	②	③	④	⑤	⑥
11 My department head does a good job of running this department.	①	②	③	④	⑤	⑥
12 My job is challenging enough to suit me.	①	②	③	④	⑤	⑥
13 I am satisfied with this organization's sick leave policy.	①	②	③	④	⑤	⑥
14 I am happy with my current workload.	①	②	③	④	⑤	⑥
15 My supervisor discusses my productivity with me.	①	②	③	④	⑤	⑥
16 In my department, employees are well utilized.	①	②	③	④	⑤	⑥
17 My supervisor does a good job of running my area.	①	②	③	④	⑤	⑥
18 Absenteeism is no problem in my department.	①	②	③	④	⑤	⑥

Source: Management Science Associates, Inc. © 1997, Independence, MO.

questions, and sometimes additional surveys are required to probe deeper. Survey techniques and analyses are becoming more and more sophisticated, and with their help management should be able to arrive at a solution to almost any morale problem that arises.

MANAGEMENT SCIENCE ASSOCIATES, INC.
Measure of Organizational Health Prepared for:
Anytown Community Hospital
Anytown, USA

Norm Group: National Norms

Date of Survey: 1 /97

Organization Total

Number of Respondents: 1314

Attitude Area/Question	Ind. Norm	Org. Norm	% Diff.	Very Pos. 1	Mod Pos. 2	Slgt Pos 3	Slgt Neg 4	Mod Neg 5	Very Neg 6	# Resp.
A. JOB SATISFACTION	2.2	2.3	-2							
1. Proud to Work for Hospital	1.7	1.6	2	56%	31%	9%	2%	1%	1%	1314
2. Job is Challenging	2.1	2.1	0	41%	32%	13%	7%	4%	3%	1310
3. Feeling of Satisfaction	2.6	2.8	-4	17%	32%	25%	12%	7%	6%	1313
4. Opportunity to Use My Abilities	2.5	2.6	-2	23%	34%	22%	11%	5%	5%	1295
B. JOB MOBILITY	3.2	3.4	-4							
1. Opportunities to Transfer	3.0	3.2	-4	13%	24%	25%	14%	11%	13%	1268
2. Chances for Advancement	3.4	3.7	-6	7%	16%	25%	23%	14%	15%	1288
C. ADMIN/SR MANAGEMENT	3.0	3.0	0							
1. Resolves Employee Complaints	3.3	3.4	-2	8%	20%	29%	19%	11%	12%	1257
2. Overall Management of Hospital	2.8	2.7	2	16%	35%	25%	13%	6%	4%	1284
3. Interest in Employees	3.2	3.2	0	14%	22%	24%	18%	11%	12%	1287
4. Communicates Hospital Objectives	2.7	2.7	0	18%	29%	30%	14%	5%	4%	1302
5. Use of Survey by Administration	2.9	3.1	-4	16%	25%	26%	13%	9%	11%	1299
D. DEPARTMENT HEAD	2.6	2.7	-2					6%		
1. Understand How Dept/Unit Success Meas.	2.5	2.7	-4	20%	34%	23%	13%	8%	5%	1303
2. Sets Clear Goals for Department/Unit	2.6	2.7	-2	24%	28%	21%	13%	9%	6%	1301
3. Good Job of Running Department/ Unit	2.6	2.6	0	28%	28%	19%	9%		7%	1305
E. SUPERVISION	2.7	2.9	-4							
1. Gives Clear Instructions	2.3	2.4	-2	31%	32%	17%	9%	6%	4%	1306
2. Overall Management of Area	2.5	2.6	-2	32%	25%	16%	8%	9%	9%	1302
3. Handling Complaints	2.9	3.2	-6	20%	22%	18%	14%	9%	16%	1298
4. Administering Discipline	3.0	3.2	-4	18%	23%	20%	15%	11%	14%	1283
5. Feel Free to Tell What I Think	2.6	2.7	-2	33%	24%	16%	8%	8%	12%	1305
6. Does Not Play Favorites	3.0	3.2	-4	23%	22%	15%	12%	8%	19%	1299
7. Discusses Productivity with Me	2.7	2.7	0	28%	26%	19%	11%	8%	8%	1305
8. Communications with Employees	2.8	3.0	-4	21%	27%	19%	12%	8%	13%	1303
F. COMMUNICATIONS	3.3	3.3	0							
1. Among Departments	3.5	3.4	2	6%	19%	31%	23%	13%	8%	1289
2. Among Shifts	3.2	3.1	2	9%	29%	28%	15%	9%	8%	1251
G. PERSONNEL/HR POLICIES	3.0	2.9	2							
1. Administered Consistently	3.0	2.9	2	13%	33%	25%	14%	8%	7%	1273
2. Fairness of Promotion Policies	3.2	3.2	0	9%	27%	27%	16%	11%	10%	1273
3. Satisfied with Personnel Policies	2.7	2.6	2	16%	40%	25%	11%	5%	4%	1292
H. JOB SECURITY	2.6	3.1	-10							
1. Takes a Lot to Lose Job	2.6	3.0	-8	22%	23%	21%	14%	10%	10%	1300
2. Feeling of Security	2.7	3.2	-10	16%	25%	21%	15%	10%	13%	1307
3. I Can Be Sure of a Job	2.5	3.1	-12	20%	26%	17%	14%	11%	12%	1309

Source: © 1997, Management Science Associates, Inc., Independence, MO

SUMMARY

Morale is a state of mind and emotion affecting the attitudes, feelings, and sentiments of groups of employees and individuals toward their work environment, colleagues, supervision, and the enterprise as a whole. Morale is always present, and it can range from high to low. The level of morale varies considerably from day to day. Morale is contagious; that is, favorable attitudes spread quickly, and unfavorable attitudes spread even more quickly. High morale is not only the concern of the supervisor; the employees are just as interested in a satisfactory level of morale. Moreover, the effect of high or low morale is felt not only by insiders but also by outsiders such as patients and visitors.

Morale can be influenced by many factors, which can be classified into two broad groups: those factors affecting the employee's activities that arise outside the enterprise and those factors originating within the job environment. The supervisor can do little to directly change the effects of outside factors on the subordinates' morale, but many internal factors, such as incentives, working conditions, and quality of work life, are within the supervisor's power to control. These factors, coupled with an attentive supervisor, willing to listen to employee concerns, can be used to significantly raise the level of subordinates' morale. If the supervisor succeeds in maintaining high morale, good teamwork and increased productivity will likely result. Research indicates that some interesting correlations exist between morale and productivity, turnover, and absenteeism.

An astute supervisor can sense changes in the level of morale by keenly observing the subordinates, but this is difficult. Often supervisors do not realize that a change has taken place until performance has been detrimentally affected. Attitude surveys are primarily used as a way of finding out how employees view their jobs, coworkers, wages, benefits, supervisors, working conditions, and so on. Surveys requested by management are often instituted by outside consultants or by the institution's human resources department.

Surveys take the form of questionnaires submitted to the employees. Once a morale survey has been performed and properly analyzed, it is absolutely necessary that management do something about those areas of dissatisfaction that appear to contribute to a lowering of morale. It is also advisable to report the results to all those who participated and to discuss them in workshops throughout the organization to find solutions to the problems.

NOTES

1. Anita Baker, "Growing Talent is Everybody's Business," *Journal of Accountancy*, 200, no. 3 (September 2005): 91.

2. Stephanie Armour, "Dust Off Those Ties and Pumps: Dress Codes Gussy Up," *USA Today*, 1B, October 26, 2005.

Beach, D. S. 1985. *Personnel: The Management of People at Work, Fifth Edition*, 307. New York: Macmillan Publishing Co.

Ceridian Corporation. 2005. "The Flip Side of Productivity." [Online article; retrieved 9/29/05.] www.ceridian.com/myceridian/article/printerfriendly/1,2723,11337–53923,00.html.

Gemignani, J. 2000. "American Workers Are Sleep Deprived." *Business and Health*. [Online article.] http://www.findarticles.com/cf_dls/m0903/5_18/62276351/p1/article.jhtml.

Journal of Accountancy. 2001. "The Best Survey Question." *Journal of Accountancy* 191 (2): 120.

Kaplan, S. 2005. "What to Do When Morale is Low." *CIO Magazine*. [Online article; retrieved 9/28/05.] http://www.cio.com/archive/050102/morale.html.

Kelly, P. M. 1998. "How to Identify and Deal with 'Whining Cry Baby (WCB) Syndrome'." *Beretta USA Leadership Bulletin* 3 (9).

Mercer Human Resources Consulting. 2001. "Healthcare Trends and Commentary—An Annual Check Up," 6–8. [Online article; viewed 4/22/06.] www.imercer.com/us/mercercommentary/healthcaretrendscommentary.pdf.

Perry, B. 2000. "Companies Rethink Casual Clothes." *USA Today* [cover story], June 27, pp. 1A-2A.

Poole, D. 2004. *"Incentives as Tools to Improve Efficiency."* [Online article; viewed 4/26/06.] Terre Haute, IN: Indiana State University School of Nursing www.IndState.edu/mary/gradpapers/orstudy.doc.

Singer, I. D. 1999. "Work-Life Benefits Can Lighten the Load." *Business & Health* 17 (10): 25.

Spath, P. L. 2002. "Upgrade Skills with Competency-Based Training." *For the Record Magazine* 14 (2): 21–22.

York, D. R. 1985. "Attitude Surveying." *Personnel Journal* (May): 70–73.

Exhibit 25.1

HOW TO IDENTIFY AND DEAL WITH "WHINING CRY BABY (WCB) SYNDROME"

By Chief Patrick M. Kelly, Medley Police Department

Hear it? That high-pitched, annoying, constant background noise? Maybe it's coming from the office next to yours, or from that little knot of people who have stopped to gossip in the hallway. Maybe it's even coming from—could it be?—you. One thing's for sure: It's getting louder and more persistent, and there's no getting away from it. If you can make out some of the words, they sound like: The department doesn't appreciate me. The department won't help me plan my career. Nobody ever tells me what's going on around here. The Chief is a jackass. My evaluation wasn't fair. My last raise was too long ago and too small. Everything's changing too fast, and not for the better. It's not fair. This place stinks. And the granddaddy of them all, morale is lower than it's ever been. Waaaaaaaaaaah. . . .

After discussion with many chief executive officers, in both private and public sectors, it is amply clear that Whining Crying Baby (WCB) Syndrome is alive and well. WCBs—employees suffering from WCB Syndrome—must be identified and managed effectively. Unidentified and/or poorly managed WCBs can affect organizational productivity, employee morale and motivation, customer service levels, and, most importantly, the entire organizational culture. WCBs possess many, if not all, of the following attributes.

WCB Attributes

Victim's Mentality—WCBs have acute victim's mentality. They are not responsible for their own negative behavior. Every negative outcome in their life is attributable to some other person(s) or some circumstance(s) beyond their control. When WCBs are challenged about questionable behavior, their reactions have become incredibly predictable and almost Pavlovian in nature. First, of course, the accused will deny being at fault and then, second, cleave almost immediately to the sequential steps of the "WCB's Defense:" (1) I didn't do it; (2) Okay, I did it, but it wasn't a violation of policy, or there is no written policy; (3) Well, yes, I know it was a violation of policy, but everyone else was doing it too; and besides, I was doing less of it; (4) Yes, I did it, but the means you used to catch me were inappropriate; (5) You are only picking on me because I'm (fill in the blank). These forms of rationalization work very well, because WCBs do not have to accept responsibility for anything that goes wrong in their personal and professional lives. Conversely, they take full credit for all positive outcomes or successful results they are associated with. Simply put, WCBs believe other people are totally responsible for their failures, while WCBs are totally responsible for all their successes.

Tuned into Radio Station WIFM—WCBs are tuned into What's In It For Me? (WIFM) 24 hours a day. They see themselves as the center of the universe and seldom consider how their actions impact others. This often manifests itself in their suggestions for organizational improvement, which are usually self-serving or loaded with hidden agendas. WCBs continuously assert their individual rights, even if those rights trample on the rights of others, or most importantly on what is best for the entire organization. WCBs often believe that seniority or "time in grade" should be the criteria assigned the greatest weight in personnel decisions. They often say, "I've been here the longest, so I've earned the assignment or promotion."

Apathetic—WCBs don't get involved and always approach their duties and tasks in a reactive mode. They initiate little, if any, work activity. WCBs prefer traditional policing methodologies and will often spend more time looking for ways to avoid work, than to simply complete the tasks as assigned. You will hear them saying, "It's not my job," "That's not in my job description," or "The only way to stay out of trouble around here is to do nothing." WCBs are usually the least productive employees. They despise community-policing initiatives and may even sabotage these proactive problem-solving efforts.

Complaining Critics—WCBs are organizational critics. They are able to identify what is wrong with everything and everyone else but spend no time assessing the individual they see in the mirror. Once WCBs complain about and/or criticize some issue or person, and place blame on it, they feverishly move to another issue. The only level of satisfaction they ever get is bringing people down to their level of anger and unhappiness. After doing this, they celebrate their hard-won battle and quickly step over the lives they have ruined.

Why Do WCBs Exist?

First, many WCBs began their behavior as children. It began with the words "Mommy and Daddy, I want. . . ." and goes on and on and on. Of course, it usually takes place in public, before the largest number of strangers possible. A Kansas State University professor, who specializes in parent-child relationships, says that whining is what's called an irrelevant behavior that parents are responsible for creating. Dr. Charles Smith says, "A child whines because they have learned that kind of repetitious, aggravating behavior gets them what they want. Parents have to realize they created this behavior and now they're going to have to suffer through it."

Unfortunately, this irrelevant behavior can continue through adolescence and into adulthood. And just like the parent, the organization is responsible if this irrelevant whining behavior continues to persist. Remember basic psychology. When a person repeats a behavior pattern, that person is getting a payoff. You must avoid the old cliche, "The squeaky wheel gets the most oil." This "oil," or payoff is simply reinforcing the WCB and his or her negative, irrelevant behavior.

It is important to note that not all WCBs are genetic, or environmental as a child, but rather rookie copies who are unfortunately paired with these individuals (veteran WCBs) and thus just don't know any better.

Second, we are a society that values individuals "rights" above all else. Psychologist Carol Tavris, in her landmark book, *Anger: The Misunderstood Emotion*, explains our tendency to whine: "The individualism of American life, to our glory and despair, creates anger and encourages its release. For when everything is possible, limitations are irksome. When the desires of the self come first, the needs of others are annoying. When we think we deserve it all, reaping only a portion can enrage." Ah, "reaping only a portion," you may say, misstates the case. WCBs don't want the whole pie, just a few more crumbs.

American organizations are simply microcosms of American society. All employees come to work with unique "individual" personalities, interests, preferences and rights. Successful employees recognize the need to balance their individual rights with the rights of the organization's internal and external stakeholders. Unfortunately, WCBs have not recognized the need to sacrifice some individual "rights" for the good of the collective organization and its customers. Those folks whom New York City behavioral scientist Deborah Bright calls "entitlists"—a polite word for WCBs—often express their outrage in passive-aggressive ways, including being chronically late or absent, stealing from the company, backstabbing coworkers or bosses, or simply withdrawing—not taking risks, not suggesting solutions, not going the extra mile—in effect just waiting around to be fired. Need we point out that these DDFO are not great career-building strategies?

Finally, our level of self-esteem affects virtually everything we think, say and do. It affects how we see the world and our place in it. It affects how others in the world see and treat us. It affects the choices we make—choices about what we will do with our lives and with whom we will be involved. It affects our ability to both give and receive praise and recognition. And, it affects our ability to take action to change things that need to be changed. WCBs, like many people in American society, suffer from low self-esteem. What separates WCBs from others suffering from low self-esteem? WCBs do not understand or have not yet accepted their low self-esteem. In fact, WCB attributes, described earlier in this article, are all manifestations of low self-esteem. They don't have time to look into the mirror objectively, because they are so busy criticizing and condemning others. Unfortunately, WCBs surround themselves with other WCBs. There is truth to the old adage, "misery loves company." WCBs commiserate with each other on a daily basis. In fact, it was from the depths of this WCB commiseration that this author broke free from the chains of this life and career-crippling syndrome.

How to Effectively Deal with WCBs

One day two frogs were playing together, hopping over each other on a park bench. Suddenly, as they neared the edge of the bench they both fell off and into a pail of milk, which was on the ground. The pail was only filled halfway, so the two frogs had a difficult time trying to get out. Eventually their commotion and cries for help drew a crowd of other frogs who gathered at the edge of the bench. When the crowd saw how hopeless their situation was, they began to jump up and down, swinging their legs and yelling, "Give up! Give up! You will never make it out! It's hopeless!" When one of the frogs in the pail saw them and heard what they were saying; he knew they were right. He didn't see the point of trying any longer, so he laid back and slowly disappeared into the pail of milk and drowned. The other frog looked up and saw the crowd jumping up and down and yelling, and this made him more determined to get out. So he started to swim around and around, faster and faster. Eventually his churning around made the milk begin to harden. He was able to get a foothold and jump out of the pail of milk and save his life.

Oh . . . by the way . . . I forgot to tell you that the second frog . . . the one that triumphed and saved his life . . . was DEAF! You see, because he was deaf, he did not hear all the negative remarks from the crowd. He saw the other frogs jumping up and down, waving and yelling to him, and he thought they were encouraging him to try harder!

The first, and most important, strategy for dealing effectively with WCBs is in this story. If you and your organization are going to succeed, you need to be like the second frog. You need to ignore the WCBs and their comments, because they will discourage you and drag you down. Getting sound advice from people who have achieved success is one thing. Listening to WCBs is another. Remember basic psychology. Ears, or people listening, is a payoff for WCBs. As long as there is an audience (payoff) for their negativity, they will continue to cry, "Waaaaaaaa. . . ." A more diplomatic way of utilizing this strategy is to become "selectively impolite." Be remote when the WCB complains. Only show interest when he or she stops complaining or says something positive.

The second strategy is to dismiss the WCB's negative comment. Say something like "You may be right," and change the subject. A leading management psychologist says that often the best way of handling something that really bothers you is not to oppose it, but to align yourself with it. This will totally confuse and disorient the WCB. Of course, it will be YOUR fault when the WCB becomes confused and disoriented.

Third, don't get flustered. If the WCB appears to enjoy upsetting you, keep your cool. Any emotional reaction from you becomes a payoff for the WCB.

Next, be direct. Tell the WCB, "Your complaining bothers me. I can't handle that kind of talk right now." Or, "It bothers me when you only talk about the negative side of things." Interestingly, as much as WCBs complain, they never seem to leave. This is because subconsciously they realize how great things really are in their current organization, or because no one else will hire them. If things are really that bad, invite them to apply elsewhere. Be cautious though; they will view this as a threat in their negative mindsets.

Fifth, jump in first. There was an office manager who had to deal with a WCB's constant complaining about her husband. One Monday morning, he asked her, "What did the MORON do to you this weekend?" Startled, she replied, "Why are you saying that about my husband?" He said he'd listened to her complaints for years and decided the man had to be a sadistic monster. She responded, "He's not that bad," and stopped complaining.

Sixth, pay attention to results. The supervisor in a printing shop said an old-time printer was always pessimistic about special printing jobs, insisting that each job was impossible. The supervisor would tell him to go ahead anyway, and in every case the job worked out. If negativity is a good employee's security blanket, let it be.

Seventh, ask for the complaints in writing. Then read them back to the WCB. Some WCBs don't know how negative they sound. Of course, many WCBs will refuse to reduce their complaints to writing, because they don't want to spend time looking for solutions. They fear formal documentation of their complaints, because then they may be asked, "How do you think we can address your complaint(s)?" This question leads to the final strategy for dealing with WCBs.

Finally, ask for clarification and empower the WCB to propose viable solutions to their complaints. Tell the WCB to describe the problem and clarify the desired outcome(s). Ask what plans the WCB has for handling the situation. Such questions will slow pathological WCBs down and force them to think about positive actions. Then again, they may respond with, "It's not my job!"

Closing Comments

One of life's greatest frustrations is dealing with WCBs who absorb your energy and drag you down. Most managers find constantly complaining, whining employees more difficult to work with than incompetent employees. "Basically, most people with positive attitudes have a negative attitude about negative attitudes," says psychologist Al Siebert, who teaches executives how to deal with difficult people on the job. "Negative people catch the blind spot of your basic optimist managerial type. These upbeat executives are very judgmental and feel negative people are defective human beings who have flawed personalities. Their position is that everything would work out if only those negative people would get an attitude transplant." Reality dictates, however, that most WCBs are not going to change as long as there are organizational "payoffs" (i.e., specialized assignments, promotions, and training opportunities) for their behavior. Eliminate rewards for inappropriate behavior and become selectively "DEAF" around WCBs, and you will become the organizational cure for "WCB Syndrome."

Source: Reprinted with permission of Jeff Reh, General Counsel. This article appeared in *Beretta USA Leadership Bulletin*, Sept. 1998, Vol. 3, Issue 9.

CHAPTER TWENTY-SIX

Discipline

CHAPTER OBJECTIVES

After you have studied this chapter, you should be able to:

1. Define the term discipline.
2. Discuss different techniques of administering discipline.
3. Describe different types of disciplinary actions.
4. Review the supervisor's role in disciplinary actions.
5. Outline the rights of employees in the disciplinary process.

T HE TERM DISCIPLINE is used to express many different ideas and is understood in several different ways. To many, discipline carries the disagreeable connotation of punishing wrongdoers. When one hears the word, one is often inclined to think immediately of authority enforcing obedience. There is a positive way of considering discipline, however, a way that is far more in keeping with good supervisory practices. Maintaining positive, sometimes also known as constructive, discipline and good influence go hand in hand.

ORGANIZATIONAL DISCIPLINE

For our purposes, *discipline* can be defined as a state of affairs or a condition of orderliness in which the members of the enterprise behave sensibly and conduct themselves according to the standards of acceptable behavior as expressed by the needs of the organization. Discipline is said to be good when the employees willingly follow the rules of the enterprise, live up to or exceed standards, and practice good self-judgment. Discipline is said to be poor when subordinates follow regulations reluctantly or refuse to follow them, violate the standards of acceptable behavior, and require constant surveillance by their supervisors. Positive discipline thrives in an organizational climate in which management applies positive motivation, sound leadership, and efficient management.

Positive Discipline and Morale

A direct correlation exists between morale and discipline. Normally, fewer problems of a disciplinary nature can be expected when morale is high, and low morale brings about increased problems of discipline. A high degree of discipline can exist despite a low level of morale. Under these conditions, discipline is probably controlled by fear and sheer force. On the other hand, it is not usually possible to maintain a high level of morale unless there is also a high degree of positive discipline.

SELF-DISCIPLINE

The best discipline is self-discipline—meaning the normal human tendency to do what needs to be done. In the healthcare setting, this is doing one's share, assisting coworkers when appropriate, and subordinating some of one's own needs and desires to the standards of acceptable behavior set for the enterprise as a whole. From early childhood, people are trained to respect rules, accept orders from those legitimately entitled to issue them, and realize that all activities set limits on the behavior of the organization's members.

Experience shows that most employees want to do the right thing. Even before they start to work, most mature people accept the idea that following instructions and fair rules of conduct is a normal responsibility that goes with any job. Thus, most employees can be counted on to exercise a considerable degree of self-discipline. They believe in coming to work on time, following the supervisor's instructions, and signing the time sheet as well as refraining from fights, drinking at work, stealing, and so forth. In other words, self-imposed discipline is based on the commitment of employees to conform to the rules, regulations, and orders that are necessary for the proper conduct of the institution.

Once the employees know what is expected of them and believe that the rules by which they are governed are reasonable, they usually observe them without problems. The supervisor must check the rules and regulations periodically to ensure they continue to be reasonable. For example, the dress codes and codes of general appearance have most certainly undergone changes in the past decade. It is unreasonable to request subordinates to comply with a dress and appearance code set up years ago that dictates that women wear dresses and men may not have facial hair. Some rules may need to be altered to address medical concerns, for example, a healthcare organization with a "no beard" policy may allow African-Americans to wear beards. Some African-Americans are prone to pseudofollicultis barbae, a painful skin condition worsened by shaving.

When new rules are introduced, the supervisor must show their current reasonableness and need to the employees. For instance, short skirts may be fashionable, but they are not conducive to a nurse's appearance and movement or functioning on the job. Instead of simply outlawing short skirts, however, a rule giving nurses a choice between wearing a certain length of hemline or uniforms with long pants might be considered a more reasonable dress code. Rules regarding hair length are relevant in some job settings, as in the surgical suite, but are irrelevant in others. Therefore, because hair is a danger to asepsis, the supervisor and possibly the chief of surgery, infection committee, and director of nursing may need to work out rules that make hair caps mandatory for operating room personnel.

The supervisor must be alert to changing styles and mores. *Mores* are culture-driven expectations. For example, in an orthodox Jewish community, married women are expected to cover their hair and wear blouses that cover their upper body to the elbow. Supervisors must make certain that the rules and regulations truly respect the diverse cultures that are represented in the work team. Otherwise, rules are not enforceable, and many unnecessary disciplinary problems may arise.

If present, mores, as well as the employees' strong sense of self-imposed discipline (norms), exert group pressure on any possible wrongdoer, further reducing the need for the supervisor's disciplinary action. *Norms* are a set of standards that regulate behavior within an organization. For example, it may be the norm in a department meeting to just listen to whatever the supervisor says and not ask questions. After the meeting, the staff will privately discuss the issues at lunch. Work groups also set norms, or standards for conduct, and standards for performance; for example, fellow employees are expected by the group to carry their fair share of work and be at work on time. Group discipline reinforces self-discipline and exerts pressure on those who do not comply with group norms and standards.

Employees must also know that they have the supervisor's unqualified support as long as they stay within the ordinary rules of conduct and their activities are consistent with what is expected of them. Proper discipline makes it necessary for the supervisor to give positive support to the right action and criticize and punish the wrong action. The subordinate must know that failure to live up to what is expected results in "punishment."

Administration cannot expect employees to practice self-discipline unless it starts at the top. Similar restrictions must be imposed on all managerial personnel to remain within the acceptable patterns of behavior. Proper conduct with respect to the needs of the organization requires the supervisor also to comply with the necessity to be on time, to observe no smoking and no drinking rules, and to dress and behave in a manner commensurate with the organizational and departmental standards.

Setting an example is a key responsibility of management. The mirror effect pervades all levels of the organization if the example is displayed by all supervisors and managers. This role modeling by management can serve to tell all staff in a nonverbal way that "I only expect of you what I expect of myself."

Regardless, employees must be informed of expectations. Supervisors should always put policies and expectations in writing and make sure they are enforced evenhandedly. These documents should be specific, including what is not acceptable, and should not be used to discriminate.

FIGURE 26.1

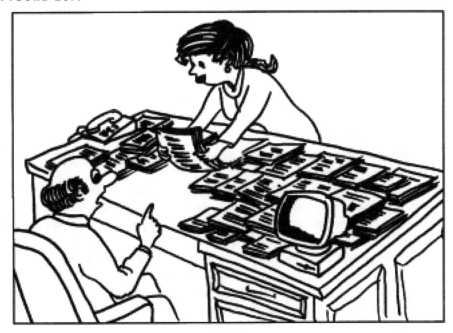

"Don't put anything there, Ms. Finkel. That spot is for my feet."

Source: Reprinted from *Hospitals & Health Networks*, by permission, June 2000, © 2000, by Health Forum, Inc.

WHEN DISCIPLINE IS WARRANTED

Although the vast majority of employees exercise considerable self-discipline, a few employees in every large organization occasionally fail to abide by established rules and standards even after having been informed of them. Some employees simply do not accept the responsibility of self-discipline. Also, a few unruly employees, probably because of their personality, background, and development, find it difficult to function within policies, rules, and regulations.

Because the job must get done, the supervisor cannot afford to let those few get away with violations. Quick and firm action is called for to correct the situation. Unless such action is taken, the morale of the other employees in the work group will be seriously weakened. At times like this, the supervisor has to rely on the power and force inherent in the managerial position, even though he or she may dislike doing so. In this situation, the supervisor must clearly realize that he or she is in charge of the department and is therefore responsible for discipline within it. If the supervisor does not correct the situation, some individuals who are merely on the borderline of being undisciplined may follow the bad example. When a defect in discipline becomes apparent, it is the supervisor's responsibility to take proper action and to resolve this employee-management conflict firmly and promptly.

When administering discipline, managers should remember that the purpose is to preserve the interests of the organization and to protect the rights of the employees. Many organizations encourage a positive discipline approach. Discipline is not for the purpose of punishment or getting even with an employee. Rather, its purpose is to improve the employee's future behavior, to correct and rehabilitate, but not to injure. Discipline corrects the subordinate's breach of the rules and carries the notice of more serious consequences in the future. Discipline also serves as a warning for other people in the department. It reminds the disciplined individual's coworkers that rules exist and that violating them does not go unnoticed or without any action from the supervisor. Moreover, discipline reassures all those employees who respect the rules out of their desire to do the right thing.

The guides and checklists provided in Figure 21.4 and Figure 21.5 may be beneficial when delivering discipline. The interests of the organization are best served when an employee understands what is expected of him or her and complies with those expectations.

Ensuring the employee has had the proper training and orientation to the work before applying discipline is one of the supervisor's principal duties. By doing so, the organization salvages a trained resource and avoids the expense of recruitment and loss of productivity resulting from a vacancy or from training a new employee.

The supervisor should administer discipline so that it motivates the employee to do what is right rather than discourages him or her from doing what is wrong. In other words, the boss must exercise positive discipline. This is not an easy task because inherently the act of punishing a subordinate for violating a rule always presupposes that the subordinate was caught violating it. Yet many others who may have done the same thing go free, so to speak, because the supervisor did not catch them. This invariably injects a note of unfairness into the disciplinary process. Administering positive discipline is also difficult because any discipline is normally resented, and it places a strain on the supervisor-subordinate relationship. Sometimes discipline only makes the subordinate double his or her efforts not to be caught again. Nevertheless, positive discipline will generally be successful and accepted if the supervisor follows a few simple rules when taking disciplinary action. Jane Boucher's book, *How to Love the Job You Hate*, offers the advice shown in Figure 26.2.

Taking Responsibility

Normally, few occasions arise that force a good supervisor to take disciplinary action. The first step is to obtain all pertinent facts. Before the supervisor does anything, it is necessary to investigate what has happened and why the employee violated the rule or failed to perform as expected. When the investigative interview is used to confront an employee about alleged acts, the skilled supervisor is observant of the employee's reactions. Reactions may expose lying and other unacceptable behavior. As Wells (2001) states, "Behaviorists tell us

If You Must Criticize Someone

Here are some suggestions for giving criticism in a way that motivates others to do a better job:

- See yourself as a teacher or coach—as being helpful. Keep in mind that you're trying to help someone improve.
- Show you care. Express your sincere concern about sharing ways the other person can boost his or her success.
- Pick the right moment to offer criticism. Make sure the person hasn't just been shaken by some incident.
- Avoid telling people they "should do such and such" or "should have done such and such." "Shoulds" make you appear rigid and pedantic.
- Avoid giving the impression that you're more concerned with seeing your recommendations put into practice than in helping the other person improve.
- Show how the person will benefit from taking the actions you suggest.
- Give specific suggestions. Being vague might only make the situation worse by creating anxiety and doubt.

Tip: Be sure you can take criticism yourself. If not, you may not be perceived as a credible source.

Source: Boucher (2001). Reprinted with permission. Jane Boucher, President, Boucher Consultants, (937)294-6960.

that lying is innate to the human species and comes about for two genetically programmed reasons: to receive rewards and/or to avoid punishment. Whether we lie depends on our calculation of the reward/punishment equation. This is called 'situational honesty'." In addition, the employee's past record should be checked, and all other pertinent information should be obtained before any action is taken. When the information collected indicates that disciplinary action is necessary, the supervisor is best qualified to handle the situation because he or she knows the employee, alleged violations, and circumstances. In addition, by being in charge of the department, the supervisor has the authority and responsibility to take appropriate action.[1] Although it may be expedient for the moment to let someone in the human resources department handle such unpleasant problems, the supervisor will not only be shirking and abdicating responsibility but also undermining his or her own position if this were allowed.

The same result will occur if the supervisor were to ignore or conveniently overlook for any length of time a subordinate's failure to meet the prescribed standards of conduct. If such breaches are condoned, the supervisor is merely communicating to the rest of the employees that he or she does not intend to enforce the rules and regulations. Thus, the supervisor must not procrastinate in administering discipline. On the other hand, the supervisor must be careful not to take hasty or unwarranted action.

Maintaining Control of Emotions

Whenever taking disciplinary action, the supervisor must not lose his or her temper. Regardless of the severity of the violation, the supervisor must not lose control of the situation, thus running the risk of losing the employees' respect. If the employees do not agree with the facts on which the disciplinary action is based, the supervisor may end up arguing with the other employees over what happened. Varying eyewitness reports will probably only confuse the situation. In addition, public discipline would humiliate the disciplined employee in the eyes of the coworkers and cause considerable damage to the entire department.

This does not mean that the supervisor should face the situation half-heartedly or haphazardly. If he or she is in danger of losing control, however, action should be avoided until tempers have cooled down. Even if the violation is significant, the supervisor cannot afford to lose his or her temper. Moreover, the supervisor should follow the general rule of never laying a hand on an employee in any way. Except for emergencies, when an employee has been injured or becomes ill or when employees who are fighting need to be separated, such a gesture could easily make matters worse.

Discipline in Private

The supervisor must make certain that all disciplinary action takes place in private, never in public. A public reprimand builds up resentment in the employee, and it may permit unrelated factors to enter the situation. For instance, if in the opinion of the other workers a disciplinary action is too severe for the violation, the disciplined employee may appear as a martyr to the rest of them. A supervisor who is disciplining in public is bound to have his or her performance judged by every employee in the department. Employees expect to be treated with the same courtesy that they extend to their supervisor. Thus, just as a supervisor would expect counseling in private, so should he or she extend the same courtesy to his or her subordinates. Therefore, privacy in taking disciplinary action must be the rule. However, because of increased litigation, some organizations mandate, or encourage, the use of witnesses at disciplinary interviews. In these cases the supervisor may invite a witness to observe the counseling. Some organizations even permit the employee to invite a witness. Should this be the situation at your organization, the human resources department no doubt can outline the criteria for the use of witnesses and their roles.

PROGRESSIVE DISCIPLINARY ACTION

The question of which type of disciplinary action to use is answered differently in different enterprises. In recent years, however, most enterprises have accepted the idea of progressive discipline, which provides for an increase in the penalty with each offense. First offenders get less severe penalties than repeat offenders; more serious infractions receive more severe penalties than lesser offenses. Unless a serious wrong has been committed, the employee is rarely discharged for the first offense. Rather, a series of progressive steps of disciplinary action are taken, such as the following:

1. informal talk,
2. spoken warning or reprimand,
3. written warning,
4. disciplinary layoff,
5. demotional downgrading, and
6. discharge.

These steps, presented in ascending order of severity, are suggestions; they are not the only means of disciplinary action, nor are they all necessary. Many enterprises, however, have found the progression of these disciplinary steps to be a viable approach.

Informal Talk

If the incident is minor and the employee has no previous record of disciplinary action, an informal friendly talk, also referred to as counseling, clears up the situation in many cases. In such a talk, the supervisor will discuss with the employee his or her behavior in relation to the standards that prevail within the enterprise. He or she will try to get to the underlying reason for the undesirable behavior. If the institution has an employee assistance program, as discussed in Chapter 24, the supervisor may refer the employee to it if indications show this program can help him or her. At the same time, the boss will try to reaffirm the employee's sense of responsibility and reestablish the previous cooperative relationship within the department. It may also be advisable to repeat once more why the action of the employee is undesirable and what it may possibly lead to. If the supervisor later finds that this friendly talk was not sufficient to bring about the desired results, it will become necessary to take the next step, a spoken warning.

Spoken Warning or Reprimand

In the reprimand interview, the supervisor should again point out how undesirable the subordinate's violation is and how it could ultimately lead to more severe disciplinary action. Such an interview has emotional overtones, as the employee most likely is resentful for having been caught again and the supervisor may also be angry. The violation should be discussed in a straightforward manner as a statement of fact, however, and the supervisor should not begin with a recital of how the fine reputation of the employee has now been tarnished.

The supervisor also should not be apologetic but should state the case in specific terms and then give the subordinate a chance to tell his or her side of the story.

The supervisor should stress the preventive purpose of this disciplinary action, but the employee must be advised that such conduct cannot be tolerated. In some enterprises a record is made on the employee's personnel file that this spoken warning has taken place. The purpose of the warning is to help the employee correct the behavior and prevent the need for further disciplinary action. The warning should leave the employee with the confidence that he or she can do better and will improve in the future. Some supervisors believe that such a verbal reprimand is not very effective. If it is carried out skillfully, however, many employees will be straightened out at this stage.

Written Warning

A written warning is formal insofar as it becomes a part of the employee's record. Written warnings are particularly necessary in work settings in which unions exist so that the document can serve as evidence in case of grievance procedures. The written warning must contain a statement of the violation and the potential consequences. Typically, a duplicate copy of it is given to the employee, and another duplicate of the warning is sent to the human resources department so that it can be inserted in the employee's permanent record.

Disciplinary Layoffs and Suspension

The next disciplinary step may be a disciplinary layoff or suspension. This step occurs when all previous steps have been taken and the employee has continued the offense or when a serious offense has occurred and time is required to fully investigate the issues. In the latter situation, the employee is suspended pending a final decision in the case. This device protects management as well as the employee; it gives management a chance to make the necessary investigation and consult higher levels of administration or the human resources department, and it provides an opportunity for tempers to cool off. In cases of temporary suspension, the employee is told that he or she is suspended and will be informed as soon as possible of the disciplinary action that will be taken, if any.

When a suspension is used as described here, the suspension itself may not be punishment. If the investigation shows that there is no cause for disciplinary action, the employee has no grievance because he or she is allowed to return to work and will be compensated for work time missed. The obvious advantage of temporary suspensions is that the supervisor can act promptly without any prejudice toward the employee.

If, on the other hand, the penalty is disciplinary in nature, it will be considered a disciplinary layoff and the time during which the employee was suspended will not be compensated. Under such conditions, the supervisor must determine what length of penalized time off would be appropriate. This will depend on how serious the offense is. Disciplinary layoffs typically extend over several days or weeks and are seldom longer than a few weeks. Neither temporary suspensions nor disciplinary layoffs should be used indiscriminately; these should be invoked primarily when the offense is likely to call for at least the layoff.

Some employees may not be impressed with spoken or written warnings. In these cases, employees on disciplinary layoffs may wake up to a short layoff without pay and probably will be convinced that the organization is really serious. A disciplinary layoff may bring back a sense of compliance with rules and regulations. In some organizations, the human resources department may have a defined time for this type of disciplinary layoff and may call them suspensions as well.

There are several disadvantages to invoking a disciplinary layoff or suspension. Some enterprises do not apply this measure at all because it hurts their productivity, especially in times of labor shortages when the employee cannot be replaced with someone who is just as skilled. Also, the employee might return from the layoff in a much less pleasant frame of mind than when he or she left. Although most managers consider the disciplinary layoff or suspension a serious measure, some employees who frequently violate the rules may not regard it as such; they may even view a few days of layoff as a welcome break from their daily routine. Although many institutions use it effectively, a number of institutions no longer use these measures. Instead, they move right to discharge, or they practice the new concept of discipline without punishment discussed in this chapter.

Demotion

The usefulness of demoting an employee is seriously questioned; therefore, this disciplinary measure is seldom invoked. To demote an employee for disciplinary reasons to a lower-level, less desirable, and lower-paying job is likely to bring about dissatisfaction and discouragement. Over an extended period an employee downgrading is a form of constant punishment. The dissatisfaction, humiliation, and ill will that result may easily spread to other employees in the department. Sometimes this measure can be viewed as an invitation for the employee to quit, rather than be discharged. Many enterprises avoid downgrading as a disciplinary measure just as they avoid disciplinary layoffs or the withholding of a scheduled pay increase. If so, they have to use termination of employment as the ultimate solution. Of course, if the employee requests to step down or be demoted, for example in a case where an individual must work rotating shifts or weekends in their current job but now find themselves having to care for an aging parent, where coordination of in-home helpers is complicated by the employee's irregular schedule, then the demotion is not disciplinary but rather an accommodation.

Discharge

Discharge, or corporate capital punishment, is the most drastic form of disciplinary action, and it should be reserved exclusively for the most serious offenses. Supervisors should resort to it infrequently and only after some of the preliminary steps have been taken. Discharge is the ultimate penalty; it is costly to the organization and causes real hardship to the person who has been discharged. When a serious wrong has been committed, however, discharge should be invoked at once. For instance, when an employee falsifies patient records to obtain narcotics or releases medical records of a celebrity to a local newspaper, immediate discharge is in order.

For the employee, discharge means hardship because it eliminates the seniority standing, possibly some pension rights, substantial vacation benefits, a high pay scale, and other benefits that the employee has accumulated in many years of service. Discharge also makes obtaining new employment difficult for the worker. In regard to the enterprise, discharges involve serious losses and waste, including the expense of training a new employee and the disruption caused by changing the makeup of the work team. Discharge may also cause damage to the morale of the group. If the discharged employee is a member of a legally protected group, such as minorities or women, administration has to be concerned about nondiscrimination and hiring quotas.

Therefore, because of these possibly serious consequences of discharge, many organizations have removed from the supervisor the authority to fire. This has been reserved for higher levels in administration; in some institutions, the supervisor's recommendation to discharge must be reviewed and approved by higher administration, the human resources director, or both. With unions, management is concerned with possible prolonged arbitration procedures, knowing that arbitrators have become increasingly unwilling to permit discharge except for the most severe violations. Although situations may arise for which the only solution is to fire the employee for just cause, these cases are the rare exception and not the rule.

Time Element

In all of the disciplinary steps previously discussed, the time element is significant. There is no reason to hold an indiscretion of past years against a person forever. Current practice is inclined to disregard offenses that have been committed more than a year previously if the person has reformed. For example, an employee with a poor record because of tardiness starts with a clean slate if he or she has maintained a good record for one year. This time element varies depending on the nature of the violation.

Documentation

It is essential for the supervisor to keep detailed records of all disciplinary actions, as they have the potential of becoming the subject of further discussions, disputes, and even litigation. The burden of proof of lawful action is on the employer. The written record should cover the time of the event, details of the offense, the supervisor's decision, and action taken. It should also include the reasoning involved. If at some future time the supervisor or the institution is asked to substantiate the action taken, it is not sufficient to depend on memory alone.

At present, it is more important than ever to keep accurate detailed records because the aggrieved employee may file a lawsuit for wrongful discharge based on discrimination, harassment, or similar reasons. If a union is involved, documentation is required to justify a disciplinary measure if it is challenged by a formal grievance procedure. Regardless of any potential consequences, written documentation at the time of the event is essential for the institution and the supervisor's own records.

Other Discharge Precautions

Because the healthcare supervisor has responsibility for ensuring the security of confidential information to which an employee may have had access, when termination occurs, the supervisor must take additional steps to ensure security of protected health information. These may include changing pass codes on door locks; removing the employee's access to the organization's information system; deleting employee accounts; and retrieving keys, tokens, or other cards that allow access into the unit.

THE SUPERVISOR'S DILEMMA

Throughout, this book has stressed the importance of the relationship of trust, confidence, and help between the supervisor and the employee. Disciplinary action is by nature painful. Therefore, despite all the restraint and wisdom with which the supervisor takes disciplinary action, it still puts a strain on the supervisor-subordinate relationship. It is difficult to impose discipline without generating resentment because disciplinary action is an unpleasant experience and puts a barrier between the supervisor and the employee. The question therefore arises as to how the supervisor can apply the necessary disciplinary action so that it is given in the least resented and most acceptable form.

The supervisor must also be concerned about equity. It is imperative that discipline be equitably applied regardless of race, sex, age, or position. Sometimes exceptions are made because the employee is the son of a "high admitter" or a neighbor of the assistant director of plant operations or the daughter of a benefactor. These are not valid reasons for exceptions. Inequitable dispensing of discipline, or for that matter, praise or assignments because of associations unrelated to the work requirements, can destroy a manager's credibility and the staff's morale more quickly than any other reason.

The "Red-Hot-Stove" Approach

McGregor refers to what he calls "the red-hot-stove rule" regarding discipline (Sayles and Strauss 1981; Strauss and Sayles 1980). When one touches a red-hot stove, the resulting discipline has four characteristics: it is immediate, with warning, is consistent, and is impersonal. First, the burn is immediate, and there is no question of the cause and effect. Second, there is a warning; everyone knows what happens if one touches a hot stove, especially if the stove is red from the heat. Third, the discipline is consistent; every time one touches a hot stove, one is burned. Fourth, the discipline is impersonal; whoever touches the hot stove is burned. A person is burned for touching the hot stove, not because of who he or she is.

This comparison illustrates that the act and the discipline seem almost as one. The discipline takes place because the person did something—he or she committed a particular act. The discipline is directed against the act and not against the person. Following the four basic rules expressed in this red-hot-stove approach helps the supervisor take the sting out of many disciplinary actions. It enables the manager to achieve positive discipline and at the same time generate in the employee the least amount of resentment.

Immediacy

The supervisor must not procrastinate; a prompt beginning of the disciplinary process is necessary as soon as possible after the supervisor notices the violation. The sooner the discipline is invoked, the more automatic it will seem and the closer will be the connection with the offensive act. As already stated, the supervisor should refrain from taking hasty action, and enough time should elapse for tempers to cool and for assembling all the necessary facts.

In some instances the employee is clearly guilty of a violation, although the full circumstances may not be known or easy to prove. Here the need for disciplinary action is unquestionable, but some doubt exists as to the severity of the penalty. In such cases the supervisor should tell the employee that he or she realizes what went on, but that some time is needed to reach a conclusion. In other cases, however, the nature of the incident makes it necessary to get the offender off the premises quickly. Some immediate action is required even if there is not yet enough evidence to make a final decision in the case.

Advance Warning

To have good discipline and employees who accept disciplinary action as fair, it is absolutely essential that all employees be clearly informed in advance what is expected of them and what the rules are. There must be warning that a certain offense leads to disciplinary action. Some enterprises rely on bulletin board announcements to make such warnings. These cannot be as effective, however, as a section in the handbook that all new employees receive when they start working for the institution. Along with the written statements in the handbook, it is advisable to include verbal clarification of the rules. During the induction process shortly after new employees are hired, they should be orally informed of what is expected of them and of the consequences of not living up to behavioral expectations.

In addition to the forewarning about general rules, the employees must be told in advance how disciplinary action is taken. The various steps of disciplinary action should be clarified before employees could possibly become involved in an offense. There are considerable doubts, however, about whether a standard penalty should be provided and stated for each offense. Should there be, for example, a clear statement that falsifying attendance records carries a one-week disciplinary layoff? Those in favor of such a list suggest that it is an effective warning device and that it provides greater disciplinary consistency. On the other hand, such a list does not permit management to take into consideration the various degrees of guilt and mitigating circumstances. In general, it is probably best not to provide a schedule of penalties for specific violations but merely to state the progressive steps of disciplinary action that can be taken. It should be clearly understood that continued violations bring about more severe penalties. Some enterprises do specify that certain serious offenses bring the penalty of immediate discharge. For most violations, however, it is unwise to spell out a rigid set of disciplinary measures.

The practice of forewarning before taking disciplinary measures also applies to rules that have not been enforced recently. If the supervisor has not disciplined anyone who violated a rule for a long time, the employees do not expect this rule to be enforced in the future. Perhaps the supervisor suddenly decides that to make a rule valid, he or she is going to make an example of one of the employees and take disciplinary action. Disciplinary action should not be used in this manner. Because a certain rule has not been enforced in the past does not mean that it cannot ever be enforced. What it does mean is that the supervisor must take certain steps before beginning to enforce such a rule. Instead of acting tough suddenly, the supervisor should give the employees some warning that this rule, previous enforcement of which has been lax, will be strictly enforced in the future. In such cases it is not enough to put the enforcement notice on the bulletin board. It is essential that, in addition to a clear written warning, supplemental verbal communication be given. The supervisor must explain to the subordinates, perhaps in a departmental meeting, that from the present time on he or she intends to enforce this rule.

Consistency

A further requirement of good discipline is consistency of treatment. The supervisor must enforce discipline at each occurrence of an offense and take the same type of disciplinary action each time. By being consistent, the supervisor sets the limit for acceptable behavior, and every individual wants to know what the limits are. Inconsistency is one of the fastest ways for a supervisor to lower the morale of the employees and lose their respect. If the supervisor is inconsistent, the employees find themselves in an environment in which they cannot feel secure. Inconsistency only leads to anxiety, creating doubts in the employees' minds about what they can and cannot do. At times the supervisor may be tempted to be lenient and overlook an infringement. In reality, however, the supervisor is not doing the employees any favors, but rather only creating a more difficult situation for all of them.

Mason Haire (1964), a well-known psychologist, compares this situation to the relationship between a motorist and a traffic police officer. He says that whenever we are exceeding the speed limit on the highway, we must feel some sort of anxiety because we are breaking the rule. On the other hand, the rule is often not enforced. We think that perhaps the police department in this location does not take the rule seriously, and we can speed a little. There is always a lurking insecurity, however, because the motorist knows that at any time the police officer may decide to enforce the rule. Many motorists probably think it is easier to operate in an environment in which the police are at least consistent one way or the other. The same holds true for most employees who have to work in an environment in which the supervisor is not consistent in disciplinary matters.

In addition, the supervisor faces another problem in trying to be consistent. On one hand, the supervisor has been cautioned to treat all employees alike and to avoid favoritism, whereas on the other hand, he or she has been told again and again to treat people as individuals in accordance with their special needs and circumstances. On the surface these two requirements appear to contradict each other. The supervisor must realize, however, that treating people fairly does not mean treating everyone exactly the same. What it does mean is that when an exception is made, it must be considered as a valid exception by the other members of the department. The rest of the employees regard an exception as fair if they know why it was made and if they consider the reason to be justified. Moreover, the other employees must be confident that if any other employee were in the same situation, he or she would receive the same treatment. If these conditions are fulfilled, the supervisor has been able to exercise fair play, be consistent in discipline, and still treat people as individuals.

The extent to which a supervisor can be consistent and still consider the circumstances is illustrated as follows. Assume that three employees were engaged in horseplay at work. Conceivably the supervisor may simply have a friendly informal talk with one of the employees, who just started work a few days ago. The second employee may receive a formal or written warning, as he had been warned about horseplay before. The third employee might receive a three-day disciplinary layoff because he had been involved in many previous cases of horseplay. All three situations must be handled with equal gravity. In deciding the penalty, however, the supervisor must take into consideration all circumstances.

Impartiality

Another way that a supervisor can reduce the amount of resentment and keep the damage to future relations with the subordinates to a minimum is to take disciplinary action as impartially as possible. In recalling the red-hot-stove rule, whoever touches the stove is burned, regardless of who he or she is. The penalty is connected with the act and not with the person. Looking at disciplinary action in this way reduces the danger to the personal relationship between the supervisor and the employee. It is the specific act that brings about the disciplinary measure, not the personality.

Keeping this in mind, the supervisor can discuss the violation objectively, excluding the personal element as much as possible. The supervisor should take disciplinary action without being apologetic about the rule or about what he or she has to do to enforce it and without showing signs of anger. Once the disciplinary action has been taken, the supervisor must treat the employee as before and try to forget what happened. Understandably the person who has been disciplined will harbor some resentment, and the supervisor who meted out the discipline probably found doing it distasteful as well. Therefore, the supervisor and the employee may feel like avoiding each other for a few days. Such feelings are understandable, but it is far more advisable for the boss to find some opportunity to show his or her previous friendly feelings toward the disciplined employee. This is easier said than done. Only the mature person can handle discipline without hostility or guilt.

DISCIPLINE WITHOUT PUNISHMENT

Recently a number of organizations have tried to remove some of the shortcomings and resentment created by disciplinary action. In these entities it has been recognized that severe disciplinary action, such as unpaid suspension, does not cause the desired change in behavior. It has frequently been observed that no employee comes back from an unpaid suspension feeling better about himself or herself, about the supervisor, or about the institution. Despite our discussion on how to reduce the supervisor's dilemma, many supervisors are not satisfied with a system of discipline in which they often suffer more pain than the employee who was disciplined. Frequently the supervisor is faced with hostility, apathy, martyrdom, reduced output, a decline in trust, and an uncomfortable personal relationship with a subordinate. Organizations such as health-care institutions, with mostly white-collar professionals and highly educated technological employees, have often searched for a more palatable approach to discipline. An unpaid suspension for a staff pharmacist, for example, has been deemed inappropriate by many supervisors.

For all these and other reasons, many organizations have resorted to a non-punitive approach that is a more mature, more positive, and a better way to encourage a disciplined workforce. This approach is known as discipline without punishment. This approach is considered a positive discipline approach and appeals to the employee's sense of responsibility and refrains from implied or spoken threats of discipline. The important feature of this concept is the decision-making leave (Campbell, Fleming, and Grote 1985). Typically, it includes a series of counselings, starting with an oral meeting where the supervisor explains the rules or expectations and the rationale for them. The employee is encouraged to ask questions but is also told of the changes in his or her performance that are expected. Usually no record of this meeting is sent to the employee's personnel file. The second counseling, which reviews the employee's performance since the first interview, is documented, and often a copy of the documentation is placed in the employee's file in personnel. When counseling discussions have not produced the desired changes, management places the person on a one-day decision-making leave, during which the institution pays the individual for the day to show the employer's desire to have him or her remain a member of the organization, which removes resentment and hostility usually produced by punitive action. The employee is instructed to return the day following the leave with a decision either to change and stay or to quit the job. Remaining with the institution is conditional on the individual's decision to solve the immediate problem and make a total performance commitment. When the employee returns to the job to announce the decision to stay, his or her supervisor expresses confidence in the individual's ability to live up to the requirements but also makes it clear that failure to do so will lead to dismissal (Campbell, Fleming, and Grote 1985).

The decision-making leave with pay shows the individual the seriousness of the situation and offers an opportunity for cool reflection. It puts the burden on the employee and clearly represents the institution's refusal to make the employee's career decision. This nonpunitive approach forces the individual to take responsibility for future performance and behavior. The employee also realizes that he or she is confronted with a tougher employer's response in case of failure to meet standards. The costs connected with paying the employee for the day are far less than those associated with disciplinary suspension without pay.

The use of decision-making leave has proved as powerful in the executive suite as on the nursing floor or in the clinical laboratories. The organizations that have adopted this nonpunitive approach show good results because the responsibility for action is shifted from the supervisor to the employee. Also, the time frame changes from the past to the future. Nonpunitive discipline forces the problem employee to choose: "Become either a committed employee or a former employee" (Campbell, Fleming, and Grote 1985).

RIGHT OF APPEAL

In our society's legal environment an individual's wrongdoing is not judged by the accuser. The judge is not a party to the dispute between the accuser and the wrongdoer. In industrial and healthcare settings, however, this is not the case. The line superior decides whether a violation has occurred, how severe it is, and what the penalty should be. If a union is in place, the employee can appeal the case through a formal grievance procedure leading to binding arbitration. Nonunion organizations should also have a formal way of appealing a manager's decision because it is always possible that an individual in a position of authority might treat a subordinate unjustly. Thus, there must be a system to right such wrongs. Every enterprise must have a system of corrective justice that is concerned with maintaining a healthy organizational climate. A system for grievances must exist that enables employees to obtain satisfaction for unjust treatment and to resolve such a conflict.

This right of appeal to higher authority should exist both in an enterprise that has a union and one that does not. Following the chain of command, the immediate supervisor's boss is the one to whom such an appeal would first be directed. From there, the complaining employee can usually carry the appeal procedure through various levels, ultimately to the CEO of the organization as the final court of appeal. Unfortunately, in the contemporary organization, no system exists that serves to separate the executive functions from those functions involved in conducting a judicial review.

All healthcare organizations should have provisions for such an appeal procedure. However, great care must be taken that the right of appeal is a real right and not merely a formality. Some supervisors will gladly tell their subordinates that they can go to the next higher boss but will never forgive them if they do. Such statements and thinking merely indicate the supervisor's own insecurity in the managerial position. As a superior, he or she must permit the employee to take an appeal to the boss without resentment. It is management's obligation to provide such an appeal procedure, and the supervisor must not feel slighted in the role as manager or leader of the department when it is used. Management's failure to provide an appeal procedure may even be a chief reason why employees take recourse to local, state, or federal agencies, or pursue unionization.

Undoubtedly, a supervisor must be very mature not to see some threat from appeals that go over his or her head. Such a situation should be handled tactfully by the supervisor's boss. In the course of an appeal, the disciplinary penalty imposed by the supervisor possibly may be reduced or completely removed. Under these circumstances the supervisor understandably may become discouraged and frustrated because the boss has not backed him or her up. This usually happens in situations in which doubt remains about the actual events and the two stories do not coincide. In such cases the "guilty" employee normally goes "free." Although this is unfortunate, it is preferable that in a few instances a guilty employee goes free instead of an innocent employee being punished. In our legal system the "accused" is presumed innocent until proven guilty, and the burden of proof is on management.

Another reason for the reversal of a decision by higher-level management is that the supervisor may have been inconsistent in the exercise of discipline or that not all the necessary facts were obtained before disciplinary action was imposed. To avoid such an unpleasant situation, the supervisor must adhere closely to all that has been said in this chapter about the exercise of positive discipline. If a supervisor is a good disciplinarian, the verdict is normally upheld by the boss. Even if it should be reversed, this is still not too high a price to pay to guarantee justice for every employee. Without justice, a good organizational climate cannot exist.

SUMMARY

Discipline is a state of affairs. If morale is high, discipline probably will be good, and less need will exist for the supervisor to take disciplinary action. A supervisor is entitled to assume that most of the employees want to do the right thing and that much of the discipline will be self-imposed by the employees. In order for employees to do what is right, they must know what is expected of them and what the rules are. These should be in writing. If the occasion should arise, however, the supervisor must know how to take disciplinary action. There is usually a progressive list of disciplinary measures, ranging from an informal talk or an oral warning to discharge. The supervisor should bear in mind that the purpose of such disciplinary measures is not retribution or humiliation of employees. Rather, the goal of disciplinary action is improvement in the future behavior of the subordinate in question and in the department's other members. The idea is to avoid similar violations in the future. Using positive discipline and discipline without punishment approaches encourages the employee to rectify his or her own faults without the supervisor imposing threats or taking harsh punishment.

Nevertheless, taking disciplinary action is a painful experience for the employee as well as the supervisor. To do the best possible job, the supervisor must ensure that all disciplinary action fulfills the requirements of immediacy, forewarning, consistency, and impartiality. Furthermore, discipline should be administered in private. Moreover, the need for a good organizational climate makes necessary a system of corrective justice whereby any disciplinary action that an employee feels is unfair can be appealed.

NOTE

1. In all of our discussions we assume that the employees of the department do not belong to a union, and therefore no contractual obligations restrict the supervisor's authority in the realm of disciplinary action.

REFERENCES

Boucher, J. 2001. *How to Love the Job You Hate*, 163–66. Nashville, TN: Thomas Nelson Publishers.

Campbell, D. N., R. L. Fleming, and R. C. Grote. 1985. "Discipline Without Punishment—At Last." *Harvard Business Review* (July–August): 162–78.

Haire, M. 1964. *Psychology in Management, Second Edition*, 74. New York: McGraw-Hill Book Co.

Sayles, L. R., and G. Strauss. 1981. *Managing Human Resources, Second Edition*, 129. Englewood Cliffs, NJ: Prentice-Hall, Inc.

Strauss, G., and L. R. Sayles. 1980. *Personnel: The Human Problems of Management, Fourth Edition*, 221. Englewood Cliffs, NJ: Prentice-Hall, Inc.

"Positive Discipline: How to Turn up the Heat without the usual Threats." Law Office Administrator. May 2001. No. 5. Atlanta, GA: Ardmore Publishing Company.

Wells, J. T. 2001. "A Fish Story—Or Not?" *Journal of Accountancy* 190 (4): 114–117.

PART VII

Controlling

CHAPTER TWENTY-SEVEN

Fundamentals of Control

CHAPTER OBJECTIVES

After you have studied this chapter, you should be able to:

1. Define the managerial function of controlling.
2. Discuss different types of control systems.
3. Outline the basic requirements of a control system.

CONTROLS, A TERM that often arouses negative connotations if it is not used properly, play an important role in the life of any organization. Everyone active in an organized activity depends on controls for effective functioning of the organization. *Controlling* is an essential function for all managers in the organization by which they monitor performance and take corrective action when needed. Controlling is the process that checks performance against standards. Its purpose is to ensure that performance is consistent with plans and that the organizational and departmental goals and objectives are achieved.

The controlling function is closely related to the other four managerial functions, but it is most closely related to the planning function. When the manager performs the planning function, the direction, goals, objectives, and policies are set and become standards against which performance is checked and appraised. Many of the tools discussed in Chapter 16 are used in the controlling function. If deviations are found, the manager has to take corrective action, which may entail new plans and standards. This is how planning decisions affect controls and how control decisions affect plans, illustrating the circular nature of the management process.

THE NATURE OF CONTROL

Although this discussion of control appears last in this book, controlling is done simultaneously with the other functions. The better the manager plans, organizes, staffs, and influences, the better the supervisor can perform the controlling function, and vice versa. Controlling is often mistaken for inspection, which is a retrospective, or after-the-fact, activity. However, as Keister (2001) states, "four keys to achieving success in an organization includes (1) having accurate measurements to indicate how well the organization is performing; (2) understanding how well other organizations (competitors as well as noncompetitors) can perform similar activities; (3) understanding why others perform better than your organization; and (4) identifying any negative discrepancy between your performance and that of another organization, and taking appropriate measures to remedy those deficiencies."

A supervisor cannot expect to have good control over the department unless sound managerial principles in pursuing the other duties are followed. Well-made plans, workable policies and procedures, a properly planned organization, appropriate delegation of authority, continuous training of employees, good instructions, and good supervision all play a significant role in the department's results. The better these requirements are fulfilled, the more effective is the supervisor's function of controlling, and less corrective action is needed.

Human Reactions to Control

Another important aspect of control is how people respond to it; as mentioned earlier, the word control often carries negative connotations. Previous chapters considered work and human satisfaction, tight versus loose supervision, delegation of authority, and on-the-job freedom in connection with motivation. Although controls are an absolute requirement in any organized activity, one must keep in mind that in behavioral terms control means placing constraints on behavior so that what people do in organizations is more or less predictable. Control systems are designed to regulate behavior, which implies loss of freedom. People react negatively to loss of freedom. The amount of control determines how much freedom of action an individual has in performing the job. Complete absence of control, however, does not maximize an individual's perception of freedom because controls not only restrict a person's behavior but also the behavior of others toward him or her.

A certain amount of control, therefore, is essential for any organizational freedom to exist. Neither the extremes of tight control nor complete lack of control, however, bring about the desired organizational effectiveness. A balance between the two extremes is therefore necessary, which considers the amount of decentralization in the organization, management styles, motivational factors, situation, professional competence of the employees, and so on. In other words, to arrive at the most desirable mixture of freedom and control, the manager must try to balance the goals of organizational effectiveness and individual satisfaction. These goals must be kept in mind whenever a manager is determining the degree of control.

The Supervisor and Control

The purpose of the controlling process is to ensure that performance is consistent with plans, that plans and standards are being adhered to, and that proper progress is being made toward objectives. When supervisors set, communicate, and apply standards for performance for their staff and processes, they are exerting control. Also, if necessary, controlling means correcting any deviations from these standards that may occur. At times, the supervisor may enlist experts within the organization for assistance in obtaining control information data and counsel. It is inappropriate, however, for the supervisor to expect anyone else to perform the controlling function for him or her.

Planning, organizing, staffing, and influencing are the preparatory steps for getting the work done. Controlling is concerned with making certain that the work is properly executed. Without controlling, supervisors are not doing a complete job of managing. Control remains necessary whenever supervisors assign duties to subordinates, as the supervisors cannot shift the responsibility they have accepted from their own superiors. In other words, a supervisor can and must assign tasks and delegate authority, but, as stated throughout this book, responsibility cannot be delegated. Rather, the supervisor must exercise control to see that the responsibility is properly carried out.

The supervisor knows that the eventual success of the department depends on the degree of difference between what should be done and what is done. Having set up the standards of performance, the supervisor must stay informed of the actual performance through observation, reports, discussion, control charts, and other devices. Only then can the supervisor prescribe the necessary corrections that bring about full compliance of the standards.

Anticipatory Aspect of Control

To a large degree, controlling is a forward-looking function; it has anticipatory aspects. Management is concerned with controls that anticipate potential sources of deviation from standards. Past experience and the study of past events tell the supervisor what has taken place and where, when, and why certain standards were not met. This enables management to make provisions so that future activities do not lead to these deviations. Unfortunately, the anticipatory aspect of controlling is not always sufficiently stressed, and often supervisors are primarily concerned with its corrective and reactive aspects. Deviations from standards are detected after they have occurred and are corrected, rather than anticipated, at the point of performance.

All efforts to control, whether corrective, reactive, or anticipatory, have an effect on the future. Normally, the supervisor can do little about the past. For example, if the work assigned to a subordinate for the day has not been accomplished, the controlling process cannot correct that. Some supervisors are inclined to scold the person responsible and assume that he or she was deliberately negligent. The good supervisor, however, looks forward rather than backward and at the same time studies the past to learn what has taken place and why. This enables him or her to take the proper steps to ensure corrective and ideally preventive action for the future.

Because control is a forward-looking function, the supervisor must discover deviations from the established standards as quickly as possible. Therefore, the supervisor's duty is to minimize the time lag between results and corrective action. For example, instead of waiting until the day is over, it is more advisable for a housekeeping supervisor to check at midday to see whether the work is progressing satisfactorily. Even though the morning is already past and nothing can be done about any deviations that may have occurred, monitoring progress earlier in the day can minimize the deviation and the correction to be made.

Not all anticipatory concerns relate to whether a process is completed correctly or a piece of equipment is functioning appropriately. The supervisor must consider the use, or to be more exact, the misuse of company assets. As Wells (2001, 31) states, "Sometimes, the truth isn't very pretty. Consider, for example, the American workforce. Although regarded by many as the finest in the world, it has a dark side. According to estimates, a third of American workers have stolen on the job. Many of these thefts are immaterial to the financial statements, but not all are . . . ." Recent high-profile incidents involving executives at HealthSouth, HCA, and Tenet have led to intensified compliance and ethics monitoring programs. Stealing from the job may take many forms, including fraud, internal theft, and asset misappropriation. Therefore, when one spends an excessive amount of time surfing the Internet when he or she should have been working, assets have been misappropriated.

The inappropriate use of work time to surf the Internet is a real concern for supervisors. If the sites being visited are pornographic and other employees see them, the supervisor could have sexual harassment complaints to deal with. Some information technology departments have successfully stemmed the inappropriate use of the Internet by (1) timing out the usage period for any user, (2) restricting sites that can be visited based on site content or domain name, and (3) periodically checking the history files of the Internet user and providing reports to the area supervisor. These control techniques are both anticipatory and concurrent in nature.

However, usage of the Internet is not the only productivity waster; there is also e-mail to contend with. Today e-mail is essential to communication between staff. It provides a medium for supervisors to disseminate procedures and keep staff up to date on new events and issues, and it allows two-way communication between different shifts and physical sites. However, according to a survey quoted in *The Sunday Oklahoman*, workers stated that they spend at least two hours a day reading and responding to e-mail (Erickson 2001). In addition to the loss of time, e-mail also fuels the grapevine and can result in inappropriate distribution of department or organization proprietary information. Methods to control unwanted dissemination of information include (1) scanning the content before the e-mail is released to the Internet, (2) restricting e-mail to only individuals on an authorized list to receive messages, and (3) restricting the size of the e-mail document or not permitting attachments.

Because individuals tend to abbreviate their comments in an e-mail message, misunderstandings can arise and politically incorrect language may be used. Jokes and photos sent via e-mail can be easily shared. These documents may be inappropriate and stir concerns of racism, harassment, and other complaints from employees receiving them. Lastly, and possibly most important for healthcare organizations, is the patient confidentiality concern. Many patient documents are electronically created and sent via e-mail to physicians and other caregivers. An employee who finds a document on a friend (or enemy) can easily transmit that document to his or her home e-mail account or to others who should not have access to it, thus violating the patient's privacy.

Having a written policy on Internet and e-mail usage is essential. Policy clauses may include (Glover 2001) the following:

- Disclosure to employees prior to hiring and periodically thereafter that all e-mail, Internet access, and computer files are subject to monitoring
- Notification to employees that the technology provided by the organization is company property and is to be used for business purposes
- Explanation to employees that despite the fact that they are given passwords to access the system, they should not have an expectation that the system is private
- Notification to employees what, if any, material they are not allowed to transport into or out of the company's system, including file downloads
- Request from each employee a written acknowledgment of receipt of the written policy when issued and updated

The supervisor's role is to ensure each of his or her subordinates has read and understood the policy and to cooperate with the information technology department and others in monitoring the usage of these assets.

CONTROL SYSTEMS

Three different types of control systems are discussed: anticipatory (preventive or ahead of time), concurrent (in process or during the event), and feedback (reactive or after-the-event) controls.

These control systems assess whether deadlines and time constraints are met (time controls), whether the appropriate amounts of inventoried parts or materials have been consumed (material controls), whether the equipment functioned properly (equipment controls), and whether the product or service was delivered at the anticipated cost (cost controls). Chapter 29 discusses how budgets are used to help management control expenses associated with services and products relative to the projected or standard expense. By their nature, budgets are financial controls. Chapter 16 discusses various quality control tools, such as the use of a control chart to monitor perioperative mortality or a run chart to display patient satisfaction with new menu items. However, many healthcare organizations have established dashboards or scorecards directly tied to the strategic goals established by the board of directors. According to Griffith and Alexander (2002), four major scorecard dimensions have gained acceptance in the healthcare industry: financial, internal business processes, customer, and learning and growth. An example of a healthcare organization's dashboard appears in Figure 27.1.

Anticipatory Controls

Anticipatory (or preventive) controls are in place before the service activity or production starts. They anticipate potential problems and prevent their occurrence. *Anticipatory control* is a proactive, not a reactive, approach.

The supervisor should preview the entire process and task. In doing this, forward-looking control mechanisms will be built into the system, and mistakes are likely to be avoided. The purpose of preliminary controls is to anticipate and prevent mistakes by taking care of a potential malfunction in advance. For example, the supervisor plans and arranges for regular preventive maintenance so that the equipment does not break down when needed.

Other examples of anticipatory controls are policies, procedures, standard practices, and rules. These are designed so that a predetermined course of action is prescribed to prevent mistakes or malfunctioning. For example, every hospital has established detailed plans and precise procedures in case of an emergency such as a fire. Disciplinary rules dealing with the problem of carrying a weapon on hospital premises constitute an anticipatory control mechanism because the rules serve as a deterrent. Other examples of preventive control mechanisms are warning signals on a piece of equipment and checklists for testing procedures. Consider the extensive checklist an anesthesiologist goes through before administering anesthesia to a patient. Using this anticipatory approach to control enables the supervisor to eliminate many potential daily crises.

Concurrent Controls

Another group of control mechanisms is composed of *concurrent controls,* which help spot problems as they occur. The purpose is to apply controls while the operations are in progress instead of waiting for the outcome. In these situations, the supervisor does not anticipate problems but monitors operations in process. For example, concurrent controls enable the supervisor to keep the quality and quantity of output standardized. There are numerous examples of concurrent control mechanisms all around the supervisor, such as simple numerical counters, automatic switches, warning signals, and sophisticated online computer systems. Whenever the supervisor does not have such aids available, he or she monitors the activities by observation and instruction or by that of other employees. Examples of familiar concurrent control mechanisms are the fuel gauge in the car and the parking meter. Many computer software applications have concurrent controls that may require entry of data in a certain field or flagging a discrepancy. The software alerts the user immediately so corrective action can be taken at that time.

FIGURE 27.1 PERFORMANCE DASHBOARD

	Key Metrics	July, 05	Aug, 05		10 - Stretch	9	8	7 - Goal	6	5	4	3	2	1	Raw Score	Weight (%)	SubTol Score
SERVICE	Emergency Dept.Sat. Mean	83.9	84.4	☺	84.5	83.9	83.3	82.7	82.2	81.7	81.2	80.7	80.2	79.5	9	0.040	0.36
SERVICE	Clinic Pt Satisfac Mean (bi-annual)	88.9	88.9		91.2	90.7	90.2	89.7	88.9	88.0	87.1	86.3	85.5	84.7	6	0.040	0.24
QUALITY	Amb. Surg Pain Mean	93.0	92.6	☹	92.1	92.0	91.8	91.6	91.1	90.6	90.1	89.6	89.1	88.6	10	0.033	0.33
QUALITY	Core Measure AMI (qrtly)	92.1%	94.7%	☺	100%	96%	93%	90%	86%	83%	80%	70%	60%	50%	8	0.033	0.26
FINANCIAL	Days in AR	48.30	46.61	☺	42.00	43.00	44.00	45.00	47.00	50.00	52.00	55.00	57.00	60.00	6	0.068	0.41
FINANCIAL	Financial Strength Index	0.99	1.30	☺	1.94	1.73	1.52	1.31	0.94	0.57	0.20	0.15	0.10	0.05	6	0.068	0.41
PEOPLE	Empl.Satisfaction (Annual)	3.72	3.72		3.80	3.77	3.74	3.72	3.67	3.62	3.57	3.52	3.47	3.42	7	0.040	0.28
PEOPLE	Qrtly.Emp.Satis. w Benefit pkg.	2.5	2.5		3.31	3.29	3.27	3.25	3.15	3.05	2.96	2.90	2.84	2.78	0	0.040	0.00
PEOPLE	Phy Recruitment (qrtly)	0.82	0.82		1.23	1.15	1.07	1.00	0.92	0.84	0.76	0.69	0.61	0.54	4	0.040	0.16
GROWTH	Cancer Center Visits	400	514	☺	455	447	440	433	428	423	417	412	407	402	10	0.027	0.27
GROWTH	Births	69	81	☺	65	64	63	62	60	58	55	52	49	47	10	0.028	0.28
GROWTH	Cardiac Cath Procedures	150	191	☺	156	153	151	149	144	139	135	131	127	123	10	0.027	0.27

☺ improvement since previous month   ☹ decline since previous month   Total Score **7.05**

Sept	Oct	Nov	Dec	Jan	Feb	March	April	May	June	July	Goal	7
5.12	4.56	4.93	5.31	5.31	5.21	6.27	6.08	5.31	5.9	5.2	Stretch	10

Feedback Controls

A third group of control mechanisms, *feedback controls*, alerts the supervisor after the event is completed. For example, an insurance company's benefits supervisor reviews an abandoned-call report and finds callers abandoning the "wait to speak to a customer service representative" option at the rate of 60 percent on Wednesday, but during the rest of the week the abandonment rate is under 10 percent. With this data in hand, the supervisor can implement changes to prevent future abandonment during Wednesday calls. The feedback control system is the most widely used category. It takes place after the process is finished and the mistake or damage is done. The purpose of this type of control is to improve from the point of damage and to prevent any future deviation and recurrence.

Feedback controls are most helpful in planning process improvements. Examples of feedback controls are quality and quantity reports, opinion surveys or service surveys, and accounting reports. The quality dashboard is such a control (see Figure 27.1). A common human resources feedback control is the exit interview performed with employees leaving the organization (see Figure 27.2). The interview is performed to determine why the employee has chosen to look elsewhere for employment or to resign from his or her position. The feedback and

FIGURE 27.2 AN EXIT INTERVIEW

Anywhere Surgi-Center Exit Interview

Our human resources department is interested in your comments about your employment here. By sharing your constructive criticism, concerns, and problems encountered during your employment we will be able to plan changes to our programs, procedures, and compensation and benefit plans. Your comments are confidential, do not become part of your personnel record, and are not shared with your past supervisor.

Tell us about the position you held with our Center:

* What position did you hold? _____ Department: _____

Tell us about your new position:

* Name of the Company: _____ Position: _____

* Compensation: _____ Did this company offer any benefits or perks that were particularly appealing? _____

Please share your comments and suggestions:

* What is the principal reason for your leaving our Center?

* How do you feel about Anywhere as a place to work?

* What changes or improvements would you suggest that we should make at the Center and/or in the department where you worked?

* Were your training, skills, and experience utilized?

* Did you feel you were a contributing member of the team?

* Were your opinions or suggestions given consideration?

* Was your salary appropriate for your position and duties?

* Were you informed of promotional opportunities?

* While you were employed here, did you notice any violations of our Code of Conduct, procedures, or regulatory requirements? ___ No; ___ Yes: If so, did you discuss the situation(s) with anyone outside of the Center? ___ No; ___ Yes: If so, who? _____

* If you reported these violations to someone in the Center, was the issue(s) resolved to your satisfaction? ___ Yes; ___ No: Why not? _____

* Would you recommend Anywhere Surgi-Center as an employer to others? ___ Yes; ___ No; If not, please explain: _____

* Is there anything else you would like us to know? _____

Thank you.

information should go to the departing employee's supervisor, who in turn will translate the comments into process corrections for the remaining employees.

Because control after the fact is the least desirable control mechanism, the supervisor should make every effort to devise as many anticipatory and concurrent control mechanisms as possible. The supervisor should be able to convert many of the feedback controls into concurrent mechanisms or even into anticipatory controls with the help of up-to-date information systems and by encouraging employee involvement in problem resolution. Brainstorming is a good technique to encourage employee input. By empowering employees to take corrective action or, at a minimum, encouraging employees to contribute ideas and comments, some feedback controls become unnecessary.

The Closeness of Control

Knowing how closely to control or monitor the work of a subordinate is a real test of any supervisor's talents. The closeness of follow-up from the subordinate's point of view is based on such factors as the experience, initiative, dependability, and resourcefulness of the employee who is given the assignment. Giving an employee an assignment and allowing him or her to do the job is part of the process of delegation. This does not mean, however, that the supervisor should leave the employee completely alone until it is time to inspect the final results. Delegation also does not mean that the supervisor should watch over every detail. Rather, the supervisor must be familiar enough with the ability of the subordinate to determine accurately how much leeway to give and how closely to follow through with the control measures.

Basic Requirements of a Control System

For any control system to be workable and effective, it must fulfill certain basic requirements. Controls should (1) be understandable; (2) register deviations quickly and be timely; (3) be appropriate, adequate, and economical; (4) be somewhat flexible; and (5) indicate where corrective action should be applied. These requirements are applicable to all services in all organized activities and to all levels within the management hierarchy. They are discussed below in general terms; it would be impossible to spell out the specific characteristics of controls used in each department or service of a healthcare enterprise.

Understanding of Controls

The first requirement of a workable control system is that the control mechanisms must be understandable and fit the people involved, the tasks, and the environment. Both the manager and the subordinates must understand the data and what type of control is to be exercised. This is necessary on all managerial levels. The farther down the hierarchy the system is to be applied, the less complicated it should be. Thus, the top-level administrator may use a complicated system of controls based on mathematical formulas, statistical analysis, and complex computer printouts that are understandable to top-level administration. The control system for the lower supervisory level, however, should be less sophisticated. It must be designed to the level of the user. If the control system is too complicated, the supervisor will frequently have to devise his or her own control system that fulfills the same need and can be understood by the employees as well.

Prompt Indication of Deviations

To have a workable control system, controls must indicate deviations quickly so that trends can be corrected without delay. As pointed out, controls are forward looking, and the supervisor cannot control the past. The sooner the supervisor is aware of deviations, however, the sooner he or she can take corrective action. It is more desirable to have deviations reported quickly, even if substantiated only by partial information, approximate figures, and estimates. In other words, it is far better for the supervisor to have prompt approximate information than highly accurate information that arrives too late to be of much value. This does not mean that the supervisor should jump to conclusions or take corrective action hastily. The supervisor's familiarity with the job to be done, knowledge, and past experience help him or her quickly sense when something is not progressing as planned and requires prompt supervisory action.

Appropriateness and Adequacy

Controls must always be appropriate and significant for the activity they are to monitor. Control tools that are suitable for the dietary department are different from those used in accounts payable. Even within nursing, the tools used by the director of nursing services are different from those the head nurse uses on the floor. An elaborate control system required in a large undertaking is not needed in a small department; however, the need for control still exists, only the magnitude of the control system is different. Whatever controls are applied, it is essential that they be appropriate for the job involved. They must be consistent with the organizational structure so that the person with authority to act will obtain the data.

Economics of Controls

Controls must be worth the expense involved—that is, they must be economical. At times, however, it may be difficult for management to ascertain how much a particular control system is worth and how much it really costs. One important criterion might be the consequences that would follow if the controls did not exist. The nurses' control of narcotics is stringent and exact, for example, whereas no one is too concerned with close control of bandages.

Flexibility

Because all undertakings work in a dynamic situation, unforeseen circumstances could play havoc even with the best-laid plans and standards. The control system must be built so that it remains flexible. It must be designed to keep pace with the continuously changing pattern of a dynamic setting. The control system must permit change as soon as the change is required, or it is bound to fail. If the employee seems to run into unexpected conditions early in the assignment, through no fault of his or her own, the supervisor must recognize this and adjust the plans and standards accordingly. The control system must leave room for individual judgment and changing circumstances.

Corrective Action

A final requirement of effective controls is that they must point the way to corrective action. It is not enough to show deviations as they have occurred. The system must also indicate where they have occurred and who is responsible for them. A common problem in many healthcare organizations is having more than one patient unit number for the same patient. This can cause havoc in health information as well as the blood bank and radiology. By developing reports to identify who is assigning new numbers to existing patients, management can follow up with in-service sessions and reeducation of appropriate staff members. Supervisors must make it their business to know precisely where the standards were not met and who is responsible for not achieving them. If successive operations are involved, it may be necessary for the supervisor to check the performance after each step has been accomplished and before the work is passed on to the next employee or to another department.

SUMMARY

Controlling is the managerial function of monitoring performance; the manager checks performance against standards and takes corrective action if deviations exist. Control is most closely related to the planning function, but it is interwoven with all the other managerial functions as well. Control is essential in every organized activity, although in behavioral terms control means placing constraints on people. A good control system must be designed so that it brings about organizational effectiveness without infringing on individual satisfaction.

In relation to time, one can distinguish among anticipatory, concurrent, and feedback control mechanisms. There are several basic requirements for a control system to be effective. The supervisor must make sure that the subordinates fully understand the controls and that the controls are appropriate for the situation. Because control is anticipatory, a control system should be designed to report deviations as promptly as possible. Controls must also be worth the expense involved and the effort put forth. A good control system also must allow sufficient flexibility to cope with new situations and circumstances in a dynamic setting. Finally, a viable control system must clearly indicate where and why deviations have occurred so that the supervisor can take appropriate corrective action at the proper place.

REFERENCES

Erickson, P. B. 2001. "Study Shows E mail Eating Up Workdays." *The Sunday Oklahoman*, July 1, p. 1-C.

Glover, R. H. 2001. "Monitoring of Employee's Use of Company-Owned Technology and the Privacy Issues it Creates in the Workplace." Gardner, Carton & Douglas Client Memorandum. *Technology and HR Law* (June): 4–5.

Griffith, J. R., and J. A. Alexander. 2002. "Measuring Comparative Hospital Performance." *Journal of Healthcare Management* 47 (1): 42.

Keister, J. 2001. "Benchmarking: Healthcare's Invaluable Measuring Stick." *For The Record* 13 (26): 19.

Wells, J. T. 2001. "Enemies Within." *Journal of Accountancy* 192 (6): 31–33.

CHAPTER TWENTY-EIGHT

The Control Process

CHAPTER OBJECTIVES

After you have studied this chapter, you should be able to do the following:

1. Discuss the steps in the control process.
2. Review the purposes for measuring and comparing performance.
3. Describe corrective action techniques.
4. Review the basic managerial steps of setting standards, measuring performance, and taking corrective action.

THE FEEDBACK MODEL OF CONTROLS

The organizational control system can be viewed as a *feedback model.* Information on how the system is doing is obtained by the supervisor, or the sensor, who then monitors the system by comparing the actual results with the desired performance. Whenever the actual performance deviates from the standards set, the system triggers corrective action in the form of an input (see Figure 28.1). This closed-loop feedback system works the same way a thermostat in the home functions. The thermostat is set at the desired degree of temperature. Whenever the room temperature falls below or rises above that temperature, the thermostat, continuously comparing room temperature to the desired temperature, corrects the variation by turning on or shutting off the furnace or air conditioner. This type of control is known as cybernetic because it monitors and manages a process with the help of a self-regulating mechanism.

In performing the controlling function, the supervisor must follow three basic steps. First, he or she sets the standards. Second, the supervisor must check and appraise performance and compare it against these standards to determine whether it meets the expected standards. Third, if standards are not met, the supervisor must take corrective action (see Figure 28.2). This sequence of steps is necessary for effective control. The supervisor could not possibly check and report on deviations without having set the standards in advance, and corrective action cannot be taken unless deviations from these standards are discovered.

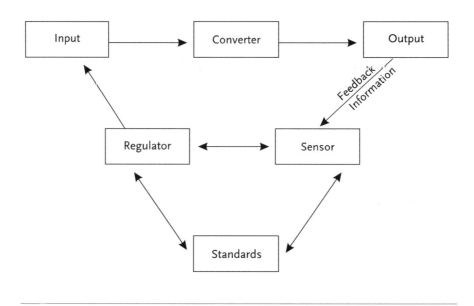

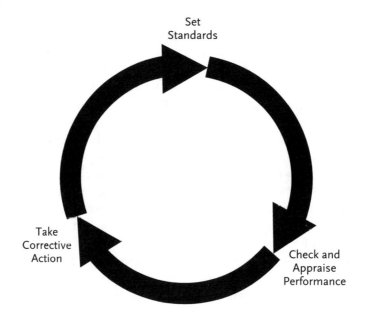

ESTABLISHING STANDARDS

The establishment of standards is the first step in the control process. Standards are criteria against which subsequent performance or results can be judged. Standards also are known as performance metrics. *Performance metrics* are any performance-related measurement of activity or resource utilization (Performance Co-Pilot Tutorial Glossary 2005). Standards state what should be done; they are derived from organizational goals and objectives, and they should be expressed in measurable terms. Occasionally, goals are established by comparing one's organization to the performance of others, which is known as benchmarking. Control standards can be as broad or as narrow as the level to which they apply. In planning, the CEO sets the overall objectives and goals that the healthcare center is to achieve. These overall objectives are then broken down into narrower objectives for the individual divisions and departments.

The supervisor of a department establishes even more specific goals that relate to quality, quantity, costs, time standards, quotas, schedules, budgets, and so forth. These goals become the criteria, the standards, for exercising control. Good performance measures should be responsibility-linked, customer-focused, balanced, timely, credible, comparable, and simple (Henderson, Chase, and Woodson 2002). These examples are tangible; however, many standards are intangible. Although the latter are much more difficult to set and work with, a healthcare institution has to consider many intangible standards, especially concerning patient care.

Tangible Standards

The most common tangible standards are physical standards that pertain to the actual operation of a department in which goods are produced (e.g., the dietary department) or services are rendered (e.g., nursing services, laboratories, and laundry). Physical standards define the amount of work to be produced within a given time span. Cost standards are also tangible standards and define direct and indirect labor costs, costs of materials and supplies used, overhead, and many other items.

These standards are quantitative and qualitative. Not only do they define, for example, how much money can be spent per patient on food, supplies, and materials for three meals a day, but they also state what quality these meals are to have as far as nutritional value, taste, and aesthetic appeal are concerned. Likewise, standards dictate how much one pound of laundry should cost and how many pounds are to be processed in a certain time, taking into consideration the state of mechanization and automation of the laundry. Furthermore, the laundry has qualitative standards in terms of sanitation and sterilization, cleanliness of the linens, color, and absence of stains. In another example, standards specify the number of nursing personnel on a floor in relation to the number of patients to be cared for. Such standards vary depending on the time of day, the nursing unit in question (e.g., an intensive care unit versus a regular floor unit), and many other factors. Standards also exist for the patient's comfort, physical needs, and safety and for the room's cleanliness and orderliness.

Intangible Standards

In addition to tangible standards that can be expressed in physical terms, there are also standards of an intangible nature. In a hospital or related healthcare facility some intangible standards are the institution's reputation in the community; the quality of medicine practiced; the excellence of patient care; and the degree of "tender loving care," the level of commitment to values, and the level of morale of the employees. It is exceedingly difficult, if not impossible, to express the criteria for such intangible standards in precise and numerical terms. It is much simpler to measure performance against tangible standards, such as number of nursing personnel in relation to the number of patients or days of revenue in unbilled accounts.

Nevertheless, a supervisor should not overlook the intangible achievements even if it is difficult to set standards for them and measure the performance of them. Tools for appraising some of these intangible standards come in the form of attitude surveys, questionnaires, and interviews. Although these tools are not exact, they can be helpful in determining to what extent certain intangible standards are being achieved. They also provide the manager with a sketch of the customers' expectations or perception of service quality. When patient questionnaires are returned indicating that the housekeeping service was poor, yet the housekeeping supervisor knows the room was cleaned daily, it may be necessary to take other actions such as having the housekeeper ask the patient before leaving the room whether the room is cleaned to the patient's satisfaction.

Approaches to Establishing Standards

In setting standards, the supervisor is aided by experience and knowledge of the various jobs to be done within the department. A supervisor has a general idea of how much time it takes to perform a certain job, what resources are required, what constitutes good performance, and what is a poor job. Job knowledge and experience are the resources the supervisor uses to establish the standards against which to judge the performance and results of the department.

Motion and Time Studies

There are also more scientific and systematic ways of establishing objective standards. In some activities the supervisor can call on industrial engineers who use work-measurement techniques to help determine the amount of work an average employee should produce within a given time period. In many departments in a healthcare organization, such as housekeeping, laundry, laboratories, courier, and dietary service, this approach is worth the effort and cost. Standards determined through work-measurement techniques help the supervisor distribute the work more evenly and judge fairly whether an employee is performing satisfactorily.

The supervisor, however, rarely conducts work-measurement analyses. They are usually assigned to an industrial engineer or perhaps to an outside consultant trained in doing motion and time studies. Motion study involves an analysis of the elements of the job and of how the job is currently performed with a view to changing, eliminating, or combining certain steps and devising a method that will be quicker and easier. Often flowcharts are drawn up that analyze the steps taken in performing the job. After a thorough analysis of the motions and workflow arrangements, the engineer will come up with what is considered the best method for doing the job in question. For example, the workplace layout may be redesigned and hand motions may be revamped.

Once the best method has been designed, time studies are performed to determine the standard time required to do the job using this method. One or more qualified workers are timed with a stopwatch as they perform the prescribed work methods. Time studies are done scientifically and systematically by selecting an average employee for observation; measuring the times used for the various elements of the job; applying leveling and other corrective factors; and making allowances for fatigue, personal needs, contingencies, and delays. The combined result leads to a standard time necessary to perform the job. Although this method is scientific, one must keep in mind that considerable judgment and many approximations are used to arrive at the standard time. Decisions involving judgment and discretion still must be made. Standard times, however, are a sound basis on which to determine objective standards. They also enable the supervisor to predict the number of employees required and the probable cost of the job to be done. In many activities outside the healthcare field, standards of this type serve as a basis for cost estimates and incentive plans.

If industrial engineers are not available, the supervisor can perform some of the studies simply by observing and timing the various operations and making the necessary adjustments previously stated. If the job to be performed in the department has never been done there before, the supervisor should try to base tentative standards on similar operations. If the new job has no similarity to any previous function, the best the supervisor can do (unless the help of industrial engineers is available) is to observe the operation while it is being performed the first few times. The supervisor has to make approximate time and motion studies to arrive at a standard for the new function. Sometimes the manufacturer of a new piece of equipment can be helpful to the supervisor in providing standard data—for example, how long it will take an apparatus to perform a certain task. Regardless of the approach taken, the supervisor should attempt to align the standards established to a quality measure that gauges the employee's ability to deliver the right output, the right way, the first time, and on time (Spath 2002).

Time Ladder for:	
Time	Activities or Duties Performed During This Period
0700	Turned on computer; went to front desk to obtain requisitions
0715	Sorted requisitions by patient floor
0730	Prepared tubes for each area/placed in phlebotomy cart
0745	same as above
0800	same as above
0815	same as above. Distributed phlebotomy carts
0830	Took break and picked up new requisitions
0845	Sorted requisitions by patient floor
0900	Prepared tubes for each area/placed in phlebotomy cart

Time Ladders

Another approach to collecting data on productivity is the time ladder. This technique requires the employee to note what he or she does during 5-, 10-, or 15-minute increments of time throughout a day for several days (see Figure 28.3). Employees who perform the same duties maintain separate ladders. The data tell the manager the average number of units one produces in a day and the types of interference an employee encounters, as well as nonproductive time (restroom visits, breaks, and so forth). The method places the burden of data collection on the employee but requires the supervisor to validate some of the data through other techniques such as direct observation.

Work Sampling Through Direct Observation

In the direct observation approach, supervisors periodically observe employees and note whether they are working, what they are working on, or whether they are idle or on break. The supervisor maintains a log that lists the employees along one axis and the key activities along the other. An example of an observation record form is shown in Figure 28.4.

Tick marks are made during each observation, marking the activity the employee is performing at the time of the observation. Each observation is usually brief (10–15 minutes total) depending on the number of employees in

Observation Record for
Health Information Management Services

	Jane Super-visor	Lori Tran-scribe	Tara Tran-scribe	Susan Tran-scribe	Larry File Clerk	Kent File Clerk	Kim Coder	Mel Coder	John Coder	Totals
Supervisory activities										
Technical (non-supervisory duties)										
Transcribing										
Handling transcribed work										
Filing records										
Sorting records										
Pulling records										
Coding										
Abstracting										
Idle, gone, non-productive activities										
Totals										

Date of this sampling:
Observation Times:
1.   4.   7.   10.
2.   5.   8.   11.
3.   6.   9.   12.

the work area, the size of the work area, and whether the supervisor must walk around to adequately observe the staff. The observations occur several times a day (known as sampling).

Because the observation times are randomly selected, they could occur at virtually any time during the workday. After several days of the observation sampling, adequate data are compiled to indicate what percentage of the time employee X was engaged in each of his or her key activities. This information provides the manager with information against which to compare production data. One might expect that if Kent files an average of 100 records a day and Larry files 250 a day and performs a comparable amount of sorting and pulling as Kent, Larry may have a better method of doing his work. If so, the manager will want Larry to show Kent this method. Alternatively, the standard could be set at 250, and Kent would be encouraged to model Larry to achieve the standard.

Although they may not be absolutely scientific, standards are more likely to be effective if they are set with the participation of the supervisor and the subordinates instead of being handed down by a staff engineer, a manager, or an outside consultant. The purpose of any standard is to establish a specific goal for the employees to strive toward, and, as with all directives, employees are likely to be more motivated to achieve those standards in which they have had some part. Furthermore, none of the above methods should be used without advising the staff in advance that the analysis is planned. Morale could be affected negatively if employees feel they are being watched and do not know why.

How to Select Strategic Standards

The number of standards or metrics that can be used to ascertain the quality and quantity of performance within a department is very large and increases rapidly as the department expands. As the operations within the department become more sophisticated and complex and the functions of the department increase, it becomes more difficult and time consuming for supervisors to check against all the conceivable standards. Therefore, they need to concentrate on certain standards by selecting some of them as the strategic ones; those that best reflect the goals and whether they are being met.

For example, a billing manager knows which strategic points to check first. He or she probably checks the bill lag or accounts receivable report and makes certain that the lag between discharge and bill drop has not lengthened, the accounts receivable are within expected limits, and the lag between discharge and coding has not significantly changed. He or she also observes where the billing personnel are and what they are doing. Each of these areas constitutes a strategic point of control for the billing manager. Unfortunately, there are no specific guidelines on how to select these strategic control points. The peculiarities of each departmental function and the makeup of the supervisor and employees are different in each situation. Thus, only general guidelines can be suggested for selecting strategic standards.

One of the first considerations in choosing one standard as more strategic than another is timeliness. Because time is essential in control and controls are anticipatory, the earlier the deviation can be discovered, the better. This helps to correct problems early before errors begin to compound. Keeping this in mind, the supervisor can determine at what point in time and in the process activities should be checked. For example, in the maintenance department, the strategic control point may be after a crack has been repaired, but before it has been repainted.

Another consideration in choosing strategic control points is whether they permit economic observations. Chapter 27 mentions that a control system must be worth the expense involved; it must be economical. The same applies to the strategic control points. A further consideration is that the strategic standards should allow comprehensive and balanced control. The supervisor must be aware that the selection of one strategic control point might have an adverse effect on another. Excessive control on the quantity of achievements often has an adverse effect on the quality. On the other hand, if expenses are selected as a strategic control point, the quality or quantity of the output may suffer. For example, the executive housekeeper must not sacrifice quality standards that have been designed to prevent infections in order to cut expenses. All these decisions depend on the nature of the work within the department. What serves well as a strategic control point in one activity does not necessarily apply in another.

A supervisor may find it simpler to choose among many strategic control point options by identifying and prioritizing those that represent a majority of the work performed in the department (recall the Pareto Principle described in Chapter 16); those that, if not monitored, could place the department or organization at risk; and those that could affect the safety or security of the organization, its resources or assets, its staff, or patients. For example, the following is a list of strategic control options available for the administrator of Small Town Hospital. Small Town is located in an agricultural community.

Daily
- Number of patients hospitalized
- Number of patients scheduled for surgery
- Percentage (semi-annual) of patients treated from service area zip codes
- Total admissions by physician
- Total surgeries by physician
- Cash taken in today
- Accounts receivable today
- Cleanliness of hallways and public areas
- Number of in-service sessions occurring throughout the hospital

Weekly
- Legislative action planned at the state capitol
- Current corn and cattle prices
- Openings or closures of businesses in the service area

This administrator could monitor a number of variables as strategic control points, but many of those listed are of little value to a supervisor. However, strategic control options for you based on this list may be knowing (1) the number of patients the hospital will serve in that day and whether there is adequate staff in your department to tend to the patients' needs or (2) the accounts receivable balance and age and cash taken yesterday. The first set of control points represents the majority of services performed, while the second set speaks to protecting the hospital's assets.

COMMUNICATING AND MONITORING STANDARDS

For control to have an effective influence on performance, the supervisor must ensure that the goals and standards are known to all the employees within the department and clarify who is responsible for their achievement so that he or she knows whom to contact for deviations if the results are not achieved and whom to praise if they are exceeded. After all, the supervisor is interested in having the standards and objectives reached. Only if each employee knows exactly what is expected concerning his or her own work can the subordinate try to achieve it. This is why the supervisor must link the standards with the individual responsibilities of each employee.

The second step in the process of control is to check on actual performance and compare measured performance against the standards. Observing and measuring performance is an ongoing activity for every manager. Work is observed, output is measured, and reports are compiled. The checking of activities is usually done by the supervisor after the subordinate has completed the function. Because the supervisor does not shift responsibility when assigning a duty to a subordinate and when delegating authority, he or she must make certain that enough controls are available to take corrective action in case the performance does not meet the standards.

Some ways for a supervisor to check on and measure performance are (1) comparing performance with standards; (2) directly observing the work and personally checking on the employees; (3) measuring work in, out, and remaining to do; and (4) studying various summaries of reports and figures that are submitted to the supervisor.

Comparing

As the manager observes and measures performance, it must be compared with the standards developed in the beginning of the control process. Such comparisons are an ongoing activity of the supervisor daily, weekly, and monthly. The observed performance may be higher, the same as, or lower than the standards. In the first two situations, the supervisor obviously does not have any problems. If the performance does not meet standards, however, corrective action is required.

Because some deviation is expected in some activities, the question is how much deviation is acceptable before taking remedial action. This depends on the activity; in some activities, minor deviations may be acceptable. In other activities, such as nursing, deviations can be critical, and even a small one may not be tolerated. Furthermore, in some activities it is easy to measure performance, as in controlling sales and production; in other activities, as in many healthcare activities, measuring performance is not easy and comparisons are sometimes less clear-cut. (See the discussion on performance appraisal in Chapter 21.) It is the supervisor's job to develop valid performance measures to control effectively and take corrective action when necessary.

Direct Personal Observation

Observation is probably the most widely used technique for measurement. There is no better way for a supervisor to check performance than by direct observation and personal contact. Unfortunately, personal observation is time consuming, but every manager should spend part of each day away from his or her desk observing the performance of the employees. For example, regular rounds are not only necessary for the head nurse; they are just as important for the director of housekeeping, the chief dietitian, and the hospital administrator.

The nursing home administrator may make rounds in the resident areas less frequently, but even he or she should make some personal observations. For the supervisor, direct observations are the most effective way of maintaining close contact with employees as part of their constant training and development. This opportunity for close personal observation is one of the great advantages of the supervisor's job; it is something that the top-level administrator cannot do to any great extent. The farther removed a manager is from the firing line, the less he or she can observe personally and the more he or she has to depend on reports. However, regardless of your level in the management ladder, you should attempt to visit all areas for which you have responsibility. Also, supervisors should encourage their superiors to participate in team or department activities (e.g., Respiratory Therapy Week luncheon, promotion parties). All employees, no matter the level, like their superiors and the higher-ups to "show their faces," especially on weekends, nights, and holidays. Employees who work at these times feel left out of the mainstream activities. Being given some attention during these off-hours can be a morale booster.

Whenever supervisors observe their employees at work, they should assume a questioning attitude and not a fault-finding one. Supervisors should not ignore mistakes, but the manner in which they question is essential. They should ask themselves whether there is any way they could help the employees do the job better or more easily, safely, or efficiently. They should notice the way the employee is doing the job, whether it is up to par or substandard. Such observations can verify lack of acceptable performance in specific areas, such as inadequate patient care, lack of orderliness, not meeting the physical needs of the patient, or sloppy work.

At times, it may be difficult to convince an employee that his or her work is unsatisfactory. If reference can be made to concrete cases, however, it is not easy for the subordinate to deny that the inadequacies exist. It is essential for the supervisor to make specific observations because without being specific, one cannot realistically appraise performance and take appropriate corrective action.

As stated, measuring performance through direct personal observation has some shortcomings; it is time consuming and means being away from the desk and office. Some other limitations also exist. The employee may perform well while the boss is around but drop back to a lower-level performance shortly after the boss is out of sight. Furthermore, it may be difficult to observe some of the activities at a critical time. Also, the supervisor should make an effort to see what is really happening and not only what he or she wants to see. Still, direct observation is practiced widely and is probably the best way of checking performance.

Reports

Written and oral reports are good means of checking on performance if a department operates around the clock, if it is large, or if it operates in different locations. When a department operates around the clock and one supervisor is responsible for all shifts, each day of the week, this person depends on reports to cover those shifts during which he or she is absent. Even with reports, the supervisor should get to work a little earlier and stay a little later in the day so that there is some overlap with the night supervisor in the morning and with the afternoon supervisor later in the day. This gives the supervisors a chance to add some spoken explanations to their written reports. Reports should be clear, complete, concise, and correct. They must be brief but still include the important details.

As the departmental supervisor checks these reports, he or she probably will find many activities that have been performed up to standard. The supervisor should concentrate on the exceptions—namely, those areas in which the performance significantly deviates from the standard. Only the exceptions require the supervisor's attention. For example, in Figure 27.1 if the pain measurement in ambulatory surgery fell to 90 percent, management would definitely want to investigate why. In fact, if the supervisor depends on reports from the various shifts, the subordinates may have been requested not to send data on those activities that have reached the preestablished standards but to report only on those items that do not meet the standards or exceed them. In this way, the supervisor can concentrate all his or her efforts on the problem areas. This is known as practicing the exception principle. In such situations, however, a climate of trust must exist between the supervisor and subordinates so that they can freely report the deviations. Subordinates should know that the boss has full confidence in the rest of their activities even though there is no report on them.

If the supervisor does depend on reports for information, it is essential that they be reviewed immediately after they are received and that action is taken without delay when needed. It is demoralizing to send reports to a supervisor who does not even read them.

The nature of healthcare activities calls for reports that are accurate, complete, and correct, especially when patient care is involved. In all other areas as well, most employees submit truthful reports, even if they are unfavorable to the employee; much depends on their relationships and the supervisor's reaction. The supervisor must check into the matter and correct any shortcomings. As long as the supervisor handles these reports constructively, stressing their honesty, the employees will continue to submit reliable reports instead of stretching the truth. The supervisor must remember the importance of upward communication, and this is one opportunity to keep the channel open and flowing (see Chapter 5).

TAKING CORRECTIVE ACTION

The third stage in the control model is taking corrective action. If there are no deviations in performance from the established standards, the supervisor's process of controlling is fulfilled by the first two steps—setting standards and checking performance. If a significant and worthwhile discrepancy or variation is found, however, the controlling function is not fulfilled until and unless the third step, appropriate corrective action, is taken. If the deviation is minor and acceptable and within a non-critical activity, it may be appropriate to do nothing except call it to the employee's attention. As always, data must be examined as quickly as possible after the observations are made so that timely corrective action can be taken to curb undesirable results and bring performance back into line.

The supervisor must first make a careful analysis of the facts and look for the reasons behind the deviations. This must be done before any specific corrective action can be prescribed. The supervisor must bear in mind that the performance standards were based on certain prerequisites, forecasts, and assumptions and that some of these may have been faulty or may not have materialized. A check on the discrepancy may also point out that the trouble was not caused by the employee in whose work it appeared but in some preceding activity. For instance, a patient's infection might not be caused by the nursing activities or conditions on the nursing floor, but rather by conditions or actions in the recovery room or the surgical suite. In such a situation, the corrective action must be directed toward the real source. In this case, the corrective action will emanate from the nursing director's office, assuming that the latter is the common line superior to all the departments concerned.

The supervisor might also discover that a deviation may be caused by an employee who is not qualified or who has not been given the proper directions and instructions. If the employee is not qualified, additional training and supervision might help, but in other cases finding a replacement might be in order. In a situation in which directions have not been given properly and the employee was not well informed of what was expected of him or her, it is the supervisor's duty to explain again the standards required.

Only after a thorough analysis of the reasons for a deviation will the supervisor be in a position to take appropriate corrective action concerning the employee in question. Again, it is not sufficient merely to find the deviation; controlling means to correct the situation. The supervisor must decide what remedial action is necessary to secure improved results in the future. Corrective action may require revising the standards, a simple discussion, a reprimand or other disciplinary action, transferring or even replacing certain employees, or devising better work methods. Corrective action, however, is not the final step. The supervisor must follow up by studying the effect of each corrective action on future control. With further study and analysis the supervisor may find that additional or different measures may be required to produce the desired results, keep operations on line, or get them back on track.

However, Advisory Publications cautions supervisors to not assume that all deviations are the result of an employee or team. Deviations can be the result of process flaws. Consider excessive overtime. If a supervisor notices that overtime expense is exceeding the budget or becoming excessive, he or she should exhaust other approaches before authorizing extra hours. Although overtime may be necessary occasionally, it can be wearing on employees, and you may find that productivity actually decreases per paid hour. As with other deviations, you should consider alternatives. If overtime is routinely used, there may not be sufficient employees to meet the work demands. Pulling together a work redesign team may identify steps or activities that have low or no value that can be eliminated, or tasks that could be automated. After these options are considered, the supervisor may determine it is better to add another full-time or part-time employee at the times that overtime is often used. The extra staff will be paid less than the direct cost of overtime. The additional person(s) can add flexibility, too. Alternatively, the team may discover the overtime only occurs during the summer months and therefore justify hiring temporary staff to fill in for the vacancies.

Supervisors must be careful not to jump to conclusions when variations are identified and consider as many causes as possible. However, do not take so much time in the analysis that the variation continues without any corrective action occurring.

BENCHMARKING

As mentioned earlier, an effective approach to improving an organization's operational performance is to identify similar organizations that seem to be performing better, visiting with the managers at those organizations, and discussing how they are able to achieve optimal performance. This process is known as benchmarking. Benchmarking allows organizations to assess their operations, become knowledgeable about competitors, and incorporate what they learn about the best practices used by these industry leaders. Using the wisdom of the optimally performing organization, the managers can attempt to implement the same or similar practices or processes at their own enterprise and hopefully experience some improvement in performance.

Benchmarking can begin at a macro level by comparing one's key statistics to those published by local, regional, or national organizations (see Figure 28.5). If your organization's length of stay falls within the first quartile but your costs fall into the third quartile, the source of the survey may be contacted for further information, or a performance improvement team may be convened to evaluate the situation.

Benchmarking is really the seeking of best practices so that your organization remains competitive in the marketplace. Other sources of best practices

NATIONAL UTILIZATION INDICATORS

	Quartile 1	Quartile 2	Quartile 3	Quartile 4
Percentage of Total Discharges	23%	42%	25%	11%
Average Length of Stay	2.79	4.81	4.86	9.26
Average Severity	0.56	1.06	1.31	2.15

NATIONAL AVERAGES FOR CHARGE, COST, AND PAYMENT, BY QUARTILE

	Quartile 1	Quartile 2	Quartile 3	Quartile 4
Average Total Charge	$9,746	$17,061	$33,943	$79,592
Average Total Cost	$4,070	$7,105	$14,079	$33,178
Average Payment	$2,517	$4,997	$10,722	$26,602

TOP 3 DRGS WITH HIGH MEDICAL/SURGICAL SUPPLY COSTS

	DRG	DRG Description	% Total DRG Cost
Quartile 3	118	Cardiac Pacemaker Device Replacement	51%
	116	Other Permanent Cardiac Pacemaker Implant	49%
	111	Major Cardiovascular Procedures w/o CC	40%
Quartile 4	515	Cardiac Defibrillator Implant w/o Cardiac Cath	70%
	514	Cardiac Defibrillator Implant w Cardiac Cath (no longer valid)	61%
	115	Permanent Cardiac Pacemaker Implant with AMI/HR/Shock or AICD Lead OR Generator	47%

Source: Reprinted with permission from *Healthcare Financial Management*, January 2005, pg. 100, by Healthcare Financial Management Association.

are professional newsletters and journals and specialty discussion groups on the Internet. Conducting some research helps you locate organizations that more closely mirror yours and allows you to compare your processes to theirs.

Benchmarking is similar to other process improvement activities. As with any activity that may require reorganizing or possibly reengineering, the customer must always be considered first, and, as noted above, the stakeholders—your employees—should always be involved in assessing the situation. According to Cashen (1999), "Furthermore, benchmarking is not a numbers-only exercise. Measuring the performance of best practice organizations only reveals that they are doing better in the chosen activities. Understanding the managerial and operational processes that allow the target organizations to achieve their results is necessary in order to create improvements in one's own activities. In other words, benchmarking is not about mimicking other organizations, it is about helping individuals learn new ways to think about existing problems."

SUMMARY

In performing the controlling function, the manager should follow three basic steps: (1) standards or metrics must be set, (2) performance must be measured and compared with standards, and (3) corrective action must be taken if necessary. In setting standards, the supervisor must be aware of both those that are tangible and those that are intangible. Many of the tangible standards can be established with the help of motion and time studies. It is much more difficult, however, to establish standards for intangible aspects of performance. Because the number of both types of standards is so large, the supervisor is the most qualified person in the department to determine its strategic control points. Using data collected from benchmarking activities may provide an indication of where standards should be established and at what level. Benchmarking data also may identify conditions that require further investigation.

After establishing the strategic metrics, the supervisor's function is to check and measure performance against them. In some instances, the supervisor has to depend on reports, but in most cases direct personal observation is the best means for appraising performance. If discrepancies from standards are revealed, the supervisor must take corrective action to bring matters back into line. An approach to improving processes and refining controls or standards is to benchmark with other organizations that have exceptional performance in areas you wish to improve. Benchmarking allows managers to build on the success of others and avoid "reinventing the mousetrap."

REFERENCES

Advisory Publications. Undated material. "A Tight Overtime Policy Provides Good Financial Control" Financial Management Strategies for Medical Offices. Conshohocken, PA: Advisory Publications.

Cashen, L. H. 1999. "Benchmarking for Competitive Improvement." QualityResource 18 (5): 15.

Henderson, D. A., B. W. Chase, and B. M. Woodson. 2002. "Performance Measures for NPOs." Journal of Accountancy 193 (1): 63.

Performance Co-Pilot Tutorial Glossary. 2005. [Online information; retrieved 10/4/2005.] http://pcp4cgl.sourceforge.net/turorial/glossary.html.

Spath, P. L. 2002. "Productivity and Quality in the HIM Department." For the Record Magazine 14 (11): 30.

CHAPTER TWENTY-NINE

Budgetary and Other Control Techniques

CHAPTER OBJECTIVES

After you have studied this chapter, you should be able to:

1. Define the approaches, types, and purposes of budgets.
2. Outline the role of the supervisor in preparing the budget.
3. Compare and contrast different budget models.
4. Review the function of budgets in cost containment.

BUDGET IS a written plan expressed in figures and numerical terms, primarily in dollars and cents, that projects revenue and expenses for a specified time. It sets the financial standards to be met by the organization. The budget is the most widely used control device not only in healthcare centers but for all phases of all other organized activities. Budgetary control is an extremely effective managerial tool, whether the manager is the CFO of an HMO or the supervisor of a department. For this reason, it is essential that every manager learn how to plan budgets, work within their boundaries, and use them properly for control purposes. Of all available control devices, the budget, especially the expense budget, is probably the one the supervisor is most familiar with and has been coping with for the longest time. The supervisor's planning and controlling of financial resources for the organization's day-to-day operations is known as operations budgeting (Dunn 2005, 9–1).

As pointed out in Chapter 10, budgeting is a planning function, but its administration is part of the controlling function. Budgets are preestablished standards to which operations are compared and, if necessary, adjusted by the exercise of control. In other words, a budget is a means of control insofar as it reflects the progress of the actual performance against the plan. In so doing, the budget provides information that enables the supervisor to take action, if needed, to make results conform to the plan.

The Nature of Budgeting and Budgetary Control

When all aspects of the institution's operations are covered by budgets and when all departmental budgets are consolidated into an overall budget, the enterprise practices comprehensive or master budgeting. Most enterprises practice comprehensive budgeting, including the overall budget for the organization and many subordinate budgets for the various divisions and departments.

Whereas the overall budget is of great concern to the CEO and the board of directors, the supervisor is mainly involved with the departmental budget, although overall budget considerations do have their effects on every departmental budget. The term budgetary control refers to the use of budgets to control the department's daily operations so that they conform to the goals and standards set by the institution. Budgetary control goes beyond merely evaluating results in relation to established goals. Such control also involves taking corrective action as needed.

The Supervisor's Concern About Budgeting[1]

Unfortunately, budgeting also has some drawbacks that management must overcome, including the following:

- *Budgeting is time consuming.* Because it is time consuming, some managers do not devote adequate time to the process. This omission must be avoided, because all parts of a budget must be sound to ensure overall effectiveness. Computerizing some aspects of budgeting can help decrease the time required. Computer-generated managerial accounting reports, which provide data on actual costs and variances, often are a byproduct of an organization's information system. In addition, electronic spreadsheets or more sophisticated decision support systems on departmental personal computers can be used to aid in budgeting. These data analysis products permit manipulation of budget variables without cumbersome recalculations. This is sometimes called what-if analysis. For example, a budget can be prepared based on volume projections, and then different levels of inflation can be programmed into the spreadsheet or decision algorithm to automatically show the effect of variable levels of inflation on the budget.
- *Budgeting is an expense in itself.* This is especially true in the case of the overly zealous manager who devotes too much time to budgeting and thus takes time away from other operational activities. For this manager, the budget often becomes an end in itself. Symptoms are treated as problems, and research may not be done to identify the real problem and develop a solution.
- *Sometimes management performance is evaluated only in monetary terms.* This is a case of quantity over quality. Although the bottom line is just as important to the viability of the healthcare organization as it is to the manufacturing firm, quality usually is considered to be even more important.

Even if a bottom-line focus is only a perception, an attitude such as this can negatively affect both budget development and compliance. The manager who is overly concerned about his or her evaluation based on budget performance may cut corners that negatively affect the quality of care or service.

Numerical Terms

The budget states the anticipated results in specific numerical terms. Although the terms are ultimately monetary, at the beginning of the budget planning process not all budgets are expressed in dollars and cents. Many budgets are stated in non-financial numerical terms, such as labor hours, hours per adjusted patient day, quantities of supplies, operations per operating room (OR), bills per hour, or lab tests per diagnosis-related group. Personnel budgets indicate the number of workers needed for each type of skill required, the number of hours allocated to perform certain activities, and so on. Although budgets may start out with numerical terms other than monetary values, ultimately every non-financial budget must be translated into dollars and cents. This is the common denominator for all activities of an organization.

MAKING THE BUDGET

Making a budget, whether it is financial or otherwise, leads to improved planning. For budgetary purposes, it is not sufficient just to make a general statement. One must quantify, date, and state specific plans in a budget. A considerable difference exists between making a general forecast and attaching numerical values to specific plans. The figures in the budget are the actual plans that become the standard of achievement. The plans are then no longer merely predictions. Rather, they are the basis for daily operations and are viewed as standards to be met.

A complete budgetary program requires the involvement of all levels of management making serious and honest considerations. Rigorous budgetary thinking is certain to improve the quality of organizational planning. Indeed, participation by all the managers and supervisors who are affected by the various budgets is a prerequisite for their successful administration. Again, this is important because it is natural for people to resent arbitrary orders. Thus, it is imperative that all budget allowances and objectives are determined with the full cooperation of those who are responsible for executing them.

Participation in Traditional Budgeting

As stated, the supervisor who must function under the departmental budget should play a significant role in preparing it. This increases the reliability, accuracy, and acceptance of the budget; the supervisor is closest to the activity, understanding all of the elements going into the budget. He or she should be requested to submit a proposed budget and participate in what is commonly known as grassroots budgeting.

For example, as the fiscal year draws to a close, the supervisor of the operating rooms should sit down and gather together those figures that will make up next year's budget. In this endeavor, the supervisor might need the assistance of his or her immediate line superior, in this case most likely the director of nursing services. The supervisor must gather all available information on past performance, expenses, salaries of nursing personnel, other wages, supplies, maintenance, and so forth. Then the supervisor should consider any possible new developments, such as increases in wages, the increased costs of supplies, and additional personnel, before he or she prepares an intelligent and realistic budget. In some smaller healthcare organizations, all budgeting may be completed by the controller or even the CEO for several reasons, including to avoid budget inflation and to save line supervisors the time because often these supervisors are working supervisors that provide day-to-day, direct patient care services.

The full responsibility for preparing the budget does not lie with the supervisor alone. It is the administrator's and every manager's duty to work on budgets. They in turn, together with the controller's and accounting department's assistance and data, give the departmental supervisor much information on past performance and future industry projections. The supervisor uses this information to substantiate future estimates and proposals in a free exchange of opinions with the line superior. After both reach a certain level of agreement, the line boss conveys the overall departmental budget to higher administration.

For example, assume that the director of environmental services supervises three areas of activity: housekeeping, dietary, and plant maintenance. The supervisors of each of these three activities work out their departmental budgets and discuss and substantiate them fully with the director of environmental services. The director combines all three budgets and produces a proposed budget for the entire environmental services division. This budget is submitted and discussed with the immediate line superior. Ultimately, the final budget is adjusted and set by top-level administration, but its effectiveness is ensured because true grassroots participation has taken place.

Such participation does not mean that the suggestions of the supervisors should or will always prevail. A careful and thorough analysis of the figures is necessary. A full discussion should take place between the supervisor and the line superior, and the supervisor should have ample opportunity to be heard and to substantiate his or her case. The budget suggestions of subordinate supervisors will not be accepted if the superior believes the figures are unrealistic, incorrect, or inadequate. Some subordinates are inclined to propose budgets with monetary levels they hope to achieve without too much effort. This is obviously done for self-protection and because the supervisor wants to play it safe. The supervisor rationalizes that, by setting the estimates of expenses high enough, he or she can be sure to stay within the allocated amount and will be praised if he or she stays well below the budget. This, however, defeats the purpose of grassroots budgeting. In those facilities following traditional management methods, the line superior should remind the supervisor that the purpose of budget participation is to arrive at realistic budgets. The superior should explain that favorable and unfavorable variances will be carefully scrutinized and that the supervisor's managerial rating will depend, among other factors, on how realistic a budget proposal he or she submits. Many discussions will be needed before the budget is completed and brought to top-level administration for final approval.

Budgeting Approaches

Most budgets cover a period of one year. These are usually submitted at one time approximately three to four months prior to the year the budget takes effect. However, some organizations have established *rolling budget* approaches. The manager initially prepares the 12 months as he or she would in the traditional approach. When the first month of the new budget ends, the manager projects that month's budget for the following year. As the second month of the new budget ends, the manager projects the second month for the next year, and so on. This allows budget planning to occur every month rather than experiencing a massive flurry of work during a few weeks of the year. Alternatively, some organizations prepare the new projections every quarter.

Another budgeting approach is the *flexible budget*. When one prepares a flexible budget, the budget is prepared with a range of activity levels (if patient volume is x, y, or z) so that adjustments can be made throughout the year if changes in activity levels occur. In flexible (or variable) budgeting, actual results are compared against the appropriate activity level. Because the flexible budget covers a range of activity, the manager can construct a new budget if actual costs are different from what was originally planned. This can be done as needed, to compare against actual results (Dunn 2005).

Although many organizations are steering away from what is known as historical or conventional budgets, they do exist. Conventional or *traditional budgeting* involves projections for the following year based on current expenditures and the previous annual budget. Under this approach, the amounts expended the prior year are increased by a certain inflation factor (or in some cases, decreased). Yet a third approach is referred to as incremental budgeting and is often coupled with the rolling or flexible budget. Because considerable effort goes into the development of these budgets, the most critical and analytical attention by top-level management is devoted to the year-over-year increment; the base is treated as though it were already authorized and requires no review. The adjusted amounts become the manager's new budget. This approach does not consider one-time purchases and encourages managers to always spend their budgets.

Under traditional budgeting, management focuses its attention on planned changes from the previous year's level of expenditures. This method assumes that the activities making up the historical base (1) are essential, (2) must be continued, (3) are being performed effectively in a cost-efficient manner, (4) are needed more than new programs, and (5) will continue to be necessary and effective next year. Although some activities meet all these criteria, it is unrealistic to assume that for the new year all of them will. Furthermore, another potential problem exists—wasteful expenditures. If the department incurs less cost than budgeted, the department may try to spend the money even if there is no real need. Although this is contrary to basic financial principles, the fear of losing the money is great if the new budget is influenced by the current level of expenditures. Another potential shortcoming arises when a department that is currently operating efficiently is faced with an across-the-board edict to cut budget amounts by a certain percentage. This penalizes the efficient supervisor and rewards the inefficiently run department.

Because of these limitations and the recent emphasis on process improvement, reengineering, and cost containment, a need for better budgeting techniques has become more important. *Zero-base budgeting* is a contemporary approach to budgeting. It was developed in the early 1970s in industrial settings and then was quickly introduced into state and federal government agencies. Today many major corporations are using zero-base budgeting, and more and more healthcare institutions are introducing it. The increase in the number of healthcare settings using zero-base budgeting is caused by changing healthcare priorities, constrained financial resources, changing technologies, available computer capabilities, and the emphasis on cost containment in particular.

Under zero-base budgeting, nothing is taken for granted; the budget for the new period ignores the previous budget. Every activity submitted for funding must be justified. This approach requires substantiation and justification of each budget item from the ground up. Zero-base budgeting gives administration an excellent opportunity to reassess all activities, departments, and projects in terms of their benefits and costs to the organization. The great advantage is that each "package" has to be planned anew and costs are calculated from scratch; this avoids the tendency to look only at changes from the previous period. Ongoing programs are reviewed and have to be justified in their entirety every budget period.

Briefly, the process involves seven steps (Cleverly 1992). First, define the outputs or services provided by the program or departmental area, such as correspondence or transcription services by the health information department. Second, determine the costs of these services or outputs, such as the cost for transcribing home health notes for the home health service. Third, identify options for reducing the cost through changes in outputs or services, such as the use of an outside contract transcription service. Fourth, identify options for producing the services and outputs more efficiently. Fifth, determine the cost savings associated with operations identified in steps 3 and 4. Sixth, assess the risks, both qualitative and quantitative, associated with the identified options of steps 3 and 4—for example, asking if the contract service will be timely. Seventh, select and implement those options with an acceptable cost-risk relationship.

All budgeting systems have some limitations, and zero-base budgeting is no exception. The additional time necessary for budget preparation and the large amount of paperwork, especially in the initial implementation year, may be viewed as offsetting the benefits. In subsequent years, however, the process will take much less time as managers become familiar with it. In the long run, the benefits of zero-base budgeting seem to far outweigh the additional work and expenditures involved. Just as each item in the budget has been examined and justified by the benefits projected, the new procedure will be fully justified and worth its costs and efforts.

Types of Budgets[2]

Each organization is different; however, three types of budgets are typically prepared. The *revenue and expense budget* is also known as the operations budget. It includes estimates of patient and non-patient revenue as well as expenses for personnel, supplies, depreciation, interest, insurance, and so on. So far this chapter has discussed the role of the supervisor in contributing to the development of this budget. In this effort, the supervisor uses volume estimates to project revenues as well as expenses.

The *capital budget* is a plan that shows the major assets to be purchased, anticipated purchase dates, and the funding sources for those purchases. It is supported by cost-benefit analyses and priority assignments that may be used to rank projects if cash or financing is inadequate to invest in all projects. You may be asked to sit on a capital expenditure committee to help assign priorities to the various projects and items requested. Often items requested are submitted on a capital request form—the organization's policies dictate when a form must be used—and this is usually linked to a dollar amount, say, $1,000. The form varies from organization to organization; however, it often includes a description of the item requested, the cost, the source of the cost estimate, the estimated life of the item for depreciation purposes, and an indication of whether any other departments may be affected by the item.

The last common budget is the *cash budget*, which is a projection of cash balances at the end of each month throughout the budget year. It is prepared by projecting when the billed charges for revenues during one period will be paid (in cash). This budget not only determines when cost-containment measures may be imperative but also whether capital items, budgeted or not, can be purchased.

Preparing the Budget

A long-standing approach to preparing and selling a budget is the *three Ps approach*: preapproach, proof, and publication (Lindo 1981).

Preapproach

1. Identify demands for your services. Determine who your customers are and assess whether they are growing in number or declining. Are there other potential new customers?
2. Evaluate your facility's economic climate. Discuss this with peer supervisors, other departments, the fiscal director, and so on.
3. Locate internal competition for funds. Consider those departments that are providing similar services or planning to do so.
4. Establish a set of realistic budget expectations. If the patient activity (e.g., number of encounters, surgeries, days) is declining 10 percent, do not submit a budget requesting 15 percent more resources.
5. Always start your budget preparation a year in advance. Do not wait until the notice arrives on your desk to begin data collection and budget preparation.

Proof

1. Provide details and sources for your budget estimates.
2. Present past performance. How well have you achieved budget expectations in the past? How successful have you been in implementing new programs and reaching the goals planned?
3. Analyze and present applicable trend data that support the activity levels projected. Remember to use written comments and graphs to enhance comprehension of your presentation.
4. Discuss the current status of prior programs implemented and/or goals assigned.
5. Prioritize new programs and/or services being proposed so you are ready, if asked to do so, to eliminate some programs and/or services proposed.

Publication

1. Once the budget is approved, summarize for your supervisor the new and ongoing key authorized programs.
2. Update the status of each of these on a regular basis, no less often than quarterly. Try to discuss your report in person as well as provide a written report to your superior.
3. Identify in your quarterly updates any enhancements being considered to the approved or ongoing programs that may appear in the next budget.
4. Well in advance of the next budget notices, meet with your superior to discuss planned enhancements or new programs being considered and to begin the pre-approach process.

Following these three steps allows the supervisor to stay ahead of others competing for funds and ensures that his or her boss is kept informed throughout the year.

Budget Director and Budget Committee

Although the authority and responsibility for the budget rest with the line officers and ultimately with the CEO and the board of directors, in some cases a team of staff accountants, headed by a budget director, the controller, or the CFO, can assist. This team of individuals (serving in an advisory capacity) can provide the line managers with advice and technical assistance but should not attempt to prepare the budgets for them. They may even prepare the initial budget letter, budget instructions and packet of forms, and data that are sent to all managers. Once all budgets have been approved by the designated superiors, the budget department staff will put the various budget estimates together in final form so that top-level administration can submit it to the board.

Some institutions also have established a budget committee that serves in an advisory and supportive capacity in coordinating the various budgets. In this instance the budget committee clearly performs a staff function. This must be distinguished, however, from those budget committees to which the board has delegated the line function of setting, rather than just coordinating, the budget. In this situation the budget committee considers all departmental budget estimates and requests, including expenses and capital expenditures and makes the final decisions. In large institutions, there may be subcommittees of the budget committee, for example, the capital expenditure committee. This form of budget committee has ultimate line authority and responsibility for determining the budget instead of a single person such as the institution's top-level administrator or executive director. The budget is approved by the committee. If budget revisions and changes are requested, it is also up to the budget committee to allow or disallow them. Several arrangements are possible within these two extremes as to where the final authority for the overall budget rests. Usually it needs the authorization of the CEO, the finance committee of the board, and eventually the board of directors.

Length of the Budget Period

Although the length of the budget period may vary, most healthcare enterprises choose one year. This period is then broken down into quarters, and many institutions even divide it by months at the time of the original budget preparation. This is usually referred to as periodic budgeting.

Healthcare institutions also typically have budgets extending over a longer term, such as three or five years. These budgets usually cover such items as capital expenditures, research programs, and expansions. Long-term or long-range budgets of this nature are used for projecting major capital needs (such as a new chemistry analyzer or a PACS system). The supervisor is asked to project capital needs for the department over a given period (3–5 years, possibly more). These needs are evaluated by senior management and as appropriate, given the long-range strategic plan of the organization, compiled into the long-term capital budget. These budgets are planning, not controlling, tools. For most healthcare organizations it is difficult to plan much beyond five years because healthcare is so heavily regulated and the regulations may vary greatly, depending on elected officials in Congress and the economy.

Flexibility of the Budgetary Process

The supervisor should keep in mind that budgets are merely tools for management and not a substitute for good judgment. Also, care should be taken not to make budgets so detailed that they become cumbersome. Budgets should always allow the supervisor enough freedom to accomplish the best objectives of the department. There must be a reasonable degree of latitude and flexibility. In fact, one of the most serious shortcomings of budgeting is the danger of inflexibility. Although budgets are plans expressed in numerical terms, the supervisor must not be led to believe that these figures are absolutely final and unalterable. Realizing that a budget should not become a straitjacket, enlightened management builds into the budgetary program a degree of flexibility and adaptability. This is necessary so that the institution can cope with changing conditions, new developments, and even possible mistakes of human error and miscalculation. Flexibility should not be interpreted to mean, however, that the budget can be changed with every whim or that it should be taken lightly.

Nevertheless, if operating conditions have appreciably changed and there are valid indications that the budget cannot be followed in the future, a revision of the budgetary program is in order. Such circumstances may be caused by unexpected events, new legislation, unanticipated wage increases, or large fluctuations in demand. Consider, for example, the budget of the nuclear medicine department, in which activities have been and are increasing constantly because of new applications and technology breakthroughs. Revenues derived from this service are increasing rapidly at the same time. It would be absurd to expect the supervisor of this department to stay within the budgeted figures for salaries and supplies if growth is significantly in excess of the budgeted volume. If the department is expected to respond and supply the increased demand for this service, the budget must be altered. In such a case the old budget has become obsolete; unless provisions are available to make the budget flexible, it will lose its usefulness altogether.

Budget Review and Revision

Increasing attention has been given to ways of ensuring budget flexibility to avoid the danger of rigidity and obsolescence. Most enterprises achieve this by periodic budget reviews and revisions. The budget is reviewed at regular intervals of one, two, or three months. In meetings between the departmental supervisor and the line superior, actual performance will be checked and compared with the budgeted figures and the supervisor will be called on to explain the causes for any variations. A thorough analysis must then be made to discover the reasons for the deviation from the budgeted amount; this may lead to budget revisions or other corrective measures.

An unfavorable variation by itself does not necessarily require a budget change; it must be studied and explained. The supervisor of nuclear medicine in the earlier example will not have any difficulties proving the need for an upward budget revision. In some organizations such a revision can be made on the departmental level, whereas in other institutions it must be carried up to the CEO or even the budget committee. If the deviations are of sufficient magnitude, it is advisable to make the necessary revisions no matter how high up in the hierarchy they have to go or how much work they may involve. If the variation is minor, it may be more expedient to let it go instead of revising the entire budget, as it has been explained and justified.

No matter what decision is made, regular budget reviews and revisions seem to be the best way of ensuring the flexibility of the budgetary process. They prevent the budget from being viewed as a straitjacket and allow the supervisor to consider it a living document and a valuable tool for control purposes.

Budgets and Human Problems

Budgets necessarily represent restrictions, and for this reason subordinates generally resent budgets. Often subordinates have a defensive approach to budgets, an approach they acquire through painful experience. Many times the subordinates become acquainted with budgets only as a barrier to spending, or the budget is blamed for failure to get or give a raise in salary. Moreover, in the minds of many subordinates the word budget has often become associated with miserly behavior rather than with planning and direction.

The line manager's job is to correct this erroneous impression by pointing out that budgeting is a disciplined approach to resolve or prevent many problems and is necessary to maintain standards of performance. The budget must be presented to the supervisor as a planning tool and not as a pressure device. Most of the problems arise at the point of budgetary control. In other words, when deviations from the budget occur, subordinates are often censured for exceeding the budget. Such budget deviations necessitate explanations, discussions, and decisions. As stated before, the budget should not be looked on lightly. The subordinate should also know that in most enterprises enough flexibility is built into the budget system to permit good common-sense departures necessary for the best functioning of the institution.

Avoiding unnecessary pressures over the budget presupposes that a good working relationship exists between the supervisor and the immediate superior. This in turn rests on clear-cut organizational lines and a thorough understanding that the line managers are responsible for control. Staff people are excluded from the process of controlling. They cannot take operating personnel to task for deviations in the budget; they can merely report the situation to the administrative officer. Effective use of budgetary procedures depends on the administration's attitudes toward the entire budgetary process, whether it will be an effective planning tool or a pressure device. Only with the planning-tool view will a supervisor believe that whatever can be done without a budget can be done much more effectively with a budget.

Cost Controls

Healthcare providers have been and still are under continuous, unrelenting pressure to keep healthcare expenditures from spiraling. It is safe to predict that the drive to control costs will increase even more because of pressures from government agencies; legislators; insurers; and purchasers of healthcare such as large corporations, managed care organizations, and even enlightened individuals. In such an environment, control of costs is an ongoing problem for everyone from the CEO to the supervisor; it is a problem that will never go away.

Cost control, also referred to as cost awareness, cost consciousness, or cost containment, should be viewed as a significant part of the supervisor's daily job. Supervisors must strive for cost consciousness with consistency. Sporadic cost-cutting efforts seldom have lasting results. Because cost awareness is an ongoing issue, the supervisor must set definite numerical objectives and make plans for containing cost. Priorities must be clarified without infringing on the quality of healthcare; this is difficult to achieve, especially if more sophistication in patient care is accompanied by general escalation of prices and wages.

To succeed in cost containment, it is essential to involve the medical staff as well as the employees of the department and make them realize that ultimately their actions will bring about results. Recall our discussion in Chapter 16 about alternatives to downsizing and in Chapter 22 about communicating change. Medical staff members, especially surgeons, have a significant impact on the cost of surgery when prosthetics and specialized instruments are required. Therefore, the physicians must be pulled into the cost-containment discussions. Sometimes this is accomplished through a medical staff committee charged with establishing clinical pathways. All employees should consider cost consciousness as a part of their job. Most physicians and employees will help cut costs and reduce waste, especially if the results of their efforts are fed back to them. Most workers are not deliberately wasteful. Many physicians and employees can make valuable suggestions and contributions to cost effectiveness. The supervisor should welcome all suggestions, investigate each one, and not fault anyone for not having thought of these changes before. Cost awareness should be an ongoing challenge in everyone's daily job and be a part of every employee's annual performance review as well as the biennial credentialing review.

Allocation of Costs

Every supervisor must see that his or her department contributes financially to the operation of the institution. However, supervisors must realize that in a healthcare center, just as in all other organized activities, some departments are revenue producing, whereas others are not. Clearly, the operating rooms and pharmacy services produce revenue, but these patient care departments could not function without the services provided by the other departments such as housekeeping, dietary services, health records, laundry, and administration. Although these are not revenue-producing departments, their costs must be carried if the healthcare facility is to function on a fiscally sound basis. As part of the Medicare-required cost-reporting function, hospitals must allocate such costs of the non-revenue-generating departments to those patient care departments that do produce revenue. The question arises as to how the costs of the many non-revenue-producing departments are allocated to the revenue-producing departments. The supervisor has no control over this portion of a department's expenses, which can make the difference between ending up with a departmental surplus or with a deficit.

A detailed discussion of the various methods of cost analysis, contribution margin approach, and other bases for allocations is beyond the scope of this book. However, the supervisor should have a general understanding of the bases on which a department is being charged for these various expenditures. This is merely for the supervisor's own information, as in reality this person is powerless to influence the costs allocated to the department. The supervisor can readily understand the direct expenses (e.g., wages, salaries, supplies, materials), as well as some of the indirect expenses (e.g., Social Security and workers compensation taxes), charged to the department. The supervisor also probably understands that the department is charged with maintenance expenses on the basis of work orders or telecommunications expenses based on the number of telephone lines, and so forth.

The overall financial performance of a department is greatly affected by how allocations for other expenditures are made—for example, administrative expenses, operation of the plant, depreciation, intern and resident service costs, in-service education, and interest expenses. Although all this is determined higher up in the administrative hierarchy, the supervisor is well advised to obtain some information on the basis for the allocation and an explanation of how it is done. The healthcare institution will try to select a basis of distribution that is fair to all departments and feasible from an accounting point of view. Understanding that this cost allocation occurs permits the supervisor to better understand how a department operates in the red (at a loss), despite the effective work of the manager and its employees.

ADDITIONAL CONTROLS

The supervisor's controlling function is closely related to and goes on simultaneously with all other managerial functions. Throughout this book many subjects are discussed as part of a particular function; now their meaning as an aid in the system of control can also be shown.

In Chapter 10, standing plans, such as policies, procedures, methods, and rules as basic tools for planning, are discussed. At this point in the book, they can also be viewed as anticipatory control devices. These tools are established with the hope and intention that they will be followed and that they work out as preventive controls. If they are violated, the supervisor, using feedback control, must take the necessary corrective action; in some cases disciplinary measures may be necessary.

We discuss positive discipline and disciplinary measures in Chapter 26 as a component of the influencing function. In the controlling context, this topic can be viewed as a preventive and reactive control technique. If a rule has been violated, the supervisor must invoke disciplinary measures, which is synonymous with taking corrective action and sending a message to the employees about proper behavior on the job.

On various occasions, we have discussed management by objectives (MBO), an agreement between the subordinate and the supervisor concerning a measurable performance objective to be achieved and reviewed within a given time period. This concept includes aspects of control. After mutually agreed on objectives have been set, results are evaluated in light of these standards, and, if necessary, shortcomings are corrected. This is another example of a control model mechanism.

Performance appraisal systems, the process of formally evaluating performance and providing feedback for performance adjustments, are discussed in Chapter 21. This process can also be viewed as part of the organizational control system. Although performance evaluation measures are presented with the staffing function, they can now be regarded as a feedback control technique in the managerial control system.

These are just a few examples, taken from discussions in previous chapters, of the various managerial control functions. They show how closely related the controlling function is to all the other functions and confirm the statement that the better the supervisor plans, organizes, staffs, and influences, the better he or she can perform the controlling function.

SUMMARY

Budgeting is planning, whereas working with the budget and budget administration fall into the manager's controlling function. Budgets are plans expressed in numerical terms, which ultimately are reduced to dollars and cents as the common denominator used in the final analysis. Budgets are also preestablished standards to which the operations of the department are compared and, if necessary, adjusted by the exercise of control. Of all control devices, the budget (primarily the expense budget) is the one most widely used and thus the one with which supervisors should be most familiar.

Because the supervisor is responsible for adhering to the departmental budget, he or she must play a significant role in its preparation. Budget making is a line responsibility shared by the supervisor and the direct line superior. Ultimately, all budgets are submitted to and approved by top-level administration, but it is essential that lower-level managers participate in making their own budgets and have sufficient opportunity to be heard and substantiate their cases.

Zero-base budgeting is a relatively new approach to budgeting. Under traditional budgeting, management's attention is primarily focused on planned changes from the previous year; under zero-base budgeting every activity and budget item must be substantiated and justified from scratch. For a budget to be a live document and not a straitjacket, the budgetary process must be flexible. There must be frequent periodic budget reviews within the normal one-year budgeting period and provisions for budget revision. Such provisions lessen the human problems that budgetary controls often cause.

In addition to budgetary controls, the supervisor should be aware of other costs that influence the overall performance of the department. Here the supervisor is concerned with how the expenditures of the non-revenue-producing departments in a healthcare institution are allocated to those departments that do produce revenues. The bases of these allocations can often make the difference between showing a departmental surplus and operating at a loss. Supervisors also play an important role in cost containment. Cost awareness, or cost consciousness, should be an ongoing consideration and part of the supervisor's daily activities.

Throughout this book, we stressed the close relationship between the controlling function and the other managerial functions. Many of the managerial duties and activities discussed previously can now be viewed as additional controls, including policies and procedures, disciplinary measures, MBOs, and performance appraisals. The most widely used control device, however, remains the budget and budgetary procedures.

NOTE

1. This section is adapted from Chapter 9 of *Finance Principles for the Health Information Manager, Second Edition,* by Rose T. Dunn.

2. Ibid.

REFERENCES

Cleverly, W. O. 1992. *Essentials of Health Care Finance, Third Edition,* 299. Rockville, MD: Aspen Publishers.

Dunn, R. 2005. *Finance Principles for the Health Information Manager, Second Edition.* St. Louis, MO: First Class Solutions.

Lindo, D. K. 1981. "How to Increase Your Budget." *Journal of Administrative Management* (October): 28–40. Used with permission. © D. Lindo, Ph.D., Burnsville, MN.

PART VIII

Labor Relations

CHAPTER THIRTY

The Labor Union and the Supervisor

CHAPTER OBJECTIVES

After you have studied this chapter, you should be able to do the following:

1. Review the history of collective bargaining and labor-related legislation.
2. Discuss the content of a typical labor contract.
3. Outline areas of concern for the supervisor.
4. Differentiate the role of the supervisor and the shop steward in organized labor environments.

ALTHOUGH LABOR UNIONS have lost membership, declining from 20.1 percent of all U.S. workers in 1983 to 12.5 percent in 2004, unions are still an influential part of the workforce. As of 2004, about 15.5 million employees are represented by unions, of which 7 percent are healthcare workers. Healthcare union membership grew by 1 percent from 2003 to 2004 (Bureau of Labor Statistics 2005a). Therefore, it is essential for supervisors to be familiar with the role labor unions play in the workplace to work with them properly.

Collective bargaining gained its major legal basis in 1935 with the enactment of the National Labor Relations Act, also known as the Wagner Act, which guaranteed workers the right to bargain collectively with their employers. In 1947, the Wagner Act was amended by the Labor-Management Relations Act, also known as the Taft-Hartley Act. By the late 1950s, union membership rose to nearly 30 percent. In 1959 the Labor-Management Reporting and Disclosure Act, sometimes referred to as the Landrum-Griffin Act, was added. In 1974, these laws were extended to cover most healthcare institutions.

Special thanks to Marc J. Leff, Esq., vice president, Human Resources, Maimonides Medical Center, Brooklyn, New York, for his update to this chapter.

The union movement was primarily a blue-collar movement because there were more blue-collar workers in the United States labor force than white-collar workers (Bureau of Labor Statistics 2005b). Since the middle 1950s, however, the number of people in white-collar occupational categories and in service industries has surpassed the blue-collar sector. As of 2004, 7.9 million union members represent white-collar employment, while 7.6 million represent blue-collar employment (Bureau of Labor Statistics 2005b). With this change, labor unions have made inroads in representing business services (e.g., computers), retail trade, finance, healthcare, government, and other sectors. A number of unions or employee associations have become the bargaining agents for teachers, college professors, nurses, airline pilots, doctors, and various other white-collar workers. However, it is beyond the confines of this book to discuss the details of labor laws or give the full history of the union movement in the United States.

THE NUANCES OF UNIONS

There is little doubt that the introduction of a union or an employee association into a hospital or related healthcare facility may be a trying experience for the supervisors, as well as for the CEO. It may bring with it tension, during which time finding constructive solutions to problems may be difficult. The issues, claims, and counterclaims are on everyone's mind and are present in the workplace, the parking lot, and even the local news media. The verbal battle may even accelerate into work slowdowns or stoppages. If the employees vote to join a union, managers are likely to believe that they have lost a battle and that their employees and union representatives have been victorious. It will take time for the ill feelings created during the organizing campaign to disappear.

Gradually, however, both the union and the administration must learn to accommodate and live with each other. Every manager must accept the fact that the labor union is a permanent force in our society. Every manager must realize that the union, just as any other organization, has the potential for either advancing or disrupting the common effort of the institution. It is in the self-interest of the administration to create a labor-management climate that directs this potential toward constructive ends. There is no simple or magic formula, however, for cultivation of a favorable climate that will result overnight in cooperation and mutual understanding between the union and management. It takes wisdom and sensitivity from every manager of the organization, from the administrator to the supervisor, to demonstrate in day-to-day relations that the union is respected as a responsible part of the institution.

In this effort to create and maintain a constructive pattern of cooperation between the healthcare institution and the union, the most significant factor usually is the supervisor of a department. Supervisors, more than anyone else, feel the strongest impact of the new situation because they make the largest number of decisions concerning unionized employees. The supervisor is the person in day-to-day employee relations who makes the labor agreement a living document, for better or for worse. To this extent, an article in *Textile World* discussed the movement away from unions and preference for cooperative labor/management committees. Of the 2,408 manufacturing employees polled, 63 percent opted for the committees, while only 22 percent chose unions. The survey also found that workers complained of a lack of participation in decisions and acknowledged the importance of management cooperating in achieving their goals (Morrissey 1995).

Supervisors are often confused as to how they should behave during an organizing campaign and after the election when the union arrives on the scene. The supervisor should realize that the subordinates usually decide for a union, not because they were gullible or naive or because the union used deceit or strong-arm methods but primarily because some of their major needs were not satisfied on the job. The supervisor should approach the union professionally and try to build a satisfactory relationship.

The supervisor should have received information and training in the fundamentals of collective bargaining and in the nature of labor agreements from the human resources department. This is essential for the development of good labor relations. The supervisor is involved in two distinct phases of labor relations: (1) the inception of unionization and (2) the day-to-day administration of the union agreement, which includes disciplining, scheduling, and reviewing performance of employees. Although the supervisor is primarily concerned with the second phase of relations with the union, he or she also plays a role in the first.

UNIONIZATION AND LABOR NEGOTIATIONS

As soon as supervisors learn that union-organizing activities are starting, this information should be passed on to higher administration and the director of human resources. (Often administration has already learned of such a campaign through other channels.) This information enables the organization to plan its strategy, usually with the help of legal counsel. Supervisors should be aware of a number of legal restrictions that must be observed during the union-organizing efforts. The following remarks are only of a very general nature; supervisors should receive more detailed instruction from their administrators and lawyers.

Labor laws restrict what managers, including supervisors, are permitted to say and do during this critical period. First, supervisors should continue to do the best possible job of supervision during this critical period. Administration should provide supervisors with information on the dos and don'ts during a union-organizing campaign (see Figure 30.1). Generally, supervisors should not make any statements in reference to unionization that could be construed as a promise if the union fails or as a threat if the union is successful. Supervisors should not question their employees privately or publicly about organizing activities. When asked, supervisors can express their opinions about unionization in a neutral manner, if this is possible, without running into the danger of having the answer interpreted as a threat or promise. The safest approach, however, is for the supervisors to avoid discussing opinions with employees in the office.

These are only a few guidelines that the supervisor should keep in mind; additional guidelines may be obtained from your legal representative or your human resources department.

Usually an election conducted by the National Labor Relations Board determines the outcome of the organizing campaign. If the union loses the election, the employees do not have a union for the immediate future. If the union wins, management has to recognize the union as the bargaining agent and begin negotiations in good faith.

On the surface, the supervisor does not appear to be significantly involved in the negotiations of a labor agreement. As stated earlier, the period during which a union first enters a department of a healthcare organization is usually trying and filled with tension. Emotions run high, and considerable disturbance can result. Under such conditions, it is understandable that the delicate negotiations of a union contract are carried out primarily by members of top-level administration, probably assisted by legal counsel.

Because a committee of employees may be participating in these negotiations, a direct line of communication exists to the other employees of the healthcare institution, but not necessarily to the supervisor. In fact, the supervisor often is less well informed about the course of negotiations than the employees. Therefore, the administrator must see that the supervisor is fully advised as to the progress and direction the negotiations are taking. In addition, the supervisor should be given an opportunity to express opinions on matters brought up during the negotiations. In other words, even though top-level management is representing the institution at the negotiating sessions, supervisors should be able to express their views through them, because ultimately it is the supervisor who bears the major responsibility for fulfilling the contract provisions.

The same necessity exists whenever renegotiations of the labor agreement take place. At that time, top-level administration should consult with the supervisors to determine how specific provisions in the contract have worked out and what changes in the contract the supervisors would like to have made. Both the administrator and the supervisors must realize that although the supervisors do not actually sit at the negotiating table, they have much to do with the nature of the negotiations. Many of the demands made by the union during the negotiations have their origin in the day-to-day operations of the department. Often the most difficult questions to be solved in the bargaining process stem from the relationship that the supervisors have with their employees.

Therefore, a great amount of communication must occur between the administrator and the supervisor before and during the negotiation of a labor agreement. To supply valuable information, the supervisor must know what has been happening in the department and have facts to substantiate his or her statements. This points to the value of documentation—that is, keeping good records of disciplinary incidents, productivity, leaves, promotions, and so forth.

Figure 30.1: Dos and Don'ts for Managers and Supervisors During a Union-Organizing Campaign

Do

1. Tell employees that the organization does not believe that they need union representation.
2. Answer employees' questions about organizational policies and discuss the union campaign issues.
3. Tell employees that if they join the union, they are expected to pay union dues and fees.
4. Assure employees that, with or without the union, management is going to continue to try to make the organization a good place to work.
5. Explain to employees that the organization will recognize the union and bargain in good faith if the majority of the employees really want it but that any improvements in wages and benefits are negotiable and not automatic, as the union might want them to believe.
6. Administer appropriate disciplinary action or terminate any employee who threatens or coerces other employees, whether for or against the union.
7. Request outside union officials to leave facility property if they try to solicit employees there. Escort them off the property or, if appropriate, call the police to have them removed.

Don't [S.P.I.T.]

S: Spy on employees or conduct surveillance of any kind to determine the level of union sentiment.

P: Promise anything. You should not do anything to suggest that you are soliciting grievances.

I: Interrogate anyone. Asking questions about union sympathies or union activity is an unfair labor practice under the law.

T: Threaten, coerce, or intimidate any employee because of his or her union activity.

Source: Abdelhak, et al. *Health Information: Management of a Strategic Resource.* 1996. Philadelphia, PA: W. B. Saunders Co. Reprinted by permission.

The supervisor should also be alert to problems that should be called to the administration's attention so that in the next set of negotiations these matters may be worked out more satisfactorily. It is in the interest of both the union and the institution to have as few unresolved problems as possible. If problems do arise, however, it is the supervisor's responsibility to see that the administration is aware of them at the time of contract negotiations.

Content of the Agreement

Once administration and the union have agreed on a labor contract, this agreement will be the basis on which both parties must operate. Virtually all collective bargaining agreements are constructed with what is called a *management rights clause*. That clause usually gives management very broad authority to manage the workforce. All other provisions in the contract are exceptions to that broad authority. Because the supervisor is now obligated to manage the department within the overall framework of the labor agreement, he or she must have complete knowledge of its provisions and how they are to be interpreted. The supervisor is the one who can cause disagreements between the union and the healthcare institution by failing to live up to the terms of the agreement. Thus, the content of the union contract must be fully explained to and understood by the supervisor.

A good way to present such explanations is at a meeting arranged for top administration and all the supervisors, which is usually chaired by the human resources or labor relations director. The purpose of the meeting is to brief the supervisors on the content of the labor contract, giving them an opportunity to ask questions about any part they do not understand. Copies of the contract and clarification of the various clauses may be furnished to the supervisors so that they may study them in advance. Because no two contracts are alike, however, it is impossible to pinpoint specific provisions that the supervisor should explore. Normally all contracts deal with matters such as union recognition, management's rights, union security, wages, conditions and hours of work, overtime, vacations, holidays, leaves of absence, seniority, promotions, and similar terms and conditions of employment. Almost certainly there are also provisions concerning complaint and grievance procedures and arbitration. In addition, many other provisions are likely to be peculiar to each institution in question.

Besides the need to familiarize the supervisors with the exact provisions of the contract, it is just as important for the administrator to explain to them the philosophy of top-level administration in reference to general relations with the union. The supervisors should understand that the intention of the administration is to maintain good working relations with the union so that organizational objectives can be achieved in a mutually satisfactory fashion. The CEO should clarify that the best way to achieve good union-management relations in a hospital or any other institution is by effective contract administration. The experts in the human resources or the labor relations department have a great deal to do with effective contract administration, but much still depends on how the supervisor handles the terms of the contract on a day-to-day basis.

The supervisors must bear in mind that the negotiated contract was carefully and thoughtfully debated and finally agreed on by both parties. Thus, it is not in the interest of successful contract administration for the supervisors to try to "beat the contract," even though they may think they are doing the institution a favor. The administrator must make it clear that to achieve satisfactory cooperation, supervisors may not construct their own contractual clauses nor can they reinterpret clauses in their own way. Once the agreement has been reached, supervisors should not attempt to change or circumvent it.

If the administrator fails to familiarize the supervisors with the provisions and spirit of the agreement, they should insist on briefing sessions and explanations before they apply the clauses of the contract in the daily working situation of the department. The advent of the labor contract does not change the supervisor's job as a manager. The supervisor must still perform the managerial functions of planning, organizing, staffing, influencing, and controlling. There is no change in the authority delegated to the department head by the administrator or in the responsibility the supervisor has accepted. The significant change is that the supervisor must now perform the managerial duties within the framework of the union agreement. He or she still has the right to require the subordinates to carry out orders and the obligation to get the job done within the department. Certain provisions within the union agreement, however, are likely to influence and even limit some activities, especially within the areas of job assignments, disciplinary action, and dismissal. In many instances, these provisions of the contract undoubtedly make it more challenging for the supervisor to be a good manager. The only way to meet the challenge is for the supervisor to improve his or her own managerial ability as well as his or her knowledge and techniques of good labor relations.

Applying the Agreement

It is in the daily application of the labor agreement that the real importance of the supervisor's contribution appears. The manner in which the day-to-day problems are handled within the framework of the union contract makes the difference between positive labor-management relations and a situation filled with unnecessary tensions and bad feelings. At best, a union contract can only set forth the broad outline of labor-management relations. To make it a positive instrument of constructive relations, the contract must be supported by appropriate and intelligent supervisory decisions. It is the supervisor who interprets management's intent by everyday actions. In the final analysis, the supervisor, through decisions, actions, and behavior, really gives the contract meaning and life.

In many instances, the supervisor may expand on some of the provisions of the contract when interpreting and applying them to specific situations. In so doing, the supervisor sets precedents that arbitrators pay heed to when deciding grievances that come before them. Almost all labor agreements have a grievance procedure leading to arbitration. An arbitrator is a person selected by the union and management to make a final and binding decision in a grievance that the parties involved are unable to settle themselves.

It is impossible for the administrator and the union to draw up a contract that anticipates every possible situation in employee relations and specifies exact directives for dealing with them. Therefore, the individual judgment of the supervisor becomes very important in deciding each particular situation. This again illustrates the significance of the supervisor's influence on the interpretation of the labor agreement.

As a representative of administration, any error in the supervisor's decision making is the administration's error. The immediate supervisor has the greatest responsibility for seeing that the clauses of the agreement are carried out appropriately. This includes the supervisor's duty to ensure that the employees comply with the provisions, just as supervisors have to operate within them. Therefore, the administrator must realize how significant a role the supervisor plays in the contract administration. Likewise, it is just as essential for the supervisor to realize how far reaching his or her decisions and actions can become.

Problem Areas

The supervisor is likely to run into difficulties in the administration of a labor agreement in two broad areas. The first covers the vast number of complaints that are concerned with single issues, such as those involving a particular disciplinary action; assignment of work; distribution of overtime; and questions about promotion, transfer, and downgrading. In each situation, the personal judgment of the supervisor is of great importance. As long as the contract provisions are met, the supervisor should feel free to deal with grievances as he or she sees fit. He or she must make certain, however, that the actions are consistent and logical even though they are made on the basis of personal judgment rather than on specifically documented rules.

The second area of difficulty in contract administration covers those grievances and problems in which the supervisor is called on to interpret a clause of the contract. The supervisor is placed in a situation in which an attempt must be made to carry out the generalized statement of the contract but finds that it is subject to varying interpretations. In such instances, he or she would be wrong to handle the problem without consulting the human resources department first. Whenever an interpretation of the contract is at issue, any decision is likely to be long lasting. Such a decision may set a precedent that the institution, the union, or even an arbitrator would want to make use of in the future. By referring these situations to human resources, management ensures that the contract is interpreted consistently throughout the healthcare organization.

Therefore, if interpretation of a clause is in doubt, the question should be brought to the attention of the human resources director. Although the supervisor may have been well indoctrinated in the meaning, philosophy, and clauses of the contract, his or her perspective is probably not broad enough to make a potentially precedent-setting interpretation. Because the supervisor did not attend the bargaining meetings, he or she cannot know the intent of the parties nor the background of this provision. For these and other reasons the supervisor should consult with human resources staff.

In non-precedent-setting situations and in the daily administration of the labor agreement, the supervisor must bear in mind that as a member of management, he or she has the right and even the duty to make a decision. The union contract does not abrogate management's right to decide; the union does, however, have a right to grieve.

For example, the supervisor's job is to maintain discipline, and if disciplinary action is necessary, he or she should take action without discussing it with the union's representative. The supervisor should understand that usually there is no duty to negotiate, and he or she should not set any precedent of determining together with the union what the supervisor's rights are in a particular disciplinary case. Of course, before any disciplinary measures are taken, a prudent supervisor will examine all the facts in the case, fulfill the preliminary steps, and think through the appropriateness of the action. This process is more fully discussed in Chapter 31.

In a few cases, the union contract will call for consultation or advance notice before the supervisor can proceed. Advance notice or consultation, however, does not mean agreement or negotiation on the final decision. Repercussions or protests from the union can still occur, although prior communication on anticipated action can prevent them somewhat. In any event, the right to decide on day-to-day issues of contract administration still rests with the supervisor and not with the union.

THE SUPERVISOR AND THE SHOP STEWARD

The supervisor probably has the most union contact with the *shop steward*, who is the first-line official of the union and is sometimes referred to as union representative or delegate. The union representative is not the same as a union business agent or business representative; these are normally full-time union officials who are employed and paid by the local or national union. At times, the supervisor is also required to interact with them.

The shop steward normally remains an employee of the healthcare facility and is subject to the same regulations as every other employee. He or she is expected to put in a full day's work for the employer, regardless of having been selected by fellow workers to be their official spokesperson with both the institution and the union. This obviously is a difficult position, as the shop steward has to serve two masters. As an employee, he or she must follow the supervisor's orders and directives; as a union official, though, he or she has responsibilities to coworkers.

Just as individuals vary in their approach to their jobs, shop stewards vary in their approach to their positions. Some are unassuming; others are overbearing. Some are helpful and courteous, whereas others are difficult. Unless special provisions exist, the shop steward's rights are the same as those of any other union member. Moreover, the shop steward is subject to the same regulations regarding quality of work and conduct as the other employees of the department. However, shop stewards are entitled to time off from their job responsibilities to conduct union business, such as representing employees at grievances.

The role of the shop steward depends considerably on the makeup of the individual and the philosophy of the union. The supervisor should always remember that the shop steward is an employee of the organization and should be treated as such. The supervisor should also remember, however, that the shop steward is the representative of the other employees; in this capacity, he or she learns quickly what the other employees are thinking and what is being said in the grapevine. Thus, the supervisor will come to understand and take advantage of the fact that the dual role can make the shop steward a good liaison between management and employees.

Although shop stewards perform a number of union functions, such as collecting dues, soliciting membership, and promoting political causes, the supervisor should realize that the shop steward's most important responsibility probably concerns employees' complaints and grievances. The shop steward's job is to bring such complaints and grievances before the supervisor. The supervisor's job is to settle them to the best of his or her ability, using the grievance procedures described in great detail in every union contract. Throughout these procedures, discussed more fully in Chapter 31, the supervisor represents management and the shop steward represents the employees for the union.

In most cases, the shop steward is sincerely trying to redress the aggrieved employee by winning a favorable ruling. At times, however, the supervisor may be under the impression that he or she is out looking for grievances merely to stay busy. Supervisors should keep in mind that the union has a legal responsibility to represent the employee, even if they believe the discipline that the supervisor administered was just. Employees can sue the union for failure to provide proper representation. This may be partly true, as the shop steward does have a political assignment, and it is necessary to assure the employees that the union is working on their behalf. The shop steward must be able to convince the employees that they can rely on him or her and therefore on the union to protect them. On the other hand, an experienced shop steward knows that normally real grievances are settled. He or she sees no need to look for complaints that do not have a valid background and would be rightfully turned down by the supervisor.

Most unions ensure that the shop steward is well trained to present the complaints and grievances so that they can be carried to a successful conclusion. The shop steward is usually well versed in understanding the content of the contract, management's obligations, and employees' rights. Before presenting a grievance, the shop steward should determine such matters as whether the contract has been violated, the employer acted unfairly, the employee's health or safety has been jeopardized, and so forth. In grievance matters, management has the obligation to prove its actions were not in violation of the contract between the union and the healthcare facility. The shop steward will challenge the management decision or action, and the supervisor must justify what he or she has done.

Because the shop steward's main interest is in the union, at times this may antagonize the supervisor. In some instances, it will be difficult for the supervisor to keep a sense of humor and remain calm. Often the supervisor also will have difficulty discussing a grievance with a shop steward on an equal footing because the shop steward is a subordinate within the normal working situation. When assuming the role of shop steward, however, the position as representative of the union members gives him or her equal standing. The supervisor should always bear in mind that the shop steward's job is political and legal and as such carries certain weight. At the same time, the supervisor should understand that a good shop steward keeps any supervisor on the alert and forces him or her to be a better manager.

SUMMARY

Approximately 12 percent of the labor force in the United States are members of an employee association or a labor union. Because unions are attempting to represent more and more employees from the service industries, it is essential that supervisors in healthcare undertakings are familiar with some basic aspects of labor union relations.

The supervisor's role in the union relations of a healthcare facility cannot be minimized. Although the supervisor is not normally a member of the management team that sits down with union negotiators to settle the terms of the labor contract, he or she does play an important indirect role in this meeting. Many of the difficulties and problems discussed at a negotiating meeting can be traced back to the daily activities of the supervisor. At best, the union contract resulting from the negotiations can set forth only the broad outline of labor-management relationships. It is the day-to-day application and administration of the agreement that makes the difference between harmonious labor relations and a situation filled with unnecessary tensions and bad feelings.

The supervisor is the person who, through daily decisions and actions, gives the contract real meaning. He or she must therefore be thoroughly familiar with the contents of the contract and with the general philosophy of management toward the union. He or she must understand the difficult and important political and legal role of the union shop steward, who serves in a dual capacity as one of the regular employees and as the representative of the union members. In grievance cases, the supervisor must learn to regard the shop steward as an equal, as one who is trained to present the complaints of union members as effectively as possible. The shop steward will challenge management's decisions, and the supervisor must justify them. Although at times it may be difficult to keep a balanced perspective, the supervisor should always remember that an alert shop steward can serve to force him or her to be a better manager.

REFERENCES

Abdelhak, M., S. Grostick, M. A. Hanken, and E. Jenkins. 1996. *Health Information: Management of a Strategic Resource.* Philadelphia, PA: Saunders.

Bureau of Labor Statistics. 2005a. "Union Members Summary." [Online information; retrieved 10/3/05.] www.bls.gov/news.release/union2.nro.htm.

————. 2005b. "Union Affiliation of Employed Wage and Salary Workers by Occupation and Industry [Online informationl; retrieved 10/3/05.] www.bls.gov/news.release/union2.to3.htm.

Morrissey, J. A. 1995. "Manufacturing Employees Believe Unions Ineffective." *Textile World Magazine* 146 (12): 63.

CHAPTER THIRTY-ONE

Handling Grievances

CHAPTER OBJECTIVES

After you have studied this chapter, you should be able to do the following:

1. Define the term grievance.
2. Differentiate between the roles of the shop steward and the supervisor in responding to a grievance.
3. Review the process of handling a grievance.

GRIEVANCE CAN be defined as a complaint that usually results from a misunderstanding, misinterpretation, or violation of a provision of the labor agreement. This complaint has been formally presented to management by the union. Almost all union contracts contain provisions for a grievance procedure. The first step of the procedure begins at the departmental level—with the supervisor or the manager and the shop steward. If the grievance is not settled there, it can be appealed to the next higher level of management; at this point usually a chief steward or a business agent of the union will enter into the picture. Contracts typically provide for an appeal to the human resources director.

The grievance procedure usually sets a time limit for each of these steps to be finished. If the dispute cannot be settled by the first two or three steps to the mutual satisfaction of both parties, the agreement usually has an arbitration provision. This means that the issue may be submitted to an impartial outsider—an *arbitrator*. After hearing testimony and evidence, the arbitrator renders a final decision, which is binding on both parties.

The supervisor thus needs to be well qualified in handling complaints and settling grievances. Indeed, in a unionized setting one of the supervisor's most important duties is to make certain that most complaints and grievances are properly disposed of during the first step of the grievance procedure. Most organizations require that supervisors consult with a labor relations specialist in the

Special thanks to Marc J. Leff, Esq., vice president, Human Resources, Maimonides Medical Center, Brooklyn, New York, for his update of this chapter.

human resources department when handling complaints. This is important because many complaints could have organizationwide implications. Grievances that refer to discrimination and equal employment opportunities could have legal implications for the entire organization.

The supervisor is not shirking responsibility or admitting ignorance by consulting with specialists in the human resources department. In some organizations, management even has conferred on the labor relations staff (a division of the human resources department) the final authority to adjudicate grievances by giving them functional authority, as discussed in Chapter 15.

The following discussion is based on an organizational setup in which the human resources and labor relations experts are in a strictly staff position and the initial formal authority and responsibility to handle grievances rest with the line supervisor. In every unionized organization, line supervisors know that handling grievances is part of their job and that it takes judgment, tact, and often more patience than comes naturally to most people.

Supervisors should not feel threatened by grievances. They frequently may think that too much of their time is spent discussing complaints and grievances instead of getting the job done in the department. They may also believe that they perform more as labor lawyers than as supervisors. Supervisors should also realize, however, that higher management regards the skill in handling grievances to be an important index of supervisory ability. The number of grievances that arise within a department is considered an indication of the state of employee-management relations.

A fine distinction can be made between the terms complaint and grievance. From the supervisor's point of view, however, a *grievance* simply means a complaint that has been formally presented either to the supervisor as a management representative or to the shop steward or any other union official. As mentioned, a grievance usually is a complaint resulting from a misunderstanding, misinterpretation, or violation of the provisions of the labor agreement. The supervisor must learn to distinguish between those grievances that are admissible and those that are gripes and merely indicate that the employee is unhappy or dissatisfied. In every case, the supervisor should listen carefully to what the employee has to say to decide what action can be taken to correct the situation.

THE SHOP STEWARD'S ROLE

As discussed briefly in Chapter 30, the *shop steward* (or union delegate) is usually the spokesperson for the employee in a grievance procedure. A grievance is the result of a disciplinary action taken against an employee after the supervisor has made a thorough investigation of the incident. The union has a legal obligation to fairly represent an employee at a grievance. Failure to do so could lead to a lawsuit by a union member against the union. The shop steward is familiar with the labor agreement and has been trained to present the employee's side of the grievance. What should the supervisor do if an employee approaches him or her without having consulted the shop steward? In such a case, it is appropriate for the supervisor to listen to the employee's story to see if it involves the union or may be of interest to it. If the contract or the union appears to be involved, the supervisor should call in the shop steward to listen to the employee's presentation. Although it is unlikely that a union member would present a grievance without the shop steward, the supervisor must notify the shop steward if this should happen.

Similarly, if the shop steward submits a grievance on behalf of the employee without that employee present, the supervisor should again listen carefully and with understanding. It is always preferable, however, to listen to complaints when both the shop steward and the complaining employee are present. Nothing can keep the supervisor from speaking directly to the employee. The hospital must negotiate any issue that is a term and condition of employment with the union as the employee's legal representative. If the shop steward is not present, the supervisor should take great care not to give the impression that he or she is undermining the shop steward's authority or relationship with the union members. There should always be free and open communication between the supervisor and the shop steward, even though the shop steward's job is to represent employees and to fight hard to win their cases.

THE SUPERVISOR'S ROLE

One of the supervisor's primary functions is to attempt to dispose of all grievances at the first step of the grievance procedure. This means that part of the supervisor's job, usually with help from staff people in the labor relations department, is to explore fully the details of the grievance, deal with the problems brought out, and try to settle them. To achieve prompt and satisfactory adjudication of grievances at this early stage, the supervisor should observe the following points in dealing with the grievance procedure.

Being Available

The supervisor must be readily available to the shop steward and to the aggrieved employee. Availability does not only mean being physically present. It also means being approachable and ready to listen with an open mind. The supervisor must not make it difficult for a complaining employee to see him or her. This does not mean that the supervisor must stop immediately what he or she is doing, but every effort must be made to set a time as quickly as possible for the first discussion. An undue delay could be interpreted by the employee and the union as managerial stalling, indifference, or resentment.

Listening

Everything stated about communication (see Chapter 5) and interviewing (see Chapter 20) is applicable to the grievance procedure as well. When a complaint is brought to the supervisor, the shop steward and the employee should be given the opportunity to present their case fully. Sympathetic listening by the supervisor is likely to minimize hostilities and tensions during the settlement of the case. The supervisor must know how to listen well. He or she must give the shop steward and the employee a chance to say whatever is on their minds. If they believe that the supervisor is truly listening to them and that fair treatment will be given, the complaint will not loom as large to them in the presentation of the problem. Halfway through the story, the complaining employee may even realize that he or she does not have a true complaint at all. Sympathetic listening can often produce this result. Also, sometimes the more a person talks, the more likely he or she is to make contradictory and inconsistent remarks, thus weakening the argument. Only an effective listener will be able to catch these inconsistencies and use them to help resolve the case. Frequently supervisors are so preoccupied with defending themselves or trying to justify their points of view that they simply do not listen.

Having Emotional Control

The supervisor must take great caution not to get angry at the shop steward or the employee. The shop steward's job and legal responsibility is to represent the employee even when he or she knows that the grievance is not valid. In such a situation, the supervisor's job is to point out objectively that the grievance has no merit. The supervisor cannot expect the shop steward to do this because he or she must serve as the employee's spokesperson at all times. Sometimes a union deliberately creates grievances to keep tensions elevated. Even this situation must not arouse the anger of the supervisor. If the supervisor does not know how to handle such occurrences successfully, he or she should discuss the matter with higher management and experts in the labor relations or human resources department. By no means, however, must the supervisor get upset, even if a grievance is unwarranted.

If arguments, tempers, and emotional outbursts run high and make good communication difficult, the supervisor may want to terminate the meeting and reschedule it. He or she must use caution not to participate in a shouting match. It is hoped that at the next meeting tempers will have cooled down and a calmer discussion will be possible.

Defining the Problem

Often the shop steward and the employee are not sufficiently clear in their presentations. It is then the supervisor's job to summarize clearly what has been presented and make certain that everyone understands the problem that must be resolved. Sometimes the complaint merely deals with the symptoms of the problem. The supervisor must know how deeply to delve to get at the root of the situation. It is necessary to define the employee's complaint and the extent of the problem precisely to determine whether a grievance is valid under the contract. Once the real problem is clarified and handled properly, it is unlikely that similar grievances will come up again.

Obtaining the Facts

All the facts should be obtained as quickly as possible to arrive at a solution of the problem and a successful adjudication of the grievance. The supervisor can probably get most of the facts by asking the complaining employee pertinent questions. In so doing, the supervisor should be objective and try not to confuse either the shop steward or the employee. He or she must ascertain who or what caused the grievance, where and when it happened, and whether there was unfair treatment. The supervisor must determine if there are witnesses and get written statements from all parties, including the grievant, before drawing a conclusion. He or she must also determine whether any connection exists between the current grievance and other grievances. Although it sometimes may be tempting to hide behind the excuse of searching for more facts, the supervisor must not do so. Furthermore, the information gathered in this investigation should be shared with the union for several reasons. First, the union has a legal right to the information. Second, the more facts the union has, the less likely it is to pursue the grievance. If there is patient-sensitive information or protected health information collected in the investigation, the supervisor should contact the human resources staff for guidance. He or she must make a decision on the basis of those facts that are available and that can be obtained without undue delay.

Sometimes, however, it is impossible to gather all the information at once; therefore, the grievance cannot be settled immediately. In this case, the supervisor must inform the aggrieved employee and the shop steward. If they see that the supervisor is working on the problem, they are likely to be reasonable and wait for an answer to be given at a specified future date.

Having Familiarity with the Contract and Consultation

After having determined the facts, the supervisor now must ascertain whether the grievance is legitimate in the context of the contract. As mentioned earlier, a grievance is usually not a grievance in the legal sense unless provisions of the labor contract have been violated or administered inconsistently. Therefore, it is necessary to check the provisions in the contract when any reference to a violation is made. If the supervisor has any question about this, he or she should consult with someone in the human resources or labor relations department or with higher management. Provisions in the labor agreement may not be clearly stated, and a question may exist about whether a certain provision in the contract is applicable at all. In such a situation, the complaining employee should be told that additional clarification in reference to the agreement is needed and that the answer will be delayed for a few days.

RESPECTING TIME LIMITS

Usually the grievance procedure sets a time limit within which the grievance must be answered. The supervisor must see that all grievances are settled as promptly and justly as possible. Postponing a judgment in the hope that the complaint may disappear is courting trouble and more grievances. Moreover, an unnecessary postponement is unfair because the employee and the shop steward are entitled to know the supervisor's position as quickly as the facts can be obtained.

Speed is definitely important in the settlement of grievances, but not if it will result in unsound decisions. If a delay cannot be avoided, the aggrieved parties must be informed. Waiting for a decision is bothersome to everybody concerned. In such a situation, it may be a good idea to put the grievance in writing and sign it so that the parties involved do not forget the details.

ADJUDICATION OF GRIEVANCES

Part of the supervisor's job is to try to resolve all grievances preferably at the first step of the grievance procedure. As already pointed out, this is included in the managerial aspects of the supervisory function. It is far better to settle a minor issue at this stage before it escalates into a major issue. The only cases that should be referred to higher levels of management are those that are unusual, that require additional interpretation of the union contract's meaning, that contain problems that have not shown up before, that involve broad policy considerations, or in which disciplinary action was taken inappropriately.

Consistency of Action

In the adjudication of grievances, the supervisor must ensure that the rights of management are protected and that the policies and precedents of the institution are followed. If the supervisor must deviate from previous adjudications, he or she must explain the reasons to the employee and the shop steward. The supervisor must make certain that both of them fully understand that this exception does not set a precedent. In such cases, the supervisor is always obliged to have this course of action reviewed and approved by higher-level administration, the human resources department, or both before informing the parties involved.

Consequences of the Settlement

The supervisor must check previous settlements and make certain that the current intended decision is consistent with past decisions, the institution's policy, and the labor agreement. The supervisor should avoid making an exception because this decision is likely to become a precedent. In adjudicating grievances, the supervisor must consider not only what effect the adjudication will have in this instance but also its implications for the future. Whenever the supervisor settles a grievance, the possibility exists that this settlement will show up as part of the labor contract in following years. Also, if the case goes to arbitration, the arbitrator is likely to look for precedents, consider them almost as binding as the labor agreement, and use them as a valid basis for the final decision.

Providing a Clear Answer

The supervisor must answer the grievance in a straightforward, reasonable manner that is perfectly clear to the aggrieved party. The answer must not be phrased in language that the aggrieved party cannot understand, regardless of whether the judgment is in favor of the employee. If the supervisor rules against the employee, the employee is that much more entitled to a clear, straightforward reply stating the reasons for the decision. Although the employee may disagree with such a reply, at least it will be understood.

Clarity is even more necessary if the supervisor has to reply to the grievance in writing. In that case, the answer must be restricted to the specific complaints involved, the words used must be appropriate, and any reference to a particular provision of the labor agreement or to the organization's rules must be clearly cited. Unless required, a written reply should not be rendered. If such a reply is required under the labor agreement, however, it is appropriate for the supervisor to discuss all the implications with higher management or with the human resources department so that a properly worded reply is given.

NON-UNIONIZED ORGANIZATIONS

Many healthcare facilities have implemented grievance procedures regardless of whether the facility has a union. Grievances need to be heard by management in a timely fashion to avoid the possible introduction of a third party and to ensure staff concerns are heard and given appropriate attention. To avoid the potential introduction of a third party, human resources departments in many facilities have developed detailed procedures that allow for (1) first-level supervisors to investigate and attempt to remedy the concern, (2) an appeal(s) process, and (3) an ad hoc committee of peers and management to hear and recommend final action as it pertains to the grievance or concern. Each step has an associated time frame to ensure timely response to the complainant.

RECORD KEEPING

It is essential for the supervisor to keep records and documents whenever a grievance decision is made. If the employee's request is satisfied, this decision may become a precedent. If the complaint cannot be settled in the first step, this grievance probably will go farther, possibly to arbitration or to a government agency or litigation as in cases of discrimination. The case will certainly go to higher levels of management, and the supervisor should not defend the action by depending on memory. Diligent recording of the facts, reasoning, and decisions should be available. With this documentation at hand, the supervisor is then able to substantiate the actions whenever asked.

Good records are an absolute necessity because the burden of proof is on the supervisor and management in disciplinary actions. Management has the right to discipline, but only for good or just cause. Management has the right to decide, but the union has the right to submit a grievance. Whenever the employee or the union maintains that the supervisor has violated the agreement or has administered its provisions in an unfair or inconsistent manner, the supervisor must defend the action. Without good records and documentation, this is often difficult, if not impossible.

Supervisors should familiarize themselves with all the previous points as aids in handling grievances. The supervisors' decisions and actions have some impact on employee-union relations at the healthcare facility. For this impact to be favorable, supervisors not only must be familiar with the points just covered but also must apply them during honest, face-to-face discussions with employees and the shop steward whenever grievances do arise.

SUMMARY

The labor agreement sets forth a broad, general outline of labor-management relationships. This outline must be fulfilled with intelligent supervisory decisions. Occasions to make such decisions arise mainly in the settlement of grievances. Indeed, the proper adjudication of grievances is one of the important components of the supervisory position. Whenever the supervisor settles grievances, the labor contract is referred to and interpreted. The settlements may have far-reaching implications because they set precedents. Much of what the union will discuss at the next contract negotiations originates with day-to-day supervisory decisions. If a grievance should go to arbitration, the impartial arbitrator will also attach great importance to precedents set by the supervisor.

Often it is not so much what the contract says that counts, but how it has been interpreted by management's front-line representative—the supervisor. This shows how important a role the supervisor actually plays in the adjudication of grievances and how necessary it is to gain considerable skill in the use of adjudication techniques. In most organizations, specialists in labor relations are involved in arriving at the appropriate settlement.

To apply adjudication techniques appropriately, the supervisor should always be available, listen carefully, and behave professionally. The supervisor must learn to define the problem, obtain the facts, and draw on his or her thorough knowledge of the contract's clauses. It is also important to avoid unnecessary delays and settle grievances at an early stage. Moreover, the supervisor must be fair in all decisions, protecting the rights of the institution and respecting the content and spirit of the agreement. The supervisor also must keep good records, give clear replies, and, above all, remain consistent.

Historically, unions have developed because management responded to the needs of their workforce inappropriately. Today unions are established for similar reasons or at least because employees perceive a lack of attention to their needs on the part of management. Supervisors manage a variety of resources but their most productive, costly, and visible resource is employees. Effective management yields high quality, high productivity, and high morale. Recognizing that employees are inherently good and desire the facility to succeed makes the management of other resources (such as money, materials, and machinery) much easier.

CHAPTER THIRTY-TWO

Emerging Influences in Healthcare

CHAPTER OBJECTIVES

After studying this chapter, you should be able to do the following:

1. Recognize the many different forces affecting healthcare and healthcare management today.
2. Apply traditional management principles to address a rapidly changing healthcare environment.

THE HEALTHCARE INDUSTRY is in a state of flux as a result of mergers, de-mergers, overzealous regulations, technology leaps, staffing shortages, high consumer demand, and increasingly educated consumers. All of these issues, as well as many more, affect how you manage your department, structure your work place, and achieve your goals. Heretofore, the book has discussed relatively traditional approaches to the roles of management—planning, organizing, staffing, influencing, and controlling. However, the successful supervisor is the one who can take the theories explored in this book and apply them to nontraditional settings.

THE FORCE OF CHANGE

Changing Occupations

In the coming years, one-half of college seniors will be working in jobs that do not exist today (Sena 2005). According to the U.S. Census Bureau, there were 2,076,000 railroad workers in 1920, down to only 231,000 today. Conversely, today we have 1,379,000 medical technicians; in 1910, there were none.[1] As the United States became more industrialized, occupations were created and eliminated (Federal Reserve Bank of Dallas 1992).

Our aging baby boomers will place a strain on today's healthcare system. Forty percent of today's 50-year-old women will live to be 100. Although healthcare professionals are specializing in many areas, geriatrics is not one of them.

The United States will need 36,000 geriatricians by 2030, but it has less than 7,000 today. Fewer than half of the medical schools in the United States incorporate geriatrics into their undergraduate curriculum (National Center for Policy Analysis 2005).

While occupational opportunities are unfolding in an era with technological advances and diversity, the federal government's Health Resources and Services Administration has concluded that staffing shortages, especially in the nursing and pharmacy areas, will become critical. Pharmacist rates of vacancy are up to 18 percent in certain areas (DHHS 2000). Nursing vacancies are projected to be at 20 percent by 2020 (DHHS 2001) (see Figure 32.1). College students are not entering the healthcare profession, possibly because of the high caseloads, long hours, or alternating shifts or because there are so many other, more glamorous, less stressful options available to today's youth. Healthcare management needs to aggressively promote this career option and provide worksite considerations that address the negative aspects of the job.

CHANGING CONSUMERS AND SATISFACTION

The baby boomers are now in their 50s and 60s and are (and will continue to be) the most powerful consumers of healthcare. They also are well educated, technology savvy, and demanding of service. They are taking care of their aging parents and overseeing the healthcare delivered to that generation. Ensuring customer satisfaction with the services your staff and your healthcare facility provide today is paramount in tying the boomers to your facility for future healthcare services. Training staff in customer service techniques must be a component of every orientation program. Although person-to-person skills are important, training in telephone and e-mail skills and etiquette should not be ignored. Skill building in explaining the psychology that governs upset customer behavior, strategies for successful customer encounters, and understanding attitudes and actions should be included in the training program. Remember that your customers today—patients as well as their relatives—are living in a fast-paced, but litigious, world. They expect answers and explanations that they understand, and they expect them both now. Delays of any kind may be perceived as maneuvers to hide something from them, thus creating a potentially angry and certainly dissatisfied customer.

Today's consumer is much more health conscious and "health literate." The Internet offers an abundance of sites offering health information and facility-specific comparative data to the public; no longer must individuals rely on the physician office visit to learn about their conditions or at which hospital to be treated. Consumers also are seeking quality care (see Figure 32.2). Quality is hard to define and each consumer has his or her own definition. However, entities such as CMS (HospitalCompare), HealthGrades, and LeapFrog have developed comprehensive benchmarking and performance measurement programs to inform consumers about institution and physician quality. Addressing disease outcomes, participating in community health projects, and surveying

FIGURE 32.1: NATIONAL SUPPLY AND DEMAND PROJECTION FOR FTE REGISTERED NURSES, 2000 TO 2020

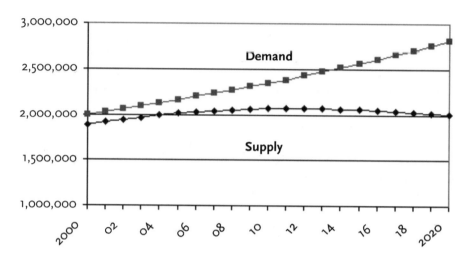

Source: U.S. Department of Health and Human Services, Bureau of Health Professionals. 2002. "Reports: Projected Supply, Demand and Shortages of Registered Nurses, 2000–2020." [Online information; retrieved 07/02.] http://bhpr.hrsa.gov/healthworkforce/reports/rnproject/default.htm.

consumers are some ways to demonstrate the facility's interest in quality and consumer satisfaction.

As for your employees, the old adage "seeing is believing" may work for or against a healthcare organization. Employees who see and believe resources are being properly channeled toward replacing and updating technology, hiring qualified staff, and staffing patient care areas with an appropriate level of staff have a better feeling about the quality of care delivered in their institution. These staff promote to friends and neighbors the advances that the organization is making in technology, patient satisfaction, outcomes, and other crucial areas. Employees who are disgruntled about any of these issues may discuss widely with friends and neighbors outside of the organization the management shortfalls by pointing to medication errors, unexpected deaths, safety issues, and so forth. Supervisors must seriously consider employee concerns and discontent and recognize that they serve as a barometer of consumer satisfaction with the organization.

Changing Technology and Medicine

A new wave of technology and medicine is on the horizon. Cloning, genetic mapping, and tissue engineering are creating the ability to design humans

FIGURE 32.2: WHAT IS THE NEW HEALTHCARE CONSUMER LOOKING FOR?

- "Patients aren't basing their decisions on medical technology or the adequacy of staffing on a nursing station. They base their decisions on things they feel qualified to judge: the room; the food; how hard it was to find a parking place; whether or not the people are smiling and friendly; the admission process; the questions they are asked and the answers they get to their questions. Those things do not necessarily have anything to do with the quality of medical care, but they are the way that healthcare providers are being evaluated.

- It seems that the new healthcare consumers simply assume that members of the healthcare fraternity will do their best to cure their ills and fix what is broken. They evaluate care and base their buying decision on the way they are treated. In a sense, it's not the care, it's the *caring*, that new consumers have on their minds."

—Dawn M. Gideon

Source: Used with permission by Transition Management Group.

---

in the future. Although this may be considered radical thinking today, in two decades or less, the use of stem cells to treat conditions like spinal cord damage, multiple sclerosis, Alzheimers, and baldness may be commonplace. A new industry of genetaceuticals will combine genetic research and pharmaceuticals. Alternative medicine using herbals, acupuncture, biofeedback, and others will grow and be a viable supplement if not alternative to traditional treatment alternatives. Access to specialists will be facilitated by technology. After all, not long ago providing healthcare services via satellite was considered unlikely, and yet today telemedicine is becoming rather commonplace. Telehealth depends on sophisticated information system technology that not only cuts through campuses and geography but also provides immediate access to critical patient care information and expert healthcare guidance from specialists across the world.

No longer does any physician believe he or she knows it all. Many seek advice from other consultants and have online access to the latest findings on drugs, treatments, and other medical advances. With patient needs becoming more complex, sophisticated medical knowledge, including human understanding and published data, and diagnostic equipment must be linked with sophisticated technology systems. Robotics in the operating room and rolling along hospital corridors has become a reality. Surgeons no longer need to touch the patient during heart bypass surgery, which according to reports is easier and less traumatic to the patient. It is not unrealistic to assume that in the next decade patients may not leave their homes for medical care. Medical care will come from remote terminal connections to home computers and use equipment currently in homes to analyze a patient's bodily functions.

Supervisors will be managing technology, and their staff must be equally technologically proficient. Fortunately, many of today's youths (Generations X and Y, and Millennials) have grown up during a period of time when technology was prevalent and the fear of using it was not present. The Internet and hand-held devices provide greater access to information, and these devices will reduce healthcare costs and improve the delivery of care (Noffsinger and Chin 2000). However, these and other technology changes will require change in work processes and even the environment. A paperless environment is inevitable. Patient records and radiological imaging as we know them today will be all online, interconnected regionally and nationally, and available to patient care providers. Access authorization will be through an ATM-like device to accommodate our mobile citizens. Robotic systems for delivering medications and other materials for the lab, pharmacy, and central supply will replace the existing human courier systems. Robots work 24 hours a day, 7 days a week and require no sick or vacation time. The need for file clerks, technicians, and couriers, as well as the equipment they use such as fax machines, will disappear. Management will need to decide if people in these roles will be displaced, retrained, or terminated.

Security will be heightened because of the accessibility of sensitive data. Thus, we should expect higher surveillance levels, card accesses, biometrics, and other similar approaches to control who has access to what, when, and where. Some employees may find biometric approaches distasteful or possibly in conflict with their religious or cultural mores. The supervisor will be required to address these concerns.

Changing Economics

A growing number of hospitals and health systems may be forced into mergers, bankruptcy, or closure because of declining Medicare and other payor revenues. Congress will look to cutting reimbursement for healthcare, now representing 15 percent of the gross domestic product, to offset significant deficits in the federal budget. The rising number of uninsured individuals (45 million) adds to the financial pressures of healthcare providers who serve these individuals for little or no compensation. Such was the case of one hospital in Washington, DC, that was forced to close because of declining reimbursement. The future for the uninsured looks bleak, and 25 percent of U.S. workers are predicted to be uninsured in 2013 (California Healthcare Foundation 2005).

Mergers, once thought to be the cure-all for providing cost-effective healthcare to a region, have had relatively high failure rates in major cities. Instead of reducing costs, a new layer of management was often created. The merger of University of California, San Francisco and Stanford University added nearly 1,000 employees to the combined organization. For the rank-and-file staff, this new layer was seen by some as nothing more than additional bureaucracy stifling the actual delivery of healthcare. When mergers failed to yield the cost savings anticipated, outsourcing gained acceptance with healthcare organizations and payors outsourcing to on- and off-shore business services, including claims processing, utilization management, collections, transcription, radiology reading, coding, and information systems management.

As mergers, closures, and outsourcing occur, the supervisors will be confronted with grapevine rumors predicting budget cutting, downsizing, and other staff apprehensions. Morale is likely to deteriorate. Following the guidance discussed in prior chapters, incorporating regular, truthful, and complete communication into the culture will be imperative. Furthermore, encouraging staff to voice their fears will serve as a buffer between them and a union organizer, especially at a time when healthcare union membership is growing. Listening and empathizing will be your best attributes. The first-line supervisor will be the agent who will make sense of, unite, and transmit the organization's culture (Valentino 2004).

Changing Policies and Regulations

The number of organizations that have some part in regulating healthcare organizations is astonishing. Figure 32.3 identifies many but does not include organizations that healthcare facilities voluntarily invite to evaluate their activities, such as the National Committee on Quality Assurance, the International Organization for Standardization, the Malcolm Baldrige National Quality Program, and the Healthcare Facilities Accreditation Program. Hospitals and other healthcare providers are so overregulated that it is a wonder how any can continue to exist. Regulations that allegedly were intended to bring administrative simplification to the forefront for healthcare, such as HIPAA, have placed significant financial and administrative burdens on all providers. Supervisors will continue to be asked to enforce security, privacy, safety measures, error prevention, documentation enhancement, and process improvement, and accomplish this demand with fewer staff. Delegation and team empowerment may not be optional but rather a necessity for tomorrow's managers to be able to do everything that is required of them in this regulated environment.

Changing Staff Issues

Specialization will continue. A new title in nursing is surfacing—clinical nurse leader (CNL). CNLs are master's-prepared nurses who assume accountability for healthcare outcomes for a specific group of clients within a unit or setting through the assimilation and application of research-based information to design, implement, and evaluate client plans of care (Begun, Tornabeni, and White 2006). Other professions are following suit. Securing education, even in the most sophisticated fields, is easier through distance learning programs. The additional education and specialization will force wages to rise, thus creating additional fiscal burdens for the organization and a class of employees who will earn more than their supervisors, known as "gold collar" workers (Cornish 2005.) A study entitled, "The Next Generation: Today's Professionals Tomorrow's Leaders," explored changes in working habits of young professionals

FIGURE 32.3: WHO REGULATES HOSPITALS?

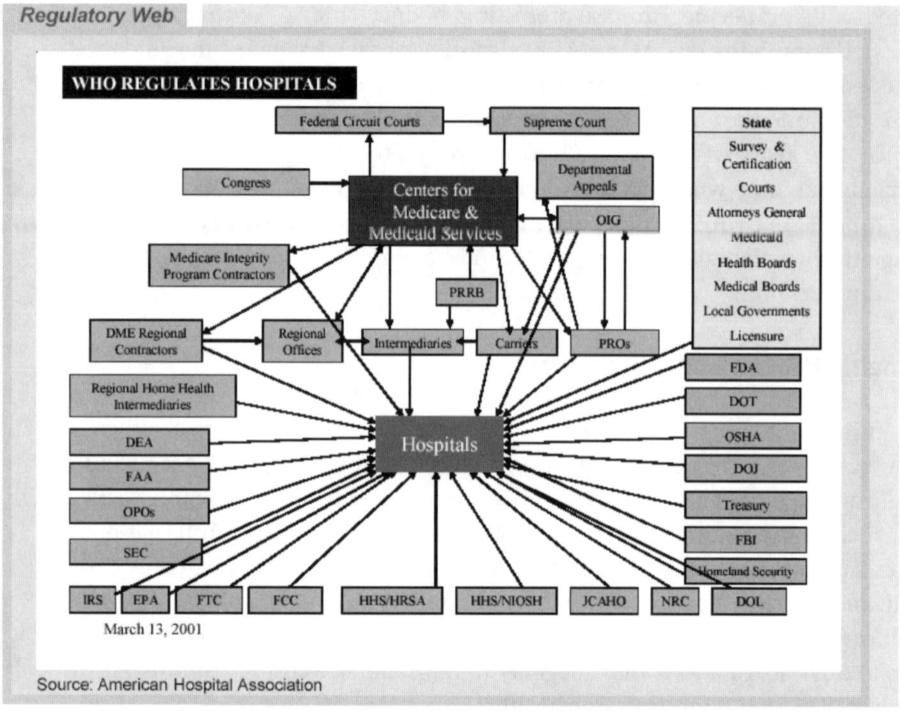

Source: American Hospital Association

Source: Reprinted from *AHA News*, Vol. 36, No. 21, by permission., May 29, 2000, © 2000, by Health Forum, Inc.

since the September 11, 2001 terrorist event. Nearly two-thirds of the respondents stated they are working differently in some way, with more than 20 percent indicating they are (1) working fewer hours, (2) limiting business travel, (3) rethinking career plans, (4) working from home more often, and (5) devoting more time to community service. Only one of the respondents lived in New York (Catalyst 2001).

Supervisors will be challenged to recruit employees and, once hired, to retain them by ensuring that the workplace is safe and secure and does not need further modifications. These conditions may lead more managers to consider tailoring work and work settings to align with the employees' life interests. By doing so, the supervisor will reduce stressors for the employee such as travel time and driver rage as well as workplace annoyances such as bad hygiene, excessive social chatter, strife over desk and chair sharing, and personal use of company copy and fax machines.

Obviously, these approaches cannot work for all healthcare organizations' staff because someone must stay at the facility to care for patients. Supervisors may, however, need to involve their patient care staff in rethinking how work is done. Using audio and video conferencing and conducting what-if brainstorming scenarios where staff are active participants will help build a more efficient and effective patient care environment and one that is more rewarding to the staff. Borrowing models from other industries will help identify options that fit in healthcare.

Workforce diversity will create unique situations for a healthcare facility, including language and cultural differences and communication concerns. It is hard to tell an employee what is expected of him or her if he or she does not speak your language, both metaphorically and literally. Similarly, your patients are encountering the same frustrations if they cannot communicate to healthcare providers in a language that is mutually understood. Supervisors may find the need to send staff members to special training courses to teach them to speak, read, and write in English. Meanwhile, you may find the diversified labor pool advantageous and an alternative to hiring translators to meet the needs of patients who speak another language.

Finally, ethics, ethical issues, and compliance will continue to be front and center. Employees, boards, and the public will expect the highest ethical conduct from healthcare leaders and employees, and patients will be encouraged to report anything to the contrary. We should question ourselves regularly if we are in the slightest way tempted to answer the question, "why shouldn't we do what is right and moral?" Ethical dilemmas, such as what the public experienced with the Terri Schiavo case, will surface more frequently as technology rather than human organs keeps people alive and will be further complicated by the battle between right-to-life groups and right-to-die organizations. As supervisors, we will be faced with these issues and the burden they place on those who serve the patient directly. Guiding our staff through these challenges will be paramount.

A FINAL WORD

Supervisors have a challenging job in any organization but particularly in healthcare, where the product of the organization can result in life or death. As a summary to this book, Exhibit 32.1 includes a list of the potential pitfalls that supervisors face daily. May you be successful in your career.

NOTE

1. "Destruction and Creation. (President's Letter)" Long Island Association, Inc. as viewed on the Internet on 2/23/06 at http://www.longislandassocia tion.org/presidents_arch.cfm?num=Pres23461111106&old=Pres5905150228 AND *The Churn—The Paradox of Progress*. Federal Reserve Bank of Dallas, 1992 as viewed on the Internet on 2/23/06 at http://oak.cats.ohiou.edu/ ~shambora/The%20Churn.pdf

Begun, J., J. Tornabeni, and K. White. 2006. "Opportunities for Improving Patient Care Through Lateral Integration: The Clinical Nurse Leader." *Journal of Healthcare Management* 51 (1): 19–25.

California HealthCare Foundation. 2005. "Health Affairs: 25 Percent of U.S. Workers Will Be Uninsured in 2013." [Online report; 10/6/05.] www.chcf.org/print.cfm?itemID=109910&currentURL=http://www.chcf.org//topics.

Catalyst. 2001. Sponsored by Ernst and Young and GE Fund. New York: Catalyst.

The Center for Health Affairs. 2005. "Industry Brief: Is Inefficiency Ailing the Healthcare System?" [Online information; retrieved 10/6/05.] http://chanet.org/Inefficiencies_in_Healthcare.pdf.

Cornish, E. 2005. "Special Report: Trends and Forecasts for the Next 25 Years." In *The Futurist*, 7–8. Bethesda, MD: World Future Society.

Federal Reserve Bank of Dallas. 1992. "The Churn—The Paradox of Progress."1992 Annual Report, 8. [Online report; retrieved 12/29/01.] http://www.dallasfed.org/htm/pubs/pdfs/anreport/arpt92.pdf.

National Center for Policy Analysis. 2005. "Where Have All the Geriatricians Gone?" *National Policy Digest*. [Online article; retrieved 9/2/05.] www.ncpa.org/newdpd/dpdarticle.php?article_id=2201.

Noffsinger, R., and S. Chin. 2000. "Improving the Delivery of Care and Reducing Healthcare Costs with the Digitization of Information." *Journal of Healthcare Information Management* 14 (2): 29.

Sena, J. 2005. "Managing Sustainable Change." Seminar. September 14, St. Louis, Missouri.

U.S. Department of Health and Human Services (DHHS). 2000. "The Pharmacist Workforce: A Study of the Supply and Demand for Pharmacists." [Online report] ftp://ftp.hrsa.gov/bhpr/nationalcenter/pharmacy/pharmshort.pdf.

———. 2001. "National Sample Survey of Registered Nurses—March 2000. Preliminary Findings, February 2001." [Online report; retrieved 2/21/01.] http://www.bhpr.hrsa.gov.

———. 2002. "Reports: Projected Supply, Demand and Shortages of Registered Nurses, 2000–2020. [Online report; retrieved 10/6/05.] http://bhpr.hrsa.gov/healthworkforce/reports/rnproject/default.htm.

Valentino, C. L. 2004. "The Role of Middle Managers in the Transmission and Integration of Organizational Culture." *Journal of Healthcare Management* 49 (6): 393.

Exhibit 32.1

FIRST-TIME MANAGEMENT BLUNDERS

by Danny Pancho

It's a heady feeling to finally get that new title, but fresh-faced managers will do well to bone up on the skills set and mind frame crucial to a successful transition from being one of the boys to becoming The Boss.

So you have finally gained that much-coveted position—you are now a manager. But if you think you have it made, think again. Like Humpty Dumpty, many a new manager has suffered a great fall, largely due to missteps and miscues in climbing the high wall of success.

So how do you avoid becoming one of the casualties of managerial unpreparedness? How do you ensure a smooth and successful transition? Here are a few tips:

Think like a manager. Many dewy managers encounter transition difficulties because they retain their rank-and-file mentality. They should be prepared to make the necessary mindset switches to cope with the higher responsibilities:

- Have the perspective of an eagle, not an ant. See the forest, not the trees—Your thinking should now take on a broader perspective. Evaluate the effect of your actions or decisions not only on your unit, but on the whole organization. Your problem solving approach should now be strategic rather than merely straightforward. (You'll learn that sometimes, it may be necessary to lose a battle to win the war.) You should begin steering a course along the company's vision.
- Analyze deeply if you have the time, but decide quickly when needed—One weakness of new managerial appointees, especially those fresh from graduate business school, is a tendency to be wishy-washy. After going through endless case studies in school, they have become so good at analyzing situations that they tend to develop analysis paralysis. They cannot decide without first making a thorough study.

  A manager must have enough self-confidence to size up situations quickly, and then, even with the barest of information available, make hard and fast decisions when called for. You must learn to develop your "gut feel" and to rely on it at crunch time.
- Think ahead: be proactive, not reactive—Often, new managers are so afraid of failure that they defer making risky decisions, waiting instead for things to come to a head and then reacting to them. A good manager is one who trains himself or herself to look ahead, weigh all possible scenarios, decide on the most probable outcome and proact accordingly.
- Be organizationally aware—Understand how the organization works—its systems, situations, pressures, culture, etc.—and how these factors combine to influence

your unit. Also, study how your own unit impacts on the other components of the organization.

A newly promoted purchasing manager I once knew paid a dear price for not heeding this advice. To win his subordinates over, he solicited assistance from the suppliers in treating them to an excursion. His objective was laudable, but his method was questionable. He violated the organization's stand against soliciting from suppliers and stirred envy in other departments. The resulting fallout was so bad that he had to leave the company.

Behave like a manager. Another managerial pitfall is failing to act appropriately. You should know that, as a manager, you are a company role model, expected to act in a certain manner reflective of your stature in the organization.

- Integrity is very important—As a role model, you must maintain and promote so-cial, ethical and organizational norms in conducting your internal and external busi-ness activities. Bear in mind that you now represent the company inside and out-side its walls, and how you behave reflects on the company.

    There was once a marketing service officer who was good at his job and was promoted to manager. Part of his new function was to manage the agency promo girls assigned to different department stores. Unfortunately, he found these pretty ladies so alluring that he was soon into relationships with some of them, and ru-mors of these liaisons eventually reached the higher echelon. Unable to fire him due to lack of solid proof, they decided to transfer him to a far-flung post where his reputation could do no harm. He ended up resigning from the company.
- Be a leader, not a boss—A few years back, I encountered a situation where the En-gineering Department, once performing well, suddenly became a problem area. It turned out that the people had a beef against the newly promoted engineering manager. Some of their feedback: "Mabuti pa noong 'bisor siya, ang bait. Nang maging manager, naging mayabang!" "Grabe maka-utos.Ora-orada! Pag di agad nasunod, nagagalit." ("It was better when he was supervisor. As manager, he has become swell-headed!" "He's too bossy. He wants things done at once, and gets angry otherwise.")

    Several coaching sessions with the manager and a teambuilding workshop with his staff were conducted, and the situation was rectified.

    To be an effective manager, you should be a leader, not a boss. You must earn your subordinates' respect, not demand it. You must also delegate properly rather than give orders. You must be sensitive to their needs and assist them when the sit-uation demands it. And most of all, develop them to be better employees, because your success depends on their success.

Work like a manager. Your new post will necessitate a change in work style and a sturdy stomach to withstand the increased pressure.

- Observe flexible work hours—A manager cannot afford to be tardy or even knock off early. Otherwise, you will have a difficult time enforcing time discipline among your subordinates.

Also, do not observe a regular "eight-to-five" routine simply because you are not paid overtime. Remember that your performance is no longer measured in work hours, but in work output. Oftentimes, this calls for putting in long and hard hours, especially if you have deadlines to meet.

- Learn to live under pressure and to avoid burnout—The major reason why the engineering manager mentioned earlier developed staff problems was his difficulty in coping with pressure. He wanted to prove himself so badly that he took on more jobs than he could possibly handle, and the demands of these simply overwhelmed him. As a result, he vented his exasperation on his hapless subordinates.

  Learn to prioritize your tasks based on their perceived importance to the organization or, equally important, to your boss. Tackle the big ones immediately and try to squeeze in the small tasks afterward. If you fill a container with sand, there is no way you can add the pebbles and stones anymore. But put in the stones first, and you can push the pebbles between the gaps, and then squeeze sand into whatever gaps still remain.

  Master the art of pacing yourself and conserving your energy for the long grind ahead. It is useless to expend all your energy at the start, only to falter at the end because you've run out of gas.

  Finally, learn to handle pressure. You should be able to tolerate stress and relieve it in a manner acceptable to the people around you. There are many articles and self-help books that can teach you how to do this.

- Be tenacious but resilient—As a manager, you should be determined to succeed. Stay on course until you have achieved your objective, or until it is no longer reasonably attainable. However, be resilient as well. You are not Superman and should expect some disappointments and failures along the way. But you should be able to handle these setbacks well and maintain your effectiveness.

There are many more expectations from you as a manager than can be mentioned in this article. Your success will depend on how well you cope with these expectations. Most important, however, is that you learn to think out of the employee box and acknowledge that you still have a lot to learn to become an effective manager. Adopt this frame of mind, and you are halfway there.

Source: Courtesy of JobStreet.com Philippines, Inc. as viewed at http://ph.jobstreet.com/employers /mot13.htm.

Index

Ability, 402–3
Acceptance authority theory, 29, 192, 194–95, 204
Accounting systems, 433
Accrued depreciation, 145
Achievement needs, 454–55
Achievement theory, 454–56
ADA. *See* Americans with Disabilities Act
Ad hoc committee, 296
Administrative management theory, 26, 28, 35
Administrative pyramid, 7f
Administrator, 120
Advance warning, 514–15
Advisory Publications, 550
Affiliation need, 454
Affirmative-action programs, 334
Aggression, 464
AHIMA. *See* American Health Information Management Association
ALCOA. *See* Aluminum Company of America
Alderfer, Clayton, 446, 450–52
Alexander, J.A., 529
Allen, Gemmy, 25–26, 45, 74
Aluminum Company of America, 151
American College of Cardiology, 286
American Health Information Management Association, 370
American Management Association, 469
Americans with Disabilities Act, 108–10
American Society of Mechanical Engineers, 173
Analyze phase, 285, 287
Anderson, Curt, 25
Anger: The Misunderstood Emotion, 498
Annual appraisal, 381
Annual review, 377
Anticipatory controls, 530
Apathy, 498
Appeal, 519–20
Appealed policy, 160
Application for employment. *See* Employment: application
Appraiser, 382–83
Arbitrator, 583
ASME. *See* American Society of Mechanical Engineers
Aspiration levels, 455–58
Assess, 274
Attending physicians, 266–67
Attitude: behavior and, 460–61; factors determining, 459–60; motivation and, 458; surveys, 490–92
Attribute theory, 435–36
Authority: acceptance theory of, 29; of attending physicians, 266–67; of committee, 299–301; decentralization, 255; definition of, 191, 204; delegation of, 190, 234–35, 243–45; direct line, 260–61; exception principle, 241; external limitations, 193; granting, 239–42; hybrid, 301; integrated approach, 196; internal limitations, 193; interpretation of, 191; legitimacy, 192; managerial, 19–20; recentralization, 291; revoking, 241–42; source of, 192; of staff, 262; of surgeons, 266–67; tapering concept, 193, 194; theories, 192–95, 204; types of, 26, 195–96; unity of command, 241

Authority relationships: coordination and, 58; definition of, 16; rules/regulations and, 192
Autocratic leadership, 439
Autocratic supervision, 417–19
Automation, 57
Availability, 585

Balanced Budget Act, 4
Baldiga, N.R., 183
Baptist Health Care System, 272
Barker, Joel, 80–81
Barnard, Chester, 29, 192, 194
BARS. *See* Behaviorally anchored rating scale
BBA. *See* Balanced Budget Act
Behaviorally anchored rating scale, 378
Behavioral management, 28–29
Benchmarking, 550–51
Benchmark jobs, 397–98
Bennis, Warren, 438
Bergquist, W.H., 34
Bertalanffy, Ludwig von, 31
Best method, 166
Body language, 76–77
Borrowed servant theory, 99–100
Boss-imposed time, 180
Boucher, Jane, 506
Bradley, Bill, 440
Brailer, David, 63
Brainstorming: formats, 308; ground rules, 277; participants in, 46;
Brandon, Nicholas, 411
Bright, Deborah, 499
Broadband, 22n
Budget: approaches, 557–59; committee, 561; cost allocation, 564–65; cost controls, 564; definition of, 553; director, 561; flexibility, 562; human problems and, 563–64; importance of, 171–72; making, 555; nature of, 554; numerical terms, 555; period length, 561–62; preparation of, 559–60; review, 562–63; revision, 562–63; supervisor concern, 554–55; 3 Ps, 559–60; traditional, 555–57; types of, 559
Budgetary control, 554
Bureaucratic management theory, 25, 26, 35
Bureau of Labor Statistics, 147
Business ethics, 47–48

Capital budget, 559
Capital expenditure request, 146
Captain of the ship doctrine, 99, 100, 267
Carnegie, Andrew, 253
Cash budget, 559
Catastrophic theory, 31
Causation, 106
Centers for Disease Control and Prevention, 112, 147
Centers of excellence, 4
Centralization-decentralization continuum, 247–49
Central tendency, 388
CEO. *See* Chief executive officer
Certified nurse assistant, 4
CFO. *See* Chief financial officer
Chain of command, 211, 235–36, 263
Chandler, Alfred, 269

About the Author

Rose T. Dunn, RHIA, M.B.A., CPA, FACHE, FHFMA, has been in healthcare management for more than 25 years. She started her career as the director of health information services at Barnes Hospital immediately following graduation from Saint Louis University and was later promoted to vice president. After 13 years at Barnes, Ms. Dunn's next position was with Metropolitan Life Insurance Company, where she was assistant vice president in MetLife's HMO subsidiary. Following this position, Ms. Dunn served as the chief financial officer of a dual-hospital system. In 1988, Ms. Dunn started a consulting firm, First Class Solutions, Inc.^{sm}, which has now grown to serve healthcare and third-party payer clients nationwide. She is chief operating officer of First Class Solutions, Inc.^{sm}

During her 25-year career Ms. Dunn has had more than 200 articles published, is a sought-after public speaker on a variety of healthcare subjects, and has authored books on legal aspects, finance, productivity, process improvement, and management. She has served as a faculty member at the University of Minnesota's Healthcare Administration Program, teaching finance; at Saint Louis University's School of Business, teaching management; and at Stephens College's Health Information Management Program, teaching legal and ethical aspects, management, and finance.

Ms. Dunn is active in several professional organizations including the Healthcare Financial Management Association (HFMA), American College of Healthcare Executives (ACHE), American Institute of Certified Public Accountants (AICPA), and American Health Information Management Association (AHIMA). She is a past-president of AHIMA and a recipient of AHIMA's highest award, the Distinguished Member Award.

Ms. Dunn received her bachelor of science (summa cum laude) and master's (cum laude) degrees from Saint Louis University.